SOCIAL NEUROSCIENCE

Social Neuroscience

INTEGRATING BIOLOGICAL AND
PSYCHOLOGICAL EXPLANATIONS
OF SOCIAL BEHAVIOR

edited by
Eddie Harmon-Jones
Piotr Winkielman

THE GUILFORD PRESS
New York   London

©2007 The Guilford Press
A Division of Guilford Publications, Inc.
72 Spring Street, New York, NY 10012
www.guilford.com

Printed in the United States of America

This book is printed on acid-free paper.

Last digit is print number: 9   8   7   6   5   4   3   2   1

Library of Congress Cataloging-in-Publication Data

Social neuroscience : integrating biological and psychological explanations of
social behavior / edited by Eddie Harmon-Jones, Piotr Winkielman.
    p. ; cm.
  Includes bibliographical references and index.
  ISBN-13: 978-1-59385-404-1 (cloth : alk. paper)
  ISBN-10: 1-59385-404-8 (cloth : alk. paper)
  1. Neuropsychology.   2. Social psychology.   I. Harmon-Jones,
Eddie.   II. Winkielman, Piotr.
  [DNLM: 1. Neuropsychology.   2. Social Behavior.   3. Nervous System
Physiology.   WL 103.5 S6775 2007]
  QP360.S594 2007
  612.8—dc22

                                                                2006032060

About the Editors

Eddie Harmon-Jones, PhD, completed his doctorate at the University of Arizona after attending the University of Kansas for his master's studies and the University of Alabama–Birmingham for his undergraduate studies. He is now an Associate Professor of Psychology at Texas A&M University. Dr. Harmon-Jones's current research focuses on emotions and motivations, their implications for social processes and behaviors, and their underlying neural circuits. His research has been supported by the National Institute of Mental Health, the National Science Foundation, and the Fetzer Institute. In 1999 he coedited *Cognitive Dissonance: Progress on a Pivotal Theory in Social Psychology*. In 2002 he received the Distinguished Award for an Early Career Contribution to Psychophysiology from the Society for Psychophysiological Research. In 2003 Dr. Harmon-Jones coedited a special issue devoted to social neuroscience for the *Journal of Personality and Social Psychology*. He has also served as an associate editor of the *Journal of Personality and Social Psychology* and is on the editorial boards of four other journals.

Piotr Winkielman, PhD, completed his doctorate at the University of Michigan and received postdoctoral training in social neuroscience at The Ohio State University after attending the University of Warsaw in Poland and the University of Bielefeld in Germany for his undergraduate studies. He is now an Associate Professor of Psychology at the University of California, San Diego. Dr. Winkielman's current research focuses on the relation between emotion, cognition, body, and consciousness using psychological and psychophysiological approaches. His research has been supported by the National Science Foundation and the National Alliance for Autism Research. He has served on the editorial boards of the *Journal of Personality and Social Psychology* and *Personality and Social Psychology Bulletin*, and is currently Associate Editor of *Emotion*. In 2005 Dr. Winkielman coedited *Emotion and Consciousness* (Guilford Press).

Contributors

Ralph Adolphs, PhD, Department of Psychology, California Institute of Technology, Pasadena, California; Department of Neurology, University of Iowa, Iowa City, Iowa

David M. Amodio, PhD, Department of Psychology, New York University, New York, New York

Bruce D. Bartholow, PhD, Department of Psychological Sciences, University of Missouri, Columbia, Missouri

Jennifer S. Beer, PhD, Department of Psychology, University of California, Davis, Davis, California

John T. Cacioppo, PhD, Department of Psychology, University of Chicago, Chicago, Illinois

Rebecca Campo, MA, Department of Psychology and Health Psychology Program, University of Utah, Salt Lake City, Utah

C. Sue Carter, PhD, Department of Psychiatry, University of Illinois–Chicago, Chicago, Illinois

Troy Chenier, MA, Department of Psychology, University of California, San Diego, La Jolla, California

Joshua Correll, PhD, Department of Psychology, University of Chicago, Chicago, Illinois

William A. Cunningham, PhD, Department of Psychology, The Ohio State University, Columbus, Ohio

Jean Decety, PhD, Department of Psychology, University of Chicago, Chicago, Illinois

Patricia G. Devine, PhD, Department of Psychology, University of Wisconsin–Madison, Madison, Wisconsin

Cheryl L. Dickter, PhD, Department of Psychology, University of North Carolina, Chapel Hill, North Carolina

Tedra Fazendeiro, PhD, Department of Psychology, University of Denver, Denver, Colorado

Gian C. Gonzaga, PhD, eHarmony.com, Pasadena, California

Eddie Harmon-Jones, PhD, Department of Psychology, Texas A&M University, College Station, Texas

Andrea S. Heberlein, PhD, Department of Psychology, Harvard University, Cambridge, Massachusetts

Dirk H. Hellhammer, PhD, Department of Theoretical and Clinical Psychobiology, University of Trier, Trier, Germany

Julianne Holt-Lunstad, PhD, Department of Psychology, Brigham Young University, Provo, Utah

Marco Iacoboni, MD, PhD, Department of Psychiatry and Biobehavioral Sciences, David Geffen School of Medicine, University of California, Los Angeles, Los Angeles, California

Tiffany A. Ito, PhD, Department of Psychology, University of Colorado, Boulder, Colorado

Marcia K. Johnson, PhD, Department of Psychology, Yale University, New Haven, Connecticut

Clemens Kirschbaum, PhD, Department of Psychology, Technical University of Dresden, Dresden, Germany

Brian Knutson, PhD, Department of Psychology, Stanford University, Stanford, California

Brigitte M. Kudielka, PhD, Department of Theoretical and Clinical Psychobiology, University of Trier, Trier, Germany

Matthew D. Lieberman, PhD, Department of Psychology, University of California, Los Angeles, Los Angeles, California

Catherine J. Norris, PhD, Department of Psychology, University of Wisconsin–Madison, Madison, Wisconsin

Kevin N. Ochsner, PhD, Department of Psychology, Columbia University, New York, New York

Maija Reblin, MA, Department of Psychology and Health Psychology Program, University of Utah, Salt Lake City, Utah

Oliver C. Schultheiss, PhD, Department of Psychology, University of Michigan, Ann Arbor, Michigan

Dennis J. L. G. Schutter, PhD, Affective Neuroscience Section, Utrecht University, Utrecht, The Netherlands

Valerie E. Stone, PhD, School of Psychology, University of Queensland, St. Lucia, Australia

Shelley E. Taylor, PhD, Department of Psychology, University of California, Los Angeles, Los Angeles, California

Bert N. Uchino, PhD, Department of Psychology and Health Psychology Program, University of Utah, Salt Lake City, Utah

Darcy Uno, PhD, Kaiser Permanente Medical Center, Roseville, California

Jack van Honk, PhD, Affective Neuroscience Section, Utrecht University, Utrecht, The Netherlands

Eve Willadsen-Jensen, MA, Department of Psychology, University of Colorado, Boulder, Colorado

G. Elliott Wimmer, BS, Department of Psychology, Stanford University, Stanford, California

Piotr Winkielman, PhD, Department of Psychology, University of California, San Diego, La Jolla, California

Contents

III. MOTIVATION PROCESSES

IV. ATTITUDES AND SOCIAL COGNITION

V. PERSON PERCEPTION, STEREOTYPING, AND PREJUDICE

VI. INTERPERSONAL RELATIONSHIPS

SOCIAL NEUROSCIENCE

I

INTRODUCTION

1

A Brief Overview of Social Neuroscience

Eddie Harmon-Jones and Piotr Winkielman

Until recently, the prevailing attitude toward biological approaches to social behavior could be described as ambivalent. On the one hand, there has long been interest in how biological variables could be used as measures of social variables and how biological variables could influence social behavior. On the other hand, the biological approaches to social psychology were seen as reductionistic and having little to contribute to "real" conceptual debates in the field. The recent years have witnessed many theoretical, methodological, and empirical breakthroughs, and now a discipline called *social neuroscience* is generating great excitement among junior and senior investigators, with a variety of journals, conferences, books, and granting agencies supporting its development. This volume aims to capture this excitement by highlighting some of the most interesting streams of social neuroscience research. In what follows, we define social neuroscience, sketch some of its historical roots, and highlight its benefits to social psychology. Finally, we describe the goals that guided us in preparing this volume and preview the chapters.

DEFINITION

The biological approach to social behavior has gone (and goes) by many definitions and names (e.g., social psychophysiology, social neuropsychology, social cognitive neuroscience, social cognitive and affective neuroscience, etc.). We prefer the relatively inclusive name *social neuroscience* and use the term rather broadly, along the lines suggested by others (Cacioppo

3

& Berntson, 2002). Social neuroscience is an integrative field that examines how nervous (central and peripheral), endocrine, and immune systems are involved in sociocultural processes. Social neuroscience is nondualist in its view of humans, yet it is also nonreductionistic and emphasizes the importance of understanding how the brain and body influence social processes, as well as how social processes influence the brain and body. In other words, social neuroscience is a comprehensive attempt to understand mechanisms that underlie social behavior by combining biological and social approaches (Cacioppo & Berntson, 2002).

HISTORICAL ROOTS

Social neuroscience has many roots. One historical root has been the continued interest in physiological responses as a window into social-psychological processes that cannot be easily accessed through self-reports or overt behavior. This interest might date back as far as the 3rd century B.C., when a Greek physician, Erasistratos, measured the heartbeat of a young man in the presence of his attractive stepmother to infer that love, not a physical illness, was the cause of the young man's malady (Mesulam & Perry, 1972). The systematic use of biological measures as a pipeline to unreportable psychological states goes back to at least the mid-1950s. It was during this time in the United States that social norms prohibiting the public expression of racial prejudice began to emerge. Being wary that participants' concerns over these norms might threaten the veracity of their self-reported racial attitudes, researchers turned to biological measures that might be resistant to overt control efforts. This research demonstrated that white U.S. participants had larger autonomic responses—for example, greater skin conductance—in response to blacks than to whites (e.g., Rankin & Campbell, 1955; Vidulich & Krevanick, 1966). Around the same time, researchers began to use psychophysiological measures to investigate processes that might be unconscious or just too subtle to capture with other methods (Lazarus & McCleary, 1951). The interest in using methods of social neuroscience to tap into social processes that might be not reported for reasons of social desirability or unawareness continues to the present.

Perhaps weightier historical roots of social neuroscience are attempts to provide a comprehensive explanation of social behavior as a function of the brain. Traditionally, psychologists have been committed to the nondualist view and sought to integrate their work with knowledge from biological scientists. Empirically, attempts to link social behavior to a specific circuit in the brain were encouraged by early neuropsychological observations of massive changes in social behavior after injury to the prefrontal cortex (e.g., Phineas Gage) and in early research on the role of the amygdala in social behavior of primates (e.g., the work on the Kluver–Bucy syndrome). Several pioneering books and papers in neuropsychology from the 1980s and 1990s discussed the idea of the *social brain* and the possible importance of certain brain functions for social behavior (e.g., Brothers, 1997; Damasio, 1994; Gazzaniga, 1985). The 1990s also witnessed some of the first calls for a comprehensive approach to social behavior by combining psychological and biological approaches (e.g., Cacioppo & Berntson, 1992; Klein & Kihlstrom, 1998). Those calls soon became a chorus as researchers from various traditions argued that various neuroscience approaches can contribute insights into central social-psychological questions and play crucial roles in solving theoretical controversies (Adolphs, 1999, 2003; Blascovich, 2000; Ochsner & Lieberman, 2001; Winkielman, Berntson, & Cacioppo, 2001). Exciting empirical investigations followed, many using the latest technologies, thus forming the field of richness and depth that we see today.

BENEFITS OF SOCIAL NEUROSCIENCE

The current excitement about and widespread recognition of social neuroscience is grounded in a growing appreciation that it can benefit social psychology in a number of ways. At first blush, some observers sometimes assume that social neuroscience simply tries to map social-psychological processes to activity in particular brain regions. Of course, this type of research exists. In fact, identifying neural correlates of psychological functions can sometimes be quite useful, as it can serve as a springboard for further theory-testing investigations (in addition to more anatomical benefits of brain mapping). On the other hand, the brain mapping of social processes is problematic. Empirically, it is very difficult to verify with certainty that a particular structure or network of structures is involved with only one psychological process, especially when the process is as complex as many discussed in social psychology (Cacioppo et al., 2003; Willingham & Dunn, 2003). Theoretically, the "mapping game" tends to produce an increasingly growing list of various functions assigned to a particular area, with little benefit for research interested in testing *psychological* propositions. Fortunately, the research on neural correlates is not the only or the most important function of a neuroscience approach to social psychology. Here are what we see as the true benefits of social neuroscience.

First, neuroscientific research and theory can inform theoretical debates in social psychology. In cognitive psychology, several theoretical debates have been greatly informed by neuroscientific studies (e.g., debates about the nature of imagery, structure of memory, early vs. late attentional selection). Similarly, in social psychology, neuroscience data can contribute such evidence. As an example, consider research by Amodio et al. (2004). Integrating ideas from cognitive neuroscience models of cognitive control (Carter et al., 1998; MacDonald, Cohen, Stenger, & Carter, 2000) with social psychological models of control of race bias, Amodio et al. (2004) predicted that when individuals confronted a conflictual situation that activated a tendency toward stereotypic thinking, as well as a belief that stereotyping is inappropriate, they would evidence heightened activity in the anterior cingulate cortex. Using event-related brain potentials, the research revealed support for the prediction, demonstrating that the activation occurred at very early stages of response execution. Such findings suggest that the detection of conflict likely operates below awareness and does not necessarily rely on conscious deliberation. The idea that conscious deliberation was necessary was previously proposed by social-psychological models of cognitive control (e.g., Monteith, 1993; Wegener & Petty, 1997; Wilson & Brekke, 1994).

Second, neuroscience methods provide powerful tools for measuring brain–body activity directly and unobtrusively and may provide information that would be impossible to assess using other techniques. For example, self-report, overt behavior, and reaction time measures are often poor indicators of affective states and are subject to alternative theoretical interpretations. Accordingly, Winkielman and Cacioppo (2001) drew on psychophysiological measures of facial electromyography to document increases in positive affective responses to fluent (easy-to-process) stimuli— a finding incompatible with alternative theoretical models that predict no affective consequences.

Third, the neuroscientific study of *social processes* can inform neuroscientific research and theory by pointing to the importance of social variables (from context to culture) in altering processes within the brain and body. For example, as discussed in this volume in chapters by Uchino and colleagues (Chapter 22), Carter (Chapter 19), and Shelley and Gonzaga (Chapter 21), manipulations of social bonds can dramatically alter neural, hormonal, and immunological processes and thus affect important health outcomes.

More generally, for social neuroscience to develop and prosper, it needs to benefit from and expand on the subdisciplines from which it arose. As such, it can benefit from the theoretical approaches of both social psychology and neuroscience and add important theoretical developments of its own (Harmon-Jones & Sigelman, 2001).

So, to summarize the benefits, good social neuroscience research integrates the theory and methods of neuroscience and social psychology to derive novel psychological hypotheses. It then tests these hypotheses using a multidisciplinary set of methods, including the behavioral measures of social psychology and the "wetter" measures of neuroscience. It goes beyond using new methods to measure existing constructs; it incorporates ideas from other domains to better understand a problem in another domain. In the end, both parent fields are benefited—theoretically, practically, and methodologically. Given these benefits, it seems that the potential of social neuroscience for addressing questions about psychological mechanisms will make it indispensable to the field.

GOALS AND ORGANIZATION OF THE BOOK

In putting together this volume, we wanted to capture the excitement of social neuroscience while pursuing three goals. First, we wanted to provide up-to-date overviews of programmatic research in social neuroscience that addresses one of the primary processes of interest to social psychologists. Of course, some chapters have implications for multiple processes, but we placed chapters into subsections based on their dominant themes. The book is thus organized with the following subsections: emotion processes; motivation processes; attitudes and social cognition; person perception, stereotyping, and prejudice; and interpersonal relationships.

Second, we wanted to highlight the theoretical and methodological richness of current research in social neuroscience. Therefore, we invited authors representing a wide variety of theoretical approaches, including social, cognitive, clinical, biological, personality, and evolutionary perspectives. We also sought to illustrate contributions of a wide range of social neuroscience methods. Thus most methods are represented. For instance, lesion methods are covered in chapters by Beer (Chapter 2), Stone (Chapter 15), and Heberlein and Adolphs (Chapter 3). FMRI methods are covered in chapters by Norris and Cacioppo (Chapter 5), Ochsner (Chapter 6), Knutson and Wimmer (Chapter 8), Cunningham and Johnson (Chapter 11), Decety (Chapter 12), Lieberman (Chapter 14), Heberlein and Adolphs (Chapter 2), and Iacoboni (Chapter 20). Hormonal methods are covered in chapters by Kudielka, Hellhammer, and Kirschbaum (Chapter 4), van Honk and Schutter (Chapter 10), Schultheiss (Chapter 9), Carter (Chapter 19), and Taylor and Gonzaga (Chapter 21). Event-related brain potential methods are covered in chapters by Amodio, Devine and Harmon-Jones (Chapter 16), Bartholow and Dickter (Chaptr 17), and Ito, Willadsen-Jensen, and Correll (Chapter 18). Regional EEG methods are covered in the chapter by Harmon-Jones (Chapter 7). Facial electromyographic methods are covered in the chapter by Fazendeiro, Chenier, and Winkielman (Chapter 13). Finally, cardiovascular methods are covered in the chapter by Uchino, Holt-Lunstad, Uno, Campo, and Reblin (Chapter 22).

Third, we wanted the volume to be widely accessible and to serve as a conceptual and methodological primer to social neuroscience. Therefore, we asked the authors to specify what theoretical advantages they get from taking a social neuroscience perspective, to explain why they use their specific methods, and to present their results and methods in a way that would be accessible to the beginner and the expert alike. We hope that the reader agrees that this approach has resulted in a cutting-edge yet accessible volume.

OVERVIEW OF THE CHAPTERS

Part II of the book, *Emotion Processes,* covers five chapters. Jennifer Beer (Chapter 2) discusses the importance of emotion–social cognition interactions for social functioning and highlights the role of the orbitofrontal cortex in such processing. Andrea Heberlein and Ralph Adolphs (Chapter 3) review research and theory on the neurobiological substrates of emotion recognition and suggest that, in order to recognize emotions in others, observers must simulate aspects of the specific emotion in the person being observed. In Chapter 4, Brigitte Kudielka, Dirk Hellhammer, and Clemens Kirschbaum review 10 years of research using the Trier Social Stress Test, an important methodological advance that provides an opportunity to study the hormone cortisol in the lab. Catherine Norris and John Cacioppo (Chapter 5) review research suggesting that social and emotional information processes are highly overlapping in both their neural substrates and psychological mechanisms. The section closes with Chapter 6, in which Kevin Ochsner reviews his research on the brain mechanisms of emotion regulation, which suggests powerful top-down influences from the cognitive onto the emotional system.

Part III, *Motivation Processes,* has four chapters. Eddie Harmon-Jones (Chapter 7) reviews research on the relationship between asymmetrical frontal cortical activity and emotional and motivational processes, which suggests new insights into theories concerned with the relationship between emotions and motivations. Brian Knutson and Elliott Wimmer (Chapter 8) propose that reward circuitry serves a broad role in social valuation and support their proposal with a variety of studies involving financial and nonfinancial rewards. In Chapter 9, Oliver Schultheiss considers theory and research on power motivation—individual differences in affective preferences for having impact on other people or the world at large—and how it interacts with social situations concerning dominance to produce differences in hormone release. Jack van Honk and Dennis Schutter (Chapter 10) also review research and theory related to dominance and submission motives and how they relate to vigilant versus avoidant responses to angry facial expressions. To investigate these important issues, their research program has used a wide variety of neuroscience tools, including steroid hormone manipulation and measurement, repetitive transcranial magnetic stimulation, and electroencephalography (EEG).

Part IV, *Attitudes and Social Cognition,* has five chapters. William Cunningham and Marcia Johnson (Chapter 11) focus on the evaluative processes that underlie attitudes and explore neural mechanisms that support their affective and cognitive components. Jean Decety (Chapter 12) proposes a social neuroscience model of human empathy. His model incorporates a number of dissociable computational mechanisms supporting affective and cognitive components of empathy. In Chapter 13, Tedra Fazendeiro, Troy Chenier, and Piotr Winkielman propose that affective and cognitive feelings can arise from the dynamics of information process-ing. They test their proposal using psychological and neuroscientific meth-ods and place it in the context of current knowledge about the neuroscience of affect and memory. Matthew Lieberman (Chapter 14) explores the neu-ral basis of automatic and controlled social cognition and argues for dissociable neural systems supporting reflexive and reflective aspects of social processing. Valerie Stone (Chapter 15) evaluates neural evidence for domain specificity in social intelligence and places this evidence in a theo-retical perspective grounded in evolutionary psychology.

Part V, *Person Perception, Stereotyping, and Prejudice*, contains three chapters. David Amodio, Trish Devine, and Eddie Harmon-Jones (Chapter 16) review research concerned with the psychological and neural mecha-nisms involved in the regulation of intergroup responses, focusing in partic-ular on the role of the anterior circulate cortex in the control of race-based responses. In Chapter 17, Bruce Bartholow and Cheryl Dickter review a number of recent experiments that have addressed important conceptual issues related to person perception using event-related potentials (ERPs) recorded noninvasively from the scalp. They also provide a sagacious dis-cussion of when it is more appropriate to use ERPs as compared with other neuroscience measures. Tiffany Ito, Eve Willadsen-Jensen, and Joshua Correll, in Chapter 18, review ERP studies examining how individuals are categorized into social groups. Their studies reveal new information regarding the timing of perceptual and cognitive processes that underlie the categorization of individuals of different social groups.

Part VI, *Interpersonal Relationships*, has four chapters. Sue Carter (Chapter 19) reviews research on the biological basis of social bonds, with a focus on the relationship between social bonding and neuropeptides (e.g., oxytocin and vasopressin). The chapter suggests mechanisms through which social experiences can be both protective and restorative in the face of life challenges. Marco Iacoboni (Chapter 20) uses his work on mecha-nisms of imitation and action understanding to suggest that social cognitive neuroscience offers a different view of a human brain. That brain needs a body to exist in a world of shared social norms in which meaning origi-nates from being in the world. In Chapter 21, Shelley Taylor and Gian Gonzaga describe a biobehavioral model of affiliative responses to stress. They suggest that oxytocin may act as a social thermostat that is responsive to adequacy of social resources, that prompts affiliative behavior when social resources fall below an adequate level, and that reduces stress responses once positive social contacts are (re)established. Bert Uchino, Julianne Holt-Lunstad, Darcy Uno, Rebecca Campo, and Maija Reblin, in Chapter 22, review research that has examined the cardiovascular conse-quences of close social relationship variables, such as the perceived avail-ability and receipt of social support and the ambivalence of the relationship ties. This research has important implications for understanding cardiovas-cular disease.

REFERENCES

Adolphs, R. (1999). Social cognition and the human brain. *Trends in Cognitive Sciences, 3,* 469–479.

Adolphs, R. (2003). Cognitive neuroscience of human social behavior. *Nature Reviews. Neuroscience, 4,* 165–178.

Amodio, D. M., Harmon-Jones, E., Devine, P. G., Curtin, J. J., Hartley, S., & Covert, A. (2004). Neural signals for the detection of unintentional race bias. *Psychological Science, 15,* 88–93.

Blascovich, J. (2000). Using physiological indexes of psychological processes in social psychological research. In H. T. Reis & C. M. Judd (Eds.), *Handbook of research methods in social and personality psychology* (pp. 117–137), Cambridge, UK: Cambridge University Press.

Brothers, L. (1997). *Friday's footprint: How society shapes the human mind.* New York: Oxford University Press.

Cacioppo, J. T., & Berntson, G. G. (1992). Social psychological contributions to the decade of the brain: Doctrine of multilevel analysis. *American Psychologist, 47,* 1019–1028.

Cacioppo, J. T., & Berntson, G. G. (2002). Social neuroscience. In J. T. Cacioppo et al. (Eds.), *Foundations in social neuroscience* (pp. 1–9). Cambridge, MA: MIT Press.

Cacioppo, J. T., Berntson, G. G., Lorig, T. S., Norris, C. J., Rickett, E., & Nusbaum, H. (2003). Just because you're imaging the brain doesn't mean you can stop using your head: A primer and set of first principles. *Journal of Personality and Social Psychology, 85,* 650–661.

Carter, C. S., Braver, T. S., Barch, D. M., Botvinick, M. M., Noll, D., & Cohen, J. D. (1998). Anterior cingulate cortex, error detection, and the online monitoring of performance. *Science, 280,* 747–749.

Damasio, A. R. (1994). *Descartes' error: Emotion, reason and the human brain.* New York: Grosset/Putnam.

Gazzaniga, M. S. (1985). *The social brain.* New York: Basic Books.

Harmon-Jones, E., & Sigelman, J. (2001). State anger and prefrontal brain activity: Evidence that insult-related relative left prefrontal activation is associated with experienced anger and aggression. *Journal of Personality and Social Psychology, 80,* 797–803.

Klein, S. B., & Kihlstrom, J. F. (1998). On bridging the gap between social-personality psychology and neuropsychology. *Personality and Social Psychology Review, 2,* 228–242.

Lazarus, R. S., & McCleary, R. A. (1951). Autonomic discrimination without awareness: A study of subception. *Psychological Review, 58,* 113–122.

MacDonald, W., III, Cohen, J. D., Stenger, V. A., & Carter, C. S. (2000). Dissociating the role of the dorsolateral prefrontal and anterior cingulate cortex in cognitive control. *Science, 288,* 1835–1838.

Mesulam, M. M., & Perry, J. (1972). The diagnosis of lovesickness: Experimental psychophysiology without polygraph. *Psychophysiology, 9,* 546–551.

Monteith, M. J. (1993). Self-regulation of stereotypical responses: Implications for progress in prejudice reduction. *Journal of Personality and Social Psychology, 65,* 469–485.

Ochsner, K. N., & Lieberman, M. D. (2001). The emergence of social cognitive neuroscience. *American Psychologist, 56*, 717–734.

Rankin, R. E., & Campbell, D. T. (1955). Galvanic skin response to negro and white experimenters. *Journal of Abnormal and Social Psychology, 51*, 30–33.

Vidulich, R. N., & Krevanick, F. W. (1966). Racial attitudes and emotional response to visual representations of the negro. *Journal of Social Psychology, 68*, 85–93.

Wegener, D. T., & Petty, R. E. (1997). The flexible correction model: The role of naïve theories of bias in bias correction. In M. P. Zanna (Ed.), *Advances in experimental social psychology* (Vol. 29, pp. 141–208). Mahwah, NJ: Erlbaum.

Willingham, D. T., & Dunn, E. W. (2003). What neuroimaging and brain localization can do, cannot do and should not do for social psychology. *Journal of Personality and Social Psychology, 85*, 662–671.

Wilson, T. D., & Brekke, N. (1994). Mental contamination and mental correction: Unwanted influences on judgments and evaluations. *Psychological Bulletin, 116*, 117–142.

Winkielman, P., Berntson, G. G., & Cacioppo, J. T. (2001). The psychophysiological perspective on the social mind. In A. Tesser & N. Schwarz (Eds.), *Blackwell handbook of social psychology: Intraindividual processes* (pp. 89–108). Oxford, UK: Blackwell.

Winkielman, P., & Cacioppo, J. T. (2001). Mind at ease puts a smile on the face: Psychophysiological evidence that processing facilitation increases positive affect. *Journal of Personality and Social Psychology, 81*, 989–1000.

II

EMOTION PROCESSES

2

The Importance of Emotion–Social Cognition Interactions for Social Functioning

INSIGHTS FROM THE ORBITOFRONTAL CORTEX

Jennifer S. Beer

How do individuals successfully navigate their social world? Social information processing theories of social adjustment suggest that social-behavioral output is a function of online processing of social stimuli (e.g., Crick & Dodge, 1994). From this perspective, people must direct their attention to particular stimuli in the social environment and interpret or give meaning to those stimuli. People then take their personal goals into account and, after calculating the outcomes associated with possible behavioral responses in the social context, decide on a particular behavioral response. Research has shown that dysfunctional online cognitive processing is more predictive of social maladjustment than global constructs such as individual differences in perspective taking, communication, and role taking (e.g., Crick & Dodge, 1994). Therefore, the study of online cognition in social situations represents an important advance in understanding the social cognitive mechanisms underlying social maladjustment.

A future direction for expanding social information–processing theories of social adjustment is suggested by previous research, which has shown that emotion has robust, predictable effects on cognition (e.g., Fiske & Taylor, 1991; Forgas, 1995; Isen & Geva, 1987; Schwarz, 1990). Emotional experience engages particular cognitive strategies that influence response selection (e.g., Levenson, 1999). For example, when people are feeling good, they are more likely to engage in automatic cognitive processes. People in good moods react quickly, underestimate risk, and focus on positive explanations when making decisions or judgments. In contrast, when people are feeling bad, they are more likely to engage in effortful cognitive processes. People in bad moods react more slowly, overestimate risk, and focus on negative explanations when making decisions or judgments. This body of research suggests that emotion should affect how people judge social stimuli and how they make decisions among possible behavioral responses in social situations. To date, this research has focused on understanding the ways in which emotion and social cognition interact; little attention has been paid to understanding whether these interactions are necessary for social adjustment.

THE ORBITOFRONTAL CORTEX: A MODEL OF EMOTIONAL INFLUENCES ON SOCIAL INFORMATION PROCESSING UNDERLYING SOCIAL ADJUSTMENT

A potential model of the relation between social adjustment and emotional influences on social information processing may be built using traditional neuropsychological and neuroscientific approaches. A host of neural areas are proposed to mediate social behavior, including the orbitofrontal cortex (Brodmann's area [BA] 11/12/parts of 47), in addition to the amygdala, anterior cingulate gyrus, and somatosensory cortices (e.g., Adolphs, 1999; Brothers, 1996; Emery & Amaral, 2000; Whalen, 1998). In particular, orbitofrontal cortex damage is associated with a host of social deficits, and, furthermore, these deficits have been theorized to reflect dysfunctional emotional influences on cognition (Beer, Shimamura, & Knight, 2004). These social deficits include risk taking and impulsivity and have been clinically characterized as socially inappropriate behavior, impaired interpersonal relationships, emotional outbursts, and personality change (Bechara, Damasio, & Damasio, 2000; Rolls, Hornak, Wade, & McGrath, 1994; Tucker, Luu, & Pribam, 1995). By examining the social deficits of these patients in relation to deficits in emotion–cognition interactions, we can begin to understand the role of these interactions for social adjustment. Additionally, neuroimaging studies of healthy orbitofrontal tissue in relation to emotion–cognition interactions and social functioning will provide complementary evidence about the importance of such interactions for social functioning. Although relatively few studies have been conducted, previous research suggests that the orbitofrontal cortex is important for various kinds of emotion–cognition interactions.

ORBITOFRONTAL CORTEX INVOLVEMENT IN EMOTIONAL MEDIATION OF DECISION MAKING

Both lesion and functional neuroimaging research have implicated the orbitofrontal cortex in emotional mediation of decision making. Lesion studies suggest that patients with orbitofrontal cortex damage fail to use emotional information to guide their decisions in a risky gambling task (Bechara et al, 2000; Rahman, Sahakian, Cardinal, Rogers, & Robbins, 2001). Patients with orbitofrontal cortex damage exhibit inadequate perception of risks and poor regulation of risky behavior. For example, patients with orbitofrontal cortex lesions fail to show an anticipatory change in skin conductance response (SCR) when deciding to make a high-risk gamble (Bechara et al, 2000). They are less likely to make decisions to maximize their chances of winning a bet and less likely to modify the monetary amount of their bets as a function of their probability of winning (Rahman et al., 2001). Another lesion study has shown that, although patients with orbitofrontal cortex damage have an intact ability to generate possible solutions to social dilemmas, they are impaired in making adaptive decisions among possible solutions (Saver & Damasio, 1991).

One functional neuroimaging study suggests that orbitofrontal cortex activity may be accounted for by emotional influences on a guessing task. Significantly more activation was found in the orbitofrontal cortex (BA 11/47) when participants were provided with feedback on gains and losses during a guessing task in comparison with a feedback condition of a planning task (Elliott, Frith, & Dolan, 1997).

ORBITOFRONTAL CORTEX INVOLVEMENT IN EMOTIONAL MEDIATION OF JUDGMENTS OF SOCIAL STIMULI

Lesion studies have also implicated the orbitofrontal cortex in emotional mediation of judgments of social stimuli. For example, orbitofrontal cortex damage was associated with difficulty in using situational context to make inferences about social scenarios involving faux pas. Patients with orbitofrontal cortex damage could accurately describe the emotional reaction of a person who had just been insulted but exhibited impaired understanding that the insult had resulted from a social faux pas and not malicious intent (Stone, Baron-Cohen, & Knight, 1998). Other research has shown that patients with orbitofrontal cortex damage are deficient at correctly judging emotional facial expressions (Beer, Heerey, Keltner, Scabini, & Knight, 2003; Hornak, Rolls, & Wade, 1996). Similarly, a functional neuroimaging study found activation in BA 47 in response to emotional facial expressions in comparison with neutral facial expressions (Sprengelmeyer, Rausch, Eysel, & Przuntek, 1998).

PREDOMINANT THEORIES OF ORBITOFRONTAL CORTEX FUNCTION

A host of studies implicate orbitofrontal cortex involvement in emotion and decision making, but what is the precise mechanism of its involvement? Three major theories have been proposed to explain the role of the orbitofrontal cortex in synthesizing emotion and cognition. The exact mechanism through which the synthesis is accomplished is somewhat different across theories.

The Somatic Marker Hypothesis

The somatic marker hypothesis suggests that poor decision making occurs when somatic information is not available to guide decision making (e.g., Bechara, et al., 2000; Bechara, Damasio, Tranel, & Damasio, 1997). From this perspective, orbitofrontal structures provide the substrate for learning associations between complex situations and the type of somatic (i.e., emotional) state usually associated with a particular situation. The orbitofrontal cortex modulates a distributed network of activity thought to reflect the brain's attempt to recreate previously experienced associations between internal physiology and external situations. Specifically, orbitofrontal structures activate in response to complex social situations and then activate somatic effectors in the amygdala, hypothalamus, and brainstem nuclei. Somatic markers are generated for the purpose of rapidly processing option–outcome associations and marking them as good or bad. Decision making can then selectively focus on option–outcome pairings that are potentially rewarding. This process should be particularly helpful when there is ambiguity in the environment and past experience is the primary source for making an informed decision (Bechara et al., 2000; Elliott, Dolan, & Frith, 2000).

Empirical support for the somatic marker hypothesis comes from a series of studies that have implemented a gambling task to examine the relation between somatic markers and decision making (e.g., Bechara et al., 1997). Over time, healthy adults, patients with damage to the dorsolateral prefrontal cortex, and patients with damage outside the prefrontal cortex gradually start to gamble in a manner that maximizes winnings. In contrast, many of the patients with orbitofrontal damage fail to implement an optimal gambling strategy on a behavioral level even though some can verbally state the optimal strategy. Furthermore, whereas normal controls show an increased SCR in anticipation of making a risky gamble, the group with orbitofrontal damage shows no anticipatory change in SCR. However, both groups do show SCR in response to winning or losing a particular gamble. These results are interpreted as indicating that orbitofrontal damage, particularly to the right side (Tranel, Bechara, & Denburg, 2002), impairs decision making because somatic markers are not triggered and therefore cannot guide their gambling decisions. Additionally, as mentioned previously, some research supports the component of the somatic marker hypothesis that states that the orbitofrontal cortex is particularly useful in ambiguous situations. Indeed, one study found that the orbitofrontal cortex was activated more in decision making in ambiguous situations than in well-understood situations (Elliott et al., 1997).

Reinforcement and Reversal

Another perspective on the role of the orbitofrontal cortex in emotion–cognition interactions focuses on reinforcement and reversal processes (Kringelbach & Rolls, 2004; Rolls, 2000). Specifically, the medial orbitofrontal cortex (BA 11/12) is theorized to be involved in computing the reward value of stimuli, and the lateral orbitofrontal cortex is theorized to be involved in computing the punishing value of stimuli that may lead to a change in behavior (Kringelbach & Rolls, 2004). From this perspective, the poor decision making and disinhibition of patients with orbitofrontal damage reflects their inability to change their behavior in response to changing stimulus–reinforcement contingencies. The orbitofrontal cortex computes the reward and punishment value of stimuli as a function of the environmental context. Furthermore, information about the stimulus–reinforcement contingencies is updated continually and allows for rapid reversal or extinction of stimulus–reinforcement associations. However, with damage to the orbitofrontal cortex, individuals are unable to alter their behavior as a function of these changing stimulus–reinforcement contingencies and presumably cannot inhibit inappropriate responses.

The empirical evidence for this position comes from research with nonhuman primates and humans. Thorpe, Rolls, and Maddison (1983) used single-unit recording in orbitofrontal neurons of three rhesus monkeys during a go/no-go visual discrimination task to examine learning and reversal of stimulus–reinforcement contingencies. The contingencies in the experiment were often reversed during the 4-hour recording session so that the previously rewarded stimuli became aversive. Some neuronal activity in the orbitofrontal cortex was associated with learning a stimulus–reinforcement contingency (e.g., responding to the presence of a reward or responding to the presence of punishment). Furthermore, activity was found (1) in response to behavior that was no longer rewarded and (2) again on the first delivery of a reward in the new paradigm. This activity was interpreted to reflect the detection of a paradigmatic shift. The involvement of the orbitofrontal cortex in reversal learning is also supported in studies with humans. Fellows and Farah (2003) found that patients with orbitofrontal damage, in comparison with control participants and patients with dorsolateral prefrontal damage, had trouble reversing associations between stimuli and rewards. Similarly, Rolls et al. (1994) tested patients with orbitofrontal damage and patients with damage outside of the orbitofrontal cortex on a visual discrimination task that examined reversal and extinction. Participants were presented with a go/no-go task involving images of patterns on a computer screen. Throughout the experiment, the reinforcement contingency changed so that previously rewarded patterns resulted in either loss of points (reversal) or no gain (extinction). The findings suggest that the group with orbitofrontal damage could learn the first pattern-reinforcement contingency in much the same way as the other patients and normal controls. However, on reversal or extinction of the previously learned contingency, patients with orbitofrontal damage were unable to stop themselves from responding to the previously rewarded patterns. As in the gambling studies, these patients could verbally report that they should no longer touch the screen for those patterns. In contrast, patients with damage outside the orbitofrontal area and normal controls did not show this type of perseveration. Staff member ratings of the social disinhibition of patients with orbitofrontal damage correlated with their error percentages from the reversal task and the extinction task. The authors interpreted these findings as indicating that patients with orbitofrontal damage experience social problems because they are unable to alter their behavior in response to changing stimulus–reinforcement contingencies that naturally occur in daily life.

Dynamic Filtering Theory

A third perspective on the role of the orbitofrontal cortex in synthesizing emotional and cognitive information is dynamic filtering theory (Shimamura, 2000). According to Shimamura and his colleagues, the prefrontal cortex is responsible for implementing a variety of gating or filtering devices in its role in the monitoring and control of information processing. In other words, the frontal lobes serve an executive function wherein neural activity from other brain regions is filtered or gated based on its relevance to the task at hand. The orbitofrontal cortex is heavily connected to sensory and limbic areas and therefore may be responsible for filtering neural activity associated with emotional response to the environments (Rule, Shimamura, & Knight, 2002). Patients with orbitofrontal damage cannot benefit from this filtering mechanism and cannot inhibit the neural activity associated with emotional processing. Therefore, the disinhibition seen in these patients may be accounted for by their inability to inhibit their response to emotional stimuli in the environment.

Empirical evidence for the dynamic filtering role of the orbitofrontal cortex for emotional stimuli comes from a study that examined event-related potentials (P300) generated in response to the novelty of unpredictable, aversive stimuli (Rule et al., 2002). Participants with orbitofrontal damage, with dorsolateral prefrontal damage, and normal control participants were presented with two kinds of novel, aversive stimuli while watching a silent movie: mild shocks and distracting noises. For both the shock and noise conditions, patients with orbitofrontal damage showed greater P300 amplitudes when compared with the other patient group and with normal controls. Additionally, patients with orbitofrontal damage did not habituate to the shocks when compared with the control group. In other words, patients with orbitofrontal damage reacted with increased novelty responses and failure to suppress a response to repeated aversive stimuli that never result in a true threat. These findings were interpreted as support for the role of the orbitofrontal cortex in regulating neural activity associated with emotional stimuli. Damage to the orbitofrontal cortex impairs the ability to recognize repeated emotional stimuli as familiar, and, therefore, reactions to the stimuli are not suppressed.

BUILDING ON CURRENT THEORY AND RESEARCH ON THE SOCIAL FUNCTIONS OF THE ORBITOFRONTAL CORTEX

Close examination of the extant theories does not permit us to point to one of the three proposed theories and name it as the correct view. It is likely that elements of all three are correct. However, it has been difficult to draw precise conclusions about the mechanisms of orbitofrontal cortex activity in relation to emotional influences on decisions and judgments for several reasons (see Table 2.1).

First, it is unlikely that physiological arousal or its mental representation is critical for enhancing cognition. Research has shown that although physiological arousal may be involved, it is too slow to account exclusively for emotional priming influences on cognition (e.g., Fiske & Taylor, 1991). Studies have also shown that patients with spinal cord injuries, bereft of physiological feedback, report subjective experiences of emotion like those of healthy control participants (Bermond, Nieuwenhuyse, Fasotti, & Schuerman, 1991; Chwalisz, Diener, & Gallagher, 1988; but see Hohmann, 1966) and do not show impaired performance on gambling tasks (North & O'Carroll, 2001). Additionally, research has shown that individuals tend to misattribute their physiological arousal (e.g., Dutton & Aron, 1974), and therefore it is unlikely that patterns of arousal (or mentally represented patterns of arousal) are all that useful for ensuring nonbiased decisions.

Other theorists have implicated the orbitofrontal cortex in updating reinforcement contingencies in rapidly changing social environments (Rolls, 2000) or in filtering the influence of emotional responses on cognition

---

TABLE 2.1. Future Directions for Research on Orbitofrontal Cortex Involvement in Emotion–Social Cognition Interactions

1. Move away from the emphasis on orbitofrontal cortex involvement in generating or representing physiological markers needed for decision making.

2. Conduct complementary studies using lesion and neuroimaging techniques. In particular, more neuroimaging studies that examine the interplay of emotion and cognition are needed.

3. Conduct more studies of emotional influences on decisions that require long-term, socially relevant knowledge.

4. Work toward understanding the orbitofrontal cortex's role in both adaptive and maladaptive emotional infuences on social cognition.

5. Adopt more standardized conceptualization and operationalization for constructs such as emotion and social behavior.

(Shimamura, 2000). More than two decades of social cognitive research suggests that emotion should influence cognition in social contexts by engaging particular cognitive strategies that ultimately influence social judgments and decisions about response selection (e.g., Fiske & Taylor, 1991; Forgas, 1995; Schwarz, 1990). Such a perspective brings together elements of extant theories of orbitofrontal cortex function and may be a more fruitful avenue toward understanding the importance of emotion–social-cognition interactions and their importance for social functioning.

Second, the small number of functional neuroimaging studies in this domain do not sufficiently complement the lesion studies. Instead of examining the interplay between cognition and emotion, functional neuroimaging studies have mostly examined orbitofrontal cortex activity in relation to either cognition (e.g., decision making vs. guessing) or emotion (i.e., presence vs. absence of punishment and reward). Although a few studies have examined orbitofrontal cortex activity in relation to mood-congruent effects on verbal fluency and memory tasks, these data have been difficult to interpret (Baker, Frith, & Dolan, 1997; Elliott, Rubinsztein, Sahakian, & Dolan, 2002; Gray, Braver, & Raichle, 2002). For example, one study did not find a behavioral mood-congruent effect of sad versus happy moods on verbal fluency (Baker et al., 1997). The absence of a behavioral effect makes it difficult to draw strong conclusions about brain activity underlying the interaction of mood and verbal fluency. Another study found orbitofrontal cortex involvement in mood-congruent processing of distracting stimuli that was of a sad nature (Elliott et al., 2002). However, this study involved participants with chronic depression, and the chronic nature of their negative mood makes it difficult to know whether these findings generalize to the influence of more temporary negative moods on attention. Finally, another study found that a more lateral portion of the prefrontal lobes was involved in emotional influences on memory for words and faces (Gray et al., 2002). However, from a social-psychological perspective, the memory task in this study is not particularly generalizable to the online social-information processing that is associated with social adjustment.

Third, emotional learning theories of orbitofrontal cortex function explain the critical involvement of the orbitofrontal cortex in *learning* novel reinforcement contingencies but do not explain why patients with orbitofrontal cortex damage in adulthood show a discrepancy between their *already acquired* knowledge and online behavior. More studies are needed that adopt paradigms that require individuals to use long-held knowledge to make decisions or judgments.

Fourth, dominant theories of orbitofrontal cortex function do not account for the robust emotion–cognition interactions found in more than two decades of behavioral research. The extant theories of the orbitofrontal cortex address only adaptive influences of task-relevant emotion on cognition. Such a claim does not account for 20 years of behavioral research

(Fiske & Taylor, 1991; Isen & Geva, 1987; Forgas, 1995; Schwarz, 1990), which has shown that a common mechanism allows emotion to sometimes enhance cognition (i.e., provide useful information that results in more adaptive decisions or judgments) and other times bias cognitive processes (i.e., provide irrelevant information that results in misguided decisions or judgments).

For example, closer examination of the one neuroimaging study that examined orbitofrontal cortex activity in relation to the interaction of cognition and feedback suggests a broader function of the orbitofrontal cortex. Orbitofrontal cortex activity was associated with the presence of feedback during a guessing task, yet this feedback provided no relevant information for success on subsequent trials (Elliott et al., 1997). Therefore, the positive and negative feedback may have acted more like an emotion induction and influenced the general mood of the participants. The increased orbitofrontal cortex activity found in the guessing task with feedback condition may have reflected the influence of participants' mood on their response selection. These findings suggest that the orbitofrontal cortex mediates the use of any emotional information, regardless of whether it is informative for the task at hand or not, when making decisions and judgments.

This field of research would benefit from the standardized measurement of the relevant constructs used by social psychologists. For example, each perspective operationalizes emotion in a different way. Is the orbitofrontal cortex important for the regulation of physiological arousal (somatic markers), for positive versus negative appraisals (reinforcement/reversal), or for a broader construct that might encompass both (filters or something altogether different)? Standard operationalizations of constructs are crucial for progress in this research field. In particular, social psychologists have standardized operationalization of emotion on the basis of empirical evidence. From this perspective, emotion is defined as a short-lived psychological–physiological phenomenon that coordinates modes of adaptation to changing environmental demands (Levenson, 1999). Although emotions can be categorized (i.e, positive, negative, or self-conscious), theorists emphasize the importance of studying specific emotions. For example, although both fear and anger are negative emotions, research has shown that each is associated with a specific phenomenological experience and facial expression (e.g., Izard, 1971; Levenson, 1999; Shaver, Schwartz, Kirson, & O'Connor, 1987), and have different consequences for decision making (Lerner & Keltner, 2000). Together these findings support the operationalization of emotion using multiple methods: self-report, physiological assessment, and/or coding of facial expression.

Finally, social psychology, perhaps more than any other scientific tradition, has a long history of strong experimental methods for studying emotion and social behavior. Paradigms that closely model real-world social interactions but that still maintain some experimental control will be critical for understanding the neural mediation of emotion and social behavior. For example, psychologists have used various methods to elicit emotions, such as showing participants emotional pictures or films (e.g., Lang, Bradley, & Cuthbert, 1995; Gross & Levenson, 1995), asking them to do behavioral tasks such as singing in public (e.g., Cohen, Nisbett, Bowdle, & Schwartz, 1996; Keltner, 1995; Miller, 1990), or asking them to recall emotional experiences (e.g., Lang, 1978; Levenson, 1999). Similar types of standardized paradigms for interpersonal interactions have also been developed (i.e., Aron, Melinat, Aron, Vallone, & Bator, 1997).

Additionally, the relevance of the typically used paradigms (i.e., gambling tasks) for everyday social behavior is not well tested. No empirical tests of social interaction (i.e., social situations involving interactions with people) have been reported. Therefore, the impact of these processes (e.g., generating somatic markers, reversing associations, and filtering emotional processing) in everyday social behavior remains an unanswered question.

MOVING TOWARD AN ANSWER: RESEARCH USING SOCIAL-PSYCHOLOGICAL AND NEUROSCIENCE APPROACHES TO STUDY ORBITOFRONTAL CORTEX FUNCTION

Many of the concerns listed herein can be addressed by careful research that focuses on standardized measurement of emotion and social cognition in paradigms that have relevance for social functioning. Our own research examining orbitofrontal cortex functioning has adopted an approach that blends a social-psychological conceptualization and measurement of emotion and social behavior with neuroscience methodology. For example, as a first step toward fleshing out the extant research on orbitofrontal function, we tested whether patients with orbitofrontal damage could experience discrete emotions and whether these emotions were elevated as might be predicted by the dynamic filtering perspective (Shimamura, 2000). Additionally, we conducted two empirical studies to test more rigorously the claim that orbitofrontal damage is associated with inappropriate social behavior. Finally, a series of studies are under way to more precisely characterize the involvement of the orbitofrontal cortex in online interactions between emotion and social cognition.

Orbitofrontal Cortex and Experimentally Induced Emotionality

Can patients with orbitofrontal damage experience discrete emotions? If so, are these emotions particularly intense, as suggested by dynamic filtering theory? After examining the extant research, it became clear that although their ability to recognize emotions in others and to respond to feedback had been tested, no thorough study of the emotionality of these patients had ever been conducted. Specifically, we extended previous research by testing orbitofrontal damage in relation to emotion using a multimethod emotion-specific assessment (Beer et al, 2001). Our findings suggest that the orbitofrontal cortex may be most important for filtering information relevant to generating self-conscious emotions (e.g., embarrassment, pride, shame, guilt). We compared patients with orbitofrontal cortex damage ($N = 6$) with age-matched controls ($N = 6$) in a series of emotion-eliciting tasks (Gross & Levenson, 1995; Keltner, 1995). Emotion was measured using self-report, autonomic nervous system physiology, and coding of facial muscle movement (Facial Action Coding System [FACS]; Ekman & Friesen, 1976). Damage to the orbitofrontal cortex was associated with increased self-reports and facial expressions of embarrassment, but no differences were found for other emotions, such as amusement (see Table 2.2). Furthermore, our findings were inconsistent with the theory that the orbitofrontal cortex is critically involved in the ability to inhibit all forms of emotion. We found no significant differences in the ability to suppress facial expressions of disgust while watching a film of an amputation. Both groups reported similar levels of disgust and displayed similar levels of facial twitching, reflecting equal effort in the suppression of facial expression (Gross & Levenson, 1993).

Orbitofrontal Cortex and Spontaneous Emotionality

Our initial study showed that patients with orbitofrontal damage could experience emotion if emotional stimuli were made explicitly salient to them. However, what kind of emotion did these patients exhibit in more typical interpersonal interactions? And was it the case that orbitofrontal damage was empirically associated with inappropriate social behavior? This study was the first empirical demonstration of the social inappropriateness associated with orbitofrontal damage. The findings suggest that in

TABLE 2.2. Comparisons between the Orbitofrontal Cortex and Control Groups for Self-Reports and Facial Expression of Emotion

	F	Eta
Embarrassment		
Self-report	5.5*	0.56
Facial expression	6.9*	0.60
Amusement		
Self-report	1.2	0.30
Facial expression	0.80	0.25
Suppression of disgust		
Self-report	0.03	0.05
Facial expression (disgust)	0.60	0.22
Facial expression (suppression)	0.28	0.15

*$p < .05$.

the context of spontaneous social interactions, patients with orbitofrontal damage tended to act inappropriately and to generate emotions that were inappropriate. That is, their emotions tended to reinforce their poor social behavior rather than correct it (Beer et al., 2003). Patients with orbitofrontal damage exhibited teasing behavior that was objectively more inappropriate than that of control participants. Rather than being embarrassed by their inappropriate teasing, the patients were more proud of their behavior.

Orbitofrontal Cortex and Self-Monitoring

The striking contrast between the objective behavior and emotional appraisals of patients with orbitofrontal damage suggested that perhaps a lack of self-insight was the real reason that these patients were not benefiting from emotional influences on their decision making. More specifically, if one is not aware that one is acting in an embarrassing manner, nothing motivates the decision to change the current behavior. In a third study, self-awareness was manipulated using a modification of the Duval and Wicklund (1972) mirror method (i.e., participants viewed their social behavior on a videotape after participating in a self-disclosure task). This study examined change in self-insight and emotional appraisals of social behavior as a function of the self-awareness manipulation (Beer, John, Scabini, & Knight, 2006). Patients with orbitofrontal damage, healthy controls, and controls with dorsolateral prefrontal damage took part in a self-disclosure task (Aron et al., 1997). This paradigm relied on participants' long-term knowledge that it is inappropriate to disclose personal information to strangers (and all three groups demonstrated equal knowledge of this social norm). In comparison with the other two groups, patients with orbitofrontal damage were judged as disclosing more personal and inappropriate information. Before viewing their videotaped behavior, patients with orbitofrontal damage had unrealistically positive self-views of their social appropriateness and were not embarrassed by their behavior. After viewing their videotaped behavior, the patients' embarrassment significantly increased. These findings suggest that the orbitofrontal cortex may support appropriate social behavior through online monitoring of behavior (e.g., in reference to social norms). In the case of orbitofrontal damage, poor monitoring or self-insight may preclude the generation of the emotions needed to motivate the correction of inappropriate behavior.

Orbitofrontal Cortex and Monitoring Emotional Influences on Decision Making

If the orbitofrontal cortex is involved in monitoring the appropriateness of behavior, does it also monitor occasions on which emotion is allowed to influence decision making and on which it is not? In a series of functional magnetic resonance imaging (fMRI) studies, we examined orbitofrontal activity in relation to emotionally primed gambles. In one study, participants were told to ignore the emotional primes when betting, and in another study they were told that the emotional prime provided useful feedback for deciding how much to risk in a subsequent gamble (i.e., a hypothetical roulette game; Beer, Knight, & D'Esposito, 2006). Increased lateral orbitofrontal activity was found in relation to inhibiting the influence of unhelpful emotional primes and in relation to incorporating the influence of helpful emotional primes in risk taking. Therefore, the orbitofrontal cortex may have many different kinds of monitoring functions (e.g., behavior in reference to norms, the influence of emotion on cognition). A remaining question is whether the orbitofrontal cortex's monitoring of the influence of emotional information on cognition is related to ensuring social appropriateness.

CONCLUSION

By adopting a blend of neuroscience and social psychological perspectives, future research will provide important information about orbitofrontal cortex mediation of social behavior. Ultimately, such research will have implications for understanding the importance of emotion–social-cognition interactions for social adjustment, in addition to potentially integrating elements of the three predominant theories of the orbitofrontal cortex.

REFERENCES

Adolphs, R. (1999). Social cognition and the human brain. *Trends in Cognitive Sciences*, 469–479.

Aron, A., Melinat, E., Aron, E. N., Vallone, R. D., & Bator, R. J. (1997). The experimental generation of interpersonal closeness: A procedure and some preliminary findings. *Personality and Social Psychology Bulletin, 4*, 363–377.

Baker, S. C., Frith, C. D., & Dolan, R. J. (1997). The interaction between mood and cognitive function studied with PET. *Psychological Medicine, 27*, 565–578.

Bechara, A., Damasio, H., & Damasio, A. R. (2000). Emotion, decision making, and the orbitofrontal cortex. *Cerebral Cortex, 10*, 295–307.

Bechara, A., Damasio, H., Tranel, D., & Damasio, A. R. (1997). Deciding advantageously before knowing the advantageous strategy. *Science, 275*, 1293–1295.

Beer, J. S., Heerey, E. H., Keltner, D., Scabini, D., & Knight, R. T. (2003). The regulatory function of self-conscious emotion: Insights from patients with orbitofrontal damage. *Journal of Personality and Social Psychology, 85*, 594–604.

Beer, J. S., John, O. P., Scabini, D., & Knight, R. T. (2006). Orbitofrontal cortex and social behavior: Integrating self-monitoring and emotion–cognition interactions. *Journal of Cognitive Neuroscience, 18*, 871–880.

Beer, J.S., Knight, R.T., & D'Esposito, M. (2006). Integrating emotion and cognition: The role of the frontal lobes in distinguishing between helpful and hurtful emotion. *Psychological Science, 17,* 448–453.

Beer, J. S., Roberts, N. A., Werner, K. H., Ivry, R. B., Scabini, D., Levenson, R. W., et al. (2001). Orbitofrontal cortex and self-conscious emotion. *Society for Neuroscience Abstracts, 27,* 1705.

Beer, J. S., Shimamura, A. P., & Knight, R. T. (2004). Frontal lobe contributions to executive control of cognitive and social behavior. In M. S. Gazzaniga (Ed.) *The cognitive neurosciences III* (3rd ed., pp. 1091–1104). Cambridge, MA: MIT Press.

Bermond, B., Nieuwenhuyse, B., Fasotti, L., & Schuerman, J. (1991). Spinal cord lesions, peripheral feedback, and intensities of emotional feelings. *Cognition and Emotion, 5,* 201–220.

Brothers, L. (1996). Brain mechanisms of social cognition. *Journal of Psychopharmacology, 10,* 2–8.

Chwalisz, K., Diener, E., & Gallagher, D. (1988). Autonomic arousal feedback and emotional experience: Evidence from the spinal cord injured. *Journal of Personality and Social Psychology, 54,* 820–828.

Cohen, D., Nisbett, R. E., Bowdle, B. F., & Schwartz, N. (1996). Insult, aggression, and the Southern culture of honor: An "experimental ethnography." *Journal of Personality and Social Psychology, 70,* 945–960.

Crick, N. R., & Dodge, K. A. (1994). A review and reformulation of social information-processing mechanisms in children's social adjustment. *Psychological Bulletin, 115,* 74–101.

Dutton, D. G., & Aron, A. P. (1974). Some evidence for heightened sexual attraction under conditions of high anxiety. *Journal of Personality and Social Psychology, 30,* 510–517.

Duval, S., & Wicklund, R. A. (1972). *A theory of objective self-awareness.* New York: Academic Press.

Ekman, P., & Friesen, W. V. (1976) *Pictures of facial affect.* Palo Alto, CA: Consulting Psychologists Press.

Elliott, R., Dolan, R. J., & Frith, C. D. (2000). Dissociable functions in the medial and lateral orbitofrontal cortex: Evidence from human neuroimaging studies. *Cerebral Cortex, 10,* 308–317.

Elliott, R., Frith, C. D., & Dolan, R. J. (1997). Differential neural response to positive and negative feedback in planning and guessing tasks. *Neuropsychologia, 35,* 1395–1404.

Elliott, R., Rubinsztein, M. B., Sahakian, B. J., & Dolan, R. J. (2002). The neural basis of mood-congruent processing biases in depression. *Archives in General Psychiatry, 59,* 597–604.

Emery, N. J., & Amaral, D. G. (2000). The role of the amygdala in primate social cognition. In R. D. Lane & L. Nadel (Eds.), *Cognitive neuroscience of emotion* (pp. 156–191). New York: Oxford University Press.

Fellows, L. K., & Farah, M. J. (2003). Ventromedial frontal cortex mediates affective shifting in humans: Evidence from a reversal learning paradigm. *Brain, 126,* 1830–1837.

Fiske, S. T., & Taylor, S. E. (1991). *Social cognition (2nd ed.).* San Francisco: McGraw-Hill.

Forgas, J. P. (1995). Mood and judgment: The affect infusion model (AIM). *Psychological Bulletin, 117,* 39–66.

Gray, J. R., Braver, T. S., & Raichle, M. E. (2002). Integration of emotion and cognition in lateral prefrontal cortex. *Proceedings of the National Academy of Sciences of the USA, 99,* 4115–4120.

Gross, J. J., & Levenson, R. W. (1993). Emotional suppression: Physiology, self-report, and expressive behavior. *Journal of Personality and Social Psychology, 64,* 970–986.

Gross, J. J., & Levenson, R. W. (1995). Emotion elicitation using films. *Cognition and Emotion, 9,* 87–108.

Hohmann, G. W. (1966). Some effects of spinal cord lesions on experienced emotional feelings. *Psychophysiology, 3,* 143–156.

Hornak, J., Rolls, E. T., & Wade, D. (1996). Face and voice expression identification in patients: The emotional and behavioral changes following ventral frontal lobe damage. *Neuropsychologia, 34,* 247–261.

Isen, A. M., & Geva, N. (1987). The influence of positive affect on acceptable level of risk: The person with a large canoe has a large worry. *Organizational Behavior and Human Decision Processes, 39,* 145–154.

Izard, C. E. (1971). *The face of emotion.* New York: Appleton-Century-Crofts.

Keltner, D. (1995). Signs of appeasement: Evidence for the distinct displays of embarrassment, amusement, and shame. *Journal of Personality and Social Psychology, 68,* 441–454.

Kringelbach, M. L., & Rolls, E. T. (2004). The functional neuroanatomy of the human orbitofrontal cortex: Evidence from neuroimaging and neuropsychology. *Progress in Neurobiology, 72,* 341–372.

Lang, P. J. (1978). A bio-informational theory of emotional imagery. *Psychophysiology, 16,* 495–512.

Lang, P. J., Bradley, M. M., & Cuthbert, B. N. (1995). *The International Affective Picture System (IAPS): Photographic slides.* Gainesville, FL: University of Florida, Center for Research in Psychophysiology.

Lerner, J. S., & Keltner, D. (2000). Fear, anger, and risk. *Journal of Personality and Social Psychology, 81,* 146–159.

Levenson, R. W. (1999). The intrapersonal functions of emotion. *Cognition and Emotion, 13,* 481–504.

Miller, R. S. (1995). Embarrassment and social behavior. In J. P. Tangney & K. W. Fischer (Eds), *Self-conscious emotions: The psychology of shame, guilt, embarrassment and pride* (pp. 322–339). New York: Guilford Press.

North, N. T., & O'Carroll, R. E. (2001). Decision making in patients with spinal cord damage: Afferent feedback and the somatic marker hypothesis. *Neuropsychologia, 39,* 521–524.

Rahman, S., Sahakian, B. J., Cardinal, R. N., Rogers, R. D., & Robbins, T. W. (2001). Decision making and neuropsychiatry. *Trends in Cognitive Sciences, 5,* 271–277.

Rolls, E. T. (2000). The orbitofrontal cortex and reward. *Cerebral Cortex, 10,* 284–294.

Rolls, E. T., Hornak, J., Wade, D., & McGrath, J. (1994). Emotion-related learning in patients with social and emotional changes associated with frontal lobe damage. *Journal of Neurology, Neurosurgery, and Psychiatry, 57,* 1518–1524.

Rule, R., Shimamura, A., & Knight, R. T. (2002). Orbitofrontal cortex and dynamic filtering of emotions. *Cognitive, Affective, and Behavioral Neuroscience, 2,* 264–270.

Saver, J. L., & Damasio, A. R. (1991). Preserved access and processing of social knowledge in a patient with acquired sociopathy due to ventromedial frontal damage. *Neuropsychologia, 29,* 1241–1249.

Schwarz, N. (1990). Feelings as information: Informational and motivational functions of affective states. In E. T. Higgins, & R. M. Sorrentino (Eds.), *Handbook of motivation and cognition: Foundations of social behavior* (Vol. 2, pp. 527–561). New York: Guilford Press.

Shaver, P. R., Schwartz, J., Kirson, D., & O'Connor, C. (1987). Emotion knowledge: Further exploration of a prototype approach. *Journal of Personality and Social Psychology, 52,* 1061–1086.

Shimamura, A. P. (2000). The role of the prefrontal cortex in dynamic filtering. *Psychobiology, 28,* 207–218.

Sprengelmeyer, R., Rausch, M., Eysel, U. T., & Przuntek, H. (1998). Neural structures associated with recognition of facial expressions of basic emotions. *Proceedings of the Royal Society of London, 265,* 1927–1931.

Stone, V. E., Baron-Cohen, S., & Knight, R. T. (1998). Frontal lobe contributions to theory of mind. *Journal of Cognitive Neuroscience, 10,* 640–656.

Thorpe, S. J., Rolls, E. T., & Maddison, S. (1983). The orbitofrontal cortex: Neuronal activity in the behaving monkey. *Experimental Brain Research, 49,* 93–115.

Tranel, D., Bechara, A., & Denburg, N.L. (2002). Asymmetric functional roles of right and left ventromedial prefrontal cortices in social conduct, decision making and emotional processing. *Cortex, 38,* 589–612.

Tucker, D. M., Luu, P., & Pribram, K. H. (1995). Social and emotional self-regulation. *Annals of the New York Academy of Sciences, 769,* 213–239.

Whalen, P. J. (1998). Fear, vigilance, and ambiguity: Initial neuroimaging studies of the human amygdala. *Current Directions in Psychological Science, 7,* 177–188.

3

Neurobiology of Emotion Recognition
CURRENT EVIDENCE FOR SHARED SUBSTRATES

Andrea S. Heberlein and Ralph Adolphs

Models of emotion recognition that emphasize simulation processes have been gaining in popularity in recent years (e.g., Adolphs, 2002; Gallese, Keysers, & Rizzolatti, 2004; Goldman & Sripada, 2005). According to such models, recognizing another person's emotional expression depends at least in part on a subset of the same neural structures that would be engaged if one were expressing the emotion oneself. A closely connected idea is that observing another's emotion would engage a subset of the structures that would be engaged if the same emotion were *experienced* (and not just expressed) in the observer. In other words, the process of recognizing an emotional expression includes *simulating* the observed emotion in one's own emotion circuitry; *shared-substrates* models emphasize this dual purpose. Because such a simulation appears to be automatically generated whenever we observe someone expressing (and presumably experiencing) an emotion, it has also been termed *vicarious responding* (Morrison, in press); such responding is often discussed in the context of empathic responses (Preston & de Waal, 2002). Although a simulation model might go so far as to posit an emotional resonance—that is, that the observer, in observing an emotional expression, comes to feel the observed emotion in him- or herself—most models agree that the response can stop short of such a resonance. An open question, therefore, concerns the extent of the simulation: Are we simulating aspects of the premotor/motor activations that would normally cause the observed emotional expression? Are we simulating also the sensory activations resulting from perceiving such an emotion were we to express it in ourselves? Or are we simulating whatever activations are responsible for the conscious experience of the emotion (perhaps a combination of subsets of the first two components)? These important distinctions leave a lot of room for different accounts of simulation and are often not sufficiently distinguished in the literature.

Experimental support for a simulation model of emotion recognition comes from multiple quarters. In electromyography studies, the facial muscles that create emotional expressions contract in emotion-specific ways as people view photographs of emotional faces (Dimberg, 1982; Dimberg et al., 2000). Because the latter study used subliminally presented images of facial expressions, it also provides evidence for the idea that simulation can occur in the absence of conscious awareness of the stimulus. As we discuss in detail later, functional neuroimaging studies have found overlapping patterns of activation when people experience emotions and observe others expressing the same emotions, and lesion studies have implicated certain structures both in expression and in experience. Specifically, two basic emotions have been associated with specific neural structures via functional imaging and lesion studies: fear with the amygdala and disgust with the insula. These observations make a compelling case for the involvement of a simulation process in which recognition relies on neural representations of one's own emotional experience.

However, recent data challenging the specificity of the involvement of the amygdala in recognizing fear have thrown into question at least some versions of shared-substrates models. Furthermore, several recent studies have implicated right-hemisphere somatosensory cortices in emotion recognition based on a variety of nonverbal cues. These cortices appear to be involved in processing the expressions of multiple basic emotions, perhaps by representing the proprioceptive and/or gut feelings associated with the perceived emotional expressions. Although the involvement of somatosensory cortices in the recognition of multiple emotions is broadly consistent with the idea of simulation, namely, that we use internal representations of our own emotional experience in order to associate labels with others' expressions, it has been unclear how to relate this involvement to the emotion-specific shared-substrates models. In this chapter, we review the evidence for simulation-based models of emotion recognition, focusing on evidence for amygdala involvement in the experience and recognition of fear, insula involvement in the experience and recognition of disgust, and right somatosensory cortex involvement in the recognition of multiple emotions. We discuss the inadequacies of simple shared-substrate models and sketch what a revised model incorporating newer data on these regions might look like.

ANATOMY OF THE AMYGDALA

The amygdala is a small, paired, almond-shaped (*amygdala* = Greek; "almond") collection of nuclei buried in the anterior medial temporal lobe. Its multiple nuclei (over a dozen in primates) have diverse connectivity,

leading some to argue that it should not be conceived of as a unitary structure at all (Swanson & Petrovich, 1998). Nonetheless, most investigators
believe it reasonable to refer to the "the amygdala," for several reasons.
First, the heterogeneous connectivity of different amygdala nuclei notwith-
standing, there is in fact substantially more connectivity among amygdala
nuclei than between a given nucleus and extra-amygdalar structures. The
flow of information through the amygdala further corroborates the view
that this is a collection of nuclei that participate in a set of related functions. Roughly, this information flow begins with input from higher order
sensory neocortices to the lateral amygdala, then on to the basal amygdala,
from which feedback projections to sensory cortical regions originate, and
to the central nucleus, the main output from the amygdala to autonomic
control structures that can trigger changes in skin conductance, heart rate,
and other aspects of emotional response. A final reason for treating the
amygdala as a single structure without decomposition into its nuclei for
studies in humans is that the spatial resolution of lesion studies, and also of
most fMRI studies, does not allow conclusions about individual nuclei.

The amygdala receives input from all sensory modalities. Except for
the case of olfaction, which is provided directly from the olfactory bulb to
the medial amygdala, highly processed sensory information comes from
higher order sensory neocortex. However, there are important exceptions
even here: There appear to be rapid, coarse subcortical sensory inputs to
the amygdala via other nuclei in the thalamus. This has been studied most
intensively in the case of auditory stimuli by Joseph LeDoux and others,
but there is evidence for such an architecture also in the case of vision.
Subcortical visual information from the superior colliculus projects to the
pulvinar thalamus and hence may project to the amygdala to provide rapid
information about the emotion signaled by visual stimuli (Jones & Burton,
1976).

THE AMYGDALA IN FEAR EXPERIENCE

Shared-substrates models of emotion recognition, by definition, require
that a given structure is critical for experience or expression as well as recognition. Early ablation studies in nonhuman primates showed changes in
behavior toward both inanimate objects and conspecifics after amygdala
damage (Kluver & Bucy, 1939/1997), and although many of these results
were subsequently shown to be due to disruptions of fibers passing through
the amygdala, subsequent lesion studies with such fibers spared have
shown circumscribed changes in apparent emotion experience (Amaral,
2002). For example, monkeys normally display fear toward snakes, even
rubber ones, but amygdalectomized monkeys do not (Kalin, Shelton,
Davidson, & Kelley, 2001; Amaral, 2002).

Classical (or Pavlovian) conditioning provides a time-honored method
for assessing the ability to represent the emotional value of sensory stimuli

independently of their perceptual properties. Though we are unable to measure the internal experience associated with the physiological response in nonhuman animals, aversive conditioning is widely referred to as "fear conditioning," presumably because the physiological responses to the aversive stimuli (and eventually to the conditioned stimuli) are similar to those associated with subjectively reported fear in humans. The amygdala is widely known to play a key role in aversive conditioning in animal models (Fanselow & LeDoux, 1999), as well as in humans (Bechara et al., 1995; LaBar, LeDoux, Spencer, & Phelps, 1995; Buchel, Morris, Dolan, & Friston, 1998; Buchel & Dolan, 2000).

Studies using multiple methods have linked the amygdala to feelings of fear and anxiety in human participants. Intracranial stimulation in the amygdala evokes the feeling of fear in patients about to undergo surgery for epilepsy (Halgren, Walter, Cherlow, & Crandall, 1978). Ketter and colleagues demonstrated a correlation between the intensity of anxiety induced by procaine, an anesthetic, and amygdala activation in an imaging study (Ketter et al., 1996), and amygdala activation is also observed when neurologically intact participants view negative or aversive stimuli (Irwin et al., 1996). However, lesion studies in humans do not support a critical role for the amygdala in the experience of fear: Participants with unilateral or bilateral amygdala damage report normal affective states, both in a retrospective consideration of the past month of experience and in a day-by-day measure over the course of a month (Anderson & Phelps, 2002). This was the case even for affective states associated with fear and anxiety, implying that the amygdala is not critical for normal experience of a range of emotional feelings, even though it may be recruited during such experience in intact brains. There are also differences in amygdala involvement in different fear behaviors in nonhuman primates depending on when damage is incurred, implying changing roles for the amygdala in fear-related behaviors during development: Whereas monkeys with adult-acquired amygdala lesions show decreases in fear toward both snakes and conspecifics, neonatally amygdalectomized monkeys show decreases in fear toward inanimate objects and snakes but *increases* in fearful responses toward conspecifics (Prather et al., 2001; Bauman, Lavenex, Mason, Capitanio, & Amaral, 2004). At a minimum, these findings indicate that the amygdala is not essential for the expression of fear responses as such, but rather that it modulates the way in which the perception of sensory stimuli can trigger such responses (Amaral, 2003).

Not only is the role of the amygdala in fear experience complex, but it has also been linked to processing of *positive* stimuli, especially highly arousing positive visual stimuli (Hamann, Ely, Grafton, & Kilts, 1999; Hamann, Ely, Hoffman, & Kilts, 2002), and appears to be important for appetitive conditioning (i.e., with pleasurable stimuli; Johnsrude, Owen, White, Zhao, & Bohbot, 2000). The activation in Hamann and colleagues' (2002) study included not only the amygdala but also the ventral striatum and ventromedial prefrontal cortex, structures closely connected to the amygdala and also previously implicated in reward processing. Thus the amygdala itself appears to participate not only in the processing of threat and negative emotions but also in circuits critically involved in processing positive emotion-relevant stimuli. This pattern of involvement may be clarified by positing a role for the amygdala in the processing of multiple types of arousing stimuli (Adolphs, Russell, & Tranel, 1999; Hamann et al., 2002).

THE AMYGDALA IN FEAR RECOGNITION

Though ablation studies in nonhuman primates had shown impaired social behavior after amygdala damage (Kluver & Bucy, 1939/1997; Amaral, 2002), it was studies of rare individuals with selective bilateral amygdala damage that initially showed a specific deficit in fear recognition consequent to amygdala damage in humans (Adolphs, Tranel, Damasio, & Damasio, 1994; Adolphs, Tranel, Damasio, & Damasio, 1995; Young et al., 1995; Calder, Young, Perrett, Hodges, & Etcoff, 1996; Broks et al., 1998; Sprengelmeyer et al., 1999). These studies primarily used standardized sets of emotional faces (e.g., Ekman & Friesen, 1976) in two task variants: labeling tasks, in which participants chose from a list of emotion words the one that best described the stimulus, and rating tasks, in which participants rated each face for the level of multiple emotions present (i.e., given a "happy" face, rating the level of happiness, sadness, fear, anger, disgust, etc.). When viewed in light of aversive conditioning studies, these initial findings supported a model in which the amygdala was characterized as a "convergence zone" (Damasio, 1989) for fear, in which cortical and subcortical regions associated with fear-related stimuli, including fearful faces, are coordinated by projections to and from the amygdala (Adolphs et al., 1995).

Functional neuroimaging studies of people with intact brains corroborated the results of the lesion studies, though they for the most part did not directly address emotion recognition; participants' tasks most commonly involved passive viewing of emotional faces or performing a task that required attention to the faces but not to their expressions (e.g., gender categorization). Participants who viewed emotional faces showed greater amygdala activation when viewing fearful as compared with neutral faces (Breiter et al., 1996; Morris et al., 1996; Pessoa, McKenna, Gutierrez, & Ungerleider, 2002; Lange et al., 2003) or happy faces (Morris et al., 1996; Phillips et al., 1998; Pessoa et al., 2002; see Phan, Wager, Taylor, & Liberzon, 2002, for a review). Though findings in this regard are mixed, amygdala activity in response to fearful faces has been found even when participants did not consciously perceive the faces: when they were presented subliminally (Whalen et al., 1998; but see Phillips et al., 2004) or during but incidental to an attention-demanding task (Vuilleumier, Armony, Driver, & Dolan, 2001; but see Pessoa et al., 2002). This activation may be due to input from the subcortical pathway, that is, from the superior colliculus to the pulvinar and thus to the amygdala (Morris, Ohman, & Dolan, 1999; Morris, de Gelder, Weiskrantz, & Dolan, 2001; Pegna, Khateb, Lazeyras, & Seghier, 2005).

As summarized previously, the amygdala is known to receive input from the visual cortex and to project back to temporal and occipital visual cortices, including the striate cortex, in primates (Amaral & Price, 1984; Amaral, Price, Pitkanen, & Carmichael, 1992), probably including humans (Catani, Jones, Donato, & ffytche, 2003). A possible functional role for this anatomical connectivity is suggested by electrophysiological data: Intracranial recordings from the human brain show that field potentials in both the amygdala (Oya, Kawasaki, Howard, & Adolphs, 2002; Krolak-Salmon, Henaff, Vighetto, Bertrand, & Mauguiere, 2004) and in the temporal visual cortex (Puce, Allison, & McCarthy, 1999) are modulated by emotional and/or social information. The time course of this field potential modulation—amygdala first, visual cortex next—is consistent with amygdala input giving rise to emotional modulation seen in the visual cortex. Further convincing evidence for the amygdala's role in the emotional modulation of the visual cortex comes from lesion studies: People with hippocampal lesions that spare the amygdala show modulation of brain activation in the visual cortex by fearful faces, but people with amygdala lesions do not show such visual cortex modulation in response to fearful faces (Vuilleumier, Richardson, Armony, Driver, & Dolan, 2004).

Although both functional imaging and lesion studies indicate a connection between fearful-face processing and the amygdala, this picture is not as simple as had initially been thought. Amygdala activity is observed not just during viewing of fearful faces but also when participants view happy as compared with neutral faces (Breiter et al., 1996; Pessoa et al., 2002). Though many studies had found impaired fear recognition after amygdala damage, not all did; patterns of impairment appeared to depend in part on the task used (Adolphs et al., 1995; Calder et al., 1996; Hamann et al., 1996; Broks et al., 1998; Schmolck & Squire, 2001). To address the difficulty in drawing conclusions about discrepant findings across multiple individuals tested using different emotion-recognition tasks, Adolphs and colleagues (Adolphs, Tranel, et al., 1999) compared nine people with bilateral amygdala damage on the same sensitive emotion rating task. Although fear was the most commonly and most severely impaired emotion, only four of the nine were impaired on fear recognition, and some were impaired on other emotions (three each were impaired on sadness, disgust, and surprise and four on anger). This result clearly showed that bilateral amygdala damage does not always lead to fear-recognition deficits from faces, nor does it lead to deficits in the recognition only of fear. However, there was no satisfying explanation for the variance between individuals. Since the publication of that study, several neuroimaging studies have taken up this challenge and explicitly examined individual differences. Perhaps not surprisingly, it has turned out that variance in personality traits and in gene polymorphisms has a large effect on amygdala activation to emotional faces (e.g., Canli, Sivers, Whitfield, Gotlib, & Gabrieli, 2002; Hariri et al., 2002; Bishop, Duncan, & Lawrence, 2004; Pezawas et al., 2005). We consider it a high priority to include comprehensive measures of individual differences (from personality questionnaires, as well as genetics) in future studies of the functions of the amygdala.

A recent examination of the parts of facial expressions used to make emotion categorizations sheds new light on the amygdala's role in facial expression recognition (Adolphs, Gosselin, et al., 2005). Adolphs and colleagues retested one of the individuals who had been tested earlier, S.M., using a careful technique in which participants make two-alternative emotion judgments based on viewing only small variably placed and variably sized regions of the face at once (Schyns, Bonnar, & Gosselin, 2002). Normal control participants use information from the eye region to make judgments of happiness, fear, sadness, and anger, and especially the latter three of these (Smith, Gosselin, & Schyns, 2004). In contrast, Adolphs and colleagues showed that S.M. does not rely on information from the eye region when judging either fear or happiness. The authors posit that, though happiness can be reliably identified without using the eye region, S.M.'s previously shown impairment in fearful-face recognition follows from her failure to pay attention to the eyes. In a direct test of this, S.M.'s fear recognition was "rescued" when she was instructed to attend to the eyes in a free-viewing emotion-recognition task (Adolphs, Gosselin, et al., 2005).

These findings fit nicely with a recent study by Whalen and colleagues (2004) in which amygdala activity was compared when participants viewed backward-masked stimuli consisting of the isolated whites of eyes against a black background. "Eye whites" isolated from a fearful facial expression are notably larger than those isolated from a happy expression, and significantly greater activity was observed in the ventral amygdala when participants viewed the fearful, as compared with the happy, eye whites (Whalen et al., 2004). No such pattern was observed when participants were tested with inverted "eye blacks" stimuli, implying that the amygdala response was not driven by shape but by the amount of white sclera visible. The authors' focus on the ventral amygdala was motivated by the location of the basolateral nuclei of the amygdala, which receive a wide range of cortical and subcortical inputs (Amaral et al., 1992; Le Doux, 1996). Thus, rather than merely responding to fearful faces in a sort of large-scale pattern recognition, the amygdala may participate in emotion recognition by responding to the presence of certain facial features, such as eyes, and directing attention for further processing to those features and the environment surrounding them. This interpretation is consistent with findings indicating that participants with bilateral amygdala damage perform poorly on other social judgments that require attention to the eyes, such as inferring intention or attention from eye gaze (Young et al., 1995) or making judgments about social emotions such as jealousy or guilt from the eye region of facial expressions (Adolphs, Baron-Cohen, & Tranel, 2002).

Our discussion so far has focused on the role of the amygdala in processing emotional faces. However, other nonverbal cues, such as vocal prosody and whole-body movements or posture, also convey emotions effectively (Scherer, 1986; Dittrich, Troscianko, Lea, & Morgan, 1996; Wallbott, 1998). There have been many fewer studies of amygdala involvement in emotion recognition using nonface cues, and at this point the evidence they have yielded is mixed. Bilaterally amygdala-damaged participant D.R., who is impaired at recognizing fear from faces, was also impaired in labeling both fearful and angry prosody (Scott et al., 1997); patient N.E., also with bilateral amygdala damage, was impaired in recognizing fear from faces, prosody, and body postures (Sprengelmeyer et al., 1999). However, three different participants, S.P., S.M., and R.H., showed no selective impairment for fear in prosodic stimuli (Anderson & Phelps, 1998; Adolphs & Tranel, 1999). Although the exact regions of extra-amygdaloid damage differ between these participants, the anatomical differences do not line up with the differences in their impairments (Calder, Lawrence, & Young, 2001), and so it is hard to draw conclusions about the importance of the amygdala in recognition of fear or any other emotions from vocal prosody. Imaging studies have also yielded mixed results: Hearing either fearful vocal expressions or laughter and crying activated amygdalar nuclei in two studies (Phillips et al., 1998; Sander & Scheich, 2001), but another study found a *decrease* in amygdala activation while participants listened to nonverbal expressions of fear (Morris, Scott, & Dolan, 1999). It should be noted that these discrepancies may be due to the limitations of temporal resolution inherent in blood-oxygen-level-dependent (BOLD) fMRI, which we discuss further.

An fMRI comparison of participants passively viewing fearful body postures, as compared with neutral postures (faces were blurred so that facial expression information was not available) yielded unilateral amygdala activity (Hadjikhani & de Gelder, 2003), implying a role for the amygdala in the processing of fearful visual expressions other than faces. However, whereas one lesion study (Sprengelmeyer et al., 1999, described earlier) complements this finding, other lesion data do not: S.M. recognizes fear normally from movie stills with the faces blanked out (Adolphs & Tranel, 2003) and also recognizes fear normally from photographs of posed emotional postures (with faces blurred) and movies of body movements, shown in either full light or point light (Atkinson, Heberlein, & Adolphs, 2006).

In summary, the model built by the early lesion and functional imaging results, in which the amygdala was critically involved in the recognition of fear but much less so, if at all, in the recognition of other emotions, has given way to a more complex picture in which fear is but one example of a broader category of stimuli that can recruit the amygdala. The amygdala's involvement in fear recognition may depend on its response to certain specific features, such as eyes or even parts of eyes—a response that may be greater for fearful faces than for other emotional expressions. Other facial expressions, and expressions in other nonverbal channels such as prosody or body posture, may also elicit but not require amygdala activation for emotion recognition; these activations may be prompted by different amygdala pathways from those that direct attention to fearful eyes. Thus the amygdala cannot be conceived as a simple "fear generator" or even as a "fear processor"; it plays roles in both the experience and the recognition of a range of negative emotional stimuli, as well as in certain highly arousing positive stimuli. As Sander and colleagues (Sander, Grafman, & Zalla, 2003) point out, consistent findings of amygdala involvement in processing fear-related stimuli do not mean that it is *dedicated* to fear-related stimuli. These authors suggest instead that the amygdala, or parts thereof, acts as a detector of salience or relevance, an interpretation similar to that of Whalen and colleagues (e.g., Whalen et al., 2004). As such, nuclei in the amygdala that receive input from subcortical pathways quickly detect the presence of environmental cues signaling potentially important social information—such as large sclera. Via projections to sensory cortices, the amygdala then directs attention to those objects to facilitate further processing. It is easier to make sense of the varied roles ascribed to the amygdala if we keep in mind, first, that it consists of many distinct nuclei with heterogeneous connectivity and, second, that these nuclei may well play multiple roles in the processing of social stimuli. Some of these roles are likely to occur rapidly after stimulus presentation, and others later. Because fMRI BOLD signal is dependent on blood flow and thus integrates over multiple seconds, it is not possible to distinguish between early and late processes—nor, of course, is it possible to do so in lesion studies. Manipulation of the timing of data acquisition and of magnetic resonance pulse sequences, as well as attention to possible habituation effects (e.g., see Breiter et al., 1996), will enable distinctions, at least, between early and late processes in future studies.

ANATOMY OF THE INSULA

The insula is a section of cortex buried underneath the frontal operculum that represents visceral interoceptive information. It receives taste information from the parabrachial nucleus and also peripheral nociceptive and visceral afferent information from the entire body. Some recent anatomical studies have argued that primates possess a dedicated pathway for unmyelinated sympathetic afferent input to peripheral layers of the dorsal horn of the spinal cord and that this information is conveyed to the insula (lateralized perhaps especially to the right insula) to form the neural substrate of the introspective awareness of one's own body state (Craig, 2002).

Indeed, imaging studies have provided some preliminary support for the idea that the ability to perceive changes in one's own body (in one experiment, sensitivity to detect one's own heartbeat) relies on the insula (Critchley, Wiens, Rotshtein, Ohman, & Dolan, 2004).

THE INSULA AND EXPERIENCE OF DISGUST

The human emotion of disgust is hypothesized to have originated in feelings of distaste (Rozin, Haidt, & McCauley, 2000); indeed, the canonical "disgust" face is similar to the expressions made by infants or nonhuman primates rejecting bad-tasting food (Darwin, 1872). As conditioned "fear" is a stand-in for experienced fear in humans, conditioned taste aversion, an acquired dislike for a taste after experiencing it immediately prior to nausea or visceral discomfort, can be related to the experience of disgust. Lesions of the insula or globus pallidus in rats lead to impairments in conditioned taste aversion (Kiefer, 1985). The insula is not entirely unique in this regard, however; lesions of the amygdala have the same effect (Kiefer, 1985), providing further evidence that the amygala is not a "fear center," nor is the insula alone in its involvement in the processing of disgust- or distate-related stimuli. This may not be surprising when we consider that the amygdala and insula are directly connected via the internal capsule and that both regions project to and receive projections from the basal ganglia (Amaral et al., 1992).

Electrical stimulation of the insula in patients undergoing surgery for epilepsy leads to nausea, unpleasant tastes, and unpleasant throat and stomach sensations (Penfield & Faulk, 1955; Krolak-Salmon et al., 2003). In functional imaging studies, exposure to aversive odors and tastes activates both amygdala and insula (Zald, Lee, Fluegel, & Pardo, 1998; Zald & Pardo, 2000; Wicker et al., 2003), thus corroborating a link between disgust and distaste. Lesion evidence provides perhaps the strongest link between the insula and the disgust experience: A patient with unilateral insula damage reported decreased intensity of disgust experience on a questionnaire, relative to controls, but not decreased anger or fear experience (Calder, Keane, Manes, Antoun, & Young, 2000), and a patient with bilateral insula damage happily drank water so salty or sour as to be unpalatable to neurologically intact control participants (Adolphs, Tranel, Koenigs, & Damasio, 2005).

However, both amygdala and insula are also active in response to pleasant tastes and smells (O'Doherty, Rolls, Francis, Bowtell, & McGlone, 2001; Wicker et al., 2003). Wicker and colleagues note overlapping activations in the amygdala for pleasant and aversive smells but distinct activations in the insular cortex, with activations elicited by aversive stimuli in anterior insula and those elicited by pleasant stimuli in posterior insula.

THE INSULA AND RECOGNITION OF DISGUST

Studies of patients with Huntington's disease (HD) were the first to implicate a specific neural substrate for disgust recognition. HD is a neurodegen-
erative disease that initially affects primarily the basal ganglia, especially
the striatum (caudate and putamen). Using tasks such as those described
earlier for use with amygdala-damaged participants, Sprengelmeyer and
colleagues (1996) showed that people in the early stages of HD were disproportionately impaired in recognizing disgust. This deficit was also
observed even in presymptomatic carriers of the mutation that causes HD
(Gray, Young, Barker, Curtis, & Gibson, 1997).

The basal ganglia are also implicated in lesion and functional imaging
studies of disgust processing, which have also reliably found an association
between disgust recognition and the insula. Damage to these regions does
not appear to impair recognition of fear, thus putting to rest claims
(Rapcsak et al., 2000) that fear recognition was impaired in participants
with bilateral amygdala damage because it is simply a harder emotion to
recognize (and, by extension, that any neurological damage that impaired emotion recognition would impair fear recognition most strongly;
Calder et al., 2001). Functional MRI studies of participants viewing disgusted faces yielded significant activations in anterior insula and basal ganglia, especially the putamen (Phillips et al., 1997; Phillips et al., 1998;
Sprengelmeyer, Rausch, Eysel, & Przuntek, 1998), and intracranial recordings from anterior insula showed preferential responses to disgusted faces
(Krolak-Salmon et al., 2003). However, insula activity is not observed
when disgusted faces are presented subliminally (Phillips et al., 2004).

Two lesion studies and one functional imaging study directly tested for
a relationship between recognition and experience of disgust. Calder and
colleagues (Calder et al., 2000) examined patient N.K., who has a lesion
affecting the insula, putamen, globus pallidus, and part of the caudate
nucleus, all on the left side. N.K. showed a selective deficit in recognizing
disgust from both facial and auditory cues. In addition, he rated his own
experience of disgust (on questionnaires) as significantly lower than controls did, despite normal ratings of his experience of fear and anger. However, he correctly assigned disgust labels to disgusting photographs, indicating that his concept of disgust is at least superficially normal. Another
patient, B., who had bilateral damage to the insula but no basal ganglia
damage, was also severely impaired in his recognition of disgust in stimuli,
as well as in his own experience of disgust (Adolphs, Tranel, & Damasio,
2003). Interestingly, this same patient in fact showed a complete inability
to recognize aversive taste stimuli, consuming such normally aversive-
tasting substances as concentrated lemon juice (Adolphs, Tranel, et al.,
2005). In an fMRI study, Wicker and colleagues (Wicker et al., 2003),
as noted earlier, found anterior insula activity when participants were
exposed to offensive odors (as compared with neutral or pleasant odors)

while being scanned. The same participants were also shown photographs of people smelling the contents of glasses and expressing pleasure, disgust, or no emotion. Viewing disgusted expressions in this context elicited greater activity in the same region of anterior insula, as compared with viewing the other expressions (Wicker et al., 2003). Thus, despite some lack of selectivity, there is both lesion and functional imaging evidence for a shared involvement of insular cortex in disgust experience and recognition.

RIGHT SOMATOSENSORY REGIONS AND EMOTION RECOGNITION

Neuropsychological studies from more than two decades have implicated right hemisphere cortices in emotion recognition. Patients with right-hemisphere lesions were impaired relative to patients with left-hemisphere damage and/or neurologically intact controls on tasks requiring emotion recognition from visual cues, including faces (Benowitz et al., 1983; Bowers, Bauer, Coslett, & Heilman, 1985; Borod et al., 1998; Kucharska-Pietura, Phillips, Gernand, & David, 2003), as well as tasks requiring the production and/or reception of vocal prosody (Ross, Thompson, & Yenkosky, 1997; Kucharska-Pietura et al., 2003). In addition, a right-hemisphere advantage for emotion recognition has been supported via a range of studies of neurologically intact participants: The left side of the face (which is processed largely by right-side visual cortices) is used more heavily than the right in judgments of expression, as well as gender, attractiveness, and age, from chimeric faces (Burt & Perrett, 1997), and participants rely more extensively on information from the left hemispace when making fine-grained judgments about negative emotional expressions (Jansari, Tranel, & Adolphs, 2000).

Recent lesion overlap studies have narrowed the focus within the right hemisphere to the frontoparietal cortices. Adolphs, Damasio, Tranel, Cooper, and Damasio (2000) compared the lesion locations of 108 people who had been tested with tasks involving recognition of six basic emotions from facial expressions (Ekman & Friesen, 1976) and found two critical regions wherein damage was systematically associated with impaired emotion recognition: right somatosensory-related areas, including S1 (BA 1–3), insula, and underlying white matter; and left frontal operculum (Broca's area/BA 44–45). In similar analyses, damage to right somatosensory and left frontal opercular areas disproportionately impaired participants' performance on an emotional prosody task (Adolphs, Damasio, & Tranel, 2002). Emotion recognition from point-light body movements[1] also critically relied on right postcentral and supramarginal gyri (Heberlein, Adolphs, Tranel, & Damasio, 2004).

Thus, though the role of left inferior frontal regions in emotion recognition may vary between stimuli, cortices in right-hemisphere postcentral and supramarginal gyri appear to be critically involved in emotion judgments based on multiple kinds of cues. These regions may participate in a modeling of what it *feels like* to be in a given emotional state, either at a motor-proprioceptive level (i.e., what it feels like to express the state) or at a more general visceral-representation level (Adolphs et al., 2000; Adolphs, 2002). Functional imaging studies also support this role. Winston and colleagues (Winston, O'Doherty, & Dolan, 2003) found greater activity in the right postcentral gyrus when participants judged which of two gender- and emotion-morphed faces was more emotional compared with their judgments of which of the pair was more male. Ruby and Decety (2004) observed right postcentral gyrus activity when participants were assessing how they themselves would feel in a given emotion-eliciting situation relative to third-person (the participants' mothers) assessments and either first- or third-person neutral-reaction predictions. The same region of right postcentral gyrus that was implicated by lesion overlap for emotion (but not personality trait) judgments from point-light walkers was also more active when neurologically intact participants made emotion, as opposed to personality, judgments from point-light stimuli (Heberlein & Saxe, 2005). In all three of these cases, right somatosensory cortices were more active during emotion judgments than during another kind of social judgment— and in two of these cases, this difference was observed even when the stimuli were the same for both judgment conditions. This indicates that it is not the presence of emotional stimuli that drives the right somatosensory involvement but specific attention to, or processing of, this information.

Whereas these studies and the lesion-overlap studies implicate right somatosensory regions in recognizing multiple basic emotions across the board, one recent study draws a different conclusion based on temporary inactivation of cortex using transcranial magnetic stimulation (TMS). Inactivating somatosensory cortices around the frontoparietal operculum, that is, those subserving lips and tongue representations, led to impairments in recognizing emotional prosody (the tone in which neutral sentences were read) but not emotional semantics (the content of sentences read in a neutral tone; van Rijn et al., 2005). However, not all emotional prosody recognition was impaired: Recognition of happiness and anger was normal, whereas recognition of fear and sadness was impaired. The authors categorize the latter as "withdrawal" emotions and the former as "approach" emotions and hypothesize that right-hemisphere cortices are important for recognition of withdrawal, but not approach, emotions. A similar distinction was found using facial expressions: Recognition of fear, but not happiness, was impaired with TMS stimulation of right somatosensory areas (Pourtois et al., 2004). Van Rijn and colleagues (2005) draw a connection between their apparent lateralization of recognition of withdrawal (vs. approach) emotions to a similar distinction demonstrated for experience (e.g., Davidson, 1992). It is unclear how to reconcile these findings with those that implicate right somatosensory regions for all emotion recognition; further studies using TMS on right and left somatosensory regions will help to address this question.

OTHER KINDS OF SIMULATION

Systems in which a perceived action is mapped onto internal representations of the same behavior—and that use that simulation to infer meaning from the action—have been described for at least two domains in addition to emotion recognition. Viewing another person's painful experience elicits activity in the same regions of anterior cingulate cortex that are active when the observers experience pain themselves, even in the absence of facial expressions or sounds—that is, evidence that the observed person is experiencing pain (Morrison, Lloyd, di Pellegrino, & Roberts, 2004; Singer et al., 2004; Jackson, Meltzoff, & Decety, 2005). Intracranial recordings in monkeys and functional imaging and TMS studies in humans have found regions in F5 or (in humans, left) inferior frontal cortex that are selectively responsive to specific actions, whether observed or performed by the observer. Cells that respond both to the sight (or sound) of an action being performed and to the performance by oneself of the action have been dubbed "mirror neurons"; this mapping has been hypothesized to facilitate imitation as well as goal recognition (Gallese, Fadiga, Fogassi, & Rizzolatti, 1996; Iacoboni et al., 1999; Jellema, Baker, Wicker, & Perrett, 2000; Kohler et al., 2002; Keysers et al., 2003). How these two types of shared-substrates mapping are related to each other and to emotion recognition is unclear, though hypotheses exist (Gallese & Goldman, 1998; Preston & de Waal, 2002; Gallese et al., 2004; Morrison, in press). Some authors also have begun to use evidence for domain-specific simulation models in discussions about simulation in mind reading or mentalizing, an ongoing debate in cognitive science and developmental psychology. Given space constraints, we do not discuss the debate here; for recent treatments of this topic, including the relationship of simulation-based models of emotion recognition and goal inferral from mirror neurons to the mentalizing debate, please see Gallese and Goldman (1998); Goldman and Sripada (2005); Saxe, (2005); and Goldman (2006).

SHARED SUBSTRATES:
A SKETCH OF A MODEL OF EMOTION RECOGNITION

If we consider the *function* of both emotional experience and the recognition of emotion in others, some level of vicarious response makes sense (Morrison, in press). For example, if fear serves to facilitate avoidance of danger, then becoming more alert to danger after viewing another's fearful expression is a good use of fear-processing circuitry. There is, in fact, evidence that watching another person undergoing aversive conditioning results in "observational conditioning," even if the only evidence of an aversive outcome that participants have is facial expressions (Olsson & Phelps, 2004). Similarly, if disgust serves to facilitate avoidance of contamination (Rozin et al., 2000), then becoming sensitized to the target of another person's disgust is also useful for avoiding such items in the future. This motivational–affective framework provides a plausible explanation for vicarious responses and also for shared substrates: Having at least a faint disgust response in response to viewing an expression of disgust would seem to be facilitated by an automatic activation of our own disgust-experience cortices. However, this explanation relies on a greater specificity of emotion–experience mapping than has been observed to date.

As our review indicates, simple shared-substrates models, in which the amygdala is specifically involved in fear recognition and experience and the insula is specifically involved in disgust recognition and experience, do not explain all of the data. The amygdala, especially, is a complex structure that plays roles in the processing of multiple types of social and nonsocial stimuli. Although it clearly plays an important role in both the experience of fear and the recognition of emotions, including fear, its involvement in those processes is not specific enough to support a simple simulation model. Amygdala activation, at least at the level at which it is measured by BOLD fMRI, does not "signal" fear. Nor does insula activation, which is observed in contexts in addition to disgust recognition and experience (e.g., Singer et al., 2004), "signal" disgust. Rather, the roles of these structures in emotion experience and recognition are more complex. In our view, the amygdala is best viewed as a structure that can produce emotional responses (emotional psychophysiological responses, for instance) in response to viewing socially relevant stimuli rather than as a structure that itself represents those emotional responses. The representation of the emotional responses takes place in somatic mapping structures that construct models of what is going on in one's own body and that can also be used to simulate what is going on in another person. These structures are varied, but both the insula and the right somatosensory cortex are two important components.

The role of the right somatosensory cortex in emotion recognition appears to be fairly broad, which is perhaps not surprising, given that it consists of multiple body maps and given that it is easy to imagine how emotion-specific representation and simulation would come about by different complex patterns within this large cortical territory. It is therefore to be expected that lesions of this region would interfere with simulation of multiple emotions. It may be involved in representing the facial (or vocal cord, or body) configuration associated with an emotional expression, and it may be involved in representing a more general body state associated with an emotional feeling (Adolphs, 2002). It remains possible, of course, that some emotion specificity would arise because of other factors, for instance because certain emotions are simply harder to recognize or require more-fine grained simulation than others (van Rijn et al., 2005).

These considerations make it difficult to sketch a complete model of the neural processes underlying emotion recognition. However, such a model is likely to have at least the following components[2]: (1) early encoding of the structure and of certain salient features of the stimulus, involving early visual structures in both cortical (lateral geniculate nucleus to striate cortex) and subcortical (superior colliculus to pulvinar nucleus to amygdala and extrastriate cortex) pathways; (2) later encoding of more complex aspects of the structure and links to representations of emotional reactions, involving extrastriate cortices, different nuclei of the amygdala, the basal ganglia, orbitofrontal cortices, and other structures important for emotional reactions, such as the hypothalamus; (3) cognitive systems that relate representations of the stimulus and of self-emotional reactions to conceptual knowledge about the emotions thus represented, including but not limited to extrastriate regions such as the fusiform face area and superior temporal sulcus/gyrus, orbitofrontal cortices, somatosensory cortices (especially on the right), and the insula.

CONCLUSIONS AND FUTURE DIRECTIONS

It seems clear that, whatever the nature of the simulation, it must simulate aspects of the specific emotion that is to be recognized sufficiently so as to distinguish the simulation of that particular emotion from the simulation of other emotions. Several additional points follow from this idea. First, the level of grain of the simulation would be expected to depend on the level of categorization engaged in by the viewer. For instance, if a viewer is asked merely whether a facial expression showed a pleasant or an unpleasant emotion, a very coarse simulation may suffice to discriminate these two superordinate categories. If the viewer is asked to distinguish among subtle shades of emotions, a more fine-grained simulation that is very emotion specific would be required. A second point is that there must be partly separable partitions of the neural model of one's own body state that are engaged in the simulation. This is so for at least two reasons: One may need to simulate what is going on in more than one other person, and one may well be experiencing an emotion different from the one being simulated. For instance, facing an angry person may make one feel afraid, yet one would need to simulate the anger in the other, and these two representations of emotional states would therefore need to be kept separate (see van Honk & Schutter, Chapter 10, this volume, for evidence on this point).

How such partitioning is achieved is one topic for future studies. We list here a few more key topics, many of which are already being addressed, that we believe will yield significant new insights into simulation models of emotion recognition. First, as briefly addressed in the section on amygdala involvement in emotion recognition, how do individual differences contribute to variability in emotion-recognition processes? Relatedly, how are these differences reflected in the differential engagement of neural structures in emotion-recognition processes? Second, how does face-based emotion recognition compare with recognition based on other cues, such as body posture, body movement, and vocal prosody? Presumably, there will be some overlap in simulation (and other) processes; both similarities and differences between such processes and face processing will be informative. Third, how do emotion-recognition processes develop? And what are the (presumably changing) roles of their neural substrates during development? Finally, what are the relationships between emotion-recognition processes and other social processes in which many of the same structures are known to play a role, such as anthropomorphizing (e.g., Martin & Weisberg, 2003; Schultz et al., 2003; Heberlein & Adolphs, 2004), attribution of personality traits or stereotyping (e.g., Adolphs, Tranel, & Damasio, 1998; Winston, Strange, O'Doherty, & Dolan, 2002; Cunningham, Johnson, Gatenby, Gore, & Banaji, 2003), moral judgment (Greene, Nystrom, Engell, Darley, & Dohen, 2004), and social contract decisions (Sanfey, Rilling, Aronson, Nystrom, & Cohen, 2003)?

NOTES

1. Such stimuli are created by attaching small lights to the major joints of a person and filming him or her walking in the dark (Johansson, 1973). From the stimuli thus created, it is easy to recognize not only human movement but also gender, emotions, intentions, and other psychological information.
2. Though we focus here on visual pathways, recognition via other modalities would be hypothesized to follow analogous routes.

REFERENCES

Adolphs, R. (2002). Recognizing emotion from facial expressions: Psychological and neurological mechanisms. *Behavioral and Cognitive Neuroscience Reviews 1*(1), 21–61.

Adolphs, R., Baron-Cohen, S., & Tranel, D. (2002). Impaired recognition of social emotions following amygdala damage. *Journal Cognitive Neuroscience 14*(8), 1264–1274.

Adolphs, R., Damasio, H., & Tranel, D. (2002). Neural systems for recognition of emotional prosody: A 3-D lesion study. *Emotion, 2*, 23–51.

Adolphs, R., Damasio, H., Tranel, D., Cooper, G., & Damasio, A. R. (2000). A role for somatosensory cortices in the visual recognition of emotion as revealed by three-dimensional lesion mapping. *Journal of Neuroscience, 20*(7), 2683–2690.

Adolphs, R., Gosselin, F., Buchanan, T. W., Tranel, D., Schyns, P., & Damasio, A.

R. (2005). A mechanism for impaired fear recognition after amygdala damage. *Nature, 433*(7021), 68–72.

Adolphs, R., Russell, J., & Tranel, D. (1999). A role for the human amygdala in recognizing emotional arousal from unpleasant stimuli. *Psychological Science, 10*(2), 167–171.

Adolphs, R., & Tranel, D. (1999). Intact recognition of emotional prosody following amygdala damage. *Neuropsychologia, 37*(11), 1285–1292.

Adolphs, R., & Tranel, D. (2003). Amygdala damage impairs emotion recognition from scenes only when they contain facial expressions. *Neuropsychologia, 41,* 1281–1289.

Adolphs, R., Tranel, D., & Damasio, A. R. (1998). The human amygdala in social judgment. *Nature, 393,* 470–474.

Adolphs, R., Tranel, D., & Damasio, A. R. (2003). Dissociable neural systems for recognizing emotions. *Brain and Cognition, 52*(1), 61–69.

Adolphs, R., Tranel, D., Damasio, H., & Damasio, A. (1994). Impaired recognition of emotion in facial expressions following bilateral damage to the human amygdala. *Nature, 372*(6507), 669–672.

Adolphs, R., Tranel, D., Damasio, H., & Damasio, A. R. (1995). Fear and the human amygdala. *Journal of Neuroscience, 15*(9), 5879–5891.

Adolphs, R., Tranel, D., Hamann, S., Young, A. W., Calder, A. J., Phelps, E. A., et al. (1999). Recognition of facial emotion in nine individuals with bilateral amygdala damage. *Neuropsychologia, 37,* 1111–1117.

Adolphs, R., Tranel, D., Koenigs, M., & Damasio, A. R. (2005). Preferring one taste over another without recognizing either. *Natural Neuroscience, 8*(7), 860–861.

Amaral, D. G. (2002). The primate amygdala and the neurobiology of social behavior: Implications for understanding social anxiety. *Biological Psychiatry, 51,* 11–17.

Amaral, D. G. (2003). The amygdala, social behavior, and danger detection. *Annals of the New York Academy of Sciences, 1000,* 337–347.

Amaral, D. G., & Price, J. L. (1984). Amygdalo-cortical projections in the monkey (*Macaca fascicularis*). *Journal Comparative Neurology, 230*(4), 465–496.

Amaral, D. G., Price, J. L., Pitkanen, A., & Carmichael, S. T. (1992). Anatomical organization of the primate amygdaloid complex. In J. P. Aggleton (Ed.), *The amygdala: Neurobiological aspects of emotion, memory, and mental dysfunction* (pp. 1–66). New York: Wiley-Liss.

Anderson, A. K., & Phelps, E. A. (1998). Intact recognition of vocal expressions of fear following bilateral lesions of the amygdala. *Neuroreport, 9,* 3607–3613.

Anderson, A. K., & Phelps, E. A. (2002). Is the human amygdala critical for the subjective experience of emotion? Evidence of intact dispositional affect in patients with amygdala lesions. *Journal of Cognitive Neuroscience, 14*(5), 709–720.

Atkinson, A. P., Heberlein, A. S., & Adolphs, R. (2006). Spared ability to recognize fear from the whole-body cues following bilateral amygdala damage. *Society for Neuroscience Abstracts.*

Bauman, M. D., Lavenex, P., Mason, W. A., Capitanio, J. P., & Amaral, D. G. (2004). The development of social behavior following neonatal amygdala lesions in rhesus monkeys. *Journal of Cognitive Neuroscience, 16*(8), 1388–1411.

Bechara, A., Tranel, D., Damasio, H., Adolphs, R., Rockland, C., & Damasio, A. R. (1995). Double dissociation of conditioning and declarative knowledge relative to the amygdala and hippocampus in humans. *Science, 269*(5227), 1115–1118.

Benowitz, L. I., Bear, D. M., Rosenthal, R., Mesulam, M. M., Zaidel, E., & Sperry, R. W. (1983). Hemispheric specialization in nonverbal communication. *Cortex, 19*, 5–11.

Bishop, S. J., Duncan, J., & Lawrence, A. D. (2004). State anxiety modulation of the amygdala response to unattended threat-related stimuli. *Journal of Neuroscience, 24*(46), 10364–10368.

Borod, J. C., Obler, L. K., Erhan, H. M., Grunwald, I. S., Cicero, B. A., Welkowitz, J., et al. (1998). Right hemisphere emotional perception: Evidence across multiple channels. *Neuropsychology, 12*(3), 446–458.

Bowers, D., Bauer, R. M., Coslett, H. B., & Heilman, K. M. (1985). Processing of faces by patients with unilateral hemisphere lesions: I. Dissociation between judgments of facial affect and facial identity. *Brain and Cognition, 4*, 258–272.

Breiter, H. C., Etcoff, N. L., Whalen, P. J., Kennedy, W. A., Rauch, S. L., Buckner, R. L., et al.(1996). Response and habituation of the human amygdala during visual processing of facial expression. *Neuron, 17*(5), 875–887.

Broks, P., Young, A. W., Maratos, E. J., Coffey, P. J., Calder, A. J., Isaac, C. L., Mayes, A. R., et al. (1998). Face processing impairments after encephalitis: Amygdala damage and recognition of fear. *Neuropsychologia, 36*(1), 59–70.

Buchel, C., & Dolan, R. J. (2000). Classical fear conditioning in functional neuroimaging. *Current Opinion Neurobiology, 10*(2), 219–223.

Buchel, C., Morris, J. S., Dolan, R. J., & Friston, K. J. (1998). Brain systems mediating aversive conditioning: an event-related fMRI study. *Neuron, 20*(5), 947–957.

Burt, D. M., & Perrett, D. I. (1997). Perceptual asymmetries in judgements of facial attractiveness, age, gender, speech and expression. *Neuropsychologia, 35*(5), 685–693.

Calder, A. J., Keane, J., Manes, F., Antoun, N., & Young, A. W. (2000). Impaired recognition and experience of disgust following brain injury. *Nature Neuroscience, 3*, 1077–1078.

Calder, A. J., Lawrence, A. D., & Young, A. W. (2001). Neuropsychology of fear and loathing. *Nature Reviews. Neuroscience, 2*, 352–363.

Calder, A. J., Young, A. W., Perrett, D. I., Hodges, J. R., & Etcoff, N. L. (1996). Facial emotion recognition after bilateral amygdala damage: Differentially severe impairment of fear. *Cognitive Neuropsychology, 13*, 699–745.

Canli, T., Sivers, H., Whitfield, S. L., Gotlib, I. H., & Gabrieli, J. D. (2002). Amygdala response to happy faces as a function of extraversion. *Science, 296*(5576), 2191.

Catani, M., Jones, D. K., Donato, R., & ffytche, D. H. (2003). Occipito-temporal connections in the human brain. *Brain, 126*, 2093–2107.

Craig, A. D. (2002). How do you feel? Interoception: The sense of the physiological condition of the body. *Nature Reviews. Neuroscience, 3*(8), 655–666.

Critchley, H. D., Wiens, S., Rotshtein, P., Ohman, A., & Dolan, R. J. (2004). Neural systems supporting interoceptive awareness. *Nature Neuroscience, 7*(2), 189–195.

Cunningham, W. A., Johnson, M. K., Gatenby, J. C., Gore, J. C., & Banaji, M. R. (2003). Neural components of social evaluation. *Journal of Personality and Social Psychology, 85*(4), 639–649.

Damasio, A. R. (1989). Time-locked multiregional retroactivation: A systems-level proposal for the neural substrates of recall and recognition. *Cognition, 33*(1–2), 25–62.

Darwin, C. (1872). *The expression of the emotions in man and animals.* London: John Murray.

Davidson, R. J. (1992). Anterior cerebral asymmetry and the nature of emotion. *Brain and Cognition, 20,* 125–151.

Dimberg, U. (1982). Facial reactions to facial expressions. *Psychophysiology, 19*(6), 643–647.

Dimberg, U., Thunberg, M., & Elmehed, K. (2000). Unconscious facial reactions to emotional facial expressions. *Psychological Science, 11*(1), 86–89.

Dittrich, W. H., Troscianko, T., Lea, S. E., & Morgan, D. (1996). Perception of emotion from dynamic point-light displays represented in dance. *Perception, 25*(6), 727–738.

Ekman, P., & Friesen, W. (1976). *Pictures of facial affect.* Palo Alto, CA, Consulting Psychologists Press.

Fanselow, M. S., & LeDoux, J. E. (1999). Why we think plasticity underlying Pavlovian fear conditioning occurs in the basolateral amygdala. *Neuron, 23*(2), 229–232.

Gallese, V., Fadiga, L., Fogassi, L., & Rizzolatti, G. (1996). Action recognition in the premotor cortex. *Brain, 119,* 593–609.

Gallese, V., & Goldman, A. (1998). Mirror neurons and the simulation theory of mind-reading. *Trends in Cognitive Sciences, 2*(12), 493–501.

Gallese, V., Keysers, C., & Rizzolatti, G. (2004). A unifying view of the basis of social cognition. *Trends in Cognitive Sciences, 8*(9), 396–403.

Goldman, A. I. (2006). *Simulating minds: The philosophy, psychology and neuroscience of Mindreading.* New York. Oxford University Press.

Goldman, A. I., & Sripada, C. S. (2005). Simulationist models of face-based emotion recognition. *Cognition, 94*(3), 193–213.

Gray, J. M., Young, A. W., Barker, W. A., Curtis, A., & Gibson, D. (1997). Impaired recognition of disgust in Huntington's disease gene carriers. *Brain, 120(Pt. 11),* 2029–2038.

Greene, J. D., Nystrom, L. E., Engell, A. D., Darley, J. M., & Cohen, J. D. (2004). The neural bases of cognitive conflict and control in moral judgment. *Neuron, 44*(2), 389–400.

Hadjikhani, N., & de Gelder, B. (2003). Seeing fearful body expressions activates the fusiform cortex and amygdala. *Current Biology, 13,* 2201–2205.

Halgren, E., Walter, R. D., Cherlow, D. G., & Crandall, P. H. (1978). Mental phenomena evoked by electrical stimulation of the human hippocampal formation and amygdala. *Brain, 101*(1), 83–117.

Hamann, S. B., Ely, T. D., Grafton, S. T., & Kilts, C. D. (1999). Amygdala activity related to enhanced memory for pleasant and aversive stimuli. *Nature Neuroscience, 2*(3), 289–293.

Hamann, S. B., Ely, T. D., Hoffman, J. M., & Kilts, C. D. (2002). Ecstasy and agony: Activation of the human amygdala in positive and negative emotion. *Psychological Science, 13*(2), 135–141.

Hamann, S. B., Stefanacci, L., Squire, L. R., Adolphs, R., Tranel, D., Damasio, H., et al. (1996). Recognizing facial emotion. *Nature, 379*(6565), 497.

Hariri, A. R., Mattay, V. S., Tessitore, A., Kolachana, B., Fera, F., Goldman, D., et al. (2002). Serotonin transporter genetic variation and the response of the human amygdala. *Science, 297*(5580), 400–403.

Heberlein, A. S., & Adolphs, R. (2004). Impaired spontaneous anthropomorphizing despite intact perception and social knowledge. *Proceedings of the National Academy of Sciences of the USA, 101*(19), 7487–7491.

Heberlein, A. S., Adolphs, R., Tranel, D., & Damasio, H. (2004). Cortical regions for judgments of emotions and personality traits from pointlight walkers. *Journal of Cognitive Neuroscience, 16*, 1143–1158.

Heberlein, A. S., & Saxe, R. (2005). Dissociation between emotion and personality judgments: Convergent evidence from functional neuroimaging. *Neuroimage, 28*, 770–777.

Iacoboni, M., Woods, R., Brass, M., Bekkering, H., Mazziotta, J., & Rizzolati, G. (1999). Cortical mechanisms of human imitation. *Science, 286*, 2526–2528.

Irwin, W., Davidson, R. J., Lowe, M. J., Mock, B. J., Sorenson, J. A., & Turski, P. A. (1996). Human amygdala activation detected with echo-planar functional magnetic resonance imaging. *Neuroreport, 7*(11), 1765–1769.

Jackson, P. L., Meltzoff, A. N., & Decety, J. (2005). How do we perceive the pain of others? A window into the neural processes involved in empathy. *Neuroimage, 24*(3), 771–779.

Jansari, A., Tranel, D., & Adolphs, R. (2000). A valence-specific lateral bias for discriminating emotional facial expressions in free field. *Cognition and Emotion, 14*, 341–353.

Jellema, T., Baker, C. I., Wicker, B., & Perrett, D. I. (2000). Neural representation for the perception of the intentionality of actions. *Brain and Cognition, 44*, 280–302.

Johansson, G. (1973). Visual perception of biological motion and a model of its analysis. *Perception and Psychophysics, 14*, 202–211.

Johnsrude, I. S., Owen, A. M., White, N. M., Zhao, W. V., & Bohbot, V. (2000). Impaired preference conditioning after anterior temporal lobe resection in humans. *Journal of Neuroscience, 20*(7), 2649–2656.

Jones, E. G., & Burton, H. (1976). A projection from the medial pulvinar to the amygdala in primates. *Brain Research, 104*(1), 142–147.

Kalin, N. H., Shelton, S. E., Davidson, R. J., & Kelley, A. E. (2001). The primate amygdala mediates acute fear but not the behavioral and physiological components of anxious temperament. *Journal of Neuroscience, 21*(6), 2067–2074.

Ketter, T. A., Andreason, P. J., George, M. S., Lee, C., Gill, D. S., Parekh, P. I., (1996). Anterior paralimbic mediation of procaine-induced emotional and psychosensory experiences. *Archives of General Psychiatry, 53*(1), 59–69.

Keysers, C., Kohler, E., Umilta, M. A., Nanetti, L., Fogassi, L., & Gallese, V. (2003). Audiovisual mirror neurons and action recognition. *Experimental Brain Research, 153*(4), 628–636.

Kiefer, S. W. (1985). Neural mediation of conditioned food aversions. *Annals of the New York Academy of Sciences, 443*, 100–109.

Kluver, H., & Bucy, P. C. (1997). Preliminary analysis of functions of the temporal lobes in monkeys. *Journal of Neuropsychiatry and Clinical Neuroscience, 9*(4), 606–620. (Original work published 1939)

Kohler, E., Keysers, C., Umilta, M. A., Fogassi, L., Gallese, V., & Rizzolatti, G. (2002). Hearing sounds, understanding actions: Action representation in mirror neurons. *Science, 297*(5582), 846–848.

Krolak-Salmon, P., Henaff, M. A., Isnard, J., Tallon-Baudry, C., Guenot, M., Vighetto, A., et al. (2003). An attention modulated response to disgust in human ventral anterior insula. *Annals of Neurology 53*(4), 446–453.

Krolak-Salmon, P., Henaff, M. A., Vighetto, A., Bertrand, O., & Mauguiere, F. (2004). Early amygdala reaction to fear spreading in occipital, temporal, and frontal cortex: A depth electrode ERP study in humans. *Neuron, 42*(4), 665–676.

Kucharska-Pietura, K., Phillips, M. L., Gernand, W., & David, A. S. (2003). Perception of emotions from faces and voices following unilateral brain damage. *Neuropsychologia, 41*, 1082–1090.

LaBar, K. S., LeDoux, J. E., Spencer, D. D., & Phelps, E. A. (1995). Impaired fear conditioning following unilateral temporal lobectomy in humans. *Journal of Neuroscience, 15*(10), 6846–6855.

Lange, K., Williams, L. M., Young, A. W., Bullmore, E. T., Brammer, M. J., Williams, S. C., et al. (2003). Task instructions modulate neural responses to fearful facial expressions. *Biological Psychiatry, 53*(3), 226–232.

Le Doux, J. (1996). *The emotional brain.* New York: Simon & Schuster.

Martin, A., & Weisberg, J. (2003). Neural foundations for understanding social and mechanical concepts. *Cognitive Neuropsychology, 20*(3–6), 575–587.

Morris, J. S., de Gelder, B., Weiskrantz, L., & Dolan, R. J. (2001). Differential extrageniculostriate and amygdala responses to presentation of emotional faces in a cortically blind field. *Brain, 124*(Pt. 6), 1241–1252.

Morris, J. S., Frith, C. D., Perrett, D. I., Rowland, D., Young, A. W., Calder, A. J., et al. (1996). A differential neural response in the human amygdala to fearful and happy facial expressions. *Nature, 383*, 812–815.

Morris, J. S., Ohman, A., & Dolan, R. J. (1999). A subcortical pathway to the right amygdala mediating "unseen" fear. *Proceedings of the National Academy of Sciences of the USA, 96*(4), 1680–1685.

Morris, J. S., Scott, S. K., & Dolan, R. J. (1999). Saying it with feeling: neural responses to emotional vocalizations. *Neuropsychologia, 37*(10), 1155–1163.

Morrison, I. (in press). Motivational-affective processing and the neural foundations of empathy. In T. Farrow & G. Woodruff (Eds.), *Empathy in mental illness.* Cambridge, UK: Cambridge University Press.

Morrison, I., Lloyd, D., di Pellegrino, G., & Roberts, N. (2004). Vicarious responses to pain in anterior cingulate cortex: Is empathy a multisensory issue? *Cognitive, Affective, and Behavioral Neuroscience, 4*(2), 270–278.

O'Doherty, J., Rolls, E. T., Francis, S., Bowtell, R., & McGlone, F. (2001). Representation of pleasant and aversive taste in the human brain. *Journal of Neurophysiology, 85*(3), 1315–1321.

Olsson, A., & Phelps, E. A. (2004). Learned fear of "unseen" faces after Pavlovian, observational, and instructed fear. *Psychological Science, 15*(12), 822–828.

Oya, H., Kawasaki, H., Howard, M. A., & Adolphs, R. (2002). Electrophysiological responses in the human amygdala discriminate emotion categories of complex visual stimuli. *Journal of Neuroscience, 22*, 9502–9512.

Pegna, A. J., Khateb, A., Lazeyras, F., & Seghier, M. L. (2005). Discriminating emotional faces without primary visual cortices involves the right amygdala. *Nature Neuroscience, 8*(1), 24–25.

Penfield, W., & Faulk, M. E., Jr. (1955). The insula: Further observations on its function. *Brain, 78*(4), 445–470.

Pessoa, L., McKenna, M., Gutierrez, E., & Ungerleider, L. G. (2002). Neural processing of emotional faces requires attention. *Proceedings of the National Academy of Sciences of the USA, 99*(17), 11458–11463.

Pezawas, L., Meyer-Lindenberg, A., Drabant, E. M., Verchinski, B. A., Munoz, K. E., Kolachana, B. S., et al. (2005). 5-HTTLPR polymorphism impacts human cingulate-amygdala interactions: A genetic susceptibility mechanism for depression. *Nature Neuroscience, 8*(6), 828–834.

Phan, K. L., Wager, T., Taylor, S. F., & Liberzon, I. (2002). Functional neuroanatomy of emotion: A meta-analysis of emotion activation studies in PET and fMRI. *Neuroimage, 16*(2), 331–348.

Phillips, M. L., Williams, L. M., Heining, M., Herba, C. M., Russell, T., Andrew, C., et al. (2004). Differential neural responses to overt and covert presentations of facial expressions of fear and disgust. *Neuroimage, 21*(4), 1484–1496.

Phillips, M. L., Young, A. W., Scott, S. K., Calder, A. J., Andrew, C., Giampietro, V., et al. (1998). Neural responses to facial and vocal expressions of fear and disgust. *Proceedings of the Royal Society B: Biological Science, 265,* 1809–1817.

Phillips, M. L., Young, A. W., Senior, C., Brammer, M., Andrew, C., Calder, A. J., et al. (1997). A specific neural substrate for perceiving facial expressions of disgust. *Nature, 389*(6650), 495–498.

Pourtois, G., Sander, D., Andres, M., Grandjean, D., Reveret, L., Olivier, E., et al. (2004). Dissociable roles of the human somatosensory and superior temporal cortices for processing social face signals. *European Journal of Neuroscience, 20*(12), 3507–3515.

Prather, M. D., Lavenex, P., Mauldin-Jourdain, M. L., Mason, W. A., Capitanio, J. P., Mendoza, S. P. et al. (2001). Increased social fear and decreased fear of objects in monkeys with neonatal amygdala lesions. *Neuroscience, 106*(4), 653–658.

Preston, S. D., & de Waal, F. B. M. (2002). Empathy: Its ultimate and proximate bases. *Behavioral and Brain Sciences, 25,* 1–72.

Puce, A., Allison, T., & McCarthy, G. (1999). Electrophysiological studies of human face perception: III. Effects of top-down processing on face-specific potentials. *Cerebral Cortex, 9,* 445–458.

Rapcsak, S. Z., Galper, S. R., Comer, J. F., Reminger, S. L., Nielsen, L., Kaszniak, A. W., et al. (2000). Fear recognition deficits after focal brain damage: A cautionary note. *Neurology, 54*(3), 575–581.

Ross, E. D., Thompson, R. D., & Yenkosky, J. (1997). Lateralization of affective prosody in brain and the callosal integration of hemispheric language functions. *Brain and Language, 56*(1), 27–54.

Rozin, P., Haidt, J., & McCauley, C. (2000). Disgust. In M. Lewis & J. M. Haviland-Jones (Eds.), *Handbook of emotions, 2nd ed.* (pp. 637–653). New York: Guilford Press.

Ruby, P., & Decety, J. (2004). How would you feel versus how do you think she would feel? A neuroimaging study of perspective-taking with social emotions. *Journal of Cognitive Neuroscience, 16*(6), 988–999.

Sander, D., Grafman, J., & Zalla, T. (2003). The human amygdala: An evolved system for relevance detection. *Reviews in the Neurosciences, 14,* 303–316.

Sander, K., & Scheich, H. (2001). Auditory perception of laughing and crying activates human amygdala regardless of attentional state. *Brain Research. Cognitive Brain Research, 12*(2), 181–198.

Sanfey, A. G., Rilling, J. K., Aronson, J. A., Nystrom, L. E., & Cohen, J. D. (2003). The neural basis of economic decision-making in the Ultimatum Game. *Science, 300*(5626), 1755–1758.

Saxe, R. (2005). Against simulation: The argument from error. *Trends in Cognitive Science, 9*(4), 174–179.

Scherer, K. R. (1986). Vocal affect expression: A review and a model for future research. *Psychological Bulletin, 99,* 143–165.

Schmolck, H., & Squire, L. R. (2001). Impaired perception of facial emotions following bilateral damage to the anterior temporal lobe. *Neuropsychology, 15*(1), 30–38.

Schultz, R. T., Grelotti, D. J., Klin, A., Kleinman, J., Van der Gaag, C., Marois, R., et al. (2003). The role of the fusiform face area in social cognition: Implications for the pathobiology of autism. *Philosophical Transactions of the Royal Society of London. Series B, Biological Sciences, 358*(1430), 415–427.

Schyns, P. G., Bonnar, L., & Gosselin, F. (2002). Show me the features! Understanding recognition from the use of visual information. *Psychological Science, 13*(5), 402–409.

Scott, S. K., Young, A. W., Calder, A. J., Hellawell, D. J., Aggleton, J. P., & Johnson, M. (1997). Impaired auditory recognition of fear and anger following bilateral amygdala lesions. *Nature, 385,* 254–257.

Singer, T., Seymour, B., O'Doherty, J., Kaube, H., Dolan, R. J., & Frith, C. D. (2004). Empathy for pain involves the affective but not sensory components of pain. *Science, 303*(5661), 1157–1162.

Smith, M. L., Gosselin, F., & Schyns, P. G. (2004). Receptive fields for flexible face categorizations. *Psychological Science, 15*(11), 753–761.

Sprengelmeyer, R., Rausch, M., Eysel, U. T., & Przuntek, H. (1998). Neural structures associated with recognition of facial expressions of basic emotions. *Proceedings of the Royal Society B: Biological Sciences, 265,* 1927–1931.

Sprengelmeyer, R., Young, A., Schroeder, U., Grossenbacher, P. G., Federlein, J., Buettner, T. et al. (1999). Knowing no fear. *Proceedings of the Royal Society B: Biological Science, 266,* 2451–2456.

Sprengelmeyer, R., Young, A. W., Calder, A. J., Karnat, A., Lange, H., Homberg, V., et al.(1996). Loss of disgust: Perception of faces and emotions in Huntington's disease. *Brain, 119 (Pt. 5),* 1647–1665.

Swanson, L. W., & Petrovich, G. D. (1998). What is the amygdala? *Trends in Neuroscience, 21,* 323–331.

van Rijn, S., Aleman, A., van Diessen, E., Berckmoes, C., Vingerhoets, G., & Kahn, R. S. (2005). What is said or how it is said makes a difference: Role of the right fronto-parietal operculum in emotional prosody as revealed by repetitive TMS. *European Journal of Neuroscience, 21*(11), 3195–3200.

Vuilleumier, P., Armony, J. L., Driver, J., & Dolan, R. J. (2001). Effects of attention and emotion on face processing in the human brain: An event-related fMRI study. *Neuron, 30*(3), 829–841.

Vuilleumier, P., Richardson, M. P., Armony, J. L., Driver, J., & Dolan, R. J. (2004).

Distant influences of amygdala lesion on visual cortical activation during emotional face processing. *Nature Neuroscience, 7,* 1271–1278.

Wallbott, H. G. (1998). Bodily expression of emotion. *European Journal of Social Psychology, 28,* 879–896.

Whalen, P. J., Kagan, J., Cook, R. G., Davis, F. C., Kim, H., Polis, S., et al. (2004). Human amygdala responsivity to masked fearful eye whites. *Science, 306* (5704), 2061.

Whalen, P. J., Rauch, S. L., Etcoff, N. L., McInerney, S. C., Lee, M. B., & Jenike, M. A. (1998). Masked presentations of emotional facial expressions modulate amygdala activity without explicit knowledge. *the Journal of Neuroscience, 18*(1), 411–418.

Wicker, B., Keysers, C., Plailly, J., Royet, J. P., Gallese, V., & Rizzolatti, G. (2003). Both of us disgusted in My insula: The common neural basis of seeing and feeling disgust. *Neuron, 40*(3), 655–664.

Winston, J. S., O'Doherty, J., & Dolan, R. J. (2003). Common and distinct neural responses during direct and incidental processing of multiple facial emotions. *Neuroimage, 20*(1), 84–97.

Winston, J. S., Strange, B. A., O'Doherty, J., & Dolan, R. J. (2002). Automatic and intentional brain responses during evaluation of trustworthiness of faces. *Nature Neuroscience, 5*(3), 277–283.

Young, A. W., Aggleton, J. P., Hellawell, D. J., Johnson, M., Broks, P., & Hanley, J. R. (1995). Face processing impairments after amygdalotomy. *Brain, 118*(Pt. 1), 15–24.

Zald, D. H., Lee, J. T., Fluegel, K. W., & Pardo, J. V. (1998). Aversive gustatory stimulation activates limbic circuits in humans. *Brain, 121*(Pt. 6), 1143–1154.

Zald, D. H., & Pardo, J. V. (2000). Functional neuroimaging of the olfactory system in humans. *International Journal of Psychophysiology, 36*(2), 165–181.

4

Ten Years of Research
with the Trier Social Stress Test—Revisited

Brigitte M. Kudielka, Dirk H. Hellhammer,
and Clemens Kirschbaum

More than 10 years ago, the Trier Social Stress Test (TSST) was introduced as a standardized protocol for the induction of moderate psychosocial stress in laboratory settings (Kirschbaum, Pirke, & Hellhammer, 1993). In this chapter, we provide an up-to-date description of the TTST protocol and review a decade of research with the TSST in healthy participants, as well as clinical populations.

The World Health Organization (WHO) concluded that stress is one of the most significant health problems in the 21st century (The World Health Report, 2001). So there is a pressing need for investigations into the biological pathways linking stress and health. Besides the sympathetic–adrenal–medullary (SAM) axis, the hypothalamic–pituitary–adrenal (HPA) axis is the major physiological stress response system in the organism. In more detail, the HPA axis is a central regulatory and control system of the organism that connects the central nervous system (CNS) with the endocrine system. Under stress, the hypothalamus secretes corticotropin-releasing hormone (CRH), which provokes the release of adrenocortico-tropic hormone (ACTH) from the pituitary. ACTH triggers the secretion of the glucocorticoid hormone cortisol from the adrenal cortex. Cortisol is predominantly (90–95%) bound to binding proteins in blood, and only 5–10% of the total plasma cortisol circulates biologically actively as unbound, "free" cortisol. The functioning of the axis is controlled by several negative feedback loops. The sequential release of CRH, ACTH, and cortisol is an attempt to ensure proper functioning of the body in times of increased demand for energy, attention, emotionality, and so forth. Because alterations in HPA axis stress responses appear to be a close correlate or even a determining factor of the onset of different diseases or disease progression (McEwen, 1998), the characterization of an individual's HPA axis response pattern to psychosocial stress appears to be of major interest.

For such a research agenda, a novel research tool was needed, because available laboratory stress protocols yielded insufficient activation of the HPA axis. In search of a laboratory stress paradigm that was potent enough to induce significant changes of endocrine and cardiovascular parameters in the majority of participants tested, we eventually developed a stress protocol termed the "Trier Social Stress Test" (TSST). Over the past decade, more than 4,000 TSST sessions were performed in many laboratories worldwide. Thus the TSST has become a standard protocol for the experimental induction of psychological stress in healthy participants, as well as clinical populations (compare Dickerson & Kemeny, 2004; Williams, Hagerty, & Brooks, 2004), investigating a wide range of different outcome variables ranging from subjective verbal stress reports to objective behavioral and biological stress responses, including parameters of the HPA and SAM axes and cardiovascular, immunological, and blood coagulation systems.

STRESSOR CHARACTERISTICS: THEORETICAL AND EMPIRICAL CONTRIBUTIONS

The pioneer of stress research, Hans Selye, defined stress as a nonspecific response of the body, characterized by the secretion of glucocorticoids, to any demand (Selye, 1936, 1983); for further definitions of stress, see Levine and Ursin (1991) and Kudielka and Kirschbaum (2001). However, Selye's idea of an unspecific stress response to very different stimuli was challenged by Mason (1968a, 1968b, 1975), who described the importance of specific emotional reactions that determine a specific endocrine stress response. Whenever a situation (or a stimulus) is perceived as novel, uncontrollable, unpredictable, or ambivalent, or if the individual anticipates negative organismic or psychological consequences, the negative feedback signals from the hippocampus and other sites will be overridden, resulting in a cascade of CRH, ACTH, and cortisol secretion. Accordingly, Henry (1992) posited that the HPA axis is activated when a sense of uncontrollability and helplessness emerges, whereas the SAM axis system (release of norepinephrine and epinephrine) is predominantly activated when an individual is confronted with a challenging situation that can be mastered actively by effort. Studies by Frankenhäuser and coworkers yielded empirical support for an endocrine stress-response model contrasting "effort without distress" (SAM axis) to "effort with distress" (HPA axis) in humans

(Frankenhaeuser, Lundberg, & Forsman, 1980; Lundberg, 1983). A review of experimental studies on psychological stress and neuroendocrine function in humans can be found in Biondi and Picardi (1999). Based on the observation that HPA axis responses to psychological stressors are extremely variable and that several studies using different types of negative situations have failed to induce significant cortisol changes, Dickerson and Kemeny (2004) recently conducted a meta-analysis of 208 laboratory studies of acute psychological stressors in order to delineate the essential situational elements capable of eliciting HPA axis responses. Their results show that motivated performance tasks elicit cortisol responses if the tasks (1) are uncontrollable, (2) create a context of forced failure in which a participant is unable to avoid negative consequences or cannot succeed despite best effort, or (3) are characterized by a social component called social-evaluative threat, in which task performance could be negatively judged by others. Tasks containing both components (uncontrollability and social-evaluative threat) were associated with the largest HPA axis stress responses and the longest recovery times. The meta-analytical findings fit to the theoretical reasoning (based on the social self-preservation theory) that "uncontrollable threats to the goal of maintaining the 'social self' would trigger reliable and substantial cortisol changes" (p. 356). Dickerson and Kemeny conclude that the TSST is one of the few available stress protocols that satisfies the criteria of a motivated performance task that combines elements of uncontrollability and high levels of social-evaluative threat. In further experimental work, it could be shown that the component of social evaluation is a crucial element of TSST-induced cortisol responses (Gruenewald, Kemeny, Aziz, & Fahey, 2004), with higher cortisol increases found in participants who experience greater increases in shame and greater decreases in social self-esteem under social-self threat.

METHODOLOGY: DETAILED DESCRIPTION OF THE TSST PROCEDURE

In this section, we provide a detailed description of the TSST protocol. The TSST is a motivated performance task consisting of a brief preparation period (3 minutes) followed by a test period in which the participant has to deliver a free speech (5 minutes) and perform mental arithmetic (5 minutes) in front of an audience. The total exposure time adds up to 13 minutes. The following description of the TSST procedure primarily applies to investigations of HPA axis responses, and, therefore, other outcome measures may require some modifications.

The test onset should be preceded by a rest period of at least 30–45 minutes to minimize effects of prior potentially stressful events or other unrelated short-term effects that might have an impact on the outcome measures under investigation. Although absolute response curves are much higher in the morning due to the circadian rhythm of HPA axis activity, comparable free cortisol net increases after TSST exposure can be assessed with equal reliability in the morning and afternoon, as reported recently (Kudielka, Schommer, Hellhammer, & Kirschbaum, 2004). However, in early morning sessions, the experimenter should ensure that the onset of a stress experiment does not interfere with the morning cortisol response to awakening (Pruessner, Wolf, et al., 1997). Also, the appropriate time window for test sessions in the morning is smaller than in the late afternoon. After providing "basal" samples for the assessment of prestress measures, the participant is introduced to the upcoming task by standardized written instructions handed over by the experimenter. Following the instructions, the participant is asked to take over the role of a job applicant who is invited for a personal interview with the company's staff managers ("selection committee"). The participant is told that, after a preparation period, he or she should introduce him- or herself to the committee in a free speech and convince them that he or she is the perfect applicant for the vacant position. After the speech, the committee might ask additional questions and will present another task later. The selection panel members are introduced as being specially trained to monitor nonverbal behavior, and participants are told to expect tape and video recordings for later analysis of their performance. It is announced that a voice frequency analysis of nonverbal behavior will be performed on the tape-recorded talk and that a video analysis of the participant's performance will also be conducted. After the participant has read the instructions and the experimenter has ensured that he or she thoroughly understands the upcoming task, the participant is guided to the business-like equipped test room. The committee, clothed in white coats and equipped with stopwatches and writing material, is already sitting at a table; a video camera and a tape recorder are installed. The selection committee is composed of two or three male and female confederates of the experimenter, unacquainted with the participant. The committee is trained to communicate with the participant in an unresponsive neutral manner and does not respond with any facial or verbal feedback. However, it has to be ensured that the committee's style of communication does not resemble harassment or evoke anger in participants. The experimenter informs the participants that the talk will be given into a microphone (pointing at a marked spot on the floor), which is positioned about 1–3 meters away from the committee's table. The experimenter briefly introduces the participant to the committee, reminds him or her that the task is to personally convince the committee, and again calls the participant's attention to the presence of the video and tape recorders. Then the experimenter leaves the room. The committee first requests the participant to sit down (unless blood pressure is measured) at a small table equipped with paper and pencil to prepare the talk (preparation period). After 3 minutes, the participant is asked to step forward to the marked spot in front of the microphone and to start the oral presentation. Participants are informed that they are not allowed to use the written notes for their speeches. Whenever a participant finishes the speech in less than 5 minutes, the managers respond in a standardized way. First they tell the volunteer, "You still have some time left. Please continue!" Should the participant finish a second time before the 5 minuts are over, the managers are quiet for 20 seconds and then ask prepared questions ("What are your personal strengths?" "What are your major shortcomings?" "Do you have enemies? Why?" "What do you think about teamwork?" "What do your boss/family/colleagues think about you? Why?" etc.). After 5 minutes, the selection committee interrupts and asks the participant to serially subtract the number 17 from 2023 as quickly and as accurately as possible. On every failure, the individual has to restart at 2023, with one member of the committee interfering: "Stop—mistake—start over at 2023, please." After 5 minutes the task is terminated, and the participant leaves the room to join the experimenter.

Samples are taken before onset and after cessation of the stress task, depending on the dynamic of the selected outcome variable (e.g., every 10–30 minutes for cortisol) and should cover prestress levels, the initial stress response, peak level, and recovery. Prestress HPA axis hormone levels should not be interpreted as baseline levels because they are substantially affected by the participants' anticipation of the upcoming challenge. At the end of the test session, the participant is fully debriefed about the goal of the study and the nature of the stressor and is informed that neither a voice frequency nor a video analysis will be performed (unless the experiment was geared to include those analyses). A full debriefing includes a visit with the confederates who took the role of the selection committee during the test.

With this protocol, salivary cortisol levels rise two- to threefold in about 70–80% of all tested participants, with peak levels around 10–20 minutes after cessation of the stress task. In addition to free cortisol, the levels of total plasma cortisol, ACTH, catecholamines (epinephrine, norepinephrine), growth hormone, prolactin, testosterone, several immune parameters (e.g., neutrophils, eosinophils, basophils, lymphocytes, IL-6, TNF-alpha), alpha-amylase, and systolic and diastolic blood pressure significantly increase following TSST exposure. Mean heart rate increases to the psychosocial stressor are about 15–25 beats per minute. Furthermore, the cortisol response to the TSST appears to be highly correlated with a transient and preceding rise in endogenous inhibitor of monoamine oxidase (MAO-AI; Clow, Patel, Najafi, Evans, & Hucklebridge, 1997). Recently, von Känel and coworkers (von Känel, Kudielka, Hanebuth, Preckel, & Fischer, 2005; von Känel, Kudielka, Preckel, Hanebuth, Hermann-Lingen, Frey, et al., 2005; Zgraggen et al., 2005) could also show that measures of hemoconcentration (hematocrit, hemoglobin, plasma volume) and blood coagulation (fibrinogen, von Willebrand factor antigen, D-dimer, clotting factors FVII:C, FVIII:C, FXII:C) are sensitive to acute psychosocial stress.

The TSST can also be employed to test children and older adults after changing the instructions slightly for the respective age group. Elderly adults are instructed to apply for a (voluntary) part-time job (e.g., child care, housekeeping, technical assistance, etc). To help a retired participant to take over the role of a job applicant, a fabricated newspaper advertisement can be presented (tested age range: 59–91 years, Kudielka et al., 1998; Kudielka, Schmidt-Reinwald, Hellhammer, & Kirschbaum, 1999; Kudielka, Schmidt-Reinwald, Hellhammer, Schürmeyer, & Kirschbaum, 2000). The adapted TSST for children (TSST-C) also consists of a preparation period, public speaking, and mental arithmetic task. In the speaking part, children receive the beginning of a story and are told that they should finish telling the story as excitingly as possible in front of a jury (tested age range: 7–14 years; Buske-Kirschbaum et al., 1997; Buske-Kirschbaum et al., 2003). The numbers used in the mental arithmetic task are adapted to the respective performance level of the respective age group.

SOURCES OF INTRA- AND INTERINDIVIDUAL DIFFERENCES

One of the most prominent features of HPA axis (and other system) responses after psychological stress is the large variation in response magnitude between participants and across test sessions. Significant differences can be observed with respect to the net hormone output, as well as the time course of hormone secretion. This section summarizes findings from studies investigating various factors that potentially contribute to differences in HPA axis responses to psychosocial stress. Considerable evidence has accumulated for a significant impact of a variety of moderating and intervening variables—including gender; endogenous and exogenous sex steroids (female menstrual cycle, administration of sex steroids); lactation and breast feeding; age; nicotine, coffee, and alcohol consumption and dietary energy supply; social support; social hierarchy; and interventions, as well as personality factors, capability of habituating to repeated stress exposures, genetic factors, and, finally, cellular mechanisms.

Gender

One of the most consistent findings from the TSST is the significantly larger salivary cortisol and ACTH response in men than in women following stress exposure. Although prestress levels are not considerably different, we have repeatedly demonstrated that free cortisol responses to psychosocial stress differ between the sexes (Kirschbaum, Wüst, & Hellhammer, 1992). Interestingly, ACTH and salivary cortisol increases in men are up to twice as high as in women. The typical mean response magnitude in men ranges from a 200 to 400% increase from baseline, whereas in women, changes of

50–150% are usually found. The same sex effect emerged for elderly individuals, with men evincing higher ACTH and free salivary cortisol responses (Kudielka et al., 1998). Meanwhile, we have observed this sex difference in adrenocortical responsivity in more than a dozen studies (for a review and meta-analysis on sex differences in human HPA-axis stress responses, see Kudielka, Hellhammer, & Kirschbaum, 2000; Kudielka & Kirschbaum, 2005; Otte et al., 2005). Moreover, in men the sole anticipation of an upcoming psychosocial stress task led to a significant free cortisol response even when they were not actually confronted with the stressor. A similar anticipatory endocrine response was absent in women (Kirschbaum, Wüst, Farg, & Hellhammer, 1992).

Endogenous and Exogenous Sex Steroids

The observed sex differences point to a possible impact of female sex steroids as potential mediators of HPA axis responses to psychosocial stress. Results from TSST studies on the effects of estrogen-containing oral contraceptives (OC) on the endocrine responsiveness to psychosocial stress are in line with this hypothesis. Several experiments revealed that women with OC medication show blunted or even absent free cortisol responses to the TSST, despite similar changes in heart rate and subjective stress ratings compared with women not using OC (Kirschbaum, Pirke, & Hellhammer, 1995). In a recent study of 81 healthy young adults, we used the TSST with men, with women in the follicular phase of the menstrual cycle, with women in the luteal phase, and with women using OC. The results disclosed that significant sex differences emerge for ACTH and free salivary cortisol but not for total plasma cortisol stress responses (Kirschbaum, Kudielka, Gaab, Schommer, & Hellhammer, 1999). Moreover, ACTH responses were elevated in men compared with women, regardless of menstrual cycle phase or use of oral contraceptives. Women in the luteal phase had comparable saliva cortisol stress responses to men, whereas women in the follicular phase or women taking OC showed significantly lower free cortisol responses. These observations point out the necessity of strictly distinguishing between the total cortisol secretion and the levels of bioavailable free cortisol.

Whereas many animal studies have directly investigated the impact of estrogens on HPA axis regulation, few experimental studies have been conducted in humans, and the empirical evidence is rather inconsistent. For example, in young men, a 48-hour estradiol application resulted in elevated free cortisol responses (Kirschbaum, Schommer, et al., 1996), whereas a 2-week estradiol treatment in postmenopausal women did not alter TSST-induced HPA axis responses. However, feedback sensitivity as measured by the combined dexamethasone–CRH test seemed to be increased in postmenopausal women after a 2-week estradiol substitution (Kudielka, Schmidt-Reinwald, Hellhammer, & Kirschbaum, 1999). To elucidate the impact of dehydroepiandrosterone (DHEA), a sex hormone precursor, we conducted a placebo-controlled double-blind study investigating HPA-axis stress responses to the TSST in 75 men and women of advanced age after a 2-week DHEA or placebo treatment (Kudielka et al., 1998). Women treated with DHEA showed ACTH stress responses similar to those of men but significantly enhanced compared with women taking placebos. No other stress response differences emerged between DHEA and placebo groups.

Lactation and Breast Feeding

Lactation in animals has been associated with attenuated hormonal responses to different kinds of stressors. It was therefore assumed that the human endocrine stress response might also be moderated by lactation in postpartum women. Heinrichs and coworkers (2001) investigated whether a blunting of endocrine stress responses in women can be ascribed to suckling as a short-term effect or to lactation in general. Lactating women were randomly assigned either to breast-feed or to hold their infants before they were exposed to the TSST. Although no significant differences in prestressor baseline hormone levels could be observed between groups, free and total cortisol responses to stress were attenuated in breast-feeding women. From these data, it can be concluded that lactation in women, in contrast to rats, does not result in a general restraint of HPA axis responses to a psychosocial stressor. Rather, suckling seems to exert a short-term suppression of the cortisol response to psychosocial stress. These results are further supported in humans by Altemus and coworkers (2001). A review of lactation and stress and the protective effects of breast feeding in humans can be found in Heinrichs, Neumann, and Ehlert (2002).

Age

Recently we performed a reanalysis of five independent studies from our laboratory in which participants from different age groups were confronted with the TSST protocol at the same time of day (Buske-Kirschbaum et al., 1997; Kirschbaum et al., 1999; Kudielka et al., 1999; Kudielka, Schmidt-Reinwald, Hellhammer, Schürmeyer, & Kirschbaum, 2000; Buske-Kirschbaum et al., 2003). In this data set, we included only those participants who were healthy (patient groups were excluded) and had received only placebo treatment. Postmenopausal women were free of any hormone replacement therapy (HRT), and, in the case of premenopausal women, only participants in the luteal phase were selected. In sum, this analysis was based on 102 healthy participants between 9 and 76 years old (Kudielka, Buske-Kirschbaum, Hellhammer, & Kirschbaum, 2004b). Results showed that the stress task induced significant HPA axis responses in all age groups in both males and females. The data revealed no sex differences in free cortisol responses in children (mean age 12.1 years) and younger adults (mean age 23.5 years) but larger free cortisol responses in elderly men than in elderly women (mean age 67.3 years). This effect did not appear to be attributable to self-reported stress level differences. For total plasma cortisol, the response patterns did not differ between age and sex groups. For total plasma cortisol, elderly women showed generally enhanced cortisol response levels compared with elderly and younger men, as well as younger women. For ACTH, the response was higher in younger adults, primarily due to an elevated response in younger men. The observed ACTH and total plasma cortisol response patterns in younger and older adults suggest that a heightened hypothalamic drive in younger men decreases with age, resulting in similar ACTH responses in elderly men and women, and that younger adult females have a higher adrenocortical sensitivity to ACTH signals. This is in accordance with earlier findings by Horrocks and coworkers (1990), who reported on greater ACTH pulses in middle-aged men, and by Roelfsema et al. (1993), who found a higher sensitivity to ACTH of the female adrenal cortex. Besides the role of sex steroids, it is also possible that some of the observed differences in HPA axis reactivity could be explained by different corticosteroid-binding globulin (CBG) levels in males and females. With respect to autonomic responses, we also observed differential heart rate responses and recovery after exposure to the TSST in healthy children, younger adults, and elderly adults, as reported by Kudielka, Buske-Kirschbaum, Hellhammer, and Kirschbaum (2004a).

Nicotine, Coffee, Alcohol Consumption, and Dietary Energy Supplies

Nicotine is a potent stimulator of the HPA axis through induction of CRH release after binding to cholinergic receptors in the locus coeruleus and hypothalamus (Fuxe, Andersson, Eneroth, Harfstrand, & Agnati, 1989; Weidenfeld, Bodoff, Saphier, & Brenner, 1989). Repeated exposure to nicotine could therefore lead to chronically elevated ACTH and/or cortisol with reduced responsiveness of the HPA axis. In fact, chronic smoking changes the HPA axis responses to stress. We repeatedly observed blunted cortisol responses to the TSST in habitual smokers (Kirschbaum, Strasburger, & Langkrär, 1993; Kirschbaum, Scherer, & Strasburger, 1994). Similar blunting of ACTH, growth hormone, and prolactin levels, as well as changes in blood pressure following stress, suggests that the alterations of the endocrine and cardiovascular systems associated with habitual nicotine use are multifaceted. Interestingly, differences in adrenocortical responses between smokers and nonsmokers have been observed only after stimulation at a suprapituitary level. Habitual smoking can therefore be considered as a potential intervening variable that could account for some of the interindividual variation observed in HPA axis responses to stress.

Besides nicotine, caffeine intake has been shown to activate important components of the pituitary–adrenocortical response in humans during resting states (Lovallo, al'Absi, Blick, Whitsett, & Wilson, 1996). In a psychological stress experiment (mental arithmetic and reaction-time task), al'Absi et al. (1998) showed evidence for combined stimulatory effects of caffeine and psychological stress on HPA axis responses.

The effects of acute alcohol intake and the role of familial risk were investigated by Zimmermann and coworkers (2004). The authors tested whether a family history of alcoholism might be associated with a greater TSST stress response and a more effective stress response dampening by oral alcohol intake. Results reveal an elevated HPA axis stress response and a stronger dampening by alcohol in sons of alcoholic fathers compared with control participants. These data suggest a mechanism by which a predisposition to develop alcohol dependence might be expressed, suggesting that a transient favorable alcohol effect may occur in participants with family histories of alcoholism but not in control participants. Stress induced by the TSST also affects drug-motivated behavior, including alcohol consumption, as investigated by de Wit and coworkers (Söderpalm & de Wit, 2002; de Wit, Söderpalm, Nikolayev, & Young, 2003).

Finally, the availability of dietary energy supplies appears to exert important regulatory functions in pituitary–adrenal stress responses, pointing to an important role of the nutritional state. In one study (Kirschbaum et al., 1997), the effects of short-term fasting and subsequent glucose administration on the free cortisol response to psychological stress were investigated. Although glucose load per se did not affect free cortisol levels, a TSST exposure induced a large cortisol response in glucose-treated participants. In contrast, fasting participants who received tap water did not respond to the psychological stressor with significant changes in cortisol levels. These data show that low glucose levels appear to inhibit adrenocortical responsiveness in healthy participants and suggest that ready access to energy is a prerequisite for HPA axis stress responses. In a second study (Gonzalez-Bono, Rohleder, Hellhammer, Salvador, & Kirschbaum, 2002), participants received either glucose, protein, fat, or water 1 hour before TSST exposure. Absolute cortisol levels and net cortisol increases were greater in the glucose group in comparison with the other three groups, and the cortisol response was positively correlated with changes in blood glucose. It can be assumed that a central mechanism, rather than peripheral mechanisms, may be responsible for regulation of energy balance and HPA axis activation. In sum, these studies show that blood glucose levels should be standardized when studying HPA axis responsiveness—for example, by standardization of the nutritional state before onset of an experiment, perhaps by consumption of standardized meals or the administration of a glucose-containing standard beverage at the beginning of a stress experiment.

Social Support

The social environment appears to exert important modulating effects on HPA axis stress responses. It has been hypothesized that one possible pathway relating the impact of social support to human well-being and health is mediated via HPA axis functioning under stress. Few data provide experimental support for the hypothesis that social support might attenuate the HPA axis response to acute stress, and effects appear to be sex specific. In a study investigating the impact of brief social support on the cortisol response to the TSST, our laboratory assigned healthy women and men to one of three support conditions: (1) no support before stress, (2) support from an opposite-sex stranger, or (3) support from the participant's partner (Kirschbaum, Klauer, Filipp, & Hellhammer, 1995). The results revealed an interesting and unexpected effect. Men showed a decreased cortisol response with increased quality of support (no support > stranger support > partner support), whereas women showed a different response pattern. There was no response difference between unsupported and stranger-supported women. However, women with partner support tended to show elevated cortisol responses to the acute stressor (no support = stranger support < partner support). Interestingly, women rated the support efficacy generally higher than men, who rate the efficacy higher when supported by their girlfriends. These results suggest that effects of social support may be gender specific. From an endocrine viewpoint, men may benefit more from opposite-sex support than women do.

The neuropeptide oxytocin is implicated both in prosocial behavior and in the central nervous system control of neuroendocrine responses to stress in animal studies, as conducted by Heinrichs, Baumgartner, Kirschbaum, and Ehlert (2003). First, they replicated the finding that salivary cortisol levels are suppressed by social support in response to stress in men and revealed an anxiolytic effect of oxytocin. Most interestingly, the combination of oxytocin and social support exhibited the lowest cortisol concentrations, as well as increased calmness and decreased anxiety during stress. In sum, oxytocin seems to enhance the buffering effect of social support on stress responsiveness, at least in men. These results concur with data from animal research suggesting an important role of oxytocin as an underlying biological mechanism for stress-protective effects of positive social support.

Social Hierarchy

Position in the social hierarchy seems to be relevant for acute HPA axis stress responses. In 63 army recruits, social status was monitored weekly over a 6-week boot camp training period (Hellhammer, Buchtal, Gutberlet, & Kirschbaum, 1997). Following exposure to psychological stress (TSST), salivary cortisol levels increased highly in socially dominant participants, whereas, only a modest elevation was observed in subordinate men. Similar group differences in HPA axis response patterns were observed under physical stress.

Interventions

Besides social support, early evidence shows that brief group-based cognitive-behavioral stress management training may reduce endocrine stress responses and cognitive appraisal to an acute stress exposure in healthy young individuals. Gaab et al. (2003) randomly assigned 48 healthy male students to receive stress management training (consisting of cognitive restructuring, problem solving, self-instruction, and relaxation training modules such as progressive muscle relaxation) either before or after the stress exposure. Participants in the treatment group (training before TSST stress exposure) showed an attenuated endocrine response compared with the group that received training after TSST stress exposure. In addition, participants in the treatment group had lower stress appraisal and higher control expectancies than the delayed-treatment group. This study shows that brief group-based cognitive-behavioral stress management training can reduce the neuroendocrine stress response to an acute stressor in healthy participants. Recently, the same group showed that attenuated cortisol stress responses appear to persist over time in both men and women (Hammerfald et al., 2006). Effects of stress management training or progressive muscular relaxation on blood pressure responses were described by Vocks, Ockenfels, Jürgensen, Mussgay, and Rüddell (2004). Finally, Khalfa, Bella, Roy, Peretz, and Lupien (2003) investigated whether relaxing music, in comparison with silence, might facilitate recovery from TSST stress exposure. It was reported that salivary cortisol levels ceased to increase after the stressor in the presence of music, whereas they continued to increase for 30 minutes in silence. In sum, stress management training and possible other interventions may prove useful in preventing detrimental effects of stress-induced neuroendocrine and cardiovascular activation in healthy participants, as well as in patients.

Personality Factors

It is tempting to speculate as to whether the HPA axis response to stress is influenced at least in part by stable trait factors, as the endocrine response to psychosocial stress can be viewed as a close interaction between situation and person variables within a given context. Applying structural equation modeling, researchers have shown that baseline measures of adrenocortical activity are indeed composed of state and trait factor variance, as well as residual error variance (Kirschbaum et al., 1990). Based on the observation that the impact of state variables appears dominant in basal cortisol levels, our laboratory, in cooperation with others, investigated the association between TSST-induced cortisol levels and 12 different personality factors. In independent studies, no close relationship between personality factors and basal cortisol levels or stress-induced cortisol increases could be observed (Brandtstädter, Baltes-Götz, Kirschbaum, & Hellhammer, 1991; Kirschbaum, Bartussek, & Strasburger, 1992). Interestingly, the result picture changes significantly when investigating the relationship between personality traits and stress responses after repeated exposures to the TSST (see the next section). As we describe, associations between personality traits and stress responses emerge only after repeated exposures to the TSST.

Habituation

After repeated exposure to (initially) stressful situations, a rapid habituation of HPA axis stress responses has been reported consistently for the TSST (Pruessner et al., 1997; Schommer, Hellhammer, & Kirschbaum, 2003; Federenko, Nagamine, Hellhammer, Wadhwa, & Wüst, 2004; Wüst, Federenko, van Rossum, Koper, & Hellhammer, 2005) and other stress protocols (Levine, 1978; Gunnar, Connors, & Isensee, 1989; Deinzer, Kirschbaum, Gresele, & Hellhammer, 1997; Gerra et al., 2000). In a large study sample, Wüst and coworkers (2005) have recently documented a substantial interindividual variability of such HPA axis response habituation patterns. Although 52% of their participants showed a well-known response habituation, almost 16% of the participants showed a response sensitization across three test sessions. It has been hypothesized that such habituation may be ascribed to a reduction in context variables across stress sessions (Mason, 1968a; Rose, 1980, 1984). Schommer et al. (2003) investigated whether peripheral catecholamines and cardiovascular parameters would show similar or different habituation patterns after repeated stress. Although HPA axis responses quickly habituated, the sympathetic nervous system showed rather uniform activation patterns with repeated exposure to psychosocial challenge. Recently, von Känel and coworkers (von Känel et al., 2004; von Känel, Kudielka, Preckel, Hanebuth, & Fischer, 2006; Mischler et al., 2005) observed that stress-related changes in blood coagulation indices, hemoconcentration, blood cells, and IL-6 levels after TSST-induced psychosocial stress and during recovery also fail to habituate to stress repeats. Based on these studies, it can be speculated that habituation to the TSST might be rather specific for HPA parameters.

To more closely investigate the relationship between personality traits and stress responses to repeated acute stress, volunteers were administered to the TSST five times on consecutive days. Results of a first investigation provided preliminary evidence that participants who showed no habituation across the five sessions tended to be lower in self-esteem and extraversion and higher in neuroticism, and they reported a greater number of physical complaints (Kirschbaum, Prüssner, et al., 1995). Pruessner, Gaab, et al. (1997) suggested that correlation coefficients between cortisol stress responses and personality factors increase with the number of test days aggregated. In agreement with the previous results, no significant correlations between personality and cortisol levels emerged on day 1. However, with two or more cortisol responses aggregated, the resulting correlation coefficients between the new dummy variables and the respective personality variable increased monotonously (e.g., "social dominance and cortisol AUC": $r_{\text{day 2}} = -.47$ to $r_{\text{aggregation days 2-5}} = -.70$). In contrast to the previously referenced studies, these data provide evidence for a relationship between personality traits and cortisol stress responses uncovered after repeated stress exposure applying data aggregation. Although novelty may mask the impact of personality on the cortisol stress response on the first exposure, differences in the ability to cope with the stressful situation may lead to different cortisol stress response patterns on subsequent stress exposures. Thus a reliable investigation of associations between personality variables and cortisol stress responses appears to require repeated TSST exposure and data aggregation.

Vital Exhaustion

The question of whether a hyper- or hyporesponsivity to acute stress may occur when an individual is chronically stressed or exhausted and no longer able to cope with environmental stress is open to debate (Kudielka et al., 2006; Kudielka, Bellingrath, & Hellhammer, 2006). Studies applying different psychological stressors seem to point at a subtle hyporeactivity in participants with higher levels of chronic stress and exhaustion or do not reveal any differences in the HPA-axis response to a single stress exposure (Pike et al., 1997; Kristenson et al., 1998; Nicolson & van Diest, 2000; Kristenson, Kucinskiene, Bergdahl, & Ort-Gomer, 2001; Matthews, Gump, & Owens, 2001). However, under repeated psychosocial short-term stress, an association between vital exhaustion and HPA axis responses emerges (Kudielka et al., 2006). Linear regression revealed a negative dose–response relationship between exhaustion and the degree of habituation. We assume that situational or psychological factors initially "mask" an existing impact of exhaustion because in this study effects of exhaustion became apparent only after repeated stress exposure.

Genetic Factors: Heritability and Polymorphisms

Besides behavioral and situational variation, HPA axis activity appears to be profoundly influenced by genetic factors, as shown in twin studies, as well as in candidate gene studies on polymorphisms in the genes that code for the glucocorticoid receptor, the mineralocorticoid receptor, the melanocortin-2 (ACTH) receptor, the melanocortin-4 receptor, the µ-opioid receptor, the GABA$_A$ (gamma-aminobutyric-acid$_A$) receptor, the α-adrenergic receptor, the 5-HT$_{2A}$ (serotonin$_{2A}$) receptor, COMT (catechol-O-methyltransferase), TNFα (tumor necrosis factor alpha) and ACE (angiotensin-I converting enzyme; for a review, see Wüst, Federenko, et al., 2004).

Earlier studies support the notion of a moderate to strong influence of genetic factors on baseline cortisol levels and the circadian rhythmicity of cortisol (Maxwell, Boyle, Greig, & Buchanan, 1969; Meikle, Bishop, Strongham, Ford, & West, 1989; Linkowski et al., 1993; Wüst, Federenko, Hellhammer, & Kirschbaum, 2000; for a review and reanalysis, see Bartels, Van den Berg, Sluyter, Boomsma, & de Geus, 2003).

A possible contribution of genetic determination on stimulated levels was studied in a sample of monozygotic (MZ) and dizygotic (DZ) twins, subjecting each individual to three different stimulation procedures (Kirschbaum, Wüst, et al., 1992), including (1) the TSST, (2) HPA axis stimulation by injection of 100μg exogenous human CRH, and (3) exhausting physical exercise (bicycle ergometry). First of all, a significant genetic influence on unstimulated cortisol levels was observed, supporting the results from other laboratories. Although the variability of salivary cortisol peak levels after hCRH administration seemed to be influenced by genetic factors (h^2 = .84), they seemed less relevant after TSST exposure (h^2 = .32) and were not detectable after stimulation with bicycle ergometry. Federenko et al. (2004) recently recruited a much larger sample of male twin pairs and subjected them to the TSST three times at 1-week intervals. In accordance with the hypothesis that "trait"-like components of the endocrine stress response may become more apparent with repeated stress exposures, it was shown that the genetic influence on HPA axis reactivity was low at the first TSST stress exposure but that it increased substantially with the repetition of the same stress protocol (area under the curve for ACTH, free and total cortisol: r_iMZ = .67–.72, r_iDZ = .10–.29). This study strongly supports the notion that genetic factors do contribute to the variability in cortisol and ACTH responses to psychosocial stress.

More recently, Wüst, Van Rossum, et al. (2004) for the first time investigated whether variants of the glucocorticoid receptor (GR) gene might contribute to the large interindividual variability of HPA axis activity and reactivity and documented a significant impact of different GR gene polymorphisms on cortisol (and maybe ACTH) responses to psychosocial stress. Besides the investigation of GR gene polymorphisms, Uhart, McCaul, Oswald, Choi, and Wand (2004) recently determined the influence of the T1521C single nucleotide polymorphism (SNP) in the GABA$_A$alpha6 receptor subunit gene (GABRA6). The authors report that ACTH, cortisol, diastolic blood pressure, and mean blood pressure responses to the TSST were significantly greater in participants who were homozygous for the T allele or heterozygous compared with participants who were homozygous for the C allele. Furmark et al. (2004) investigated a functional polymorphism in the promoter region of the human serotonin transporter (5-HTT) gene that has been related to negative affect and amygdala activity. Genotyping identified patients with social phobia who had long versus short alleles in the promoter region of the 5-HTT gene. Individuals with one or two copies of the short allele, expressing up to 50%

less transporter protein, exhibited significantly increased levels of anxiety-related traits, state anxiety, and enhanced right amygdala responding to a speaking task protocol, compared with participants who were homozygous for the long allele. In sum, we may speculate that the described variants may contribute to the individual vulnerability for HPA-related disorders. This remains a challenge for future research.

Glucocorticoid Sensitivity and Cellular Transcription

Finally, a cell's response to cortisol is predominantly determined by both the steroid level it is exposed to and its sensitivity for glucocorticoids, that is, the efficacy of glucocorticoid-mediated signal transduction (Bamberger, Schulte, & Chrousos, 1996). In a series of experiments applying the TSST stress protocol, Rohleder and coworkers (Rohleder, Schommer, Hellhammer, Engel, & Kirschbaum, 2001; Rohleder, Kudielka, Hellhammer, Wolf, & Kirschbaum, 2002; Rohleder, Wolf, Piel, & Kirschbaum, 2003) investigated the influence of age, sex, and sex hormone status on GC sensitivity of peripheral proinflammatory cytokine production (for a review, see Rohleder, Wolf, & Kirschbaum, 2003). The first study revealed that stress-induced free cortisol stress responses did not differ between men and women, although GC sensitivity and lipopolysaccharide (LPS)-stimulated cytokine production showed large sex differences (Rohleder et al., 2001). In a second study in younger, compared with elderly, healthy men treated with either placebo or testosterone, stress-induced increases in cortisol again did not differ significantly between experimental groups, but GC sensitivity increased significantly in young controls and testosterone-treated elderly men, whereas a decrease was found in placebo-treated elderly men. It was hypothesized that the increase in GC sensitivity after stress serves to protect the individual from detrimental increases of pro-inflammatory cytokines, a mechanism that is disturbed in elderly men and partly restored by testosterone treatment (Rohleder et al., 2002). A third study addressed the question of whether blunted free cortisol response of oral contraceptive users may be compensated at the level of the target tissue (Rohleder, Wolf, Piel, & Kirschbaum, 2003). Based on the results, one can speculated whether an increase in GC sensitivity of proinflammatory cytokine production may, at least in part, compensate the low cortisol levels observed in OC users after stress. This could be one mechanism to protect women using OC from chronic inflammatory and autoimmune diseases.

Bierhaus, Wolf, and colleagues (2003) employed the TSST to elucidate how neuroendocrine stress responses can mediate cellular processes, which, in the long run, can promote vascular diseases. Various genes are controlled by the transcription factor nuclear factor kappaB (NF-κB), a protein that appears to be highly sensitive to psychosocial stress. In animal and human studies, the authors showed that norepinephrine-dependent adrenergic stimulation results in a rapid up-regulation of NF-κB in vitro, as well as in vivo. Their data provide convincing evidence that the activation of the transcription factor NF-κB (nuclear factor kappaB) might represent a norepinephrine-dependent pathway converting psychosocial stress into cellular dysfunction.

CLINICAL STUDIES

Besides its use with healthy study participants, the TSST can also be used in clinical populations, with disorders ranging from psychiatric diseases to somatic complaints, as shown in several studies over the past years (Heim, Newport, et al., 2000). To date, the TSST has been successfully applied with patients suffering from, for example, major depression, anxiety disorder, social phobia, posttraumatic stress disorder (PTSD), burnout, exhaustion, chronic fatigue syndrome, fibromyalgia, recurrent abdominal pain, chronic pelvic pain, temporomandibular dysfunction (myofascial pain and dysfunction), functional gastrointestinal disorders (irritable bowel syndrome [IBS] or nonulcer dyspepsia), different manifestations of chronic atopy, atopic dermatitis, or chronic allergic asthma, with adults with a history of sexual or physical childhood abuse, and with breast cancer survivors.

In two studies, Young and coworkers (Young, Lopez, Murphy-Weinberg, Watson, & Akil, 2000; Young, Abelson, & Cameron, 2004) investigated endocrine stress responses in major depression. Results of the first study suggest that depressed patients manifest normal cortisol responses to social stress despite increased prestressor plasma cortisol levels. However, the beta-endorphin response to the TSST was significantly smaller in the depressed patients compared with a matched control group. In a second study, no diagnosis-related or gender-specific effects for plasma cortisol were found, but an exaggerated ACTH response in the depressed group with comorbid anxiety disorder appeared. Gold, Zakowski, Valdimarsdottir, and Bovbjerg (2004) and Miller, Rohleder, Stetler, and Kirschbaum (2005) used modified versions of the TSST. For a meta-analysis of depression and cortisol responses to psychological stress, see also Burke, Davis, Otte, and Mohr (2005).

In a study of peripubertal males affected by anxiety disorder and age-matched healthy controls, Gerra et al. (2000) applied a battery of psychological stress tests, including the TSST protocol, to investigate stress responses in plasma levels of norepinephrine, epinephrine, cortisol, ACTH, beta-endorphin, growth hormone, prolactin, and testosterone. Their results support the hypothesis that hyperactivity of the noradrenergic system in response to acute stress is associated with anxiety disorders in adolescents. The children's version of the TSST (TSST-C) was also applied in young patients with recurrent abdominal pain and with anxiety disorders and in a healthy control group in order to compare clinical symptoms, diagnoses, and physiological responses to stress (Dorn et al., 2003). Jezova, Makatsori, Duncko, Moncek, and Jakubek (2004) used a modified version of the TSST in healthy participants with high and low trait anxiety.

Heim and coworkers (Heim, Newport, et al., 2000) found that women with a history of childhood abuse exhibited increased HPA axis and autonomic responses to acute stress compared with controls. This effect was particularly robust in women with current symptoms of depression and anxiety. Women with histories of childhood abuse and diagnoses of current major depression exhibited a more than six-fold greater ACTH response to stress than the age-matched controls. The authors suggest that a hyperreactivity of the HPA axis and autonomic nervous system, presumably due to CRF hypersecretion, is a persistent consequence of childhood abuse that may contribute to the diathesis for adulthood psychopathological conditions.

In adults with social phobia, Condren, O'Neill, Ryan, Barrett, and Thakore (2002) observed similar baseline measures of cortisol but significantly greater stress-induced cortisol net increases in patients compared with controls, suggesting that patients with social phobia were hyperresponsive when confronted with psychological stress (see also Levin et al., 1993; Furlan, DeMartinis, Schweizer, Rickels, & Lucki, 2001). However, in adolescent girls with social phobia, Martel et al. (1999) could induce significant changes in salivary cortisol by applying a modified TSST procedure but did not observe any differences compared with a healthy control group.

Gaab et al. (2005) exposed patients suffering from chronic fatigue syndrome (CFS) and healthy controls to the TSST. Although cortisol responses to stress were normal, proinflammatory cytokine levels in patients with CFS were significantly attenuated. However, significantly blunted cortisol responses to the TSST have been observed in breast cancer survivors with enduring fatigue in contrast to nonfatigued survivors, controlling for depression and other potential confounds (Bower, Ganz, & Aziz, 2005). A modified version of the TSST was applied by Jones, Rollman, and Brooke (1997) in women suffering from temporomandibular dysfunction (TMD; myofascial pain and dysfunction).

Recently, Wiesli et al. (2005) applied the TSST in patients with type 1 diabetes. Following food intake (but not in the fasting state), a significantly delayed recovery of stress-induced glucose concentrations was observed compared with a control condition.

In several independent studies, Buske-Kirschbaum and coworkers applied the TSST to adults, as well as children, suffering from different manifestations of chronic atopy. Children with atopic dermatitis as well as chronic allergic asthma, showed a significantly blunted cortisol response to the TSST and similar heart rate responses when compared with a sex- and age-matched control group (Buske-Kirschbaum et al., 1997; Buske-Kirschbaum et al., 2003). Similarly, adult dermatitis patients showed significantly attenuated cortisol and ACTH responses to the stressor and altered immunomodulation, whereas catecholamine levels were significantly elevated in patients with atopy compared with controls (Buske-Kirschbaum, Geiben, Hollig, Morschhauser, & Hellhammer, 2002; Buske-Kirschbaum, Gierens, Hollig, & Hellhammer, 2002). No difference between experimental groups was found in basal cortisol and ACTH concentrations, whereas basal catecholamine levels were significantly elevated. These findings suggest that a hyporesponsive HPA axis response to psychological stress may represent a common feature of different manifestations of chronic atopy and that stress may be associated with atopy-relevant immunological changes in sufferers of atopic dermatitis (for reviews, see also Buske-Kirschbaum, Jobst, & Hellhammer, 1998; Buske-Kirschbaum, Geiben, & Hellhammer, 2001; Buske-Kirschbaum & Hellhammer, 2003).

CONCLUSIONS

Throughout more than a decade of research, the TSST has proven a useful tool in the fields of basic, applied, and clinical psychobiological research with a wide range of psychobiological outcome variables. Besides the direct study of different biological stress systems such as the HPA and SAM axes or the cardiovascular system, the TSST can be used to investigate biological pathways between stress and disease (Heim, Ehlert, & Hellhammer, 2000), or to study stress-related phenomena (e.g., effects of stress on memory, cognition, or approach–avoidance behavior; Kirschbaum, Platte, Pirke, & Hellhammer, 1996; Wolf, Kudielka, Hellhammer, Hellhammer, & Kirschbaum, 1998; Wolf, Schommer, Hellhammer, McEwen, & Kirschbaum, 2001; Payne, Nadel, Allen, Thomas, & Jacobs, 2002; Takahashi et al., 2004; Abercrombie, Speck, & Monticelli, 2006; Elzinga & Roelofs, 2005; Kuhlmann, Piel, & Wolf, 2005; Roelofs, Elzinga, & Rotteveel, 2005) and interactions between stress and drug effects (e.g., ascorbic acid, alcohol, metamphetamine, lamotrigine treatment; Brody & Preut, 2002; Brody, Preut, Schommer, & Schürmeyer, 2002; Söderpalm & de Wit, 2002; Söderpalm, Nikolayev, & de Wit, 2003; Makatsori et al., 2004). Because numerous moderating and intervening factors for HPA axis responses to acute psychosocial stress have been carefully described in different laboratories, the known sources of individual variability should be considered in the design of future studies. Clinical studies continue to accumulate evidence that different diseases are associated with characteristic stress-response profiles. Furthermore, biological mechanisms begin to unfold that could be helpful in explaining the stress–disease association. In a next step, the challenge to researchers will be to investigate whether the TSST protocol can be applied as a diagnostic tool for the prediction of disease susceptibility and symptom severity and/or for monitoring the efficacy of interventions.

REFERENCES

Abercrombie, H. C., Speck, N. S., & Monticelli, R. M. (2006). Endogenous cortisol elevations are related to memory facilitation only in individuals who are emotionally aroused. *Psychoneuroendocrinology, 31*(2), 187–196.

al'Absi, M., Lovallo, W. R., McKey, B., Sung, B. H., Whitsett, T. L., & Wilson, M. F. (1998). Hypothalamic–pituitary–adrenocortical responses to psychological stress and caffeine in men at high and low risk for hypertension. *Psychosomatic Medicine, 60*(4), 521–527.

Altemus, M., Redwine, L. S., Leong, Y. M., Frye, C. A., Porges, S. W., & Carter, C. S. (2001). Responses to laboratory psychosocial stress in postpartum women. *Psychosomatic Medicine, 63*(5), 814–821.

Bamberger, C. M., Schulte, H. M., & Chrousos, G. P. (1996). Molecular determinants of glucocorticoid receptor function and tissue sensitivity to glucocorticoids. *Endocrine Reviews, 17*(3), 245–261.

Bartels, M., Van den Berg, M., Sluyter, F., Boomsma, D. I., & de Geus, E. J. (2003). Heritability of cortisol levels: Review and simultaneous analysis of twin studies. *Psychoneuroendocrinology, 28*(2), 121–137.

Bierhaus, A., Wolf, J., Andrassy, M., Rohleder, N., Humpert, P. M., Petrov, D., et al. (2003). A mechanism converting psychosocial stress into mononuclear cell activation. *Proceedings of the National Academy of Sciences of the USA, 100*(4), 1920–1925.

Biondi, M., & Picardi, A. (1999). Psychological stress and neuroendocrine function in humans: the last two decades of research. *Psychotherapy and Psychosomatics, 68*(3), 114–150.

Bower, J. E., Ganz, P. A., & Aziz, N. (2005). Altered cortisol response to psychologic stress in breast cancer survivors with persistent fatigue. *Psychosomatic Medicine, 67*(2), 277–280.

Brandtstädter, J., Baltes-Götz, B., Kirschbaum, C., & Hellhammer, D. (1991). Developmental and personality correlates of adrenocortical activity as indexed by salivary cortisol: Observations in the age range of 35 to 65 years. Journal of Psychosomatic Research, *35*(2–3), 173–185.

Brody, S., & Preut, R. (2002). Cannabis, tobacco, and caffeine use modify the blood pressure reactivity protection of ascorbic acid. *Pharmacology, Biochemistry, and Behavior, 72*(4), 811–816.

Brody, S., Preut, R., Schommer, K., & Schürmeyer, T. H. (2002). A randomized controlled trial of high-dose ascorbic acid for reduction of blood pressure, cortisol, and subjective responses to psychological stress. *Psychopharmacology, 159*(3), 319–324.

Burke, H. M., Davis, M. C., Otte, C., & Mohr, D. C. (2005). Depression and cortisol responses to psychological stress: A meta-analysis. *Psychoneuroendocrinology, 30*(9), 846–856.

Buske-Kirschbaum, A., Geiben, A., & Hellhammer, D. (2001). Psychobiological aspects of atopic dermatitis: An overview. *Psychotherapy and Psychosomatics, 70*(1), 6–16.

Buske-Kirschbaum, A., Geiben, A., Hollig, H., Morschhauser, E., & Hellhammer, D. (2002). Altered responsiveness of the hypothalamus–pituitary–adrenal axis and the sympathetic adrenomedullary system to stress in patients with atopic dermatitis. *Journal of Clinical Endocrinology and Metabolism, 87*(9), 4245–4251.

Buske-Kirschbaum, A., Gierens, A., Hollig, H., & Hellhammer, D. H. (2002). Stress-induced immunomodulation is altered in patients with atopic dermatitis. *Journal of Neuroimmunology, 129*(1–2), 161–167.

Buske-Kirschbaum, A., & Hellhammer, D. H. (2003). Endocrine and immune responses to stress in chronic inflammatory skin disorders. *Annals of the New York Academy of Sciences, 992,* 231–240.

Buske-Kirschbaum, A., Jobst, S., & Hellhammer, D. H. (1998). Altered reactivity of the hypothalamus–pituitary–adrenal axis in patients with atopic dermatitis: Pathologic factor or symptom? *Annals of the New York Academy of Sciences, 840,* 747–754.

Buske-Kirschbaum, A., Jobst, S., Psych, D., Wustmans, A., Kirschbaum, C., Rauh, W., et al., (1997). Attenuated free cortisol response to psychosocial stress in children with atopic dermatitis. *Psychosomatic Medicine, 59*(4), 419–426.

Buske-Kirschbaum, A., von Auer, K., Krieger, S., Weis, S., Rauh, W., & Hellhammer, D. (2003). Blunted cortisol responses to psychosocial stress in asthmatic children: A general feature of atopic disease? *Psychosomatic Medicine, 65*(5), 806–810.

Clow, A., Patel, S., Najafi, M., Evans, P. D., & Hucklebridge, F. (1997). The cortisol response to psychological challenge is preceded by a transient rise in endogenous inhibitor of monoamine oxidase. *Life Sciences, 61*(5), 567–575.

Condren, R. M., O'Neill, A., Ryan, M. C., Barrett, P., & Thakore, J. H. (2002). HPA axis response to a psychological stressor in generalised social phobia. *Psychoneuroendocrinology, 27*(6), 693–703.

de Wit, H., Söderpalm, A. H., Nikolayev, L., & Young, E. (2003). Effects of acute social stress on alcohol consumption in healthy subjects. *Alcohol Clinical and Experimental Research, 27*(8), 1270–1277.

Deinzer, R., Kirschbaum, C., Gresele, C., & Hellhammer, D. H. (1997). Adrenocortical responses to repeated parachute jumping and subsequent h-CRH challenge in inexperienced healthy subjects. *Physiology and Behavior, 61*(4), 507–511.

Dickerson, S. S., & Kemeny, M. E. (2004). Acute stressors and cortisol responses: a theoretical integration and synthesis of laboratory research. *Psychological Bulletin, 130*(3), 355–391.

Dorn, L. D., Campo, J. C., Thato, S., Dahl, R. E., Lewin, D., Chandra, R., et al. (2003). Psychological comorbidity and stress reactivity in children and adolescents with recurrent abdominal pain and anxiety disorders. *Journal of the American Academy of Child and Adolescent Psychiatry, 42*(1), 66–75.

Elzinga, B. M., & Roelofs, K. (2005). Cortisol-induced impairments of working memory require acute sympathetic activation. *Behavioral Neurosciences, 119*(1), 98–103.

Federenko, I. S., Nagamine, M., Hellhammer, D. H., Wadhwa, P. D., & Wüst, S. (2004). The heritability of hypothalamus pituitary adrenal axis responses to psychosocial stress is context dependent. *Journal of Clinical Endocrinology and Metabolism, 89*(12), 6244–6250.

Frankenhaeuser, M., Lundberg, U., & Forsman, L. (1980). Dissociation between sympathetic–adrenal and pituitary–adrenal responses to an achievement situation characterized by high controllability: comparison between type A and type B males and females. Biological Psychology, *10*(2), 79–91.

Furlan, P. M., DeMartinis, N., Schweizer, E., Rickels, K., & Lucki, I. (2001).

Abnormal salivary cortisol levels in social phobic patients in response to acute psychological but not physical stress. *Biological Psychiatry, 50*(4), 254–259.

Furmark, T., Tillfors, M., Garpenstrand, H., Marteinsdottir, I., Langstrom, B., Oreland, L., et al. (2004). Serotonin transporter polymorphism related to amygdala excitability and symptom severity in patients with social phobia. *Neuroscience Letters, 362*(3), 189–192.

Fuxe, K., Andersson, K., Eneroth, P., Harfstrand, A., & Agnati, L. F. (1989). Neuroendocrine actions of nicotine and of exposure to cigarette smoke: Medical implications. *Psychoneuroendocrinology, 14*(1–2), 19–41.

Gaab, J., Blattler, N., Menzi, T., Pabst, B., Stoyer, S., & Ehlert, U. (2003). Randomized controlled evaluation of the effects of cognitive-behavioral stress management on cortisol responses to acute stress in healthy subjects. *Psychoneuroendocrinology, 28*(6), 767–779.

Gaab, J., Rohleder, N., Heitz, V., Engert, V., Schad, T., Schürmeyer, T. H., et al. (2005). Stress-induced changes in LPS-induced pro-inflammatory cytokine production in chronic fatigue syndrome. *Psychoneuroendocrinology, 30*(2), 188–198.

Gerra, G., Zaimovic, A., Zambelli, U., Timpano, M., Reali, N., Bernasconi, S., et al. (2000). Neuroendocrine responses to psychological stress in adolescents with anxiety disorder. *Neuropsychobiology, 42*(2), 82–92.

Gold, S. M., Zakowski, S. G., Valdimarsdottir, H. B., & Bovbjerg, D. H. (2004). Higher Beck depression scores predict delayed epinephrine recovery after acute psychological stress independent of baseline levels of stress and mood. *Biological Psychology, 67*(3), 261–273.

Gonzalez-Bono, E., Rohleder, N., Hellhammer, D. H., Salvador, A., & Kirschbaum, C. (2002). Glucose but not protein or fat load amplifies the cortisol response to psychosocial stress. *Hormones and Behavior, 41*(3), 328–333.

Gruenewald, T. L., Kemeny, M. E., Aziz, N., & Fahey, J. L. (2004). Acute threat to the social self: Shame, social self-esteem, and cortisol activity. *Psychosomatic Medicine, 66*(6), 915–924.

Gunnar, M. R., Connors, J., & Isensee, J. (1989). Lack of stability in neonatal adrenocortical reactivity because of rapid habituation of the adrenocortical response. *Developmental Psychobiology, 22*(3), 221–233.

Hammerfald, K., Eberle, C., Grau, M., Kinsperger, A., Zimmermann, A., Ehlert, U., et al. (2006). Persistent effects of cognitive-behavioral stress management on cortisol responses to acute stress in healthy subjects: A randomized controlled trial. *Psychoneuroendocrinology, 31*(3), 333–339.

Heim, C., Ehlert, U., & Hellhammer, D. H. (2000). The potential role of hypocortisolism in the pathophysiology of stress-related bodily disorders. *Psychoneuroendocrinology, 25*(1), 1–35.

Heim, C., Newport, D. J., Heit, S., Graham, Y. P., Wilcox, M., Bonsall, R., et al. (2000). Pituitary-adrenal and autonomic responses to stress in women after sexual and physical abuse in childhood. *Journal of the American Medical Association, 284*(5), 592–597.

Heinrichs, M., Baumgartner, T., Kirschbaum, C., & Ehlert, U. (2003). Social support and oxytocin interact to suppress cortisol and subjective responses to psychosocial stress. *Biological Psychiatry 54*(12), 1389–1398.

Heinrichs, M., Meinlschmidt, G., Neumann, I., Wagner, S., Kirschbaum, C., Ehlert, U., et al. (2001). Effects of suckling on hypothalamic–pituitary–adrenal axis responses to psychosocial stress in postpartum lactating women. *Journal of Clinical Endocrinology and Metabolism, 86*(10), 4798–4804.

Heinrichs, M., Neumann, I., & Ehlert, U. (2002). Lactation and stress: Protective effects of breast-feeding in humans. *Stress, 5*(3), 195–203.

Hellhammer, D. H., Buchtal, J., Gutberlet, I., & Kirschbaum, C. (1997). Social hierarchy and adrenocortical stress reactivity in men. *Psychoneuroendocrinology, 22*(8), 643–650.

Henry, J. P., 1992. Biological basis of the stress response. *Integrative Physiological and Behavioral Science, 27*(1), 66–83.

Horrocks, P. M., Jones, A. F., Ratcliffe, W. A., Holder, G., White, A., Holder, R., et al. (1990). Patterns of ACTH and cortisol pulsatility over twenty-four hours in normal males and females. *Clinical Endocrinology, 32*(1), 127–134.

Jezova, D., Makatsori, A., Duncko, R., Moncek, F., & Jakubek, M. (2004). High trait anxiety in healthy subjects is associated with low neuroendocrine activity during psychosocial stress. *Progress in Neuropsychopharmacology and Biology Psychiatry, 28*(8), 1331–1336.

Jones, D. A., Rollman, G. B., & Brooke, R. I. (1997). The cortisol response to psychological stress in temporomandibular dysfunction. *Pain, 72*(1–2), 171–182.

Khalfa, S., Bella, S. D., Roy, M., Peretz, I., & Lupien, S. J. (2003). Effects of relaxing music on salivary cortisol level after psychological stress. *Annals of the New York Academy of Sciences, 999*, 374–376.

Kirschbaum, C., Bartussek, D., & Strasburger, C. J. (1992). Cortisol responses to psychological stress and correlations with personality traits. *Personality and Individual Differences, 13*, 1353–1357.

Kirschbaum, C., Gonzalez Bono, E., Rohleder, N., Gessner, C., Pirke, K. M., Salvador, A., et al. (1997). Effects of fasting and glucose load on free cortisol responses to stress and nicotine. *Journal of Clinical Endocrinology and Metabolism, 82*(4), 1101–1105.

Kirschbaum, C., Klauer, T., Filipp, S. H., & Hellhammer, D. H. (1995). Sex-specific effects of social support on cortisol and subjective responses to acute psychological stress. *Psychosomatic Medicine, 57*(1), 23–31.

Kirschbaum, C., Kudielka, B. M., Gaab, J., Schommer, N. C., & Hellhammer, D. H. (1999). Impact of gender, menstrual cycle phase, and oral contraceptives on the activity of the hypothalamus–pituitary–adrenal axis. *Psychosomatic Medicine, 61*(2), 154–162.

Kirschbaum, C., Pirke, K. M., & Hellhammer, D. H. (1993). The Trier Social Stress Test: A tool for investigating psychobiological stress responses in a laboratory setting. *Neuropsychobiology, 28*(1–2), 76–81.

Kirschbaum, C., Pirke, K. M., & Hellhammer, D. H. (1995). Preliminary evidence for reduced cortisol responsivity to psychological stress in women using oral contraceptive medication. *Psychoneuroendocrinology, 20*(5), 509–514.

Kirschbaum, C., Platte, P., Pirke, K. M., & Hellhammer, D. (1996). Adrenocortical activation following stressful exercise: Further evidence for attenuated free cortisol responses in women using oral contraceptives. *Stress Medicine, 12*, 137–143.

Kirschbaum, C., Prüssner, J. C., Stone, A. A., Federenko, I., Gaab, J., Lintz, D., et al. (1995). Persistent high cortisol responses to repeated psychological stress in a subpopulation of healthy men. *Psychosomatic Medicine, 57*(5), 468–474.

Kirschbaum, C., Scherer, G., & Strasburger, C. J. (1994). Pituitary and adrenal hormone responses to pharmacological, physical, and psychological stimulation in habitual smokers and nonsmokers. *Clinical Investigator, 72*(10), 804–810.

Kirschbaum, C., Schommer, N., Federenko, I., Gaab, J., Neumann, O., Oellers, M., et al. (1996). Short-term estradiol treatment enhances pituitary-adrenal axis and sympathetic responses to psychosocial stress in healthy young men. *Journal of Clinical Endocrinology and Metabolism, 81*(10), 3639–3643.

Kirschbaum, C., Steyer, R., Eid, M., Patalla, U., Schwenkmezger, P., & Hellhammer, D. H. (1990). Cortisol and behavior: 2. Application of a latent state–trait model to salivary cortisol. *Psychoneuroendocrinology, 15*(4), 297–307.

Kirschbaum, C., Strasburger, C. J., & Langkrär, J. (1993). Attenuated cortisol response to psychological stress but not to CRH or ergometry in young habitual smokers. *Pharmacology, Biochemistry, and Behavior, 44*(3), 527–531.

Kirschbaum, C., Wüst, S., Faig, H. G., & Hellhammer, D. H. (1992). Heritability of cortisol responses to human corticotropin-releasing hormone, ergometry, and psychological stress in humans. *Journal of Clinical Endocrinology and Metabolism, 75*(6), 1526–1530.

Kirschbaum, C., Wüst, S., & Hellhammer, D. (1992). Consistent sex differences in cortisol responses to psychological stress. *Psychosomatic Medicine, 54*(6), 648–657.

Kristenson, M., Kucinskiene, Z., Bergdahl, B., & Ort-Gomer, K. (2001). Risk factors for coronary heart disease in different socioeconomic groups of Lithuania and Sweden: The LiVicordia Study. *Scandinavian Journal of Public Health, 29*(2), 140–150.

Kristenson, M., Orth-Gomer, K., Kucinskiene, Z., Bergdahl, B., Calkauskas, H., Balinkyniene, I., et al. (1998). Attenuated cortisol reponses to a standardized stress test in Lithuanian versus Swdish men: The LiVicordia study. *International Journal of Behavioral Medicine, 5*(1), 17–30.

Kudielka, B. M., Bellingrath, S., & Hellhammer, D. H. (2006). Cortisol in burnout and vital exhaustion: An overview. *Giornale Italiano di Medicina del Lavorio ed Ergonomia [Applied Psychology to Work and Rehabilitation Medicine], 28*(Suppl. 1), 34–42.

Kudielka, B. M., Buske-Kirschbaum, A., Hellhammer, D. H., & Kirschbaum, C. (2004a). Differential heart rate reactivity and recovery after psychosocial stress (TSST) in healthy children, younger adults, and elderly adults: The impact of age and gender. *International Journal of Behavioral Medicine, 11*(2), 116–121.

Kudielka, B. M., Buske-Kirschbaum, A., Hellhammer, D. H., & Kirschbaum, C. (2004b). HPA axis responses to laboratory psychosocial stress in healthy elderly adults, younger adults, and children: Impact of age and gender. *Psychoneuroendocrinology, 29*(1), 83–98.

Kudielka, B. M., Hellhammer, D. H., & Kirschbaum, C. (2000). Sex differences in human stress response. In G. Fink (Ed.), *Encyclopedia of stress* (Vol. 3, pp. 424–429). San Diego: Academic Press.

Kudielka, B. M., Hellhammer, J., Hellhammer, D. H., Wolf, O. T., Pirke, K. M., Varadi, E., et al. (1998). Sex differences in endocrine and psychological responses to psychosocial stress in healthy elderly subjects and the impact of a 2-week dehydroepiandrosterone treatment. *Journal of Clinical Endocrinology and Metabolism, 83*(5), 1756–1761.

Kudielka, B. M., & Kirschbaum, C. (2001). Stress and health research. In N. J.

Smelser & P. B. Baltes (Eds.), *International encyclopedia of the social and behavioral sciences* (Vol. 22, pp. 15170–15175). Oxford, UK: Elsevier.

Kudielka, B. M., & Kirschbaum, C. (2005). Sex differences in HPA axis responses to stress: A review. *Biological Psychology, 69*(1), 113–132.

Kudielka, B. M., Schmidt-Reinwald, A. K., Hellhammer, D. H., & Kirschbaum, C. (1999). Psychological and endocrine responses to psychosocial stress and dexamethasone/corticotropin-releasing hormone in healthy postmenopausal women and young controls: The impact of age and a two-week estradiol treatment. *Neuroendocrinology, 70*(6), 422–430.

Kudielka, B. M., Schmidt-Reinwald, A. K., Hellhammer, D. H., Schürmeyer, T., & Kirschbaum, C. (2000). Psychosocial stress and HPA functioning: No evidence for a reduced resilience in healthy elderly men. *Stress, 3*(3), 229–240.

Kudielka, B. M., Schommer, N. C., Hellhammer, D. H., & Kirschbaum, C. (2004). Acute HPA axis responses, heart rate, and mood changes to psychosocial stress (TSST) in humans at different times of day. *Psychoneuroendocrinology, 29*(8), 983–992.

Kudielka, B. M., von Känel, R., Preckel, D., Zgraggen, L., Mischler, K., & Fischer, J. E. (2006). Exhaustion is associated with reduced habituation of free cortisol responses to repeated acute psychosocial stress. *Biological Psychology, 72*(2), 147–153.

Kuhlmann, S., Piel, M., & Wolf, O. T. (2005). Impaired memory retrieval after psychosocial stress in healthy young men. *Journal of Neuroscience, 25*(11), 2977–2982.

Levin, A. P., Saoud, J. B., Straumann, T., Gorman, J. M., Fyer, A. J., Crawford, R., et al. (1993). Responses of "generalized" and "discrete" social phobics during public speaking. *Journal of Anxiety Disorders, 7*, 207–221.

Levine, S. (1978). Cortisol changes following repeated experiences with parachute training. In H. Ursin, E. Baade, & S. Levine (Eds.), *Psychobiology of stress: A study of coping men* (pp. 51–56). New York: Academic Press.

Levine, S., & Ursin, H. (1991). What is stress? In R. M. Brown, G. F. Koob, & C. Rivier (Eds.), *Stress, neurobiology and neuroendocrinology* (pp. 3–21). New York: Dekker.

Linkowski, P., Van Onderbergen, A., Kerkhofs, M., Bosson, D., Mendlewicz, J., & Van Cauter, E. (1993). Twin study of the 24-h cortisol profile: Evidence for genetic control of the human circadian clock. *American Journal of Physiology, 264*(2, Pt. 1), E173–181.

Lovallo, W. R., al'Absi, M., Blick, K., Whitsett, T. L., & Wilson, M. F. (1996). Stress-like adrenocorticotropin responses to caffeine in young healthy men. *Pharmacology Biochemistry, and Behavior, 55*(3), 365–369.

Lundberg, U. (1983). Sex differences in behaviour pattern and catecholamine and cortisol excretion in 3- 6-year-old day-care children. *Biological Psychology, 16*(1–2), 109–117.

Makatsori, A., Duncko, R., Moncek, F., Loder, I., Katina, S., & Jezova, D. (2004). Modulation of neuroendocrine response and non-verbal behavior during psychosocial stress in healthy volunteers by the glutamate release-inhibiting drug lamotrigine. *Neuroendocrinology, 79*(1), 34–42.

Martel, F. L., Hayward, C., Lyons, D. M., Sanborn, K., Varady, S., & Schatzberg, A. F. (1999). Salivary cortisol levels in socially phobic adolescent girls. *Depression and Anxiety, 10*(1), 25–27.

Mason, J. W. (1968a). A review of psychoendocrine research on the pituitary-adrenal cortical system. *Psychosomatic Medicine, 30*(5) (Suppl.), 576–607.

Mason, J. W. (1968b). A review of psychoendocrine research on the sympathetic-adrenal medullary system. *Psychosomatic Medicine, 30*(5) (Suppl.), 631–653.

Mason, J. W. (1975). A historical view of the stress field. *Journal of Human Stress 1*(1), 6–12, 22–36.

Matthews, K. A., Gump, B. B., & Owens, J. F. (2001). Chronic stress influences cardiovascular and neuroendocrine responses during acute stress and recovery, especially in men. *Health Psychology, 20*(6), 403–410.

Maxwell, J. D., Boyle, J. A., Greig, W. R., & Buchanan, W. W. (1969). Plasma corticosteroids in healthy twin pairs. *Journal of Medical Genetics, 6*(3), 294–297.

McEwen, B. S. (1998). Protective and damaging effects of stress mediators. *New England Journal of Medicine, 338*(3), 171–179.

Meikle, A. W., Bishop, D. T., Stringham, J. D., Ford, M. H., & West, D. W. (1989). Relationship between body mass index, cigarette smoking, and plasma sex steroids in normal male twins. *Genetic Epidemiology, 6*(3), 399–412.

Miller, G. E., Rohleder, N., Stetler, C., & Kirschbaum, C. (2005). Clinical depression and regulation of the inflammatory response during acute stress. *Psychosomatic Medicine, 67*(5), 679–687.

Mischler, K., Fischer, J. E., Zgraggen, L., Kudielka, B. M., Preckel, D., & von Känel, R. (2005). The effect of repeated acute mental stress on habituation and recovery responses in hemoconcentration and blood cells in healthy men. *Life Sciences, 77*(10), 1166–1179.

Nicolson, N. A., & van Diest, R., 2000. Salivary cortisol patterns in vital exhaustion. *Journal of Psychosomatic Research, 49*(5), 335–342.

Otte, C., Hart, S., Neylan, T. C., Marmar, C. R., Yaffe, K., & Mohr, D. C. (2005). A meta-analysis of cortisol response to challenge in human aging: Importance of gender. *Psychoneuroendocrinology, 30*(1), 80–91.

Payne, J. D., Nadel, L., Allen, J. J., Thomas, K. G., & Jacobs, W. J. (2002). The effects of experimentally induced stress on false recognition. *Memory, 10*(1), 1–6.

Pike, J. L., Smith, T. L., Hauger, R. L., Nicassio, P. M., Patterson, T. L., McClintick, J., et al. (1997). Chronic life stress alters sympathetic, neuroendocrine, and immune responsivity to an acute psychological stressor in humans. *Psychosomatic Medicine, 59*(4), 447–457.

Pruessner, J. C., Gaab, J., Hellhammer, D. H., Lintz, D., Schommer, N., & Kirschbaum, C. (1997). Increasing correlations between personality traits and cortisol stress responses obtained by data aggregation. *Psychoneuroendocrinology, 22*(8), 615–625.

Pruessner, J. C., Wolf, O. T., Hellhammer, D. H., Buske-Kirschbaum, A., von Auer, K., Jobst, S., et al. (1997). Free cortisol levels after awakening: A reliable biological marker for the assessment of adrenocortical activity. *Life Sciences, 61*(26), 2539–2549.

Roelfsema, F., van den Berg, G., Frolich, M., Veldhuis, J. D., van Eijk, A., Buurman, M. M., et al. (1993). Sex-dependent alteration in cortisol response to endogenous adrenocorticotropin. *Journal of Clinical Endocrinology and Metabolism, 77*(1), 234–240.

Roelofs, K., Elzinga, B. M., & Rotteveel, M. (2005). The effects of stress-induced cortisol responses on approach–avoidance behavior. *Psychoneuroendocrinology, 30*(7), 665–677.

Rohleder, N., Kudielka, B. M., Hellhammer, D. H., Wolf, J. M., & Kirschbaum, C. (2002). Age and sex steroid-related changes in glucocorticoid sensitivity of pro-inflammatory cytokine production after psychosocial stress. *Journal of Neuroimmunology, 126*(1–2), 69–77.

Rohleder, N., Schommer, N. C., Hellhammer, D. H., Engel, R., & Kirschbaum, C. (2001). Sex differences in glucocorticoid sensitivity of proinflammatory cytokine production after psychosocial stress. *Psychosomatic Medicine, 63*(6), 966–972.

Rohleder, N., Wolf, J. M., & Kirschbaum, C. (2003). Glucocorticoid sensitivity in humans: Interindividual differences and acute stress effects. *Stress, 6*(3), 207–222.

Rohleder, N., Wolf, J. M., Piel, M., & Kirschbaum, C. (2003). Impact of oral contraceptive use on glucocorticoid sensitivity of pro-inflammatory cytokine production after psychosocial stress. *Psychoneuroendocrinology, 28*(3), 261–273.

Rose, R. M. (1980). Endocrine responses to stressful psychological events. *Psychiatric Clinics of North America, 3*, 251–276.

Rose, R. M. (1984). Overview of endocrinology of stress. In G. M. Brown, S. H. Koslow, & S. Reichlin (Eds.), *Neuroendocrinology and psychiatric disorder* (pp. 95–122). New York: Raven Press.

Schommer, N. C., Hellhammer, D. H., & Kirschbaum, C. (2003). Dissociation between reactivity of the hypothalamus–pituitary–adrenal axis and the sympathetic–adrenal–medullary system to repeated psychosocial stress. *Psychosomatic Medicine, 65*(3), 450–460.

Selye, H. (1936). A syndrome produced by diverse nocuous agents. *Nature, 32.*

Selye, H. (1983). The stress concept: Past, present, and future. In C. L. Cooper, (Ed.), *Stress research* (pp. 1–20). Chichester, UK: Wiley.

Söderpalm, A., Nikolayev, L., & de Wit, H. (2003). Effects of stress on responses to methamphetamine in humans. *Psychopharmacology, 170*(2), 188–199.

Söderpalm, A. H., & de Wit, H. (2002). Effects of stress and alcohol on subjective state in humans. *Alcohol Clinical and Experimental Research, 26*(6), 818–826.

Takahashi, T., Ikeda, K., Ishikawa, M., Tsukasaki, T., Nakama, D., Tanida, S., et al. (2004). Social stress-induced cortisol elevation acutely impairs social memory in humans. *Neuroscience Letters, 363*(2), 125–130.

Uhart, M., McCaul, M. E., Oswald, L. M., Choi, L., & Wand, G. S. (2004). GABRA6 gene polymorphism and an attenuated stress response. *Molecular Psychiatry, 9*(11), 998–1006.

Vocks, S., Ockenfels, M., Jürgensen, R., Mussgay, L., & Rüddel, H. (2004). Blood pressure reactivity can be reduced by a cognitive behavioral stress management program. *International Journal of Behavioral Medicine, 11*(2), 63–70.

von Känel, R., Kudielka, B. M., Hanebuth, D., Preckel, D., & Fischer, J. E. (2005). Different contribution of interleukin-6 and cortisol activity to total plasma fibrin concentration and to acute mental stress-induced fibrin formation. *Clinical Science (London), 109*(1), 61–67.

von Känel, R., Kudielka, B. M., Preckel, D., Hanebuth, D., & Fischer, J. E. (2006). Delayed response and lack of habituation in plasma interleukin-6 to acute mental stress in men. *Brain, Behavior, and Immununity, 20*(1), 40–48.

von Känel, R., Kudielka, B. M., Preckel, D., Hanebuth, D., Herrmann-Lingen, C., Frey, K., et al. (2005). Opposite effect of negative and positive affect on stress procoagulant reactivity. *Physiology and Behavior, 86*(1–2), 61–68.

von Känel, R., Preckel, D., Zgraggen, L., Mischler, K., Kudielka, B. M., Haeberli,

A., et al. (2004). The effect of natural habituation on coagulation responses to acute mental stress and recovery in men. *Thrombosis and Haemostasis, 92*(6), 1327–1335.

Weidenfeld, J., Bodoff, M., Saphier, D., & Brenner, T. (1989). Further studies on the stimulatory action of nicotine on adrenocortical function in the rat. *Neuroendocrinology, 50*(2), 132–138.

Wiesli, P., Schmid, C., Kerwer, O., Nigg-Koch, C., Klaghofer, R., Seifert, B., et al. (2005). Acute psychological stress affects glucose concentrations in patients with type 1 diabetes following food intake but not in the fasting state. *Diabetes Care, 28*(8), 1910–1915.

Williams, R. A., Hagerty, B. M., & Brooks, G. (2004). Trier Social Stress Test: A method for use in nursing research. *Nursing Research, 53*(4), 277–280.

Wolf, O. T., Kudielka, B. M., Hellhammer, D. H., Hellhammer, J., & Kirschbaum, C. (1998). Opposing effects of DHEA replacement in elderly subjects on declarative memory and attention after exposure to a laboratory stressor. *Psychoneuroendocrinology, 23*(6), 617–629.

Wolf, O. T., Schommer, N. C., Hellhammer, D. H., McEwen, B. S., & Kirschbaum, C. (2001). The relationship between stress-induced cortisol levels and memory differs between men and women. *Psychoneuroendocrinology, 26*(7), 711–720.

World Health Organization. (2001). *Mental health: New understanding, new hope.* Geneva, Switzerland: Author.

Wüst, S., Federenko, I., Hellhammer, D. H., & Kirschbaum, C. (2000). Genetic factors, perceived chronic stress, and the free cortisol response to awakening. *Psychoneuroendocrinology, 25*(7), 707–720.

Wüst, S., Federenko, I. S., van Rossum, E. F., Koper, J. W., & Hellhammer, D. H. (2005). Habituation of cortisol responses to repeated psychosocial stress. Further characterization and impact of genetic factors. *Psychoneuroendocrinology, 30*(2), 199–211.

Wüst, S., Federenko, I. S., van Rossum, E. F., Koper, J. W., Kumsta, R., Entringer, S., et al. (2004). A psychobiological perspective on genetic determinants of hypothalamus–pituitary–adrenal axis activity. *Annals of the New York Academy of Sciences, 1032*, 52–62.

Wüst, S., Van Rossum, E. F., Federenko, I. S., Koper, J. W., Kumsta, R., & Hellhammer, D. H. (2004). Common polymorphisms in the glucocorticoid receptor gene are associated with adrenocortical responses to psychosocial stress. *Journal of Clinial Endocrinology and Metabolism, 89*(2), 565–573.

Young, E. A., Abelson, J. L., & Cameron, O. G. (2004). Effect of comorbid anxiety disorders on the hypothalamic–pituitary–adrenal axis response to a social stressor in major depression. *Biological Psychiatry, 56*(2), 113–120.

Young, E. A., Lopez, J. F., Murphy-Weinberg, V., Watson, S. J., & Akil, H. (2000). Hormonal evidence for altered responsiveness to social stress in major depression. *Neuropsychopharmacology, 23*(4), 411–418.

Zgraggen, L., Fischer, J. E., Mischler, K., Preckel, D., Kudielka, B. M., & von Känel, R. (2005). Relationship between hemoconcentration and blood coagulation responses to acute mental stress. *Thrombosis Research, 115*(3), 175–183.

Zimmermann, U., Spring, K., Kunz-Ebrecht, S. R., Uhr, M., Wittchen, H. U., & Holsboer, F. (2004). Effect of ethanol on hypothalamic–pituitary–adrenal system response to psychosocial stress in sons of alcohol-dependent fathers. *Neuropsychopharmacology, 29*(6), 1156–1165.

5

I Know How You Feel

SOCIAL AND EMOTIONAL INFORMATION PROCESSING IN THE BRAIN

Catherine J. Norris and John T. Cacioppo

Hominids are believed to have walked the earth for the past 7 million years, or approximately 0.1% of the earth's history. *Homo sapiens* (Latin for "wise man") were not the first bipedal creatures, nor apparently were they the first to use tools; and they have evolved only recently (100,000 years ago, or 0.15%), even within the epoch of hominids (Calvin, 2004). Of the brief span humans have roamed the earth, take less than the last 10% of this time—merely the past 3,000–5,000 years—and you find achievements unparalleled by anything before it: the engineering of the Great Pyramids, the elegance of Beethoven's Ninth Symphony, the discernment of heterotic string theory, the efficiency of mass production, the triumph of modern medicine, and the wonder of space exploration. We, apparently uniquely, contemplate the history of the earth, the reach of the universe, the origin of the species, and the genetic blueprint of life. We may take due pride in our collective achievements, cultivated tastes, and dispassionate problem solving when confronted with life-threatening challenges, but *Homo sapiens*, also apparently uniquely among species, carelessly or arrogantly extinguish species en masse, exploit essential environments and resources, wage war on one another, and concoct nuclear and biological weapons that threaten to render humans extinct. The properties of *Homo sapiens* responsible for this state of affairs continue to be debated, but big brains that make mental simulations and strategies possible, hands with fingers and thumbs that permit precise manipulations, and social bonding and language that promote complex and coordinated collective actions are commonly thought to be among those that are important.

Given their evolutionary heritage and daily currency, there is little wonder that both emotional and social processes are biologically rooted and culturally molded. Evidence of both biological and sociocultural contributions to emotions is now so plentiful that few would doubt this assertion, and evidence for biological and emotional contributions to social processes is rapidly accumulating. Altruistic reward and punishment, for instance, are thought to have been crucial for the evolution of a level of cooperation in human societies that is unparalleled (e.g., Boyd, Gintis, Bowles, & Richerson, 2003; Fehr & Gächter, 2002).

The past decade has even seen a virtual explosion of research on the neural networks underlying human emotions and, for the most part quite separately, on the neural substrates underlying social perception, reasoning, and behavior. Surprisingly little attention has been devoted to the relationship *between* these neural systems, however, despite the essential role that emotions play in social development and discourse. Our focus in this chapter is on this latter question. We begin by considering the adaptive significance of emotional and social stimuli, as well as the inherent links between them, as many emotion elicitors are social in nature and emotions are critical for the formation and maintenance of social relationships. Furthermore, we argue that social processes may have co-opted existing neural networks for affective processing to promote interactive and synergistic processing. Finally, we consider the importance of the social context for interpreting the intentions of conspecifics and for the culturally appropriate expression and experience of emotion.

EMOTIONS AS ADAPTIVE
NEUROBEHAVIORAL ORGANIZATIONS

From 1831 to 1836, Charles Darwin sailed on the naval survey ship *HMS Beagle*, invited as company for Robert FitzRoy, the ship's captain whose rank precluded his socializing with anyone but another gentleman. The observations and specimens with which Darwin returned led to the realization that all organisms compete for resources and that those that had some advantage in a habitat would be more likely to transmit this advantage to future generations via their offspring. Following the publication of *Origin of the Species* (Darwin, 1859), Darwin turned his attention to explaining the evolution of behavior. For example, pondering the nature of facial expressions, he wrote: "No doubt as long as man and all other animals are viewed as independent creations, an effectual stop is put to our natural desire to investigate as far as possible the causes of Expression" (Darwin, 1872, p. 12). Thus, Darwin observed that to understand the expression of emotion, humans must be understood as falling on a continuum of species;

observing the behavior of other animals, therefore, could shed light on the expression and function of emotion for humans.

The evolutionary approach to studying emotions has given rise to the notion of emotions as response packages, as predispositions to respond in specific, adaptive ways to environmental stimuli. Emotion theorists disagree about the number of emotions, the structure of emotions, the primacy of emotions, and the relationship between feelings and emotions, but there is general agreement that emotions have adaptive utility. Whether fleeing from a potentially harmful stimulus, such as a snarling bear giving chase, or pursuing something beneficial, such as food or a caring partner, emotions promote adaptive responses and future guidance regarding approach and avoidance behavior. Fear and disgust provide clear illustrations of the value of emotional experience—without these two emotions, an individual (whether human or a nonhuman animal) is unlikely to survive long in most environments. Both fear and disgust are emotional responses to threatening stimuli that often result in avoidance; whereas fear promotes avoidance of predators and potentially harmful encounters, the adaptive utility of disgust includes the avoidance of poisons, rancid foodstuffs, and materials that may promote disease (Curtis, Aunger, & Rabie, 2004).

Many contemporary theorists have approached the study of emotion from a cognitive but equally adaptive perspective, arguing that emotions serve as signals that provide information regarding pursuit of current goals. Positive emotions (e.g., joy, contentment, pride) are experienced when progress is made toward a goal; whereas negative emotions (e.g., fear, sadness, anger) indicate the potential or confirmed loss of a goal or otherwise thwarted efforts toward goal attainment (e.g., Carver & Scheier, 1990; Stein & Trabasso, 1992). Others have emphasized the continuity across the neuraxis of the partially separable substrates for positive and negative affect, including a focus on differences in the stimuli that trigger positivity and negativity, the behavioral responses that each guides, and the heterarchical control of these substrates (for reviews, see Berntson, Boysen, & Cacioppo, 1993; Berridge, 2004). Regardless of the different perspectives of current emotion researchers, agreement on the fundamentally adaptive nature of emotion is ubiquitous.

Views of the evolutionary advantage of emotions often focus on the benefit of an emotional response for an individual; for example, being frightened and consequently avoiding a poisonous snake has immediate benefits for the potential victim but does not necessarily affect anyone else. However, *Homo sapiens* are characteristically social beings, and emotions may therefore have adaptive significance not only for an individual but also for the social group to which an individual belongs. To this end, recent research has tested hypotheses regarding altruistic punishment, the costly punishment of social defectors in the service of the public good. Fehr and Gächter (2002) argue that when some group members fail to cooperate (e.g., by keeping all resources to themselves rather than sharing reciprocally and fairly, a behavior referred to as *defecting*), other members may, at a personal cost, punish such "defectors" to encourage socially responsible behavior in the future. Importantly, altruistic punishment occurs even when punishers can expect no benefit to themselves (i.e., they have no future encounters with defectors and cannot gain a reputation as no communication between group members is possible) and when punishment is costly for them. In a recent study using positron emission tomography (PET) to study the neural basis of altruistic punishment, de Quervain and her colleagues (2004) suggest that the anticipation of a pleasant emotional response following the punishment of a defector may motivate punishers. Consistent with this reasoning, they found activation of the caudate nucleus (a neural structure implicated in reward processing) correlated with degree of punishment levied. In other words, emotions may serve to encourage individual behaviors that promote collective over self-interests.

The question remains as to whether the evolution of behaviors that benefit the group at the expense of personal gains is viable. To address this question, Boyd and colleagues (2003) developed a set of simulation models in which the frequency of cooperation within a group over many time periods (2,000 years) was measured as a function of the presence or absence of altruistic punishment, in addition to other factors such as group size and rate of intergroup conflict. Results indicated that models of group selection in which altruistic punishment was present were more effective in maintaining high frequency of cooperation across all group sizes, suggesting that altruistic punishment is a viable solution to the evolutionary puzzle of social cooperation. In sum, research on altruistic punishment indicates that in the case of *Homo sapiens*, emotions evolved not only to protect the individual from predators and to encourage the pursuit of appetitive stimuli but also to promote reciprocity, cooperation, communication, and collective action, which allowed for the creation of organizations, institutions, and cultures in their wake.

HUMANS ARE *SOCIAL* ANIMALS

Although emotions have adaptive utility for humans as well as for animals (as Darwin originally suggested), it is important to note that human beings are fundamentally social creatures. And as emotions may have evolved to promote cooperation and communication in a social group, conspecifics are a major source of adaptive emotions in these groups, societies, and institutions. Social information is highly valued and critical for survival throughout the lifespan, as it contributes to successful attachment, reproduction, vigilance toward threatening encounters, and protection of territory and significant others. From birth, we engage in behaviors intended to ensure affiliation with other members of the species, especially caregivers (Bowlby, 1969/1982). Quality of social interactions in infancy, including maternal responsiveness and attachment style, is associated with physical growth (e.g., insufficient interactions result in failure to thrive; Ward, Lee, & Lipper, 2000); successful emotion regulation (Cassidy, 1994; Thompson, 1994); language and social cognition skills in preschool (Beckwith & Rodning, 1996); and intellectual competence in adolescence (Cohen, 1995). Healthy social relationships continue to be important for emotional and physical well-being throughout the lifespan, as evidenced by research demonstrating that social isolation is a major risk factor for morbidity and mortality (House, Landis, & Umberson, 1988) and that loneliness, an emotional response to broken or inadequate social connections, is related to cardiovascular function and sleep quality (Cacioppo et al., 2002). In fact, loneliness may be an adaptive emotional response that evolved to encourage the maintenance of pair bonds, maternal care, and the return of hunter-gatherers to dependent others even in times of dire need (Cacioppo & Hawkley, 2005).

In addition to long-standing social relationships, daily interactions with conspecifics are also critical for survival, as they provide information about the environment and are the primary elicitors of emotions designed to promote both affiliative and protective behaviors (cf. Keltner & Kring, 1998). A set of recent studies highlights the relationship between quality of everyday interactions, emotional experience, and loneliness. Hawkley, Burleson, Berntson, and Cacioppo (2003) demonstrated that lonely individuals report feeling more negative and less positive about their interaction partners than do socially connected individuals, in addition to reporting higher negative affect and lower positive affect over the course of a week. Furthermore, multilevel modeling of data collected using experiential sampling methodology (ESM; Larson & Csikszentmihalyi, 1983) provided evidence that loneliness has a pervasive influence on everyday affective experience and quality of social interactions and, importantly, that these two outcome factors have reciprocal effects on each other (Hawkley, Preacher, & Cacioppo, in press). In other words, both the chronic perception of one's social belongingness (i.e., loneliness–social connectedness) and fluctuations in the quality of social interactions appear to have effects on one's daily emotional life. In addition, loneliness relates to cardiovascular functioning and stress appraisals, such that lonely individuals exhibit greater total peripheral resistance (TPR) and lower cardiac output (CO) than their socially embedded counterparts (Cacioppo et al., 2002; Hawkley et al., 2003). Thus daily social interactions have consequences not only for emotional experience but also for cardiovascular functioning and health.

Social relationships are so fundamental for humans that nonsocial stimuli or events are often anthropomorphized, or infused with social meaning. In an historical example, Heider and Simmel (1944) developed a short film depicting geometrical figures (e.g., triangles) in motion and reported that most individuals spontaneously describe the film in terms of social interactions between three human-like characters through attribution of intentions, emotions, gender, relationships, and personality to the three shapes. Heberlein and Adolphs (2004) have recently argued that these spontaneous social attributions rely on the functioning of an intact amygdala, based on evidence that S.M., a patient with bilateral damage to the amygdala, failed to spontaneously provide a social interpretation of the film. Interestingly, S.M. performed normally on direct questions regarding the film that relied on social attributions (e.g., "What was the large triangle like?"), suggesting that her impairment lies in automatically inferring social meaning from a nonsocial stimulus and that the amygdala may play an important role in these social inferences. The tendency to spontaneously make social attributions about stimuli or events may be an adaptive mechanism for a highly social species.

SOCIAL STIMULI POSSESS
INHERENT ADAPTIVE SIGNIFICANCE

Research on emotion often focuses on responses to nonsocial stimuli, such as dangerous creatures (e.g., snakes, spiders, bears) and primary rewards (e.g., food) and, in addition, tends to treat social and nonsocial stimuli as comparable; however, most emotion elicitors in life are social. Facial expressions provide both social and emotional information, conspecifics often generate and reciprocate our own emotional reactions, and social fears (e.g., speaking in public) and triumphs (e.g., a home team victory) dominate our emotional lives. In their social-functional account of emotion, Keltner and Kring (1998) argue that emotions serve a set of functions that are critical for coordinating social interactions. A conspecific can serve either as an emotional stimulus (e.g., encountering an unknown person on a dark street late at night) or as a cue to an emotionally relevant stimulus present in the environment (e.g., a fearful individual may indicate the presence of a dangerous stimulus, such as a snake). In addition, our perception of others' emotions can elicit emotional states that are either reflective (e.g., empathy) or complementary (e.g., fear of an unknown individual expressing anger), thus providing information regarding the relationship and promoting adaptive behaviors in the context of social interactions.

Because of the inherent connections between and the relative importance of social and emotional information, we have argued that social and emotional processes may interact, as well as share some basic neural mechanisms (Norris, Chen, Zhu, Small, & Cacioppo, 2004). Specifically, we proposed that social and emotional information is interactively processed in order to produce adaptive behavior and serve regulatory functions for an individual embedded in a social environment. We suggest that because social stimuli are strong elicitors of emotion, they have the same adaptive utility as emotional stimuli and may possess inherent, latent emotional significance.

The adaptive advantage of discerning social signals and organizing flexible behavioral responses may have been achieved in part by co-opting and building on selected neural systems that evolved originally for dealing with hedonic events (threats, appetitive stimuli). This would mean that social stimuli can be processed quickly by neural regions implicated in motivational processes (e.g., medial orbitofrontal cortex) and in generating (e.g., amygdala, insula, motor cortex) and regulating (e.g., ventrolateral and medial prefrontal cortex) an emotional response.

A recent study using functional magnetic resonance imaging (fMRI) provides an appropriate illustration of this co-option hypothesis. Eisenberger, Lieberman, and Williams (2003) reported neural activation in a dorsal portion of the anterior cingulate cortex (ACC) implicated in the affective component of the pain response when participants were excluded from a social situation (i.e., a ball-tossing game). The authors argue that the similarity in activation of the dorsal ACC to physical pain (e.g., Rainville, Duncan, Price, Carrier, & Bushnell, 1997) and to social pain suggests that the experiences of physical and social pain may share a common neuroanatomical basis. Furthermore, Eisenberger and her colleagues suggest that "Because of the adaptive value of mammalian social bonds, the social attachment system . . . may have piggybacked onto the physical pain system to promote survival" (p. 291). The co-option of neural systems for purposes other than their primary function is potentially a flexible, conservative answer to challenges presented over the course of evolution.

Additional evidence for the hypothesis that the neural mechanisms contributing to the detection of social cues may have co-opted and built on existing emotion networks is provided by data implicating certain brain regions in processing both social and emotional stimuli. The amygdala, a limbic structure occasionally referred to oversimplistically as the emotional brain, is clearly involved in social behavior, as well as emotional experience. Kluver and Bucy (1939/1997) first reported disturbances in the social behavior of primates with extensive amygdala damage; research by Heberlein and Adolphs (2004) using the Heider and Simmel (1944) paradigm discussed earlier provides convergent evidence for the role of the amygdala in making social inferences in humans. Much of the research on amygdalar function has focused on judgments and responses to facial displays of emotion, either using fMRI to investigate patterns of neural activity in nondamaged individuals or examining the behavior of people with amygdala damage. These studies suggest that the amygdala is involved in processing emotional expression, particularly fear (cf. Adolphs, Tranel, Damasio, & Damasio, 1994; Breiter et al., 1996); in making judgments regarding the trustworthiness of unknown individuals (Adolphs, Tranel, & Damasio, 1998; Winston, Strange, O'Doherty, & Dolan, 2002); and in the attribution of internal states, beliefs, and desires to other people (Baron-Cohen et al., 2000). However, it is important to note that each of these studies confounds social and emotional processes; for example, as determining the emotion expressed by a conspecific requires distilling emotional information from a social context, an impairment in one necessarily affects the other.

One recent study has attempted to compare amygdalar activation in response to faces and scenes in order to examine whether the amygdala is implicated in processing only emotional stimuli that contain social cues (e.g., faces) or whether amygdalar activation generalizes to other kinds of emotional stimuli as well. Hariri, Tessitore, Mattay, Fera, and Weinberger (2002) used fMRI to measure amygdalar activation while participants viewed fearful and threatening faces and 'scenes' taken from the International Affective Picture System (IAPS; Lang, Bradley, & Cuthbert, 1999). Importantly, none of the IAPS pictures contained human faces, but rather included natural threats (i.e., dogs, snakes, spiders, sharks) and other threats (i.e., guns, car accidents, plane crashes, explosions). The authors report that the amygdala showed significant activation to both types of stimuli; however, activation of the right amygdala was significantly greater when participants viewed fearful and threatening faces than scenes. These results suggest that the amygdala is involved in processing both emotional and social stimuli, consistent with the hypothesis that social cognition may have co-opted existing neural networks underlying hedonic processes.

The study conducted by Hariri et al. (2002) contained a number of design features that limit its interpretation. For instance, the authors suggest that differences in complexity, arousal, or similarity of the stimuli across conditions could potentially account for observed differences in activation for faces and scenes (Hariri et al., 2002); none of these explanations can be ruled out. Furthermore, the study by Hariri et al. (2002) does not directly address the question of whether the amygdala is involved in processing emotional stimuli or whether activation would be observed in response to neutral stimuli, as well.

We recently conducted an fMRI study to investigate the interactive and independent effects of social and emotional processes in the brain in which we controlled for the confounding factors in the Hariri et al. study (2002) and included neutral stimuli to allow a test of effects due to emotionality (Norris et al., 2004). Participants viewed a set of IAPS pictures that varied in two dimensions, such that each picture was either neutral or emotional (pleasant or unpleasant stimuli) and was either social (i.e., contained one or more faces or bodies of conspecifics) or nonsocial (i.e., scenes, objects). Animals were excluded from the design; all four groups of stimuli were matched on complexity; and social and nonsocial stimuli were equally arousing. Results for the amygdala, one of our regions of interest, indicated two main effects, such that amygdalar activation was greater for emotional than for neutral stimuli and greater for social than for nonsocial stimuli (Norris et al., 2004; see Figure 5.1). Thus the amygdala, a central component of many neuroanatomically based theories of emotion, is also clearly implicated in social cognition. These findings suggest that the

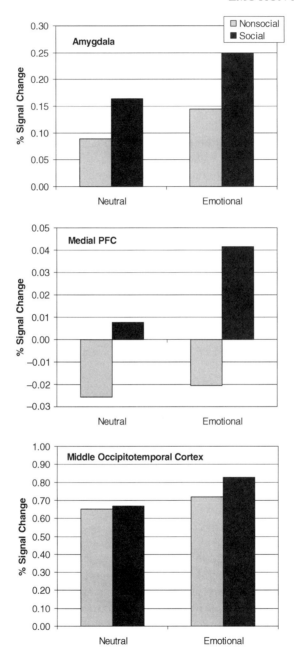

FIGURE 5.1. Patterns of neutral activation in the amygdala (top), medial prefrontal cortex (middle), and middle occipitotemporal cortex (bottom) during viewing of pictures that vary in social and emotional content. Bars represent the mean percent signal change for the peak of the hemodynamic response in a priori regions of interest. Based on Chen, Zhu, Small, and Cacioppo (2004).

amygdala may be involved in more general motivational processes, with both emotional (negative and positive) and social stimuli possessing strong motivational significance. However, social stimuli have arguably acquired motivational significance through the process of the evolution of *Homo sapiens* and their inherently social nature; whereas emotional stimuli (e.g., babies, snakes, diseased things) may be more primary motivators. Patterns of amygdalar activation to emotional and social stimuli therefore suggest that social cognition may have co-opted existing neural networks for processing stimuli with hedonic value.

The hypothesis that social information processing co-opted neural organizations that are involved in emotional information processing is also in line with our finding that the amygdala was not alone in being affected by social stimuli. Norris et al. (2004) found the medial prefrontal cortex (mPFC) and the middle occipitotemporal cortex (i.e., visual association cortex), neural regions often reported as being activated by emotional pictures, were also more active when participants viewed pictures that depicted conspecifics than those that did not (see Figure 5.1). Phan, Wager, Taylor, and Liberzon's (2002) meta-analysis indicated that the mPFC is commonly activated in studies of emotion. Specifically, they found mPFC to be active during experiences of happiness, fear, anger, sadness, and disgust, regardless of whether elicitation occurred visually, auditorially, or through guided recall. Although the specific role of mPFC in emotional processes has yet to be specified, it is noteworthy that the mPFC appears also to be more active to social than nonsocial stimuli matched for extremity, arousal, visual complexity, and luminance (Norris et al., 2004). Moreover, a good deal of research supports the claim that portions of the occipital cortex are more active to emotionally arousing pictorial stimuli than to neutral, unarousing stimuli (cf. Phan et al., 2002; Lane, Chua, & Dolan, 1999; Lang et al. 1998). We replicated this effect and further found that the middle occipitotemporal cortex was also more active to social than to nonsocial stimuli (Norris et al., 2004), suggesting that both emotional and social information garner attentional resources.

Interestingly, complementary findings suggest that neural regions implicated in social cognition (e.g., gaze pursuit, perception of biological motion, face perception and recognition) are also sensitive to emotional content. One of the first studies to demonstrate this pattern was a PET study conducted by Geday, Gjedde, Boldsen, and Kupers (2003) in which participants viewed a set of pictures that varied both in social complexity, from low (e.g., faces) to high (e.g., social situations), and in emotional valence (positive, negative, neutral). Results demonstrated that regional cerebral blood flow (rCBF) in the fusiform gyrus, a neural region previously implicated in face perception (cf. Kanwisher, McDermott, & Chun, 1997), was not only greater when participants viewed more complex versus less complex social stimuli but was also greater when participants viewed emotional (i.e., positive and negative) as compared with neutral stimuli (see also Dolan et al., 1996; Vuilleumier, Armony, Driver, & Dolan, 2001). In other words, neural structures involved in processing social signals, such as eye gaze, faces, and biological motion, may have evolved to also be sensitive to emotional content based on the fact that social stimuli have inherent emotional value for human beings and other social species.

We recently replicated the finding that the fusiform gyrus is more active to emotional than to neutral stimuli; furthermore, this pattern was driven by activation to social stimuli, consistent with the proposed role of the fusiform in social cognition (Norris et al., 2004). In addition, our results indicated that two other neural regions implicated in processing social information were also sensitive to emotional content: the superior temporal sulcus (STS) and the inferior frontal gyrus (IFG). Although the STS is most often considered to be involved in the perception of biological motion (cf. Puce & Perrett, 2003; Grossman & Blake, 2001), a growing literature supports the conclusion that the STS is also sensitive to emotional content. Narumoto, Okada, Sadato, Fukui, & Yonekura (2001) showed that selective attention to emotional expression versus to the face itself enhanced activation of the right STS. In a study examining the neural correlates of basic and moral emotions, Moll et al. (2002) reported that the STS was recruited by viewing scenes evocative of moral emotions. Kilts, Egan, Gideon, Ely, and Hoffman (2003) demonstrated that whereas dynamic emotional displays of anger expressions elicit greater activation of the STS than do static emotional displays of anger, this finding does not generalize to expressions of happiness. Thus the STS is not just activated by dynamic (i.e., moving) stimuli but is also selectively responsive to different emotional content, and particularly to emotional stimuli that may have stronger motivational significance for the observer (anger vs. happiness).

The IFG has also been implicated in social cognition, particularly face processing, as evidenced by studies examining visual imagery of famous faces (Ishai, Haxby, & Ungerleider, 2002), integration of visual faces and names (Campanella et al., 2001), viewing of unfamiliar faces (McDermott, Buckner, Petersen, Kelley, & Sanders, 1999), and performing a face-matching task (Haxby, et al., 1994). In addition, regions of the IFG in the left hemisphere are critically important for speech perception and potentially for the integration of heard speech and speech read from a moving face (Calvert & Campbell, 2003). Rizzolatti and his colleagues (cf. Rizzolatti, Fadiga, Gallese, & Fogassi, 1996) have argued that the human IFG may correspond to area F5 of the monkey premotor cortex, which contains *mirror neurons* that discharge both when an action is performed and when it is observed (cf. Rizzolatti, Fogassi, & Gallese, 2001; Gallese, Fadiga, Fogassi, & Rizzolatti, 1996; Koski et al., 2002). These findings, taken together, have led some researchers to suggest that the IFG is involved in empathy, an emotion that derives its meaning from the social context and that may function through imitative mechanisms (cf. Carr, Iacoboni, Dubeau, Mazziotta & Lenzi, 2003; Meltzoff & Decety, 2003).

In sum, converging evidence supports the notion that neural structures involved in social information processing, such as perception of faces and biological motion, are also involved in emotional processing. The fusiform gyrus, the STS, and the IFG have all been shown to be recruited both when individuals process social stimuli and when stimuli have emotional significance.

Finally, it is also possible that social and emotional information may be interactively processed in the brain such that emotional stimuli that depict or implicate conspecifics may elicit much stronger activation than either social or emotional stimuli alone. In our recent fMRI study (Norris et al., 2004), three neural regions showed evidence of the interactive processing of social and emotional information: the thalamus, the middle occipito-temporal cortex, and the STS all exhibited the same pattern, such that pictures that were emotional in nature and that contained social cues elicited greater activation than those that were either emotional, social, or neither. Importantly, these three neural regions are relatively early in the processing stream, suggesting that emotional stimuli depicting conspecifics may garner greater attentional resources. Thus emotional and social information appear to interact at very early stages of processing, consistent with the evolutionary significance of social and emotional stimuli.

ET TU, BRUTE: THEORY OF MIND

As exemplified by perhaps the most famous betrayal in history—that of Caesar by Brutus, his fellow statesman and confidante—it can be dangerous not to read correctly the motives and intentions of others. Conspecifics can be not only cooperators but also defectors; in fact, a recent article suggests that, when altruistic behavior benefits not only the group but also the contributor, selection may lead to an asymmetric stable state, in which some individuals make high levels of cooperative investment and others invest little or nothing (Doebeli, Hauert, & Killingback, 2004). Thus the achievement of a steady state in a cooperative environment may require the presence of both types of individuals. However, this is not to say that interpersonal interactions necessarily benefit from such a mixed society of givers and takers. Accurate evaluation of the motives of others and decryption of their current emotional states are skills necessary for navigating our social world.

Although every social species may possess specialized systems for the perception of social cues (e.g., biological motion, eye gaze), humans appear unique in their ability to empathize with and infer the intentions of conspecifics. Recent evidence supports the existence of neural mechanisms for these high-level social computations. Much of our emotional life relies not on reacting to simple stimuli but on sophisticated calculations that take into consideration motives, context, past experience, and relationship history. This is particularly true for emotion elicitors that are social, such as an unknown person encountered in an alley or a late-night call from a close friend.

One example of the effects of social context on emotion is that of empathy, in which the emotional meaning of an event is completely dependent on the social context and in which the experienced emotion mirrors that of a conspecific. By definition, empathy cannot occur in the absence of a social context. Recent research on the neural mechanisms underlying empathy suggests that empathic responses are accompanied by, if not generated through, imitation of facial expressions. In one such study, Carr and her colleagues (Carr, Iacoboni, Dubeau, Mazziotta, & Lenzi, 2003) argue that imitation produces an action representation in premotor areas (including the IFG) that modulates the activity of emotional networks containing the insula and amygdala, thereby eliciting an empathic response.

A recent study suggests that empathy does not rely merely on mirror neurons and activation of motor networks or imitation of emotional expression but may have also co-opted other neural structures involved in emotional processing. Singer and her colleagues (2004) conducted an fMRI study to investigate the neural networks underlying both the firsthand experience of pain and the observation of the pain of a loved one. Participants either received a painful stimulus or viewed a cue when their partners (located in the same room) received the painful stimulus. Activation of the ACC, a neural structure known to be involved in the affective experience of pain, when the partner received the painful stimulus correlated with empathy as measured by self-report. Thus the experience of empathic pain for a loved one may have co-opted the existing pain network, similar to the experience of social rejection (Eisenberger et al., 2003).

Empathy, however, is not always the adaptive response to a conspecific's emotion display; motives, intentions, and context must be taken into consideration to generate an appropriate response. Literary accounts of Brutus's betrayal of Caesar (such as Shakespeare's play *Julius Caesar*) suggest that the murderous Romans knelt before Caesar and asked his pardon moments before stabbing him. Though Darwin (1872; see Ekman, 2003) spoke little of the ability to control expression for the purpose of deception, it is clear that we cannot always take emotion displays at face value. For example, if one were to arrive late to a movie only to view a grown man weeping onscreen, one might be inclined to feel empathic toward him. If 5 minutes later, one were to discover that the character was mourning his failed attempt to murder the hero of the film, one's response would change dramatically. Thankfully, we are not dependent on blind faith attributions of the motivations that drive fellow human beings; rather, we are able to reason and make inferences about others' mental states. Such inferences constitute additional contextual (and social) influences on emotional experience. The neuroscientific study of "theory of mind" (ToM) has consistently revealed a set of neural regions involved in understanding the intentions of others, including the STS and temporoparietal junction (TPJ; Saxe & Kanwisher, 2003), as well as the mPFC and anterior paracingulate (Gallagher, Jack, Roepstorff, & Frith, 2002). Accurate assessment of conspecifics' intentions, beliefs, and motivations is critical for adaptive emotional responses in a social environment. Thus we might predict that neural regions implicated in ToM will show some evidence of an interaction between social and emotional processes. Indeed, the STS and mPFC are sensitive to both the emotional and social content of pictures; both regions also appear to interactively process social and emotional information, such that emotional stimuli depicting conspecifics recruit greater neural resources (Norris et al., 2004).

Further evidence for the influence of social context on emotional processes comes from research on autism, a neurodevelopmental syndrome thought to result in the selective impairment of theory of mind abilities. Autistic individuals show deficits in social functioning, as well as in emotion perception (Abdi & Sharma, 2004), empathy (Baron-Cohen, 2004), perception of biological motion (Blake, Turner, Smoski, Pozdol, & Stone, 2003), face processing (Dawson et al., 2002; Grelotti, Gauthier, & Schultz, 2002), gaze pursuit (Emery, 2000), and spontaneous mimicry of emotional expressions (McIntosh, Riechmann-Decker, Winkielman, & Wilbarger, in press). In addition, studies using a wide range of methods, including functional neuroimaging, postmortem measurements, and behavioral studies, have begun to examine the neuroanatomical correlates of autism. Many researchers have focused on the amygdala as a potential neural mediator of autism (Baron-Cohen, 2004; Baron-Cohen et al., 2000; Howard et al., 2000). Di Martino and Castellanos (2003) reviewed the neuroimaging literature and suggest that autism is associated with decreased neural activation in ventromedial PFC, the TPJ, and extended amygdala and with increased activation in primary sensory cortices. All of this research is consistent with a deficit in ToM that potentially has downstream consequences for emotional processes that are dependent on the social context (e.g., facial expressions, empathy). Furthermore, autistic children do not differ from normally developing children in patterns of emotional modulation of the startle response, a task that relies heavily on basic emotional responses and does not require modulation by the social context (Salmond, de Haan, Friston, Gadian, & Vargha-Khadem, 2003); and it has been argued that basic responses to emotional expressions remain intact in autism, whereas the true deficit lies in an impaired ability to represent the individual displaying the emotion (Blair, 2003). In sum, although autism is characterized by impairments in spontaneous "socio-emotional" processing, such as a lack of spontaneous activation of premotor cortex to action observation (McIntosh et al., in press), additional impairments are evident in the modulation of emotional responses as a function of interpretations of and judgments about the social context, that is, of the ability of the social context to influence emotional processes.

SOCIAL MODULATION OF EMOTIONAL PROCESSES

The immediate social context can not only provide many clues as to a conspecific's goals and intentions as intimated by theory of mind research but can also affect the emotional meaning of an event, and therefore it needs to be considered when determining an adaptive response in any environment. In other words, the emotional meaning of an event can be influenced by social context and culture. Take, for example, a standard practice on reality television programs such as *Survivor* and *The Apprentice* that involves mixing teams over the course of the competition. A victory by a single contestant can be experienced either as a triumph (if he or she is a teammate) or a defeat (if he or she is an opponent); in addition, one contestant's emotional response to another's victory can change over the course of the season as contestants are shuffled among teams. In sum, the social context of an event can modulate our emotional experience to produce even polar-opposite reactions to the same event (see Englis, Vaughan, & Lanzetta, 1982).

The social context can also modulate how one responds to the event. Appropriate emotional displays and responses in different social contexts are prescribed by display rules (e.g., cultural prescriptions for displays of emotion), which are acquired through social learning. Failure to regulate emotional expressions in the socially prescribed fashion can have significant and immediate effects. In the first presidential debate of the 2004 campaign between President George W. Bush and Senator John Kerry, President Bush was observed showing a range of unpleasant facial expressions when Senator Kerry was speaking. President Bush's immediate decline in the voter polls has been partially attributed to his inappropriate emotion displays.

In contrast to the "emotion expression view" of facial displays, which suggests that expressions of emotion are simply "readouts" of a person's internal emotional state (e.g., Buck, 1994), Fridlund (1991, 1994) has proposed that facial expressions are social signals and, as such, can be modified by the social context (the "behavioral ecology view" of emotional expression). Although the two views are clearly not mutually exclusive (cf. Cacioppo, Bush, & Tassinary, 1992) because facial expression may serve both purposes, Fridlund's research illustrates the point that emotional expression can be influenced by the social context. In one such study, degree of smiling to a pleasant film varied as a function of the social context, such that participants smiled more when a friend was present in the same room than when they were alone and had not arrived with a friend; importantly, self-reported feelings did not differ across contexts (i.e., the social environment did not simply increase enjoyment of the film; Fridlund, 1991). This finding clearly suggests that the presence or absence of a close friend can influence facial displays of happiness. However, a similar study investigating responses to sad films found that participants expressed less sadness when in the presence of a friend or a stranger (Jakobs, Manstead, & Fischer, 2001). Although this finding may seem contrary to the hypothesis that facial expressions are social signals that promote behaviors in others, it suggests that some emotions are regulated in certain social contexts; it is not often appropriate or comfortable to show signs of extreme sadness (e.g., crying) to either close friends or strangers. Thus context can also promote socially learned attempts at regulation of emotion expression.

The idea that emotional expression can be modulated by the social context, and specifically by socially learned display rules and appropriate regulation of responses, poses the question of how individuals acquire these norms. Mesquita and Frijda (1992) provide an excellent review of the cross-cultural literature on emotion, from emotion antecedents and interpretation of events (e.g., death as a loss vs. a gain) to physiological responses and facial expressions to appropriate, culturally dependent emotional experience (e.g., guilt vs. shame; acceptance of anger). New research on the development of emotion regulation suggests that infant imitation of facial acts (Meltzoff & Decety, 2003) and early caregiver relationships (Cole, Martin, & Dennis, 2004) are critical for appropriate development of empathy and emotion regulation. Furthermore, Anderson, Bechara, Damasio, Tranel, and Damasio (1999) have shown that the ventromedial prefrontal cortex (PFC) may be required for the learning of social norms and rules regarding emotion regulation and display. The authors performed detailed case studies on two individuals who had acquired large lesions of the ventral PFC during the first few months of life and compared their behavior with that of patients who acquired comparable lesions much later in life. Major differences in behavior observed between patients with early and late acquisition of ventral PFC lesions appear to stem from a difference in learned social norms regarding behavior and emotional expression, such that those who acquire lesions early in life fail to learn socially appropriate responses.

Finally, there exist a small subset of emotions that depend heavily on both the immediate social context and on acquired cultural norms; such "social emotions" include guilt, shame, pride, embarrassment, and others (Barrett & Nelson-Goens, 1997). The social emotions serve to protect and uphold cultural norms of behavior, as they promote socially acceptable behaviors while discouraging behaviors that would be harmful for the society. Pride and admiration may function as rewards for individuals who attain culturally mandated standards of excellence; guilt and shame as punishments for inappropriate, potentially detrimental behaviors. Thus culture plays an important role in determining the conditions under which social emotions are experienced, in addition to which social emotions are prominent (e.g., guilt in the United States; shame in Japan). Clearly, social emotions serve as an illustration of the interaction of social and emotional processes. Recently, Adolphs, Baron-Cohen, and Tranel (2002) conducted a study investigating the role of the amygdala, a structure implicated in both social and emotional processes, in the recognition of social emotions. Individuals with amygdala damage were impaired in recognizing social emotions, more so than in recognizing basic emotions (e.g., happiness, anger). The authors suggest that the amygdala may be involved in processing complex social stimuli. Furthermore, they suggest that, as people with autististm also are impaired in the recognition of social emotions, the deficits observed in social cognitive abilities in autism may be due to dysfunction of the amygdala.

SUMMARY

Interest in the overlap and influences between social and emotional information processes as illuminated by a neuroscience perspective, although relatively recent, is leading to new findings and insights on a weekly basis. Both emotional and social stimuli have adaptive utility for humans. To promote flexible, accurate, and efficient responding, we have suggested that social information processing may have co-opted existing structures specialized for affective processing and that neural regions that have evolved to serve social information processing may also be involved in a variety of emotional processes (Norris et al., 2004; Eisenberger et al., 2003). Emotion is critical for our social relationships (e.g., Keltner & Kring, 1998), and relationships are important for our and the collective emotional well-being (Cacioppo & Hawkley, 2005). We, therefore, reviewed evidence that social and emotional stimuli can have additive and synergistic effects on neural substrates in cortical and limbic regions, as well as evidence that social stimuli can also modulate the experience and expression of emotions.

ACKNOWLEDGMENT

This work was supported by National Institute of Mental Health Grant No. P50 MH52384-01A1.

REFERENCES

Abdi, Z., & Sharma, T. (2004). Social cognition and its neural correlates in schizophrenia and autism. *CNS Spectrums, 9,* 335–343.

Adolphs, R., Baron-Cohen, S., & Tranel, D. (2002). Impaired recognition of social emotions following amygdala damage. *Journal of Cognitive Neuroscience, 14,* 1264–1274.

Adolphs, R., Tranel, D., & Damasio, A. R. (1998). The human amygdala in social judgment. *Nature, 393,* 470–474.

Adolphs, R., Tranel, D., Damasio, H., & Damasio, A. (1994). Impaired recognition of emotion in facial expressions following bilateral damage to the human amygdala. *Nature, 372,* 669–672.

Anderson, S. W., Bechara, A., Damasio, H., Tranel, D., & Damasio, A. R. (1999). Impairment of social and moral behavior related to early damage in human prefrontal cortex. *Nature Neuroscience, 2,* 1032–1037.

Baron-Cohen, S. (2004). Autism: Research into causes and intervention. *Pediatric Rehabilitation, 7,* 73–78.

Baron-Cohen, S., Ring, H. A., Bullmore, E. T., Wheelwright, S., Ashwin, C., & Williams, S. C. (2000). The amygdala theory of autism. *Neuroscience and Biobehavioral Reviews, 24,* 355–364.

Barrett, K. C., & Nelson-Goens, G. C. (1997). Emotion communication and the development of the social emotions. In K. C. Barrett (Ed.), *Communication of emotion: Current research from diverse perspectives* (pp. 69–88). San Francisco: Jossey-Bass.

Beckwith, L., & Rodning, C. (1996). Dyadic processes between mothers and preterm infants: Development at ages 2 to 5 years. *Infant Mental Health Journal, 17,* 322–333.

Berntson, G. G., Boysen, S. T., & Cacioppo, J. T. (1993). Neurobehavioral organization and the cardinal principle of evaluative bivalence. *Annals of the New York Academy of Sciences, 702,* 75–102.

Berntson, G. G., & Cacioppo, J. T. (2000). Psychobiology and social psychology: Past, present, and future. *Personality and Social Psychology Review, 4,* 3–15.

Berntson, G. G., & Cacioppo, J. T. (in press). The neuroevolution of motivation. In J. Y. Shah & W. Gardner (Eds.), *Handbook of motivation science: The social psychological perspective.* New York: Guilford Press.

Berridge, K. C. (2004). Motivation concepts in behavioral neuroscience. *Physiology & Behavior, 81,* 179–209.

Blair, R. J. (2003). Facial expressions, their communicatory functions and neurocognitive substrates. *Philosophical Transactions of the Royal Society of London: Series B. Biological Sciences, 358,* 561–572.

Blake, R., Turner, L. M., Smoski, M. J., Pozdol, S. L., & Stone, W. L. (2003). Visual recognition of biological motion is impaired in children with autism. *Psychological Science, 14,* 151–157.

Bowlby, J. (1982). *Attachment and loss: Vol. 1. Attachment.* New York: Basic Books. (Original work published 1969)

Boyd, R., Gintis, H., Bowles, S., & Richerson, P. J. (2003). The evolution of altruistic punishment. *Proceedings of the National Academy of Sciences of the USA, 100,* 3531–3535.

Breiter, H. C., Etcoff, N. L., Whalen, P. J., Kennedy, W. A., Rauch, S. L., Buckner, R. L., et al. (1996). Response and habituation of the human amygdala during visual processing of facial expression. *Neuron, 17,* 875–887.

Buck, R. (1994). Social and emotional functions in facial expression and communication: The readout hypothesis. *Biological Psychology, 38,* 95–115.

Cacioppo, J. T., Bush, L. K., & Tassinary, L. G. (1992). Microexpressive facial actions as a function of affective stimuli: Replication and extension. *Personality and Social Psychology Bulletin, 18,* 515–526.

Cacioppo, J. T., & Hawkley, L. C. (2005). People thinking about people: The vicious cycle of being a social outcast in one's own mind. In K. D. Williams, J. P. Forgas, & W. von Hippel (Eds.), *The social outcast: Ostracism, social exclusion, rejection, and bullying* (pp. 91–108). New York: Psychology Press.

Cacioppo, J. T., Hawkley, L. C., Crawford, L. E., Ernst, J. M., Burleson, M. H.,

Kowalewski, R. B., et al. (2002). Loneliness and health: Potential mechanisms. *Psychosomatic Medicine, 64,* 407–417.

Calvert, G. A., & Campbell, R. (2003). Reading speech from still and moving faces: The neural substrates of visible speech. *Journal of Cognitive Neuroscience, 15,* 57–70.

Calvin, W. H. (2004). *A brief history of the mind: From apes to intellect and beyond.* Oxford, UK: Oxford University Press.

Campanella, S., Joassin, F., Rossion, B., De Volder, A., Bruyer, R., & Crommelinck, M. (2001). Association of the distinct visual representations of faces and names: A PET activation study. *NeuroImage, 14,* 873–882.

Carr, L., Iacoboni, M., Dubeau, M. C., Mazziotta, J. C., & Lenzi, G. L. (2003). Neural mechanisms of empathy in humans: A relay from neural systems for imitation to limbic areas. *Proceedings of the National Academy of Sciences of the USA, 100,* 5497–5502.

Carver, C. S., & Scheier, M. F. (1990). Origins and functions of positive and negative affect: A control-process view. *Psychological Review, 97,* 19–35.

Cassidy, J. (1994). Emotion regulation: Influences of attachment relationships. *Monographs of the Society for Research in Child Development, 59,* 228–283.

Cohen, S. E. (1995). Biosocial factors in early infancy as predictors of competence in adolescents who were born prematurely. *Journal of Developmental and Behavioral Pediatrics, 16,* 36–41.

Cole, P. M., Martin, S. E., & Dennis, T. A. (2004). Emotion regulation as a scientific construct: Methodological challenges and directions for child development research. *Child Development, 75,* 317–333.

Curtis, V., Aunger, R., & Rabie, T. (2004). Evidence that disgust evolved to protect from risk of disease. *Proceedings of the Royal Society of London: Series B. Biological Sciences, 271,* S131–S133.

Darwin, C. (1859). *The origin of the species by means of natural selection: Or, the preservation of favored races in the struggle for life.* London: Murray.

Darwin, C. (1872). *The expression of the emotions in man and animals.* London: Murray.

Dawson, G., Webb, S., Schellenberg, G. D., Dager, S., Friedman, S., Aylward, E., et al. (2002). Defining the broader phenotype of autism: Genetic, brain, and behavioral perspectives. *Development and Psychopathology, 14,* 581–611.

de Quervain, D. J.-F., Fischbacher, U., Treyer, V., Schellhammer, M., Schnyder, U., Buck, A., et al. (2004). The neural basis of altruistic punishment. *Science, 305,* 1254–1258.

Di Martino, A., & Castellanos, F. X. (2003). Functional neuroimaging of social cognition in pervasive developmental disorders: A brief review. *Annals of the New York Academy of Sciences, 1008,* 256–260.

Doebeli, M., Hauert, C., & Killingback, T. (2004). The evolutionary origin of cooperators and defectors. *Science, 306,* 859–862.

Dolan, R. J., Fletcher, P., Morris, J., Kapur, N., Deakin, J. F., & Frith, C. D. (1996). Neural activation during covert processing of positive emotional facial expressions. *Neuroimage, 4,* 194–200.

Eisenberger, N. I., Lieberman, M. D., & Williams, K. D. (2003). Does rejection hurt? An fMRI study of social exclusion. *Science, 302,* 290–292.

Ekman, P. (2003). Darwin, deception, and facial expression. *Annals of the New York Academy of Sciences, 1000,* 205–221.

Emery, N. J. (2000). The eyes have it: The neuroethology, function and evolution of social gaze. *Neuroscience and Biobehavioral Reviews, 24,* 581–604.

Englis, B. G., Vaughan, K. B., & Lanzetta, J. T. (1982). Conditioning of counter-empathic emotional responses. *Journal of Experimental Social Psychology, 18,* 375–391.

Fehr, E., & Gächter, S. (2002). Altruistic punishment in humans. *Nature, 415,* 137–140.

Fridlund, A. J. (1991). Sociality of solitary smiling: Potentiation by an implicit audience. *Journal of Personality and Social Psychology, 60,* 229–240.

Fridlund, A. J. (1994). *Human facial expression: An evolutionary view.* San Diego: Academic Press.

Gallagher, H. L., Jack, A. I., Roepstorff, A., & Frith, C. D. (2002). Imaging the intentional stance in a competitive game. *NeuroImage, 16,* 814–821.

Gallese, V., Fadiga, L., Fogassi, L., & Rizzolatti, G. (1996). Action recognition in the premotor cortex. *Brain, 119,* 593–609.

Geday, J., Gjedde, A., Boldsen, A-S., & Kupers, R. (2003). Emotional valence modulates activity in the posterior fusiform gyrus and inferior medial prefrontal cortex in social perception. *NeuroImage, 18,* 675–684.

Grelotti, D. J., Gauthier, I., & Schultz, R. T. (2002). Social interest and the development of cortical face specialization: What autism teaches us about face processing. *Developmental Psychobiology, 40,* 213–225.

Grossman, E. D., & Blake, R. (2001). Brain activity evoked by inverted and imagined biological motion. *Vision Research, 41,* 1475–1482.

Hariri, A. R., Tessitore, A., Mattay, V. S., Fera, F., & Weinberger, D. R. (2002). The amygdala response to emotional stimuli: A comparison of faces and scenes. *Neuroimage, 17,* 317–323.

Hawkley, L. C., Burleson, M. H., Berntson, G. G., & Cacioppo, J. T. (2003). Loneliness in everyday life: Cardiovascular activity, psychosocial context, and health behaviors. *Journal of Personality and Social Psychology, 85,* 105–120.

Hawkley, L. C., Preacher, K. J., & Cacioppo, J. T. (in press). Multilevel modeling of social interactions and mood in lonely and socially connected individuals: The MacArthur social neuroscience studies. In A. D. Ong & M. van Dulmen (Eds.), *Handbook of Methods in positive psychology.* New York: Oxford University Press.

Haxby, J. V., Horwitz, B., Ungerleider, L. G., Maisog, J. M., Pietrini, P., & Grady, C. L. (1994). The functional organization of human extrastriate cortex: A PET-rCBF study of selective attention to faces and locations. *Journal of Neuroscience, 14,* 6336–6353.

Heberlein, A. S., & Adolphs, R. (2004). Impaired spontaneous anthropomorphizing despite intact perception and social knowledge. *Proceedings of the National Academy of Sciences of the USA, 101,* 7487–7491.

Heider, F., & Simmel, M. (1944). An experimental study of apparent behavior. *American Journal of Psychology, 57,* 243–259.

House, J. S., Landis, K. R., & Umberson, D. (1988). Social relationships and health. *Science, 241,* 540–545.

Howard, M. A., Cowell, P. E., Boucher, J., Broks, P., Mayes, A., Farrant, A., et al. (2000). Convergent neuroanatomical and behavioural evidence of an amygdala hypothesis of autism. *Neuroreport, 11,* 2931–2935.

Ishai, A., Haxby, J. V., & Ungerleider, L. G. (2002). Visual imagery of famous faces: Effects of memory and attention revealed by fMRI. *Neuroimage, 17,* 1729–1741.

Jakobs, E., Manstead, A. S. R., & Fischer, A. H. (2001). Social context effects on facial activity in a negative emotional setting. *Emotion, 1,* 51–69.

Kanwisher, N., McDermott, J., & Chun, M. M. (1997). The fusiform face area: A module in human extrastriate cortex specialized for face perception. *Journal of Neuroscience, 17,* 4302–4311.

Keltner, D., & Kring, A. M. (1998). Emotion, social function, and psychopathology. *Review of General Psychology, 2,* 320–342.

Kilts, C. D., Egan, G., Gideon, D. A., Ely, T. D., & Hoffman, J. M. (2003). Dissociable neural pathways are involved in the recognition of emotion in static and dynamic facial expressions. *NeuroImage, 18,* 156–168.

Kluver, H., & Bucy, P. C. (1997). Preliminary analysis of functions of the temporal lobes in monkeys. *Journal of Neuropsychiatry and Clinical Neurosciences, 9,* 606–620. (Original work published 1939)

Koski, L., Wohlschlager, A., Bekkering, H., Woods, R. P., Dubeau, M. C., Mazziotta, J. C., et al. (2002). Modulation of motor and premotor activity during imitation of target-directed actions. *Cerebral Cortex, 12,* 847–855.

Lane, R. D., Chua, P. M-L., & Dolan, R. J. (1999). Common effects of emotional valence, arousal, and attention on neural activation during visual processing of pictures. *Neuropsychologia, 37,* 989–997.

Lang, P. J., Bradley, M. M., & Cuthbert, B. N. (1999). *International Affective Picture System (IAPS): Instruction manual and affective ratings* (Technical Report No. A-4). Gainesville: University of Florida, Center for Research in Psychophysiology.

Lang, P. J., Bradley, M. M., Fitzsimmons, J. R., Cuthbert, B. N., Scott, J. D., Moulder, B., et al. (1998). Emotional arousal and activation of the visual cortex: An fMRI analysis. *Psychophysiology, 35,* 199–210.

Larson, R., & Csikszentmihalyi, M. (1983). The experiences method. *New Directions for Methodology of Social and Behavioral Science, 15,* 41–56.

McDermott, K. B., Buckner, R. L., Petersen, S. E., Kelley, W. M., & Sanders, A. L. (1999). Set- and code-specific activation in frontal cortex: An fMRI study of encoding and retrieval of faces and words. *Journal of Cognitive Neuroscience, 11,* 631–640.

McIntosh, D. N., Reichmann-Decker, A., Winkielman, P., & Wilbarger, J. L. (in press). When the social mirror breaks: Deficits in automatic, but not voluntary, mimicry of emotional facial expressions in autism. *Developmental Science.*

Meltzoff, A. N., & Decety, J. (2003). What imitation tells us about social cognition: A rapprochement between developmental psychology and cognitive neuroscience. *Philosophical Transactions of the Royal Society of London: Series B. Biological Sciences, 358,* 491–500.

Mesquita, B., & Frijda, N. H. (1992). Cultural variations in emotions: A review. *Psychological Bulletin, 112,* 179–204.

Moll, J., de Oliveira-Souza, R., Eslinger, P. J., Bramati, I. E., Mourao-Miranda, J., Andreiuolo, P. A., et al. (2002). The neural correlates of moral sensitivity: A functional magnetic resonance imaging investigation of basic and moral emotions. *Journal of Neuroscience, 22,* 2730–2736.

Narumoto, J., Okada, T., Sadato, N., Fukui, K., & Yonekura, Y. (2001). Attention to emotion modulates fMRI activity in human right superior temporal sulcus. *Cognitive Brain Research, 12,* 225–231.

Norris, C. J., Chen, E. E., Zhu, D. C., Small, S. L., & Cacioppo, J. T. (2004). The interaction of social and emotional processes in the brain. *Journal of Cognitive Neuroscience, 16,* 1818–1829.

Phan, K. L., Wager, T., Taylor, S. F., & Liberzon, I. (2002). Functional neuroanatomy of emotion: A meta-analysis of emotion activation studies in PET and fMRI. *NeuroImage, 16,* 331–348.

Puce, A., & Perrett, D. (2003). Electrophysiology and brain imaging of biological motion. *Philosophical Transactions of the Royal Society of London: Series B. Biological Sciences, 358,* 435–445.

Rainville, P., Duncan, G. H., Price, D. D., Carrier, B., & Bushnell, M. C. (1997). Pain affect encoded in human anterior cingulate but not somatosensory cortex. *Science, 277,* 968–971.

Rizzolatti, G., Fadiga, L., Gallese, V., & Fogassi, L. (1996). Premotor cortex and the recognition of motor actions. *Cognitive Brain Research, 3,* 131–141.

Rizzolatti, G., Fogassi, L., & Gallese, V. (2001). Neurophysiological mechanisms underlying the understanding and imitation of action. *Nature Reviews. Neuroscience, 2,* 661–670.

Salmond, C. H., de Haan, M., Friston, K. J., Gadian, D. G., & Vargha-Khadem, F. (2003). Investigating individual differences in brain abnormalities in autism. *Philosophical Transactions of the Royal Society of London: Series B. Biological Sciences, 358,* 405–413.

Saxe, R., & Kanwisher, N. (2003). People thinking about thinking people: The role of the temporo-parietal junction in "theory of mind." *NeuroImage, 19,* 1835–1842.

Singer, T., Seymour, B., O'Doherty, J., Kaube, H., Dolan, R. J., & Frith, C. D. (2004). Empathy for pain involves the affective but not sensory components of pain. *Science, 303,* 1157–1162.

Stein, N. L., & Trabasso, T. (1992). The organization of emotional experience: Creating links among emotion, thinking, language, and intentional action. *Cognition and Emotion, 6,* 225–244.

Thompson, R. A. (1994). Emotion regulation: A theme in search of definition. *Monographs of the Society for Research in Child Development, 59,* 15–52, 250–283.

Vuilleumier, P., Armony, J. L., Driver, J., & Dolan, R. J. (2001). Effects of attention and emotion on face processing in the human brain: An event-related fMRI study. *Neuron, 30,* 829–841.

Ward, M. J., Lee, S. S., & Lipper, E. G. (2000). Failure-to-thrive is associated with disorganized infant–mother attachment and unresolved maternal attachment. *Infant Mental Health Journal, 21,* 428–442.

Winston, J. S., Strange, B. A., O'Doherty, J., & Dolan, R. J. (2002). Automatic and intentional brain responses during evaluation of trustworthiness of faces. *Nature Neuroscience, 5,* 277–283.

6

How Thinking Controls Feeling
A SOCIAL COGNITIVE NEUROSCIENCE APPROACH

Kevin N. Ochsner

In the movie *The Princess Bride*, a farm boy named Westley tells his beloved Princess Buttercup, "Life is pain, Highness. Anyone who says differently is selling something." Westley speaks these words disguised as the Man in Black, which befits his dark portrait of life as bleak, full of hardship and emotional distress. Like many memorable movie lines, these words have some truth to them. Indeed, there are times when our frustrations, disappointments, embarrassments, and losses can seem never-ending. For confirmation that life's woes are quite commonplace, we need look no further than the pages of any daily newspaper. In March 2005, searches on the *New York Times* website for the words "emotion" or "stress" respectively returned 7,438 and 8,510 articles since 1996. The fact that a vast majority of articles were common to both searches indicates that, when writing about emotion, the *Times* is chronicling not our joys but our sorrows.

But is life always pain? Perhaps not. In another instance of art imitating life, Westley himself sells a sunnier perspective to Buttercup—but only after having removed his Black Mask and revealing his true identity as the film's heroic protagonist. While navigating the dangers of the Fire Swamp, Buttercup despairs: "We'll never succeed. We may as well die here." Westley replies, "No, no. We have already succeeded . . . " and proceeds to recount how they already have overcome many Swamp obstacles and possess the skills necessary to avoid any others. The message here is that beneath our occasional Black Masks, we all possess the ability to look on the bright side. When faced with scary situations that we cannot escape, we can control our fears and anxieties by thinking differently.

This ability to change the way we feel by changing the way we think has long been a topic of interest for laypersons and psychologists alike, and it goes by many names. "Rationalization" is used colloquially when we doubt the rationalizer's ability or success in getting over a breakup, a loss, or a disappointment. "Spin" (or "issue framing") is used by politicians, marketers, and media to describe how they can manipulate the emotional impact of an event on the public by altering its interpretation. "Coping" is used by clinical researchers who examine the ability to carry on and even thrive in the face of trauma and loss. And "reappraisal" is used by social psychologists who study the contexts in which different cognitive strategies have different consequences for emotional responding.

For present purposes, these abilities can be referred to broadly as the *cognitive control of emotion*. Despite long-standing interest in this topic, only recently has neuroscience research begun to rigorously examine how thinking controls feeling. The goal of this chapter is to describe our approach to this issue, which employs functional magnetic resonance imaging (fMRI) to test hypotheses about the psychological and neural mechanisms of one form of cognitive control that is known as reappraisal. To achieve this end, the chapter is divided into three parts. The first describes the motivation for and nature of the social cognitive neuroscience approach that guides this research. The second describes a series of experiments that address the neural bases of reappraisal, with an emphasis on understanding how interactions between control systems and emotional appraisal systems give rise to successful emotion regulation. The third and last part places this work in a broader context and discusses future directions for research in this area.

THE SOCIAL COGNITIVE NEUROSCIENCE APPROACH

Social cognitive neuroscience integrates the theories and methods of social psychology and cognitive neuroscience to study phenomena at multiple levels of analysis (Lieberman, 2000; Ochsner, 2004; Ochsner & Lieberman, 2001). To illustrate how this approach has guided our research on the brain bases of reappraisal, it is useful to consider, first, neuroscience work on emotion and cognitive control that was available when our work began. After examining how the strengths and weaknesses of that work motivated our social cognitive neuroscience approach, this section considers the nature of the approach in more detail.

The Motivation for the Approach

Around the turn of the 21st century, when this line of research began, there were no functional imaging studies that had investigated the brain bases of reappraisal specifically and few that had examined any form of cognitive control over emotion more generally. Therefore, to inform our thinking about the neural systems supporting reappraisal, it seemed prudent to examine closely extant cognitive neuroscience work on emotion and cognitive control and social psychological work on emotion and emotion regulation.

Comparison of cognitive neuroscientific and social psychological approaches to emotion, however, revealed an important and telling difference that can be highlighted by their answers to an age-old question: Would a rose by any other name smell as sweet? For cognitive neuroscience theories (and the behavioral neuroscience theories on which they were based), the answer to this question would be *yes*, because they tend to treat emotion as a property of a stimulus, like shape, size, or color. In this view, emotions are automatic response tendencies linked to specific stimulus properties (Feldman Barrett, Ochsner, & Gross, in press). Thus, in order to generate strong or weak or positive or negative emotions, one simply needs stimuli that have "big" or "small" or "pleasant" or "unpleasant" emotional properties. The implicit assumption here is that emotions can be manipulated in much the same way that one would use big or small stimuli to examine encoding of size, blue and red or gray stimuli to examine processing of color, sweet- as compared with neutral-scented flowers to examine processing of smell, and so on.

By contrast, for some social psychological theories (and clinical theories to which they are related), the answer to the question about a sweet smelling rose is *no*: If you believed the rose was another flower (e.g., a daisy) that is not so sweet smelling, then the rose under your nose would not smell as sweet. The reason is that emotion is thought to be a context-dependent process in which emotional responses depend on an interaction between stimulus properties and the way they are interpreted, or *appraised*, in terms of their significance to one's current goals, wants, or needs (Feldman Barrett et al., in press; Lazarus, 1991; Scherer, Schorr, & Johnstone, 2001; Smith & Ellsworth, 1985). In this view, the same stimulus (e.g., a blow to the back) could elicit different emotional responses (anger or sympathy) depending on the way in which it was appraised (as an intentional strike vs. the result of someone accidentally tripping and falling into you).

Both of these views have merit. On the one hand, in some circumstances our emotional responses may be driven in a bottom-up fashion by the rapid encoding of stimulus properties that have learned or intrinsic pleasant or unpleasant properties and associations. On the other hand, in many circumstances our emotional responses are importantly shaped by the top-down influences of stored knowledge, contextual information, and our deliberate attempts to reevaluate and reinterpret the meaning of emotionally evocative situations. Emotions, therefore, may derive from the interaction of both bottom-up and top-down processes (Feldman Barrett et al., in press; Lazarus & Alfert, 1964; Ochsner & Feldman Barrett, 2001; Scherer, 1984; Scherer et al., 2001).

Using the Approach to Develop a Social Cognitive Neuroscience Model of Emotion and Emotion Regulation

With these contrasting approaches in mind, my colleagues and I developed an integrative approach that would draw on the cognitive neuroscience literature on emotion and cognitive control to identify brain systems that could be involved in the bottom up and top-down appraisal of emotional stimuli.

During the past decade, human cognitive neuroscience research has converged with a large animal literature to implicate one subcortical brain structure in particular—the amygdala—in the bottom-up processing of emotion. Prior animal work using conditioning paradigms has demonstrated that the amygdala plays an essential role in associating neutral perceptual stimuli with the physiological and behavioral responses that make up a fear response (Davis, 1998; LeDoux, 2000). Human functional imaging and neuropsychological studies similarly have demonstrated a role for the amygdala in acquiring conditioned fear responses (e.g., Buchel & Dolan, 2000; LaBar & LeDoux, 1996; Morris & Dolan, 2004; Phelps et al., 1998) and have extended the amygdala's role to the preattentive detection of arousing, ambiguous, and potentially threatening stimuli (Anderson & Phelps, 2001; Morris, Ohman, & Dolan, 1999; Whalen, Rauch, et al., 1998), consolidating episodic memories for both positive and negative arousing events (Hamann, 2001), recognizing facial expressions that signal so-called basic emotions (especially fear; Adolphs et al., 2005; Calder, Lawrence, & Young, 2001), identifying more subtle social cues that signal boredom and flirtation (Adolphs, Sears, & Piven, 2001), and guiding judgments of social targets that could be judged unfriendly or untrustworthy (Adolphs, Tranel, & Damasio, 1998; Winston, Strange, O'Doherty, & Dolan, 2002). Thus the amygdala appears crucial for perception of, memory for, and judgments about emotionally arousing stimuli, primarily potentially threatening ones. On the basis of this accumulated evidence, we reasoned that the amygdala should be an important structure for the bottom-up generation of an aversive emotional response.

That being said, two important caveats are in order concerning the amygdala's role in emotion. First, the amygdala does not appear to be crucial for generating some nonverbal behavioral expressions of emotion and may not play a direct role in emotional experience, as suggested by the fact that even bilateral amygdala lesions do not substantially affect these capacities (Anderson & Phelps, 2000, 2002). Second, the amygdala is by no means the only structure important for human emotion, and at least three other structures may play important roles depending on the stimulus and its context. As described in more detail elsewhere (Adolphs, 2003; Calder et al., 2001; Feldman Barrett et al., in press; Ochsner & Feldman Barrett, 2001; Ochsner & Gross, 2005), the ventral striatum seems essential for the bottom-up encoding of stimuli that have learned or intrinsic reward value (Delgado, Nystrom, Fissell, Noll, & Fiez, 2000; Knutson, Fong, Adams, Varner, & Hommer, 2001; O'Doherty, Deichmann, Critchley, & Dolan, 2002); the anterior insula is involved in responses to aversive, and especially, disgusting stimuli (Calder et al., 2001), which may be related to its role in interoception and awareness of the viscera (Critchley, Wiens, Rotshtein, Ohman, & Dolan, 2004); and, finally, the orbitofrontal cortex is important for linking affective associations to currently active goals and response options so that the value of stimuli can be updated flexibly in a context-sensitive manner (Bechara, Damasio, & Damasio, 2000; Beer, Heerey, Keltner, Scabini, & Knight, 2003; Beer, Shimamura, & Knight, 2004; Fellows & Farah, 2004; Hornak et al., 2004). Thus, although our own work has focused primarily on the role of the amygdala in emotion and emotion regulation, it is important to recognize that other brain systems play important roles as well.

To identify brain systems associated with top-down emotional processing my colleagues and I turned to the large literature on cognitive control that had implicated two brain systems—the anterior cingulate cortex and the dorsolateral prefrontal cortex—in the ability to control language, spatial attention, and memory. According to models of cognitive control, lateral prefrontal and cingulate systems play complementary roles in the regulation of behavior. Lateral prefrontal cortex (PFC) is important for the selection, maintenance, and application of goal-directed strategies and supports such cognitive abilities as working memory, response inhibition, and executive control more generally (Banich et al., 2000; D'Esposito, Postle, Ballard, & Lease, 1999; Jonides, Smith, Marshuetz, Koeppe, & Reuter-Lorenz, 1998; Miller & Cohen, 2001; Wagner, Pare-Blagoev, Clark, & Poldrack, 2001). Dorsal regions of anterior cingulate cortex (dACC) and the neighboring supplementary motor area are thought to monitor the extent to which current behavior is staying on track, to signal the need for ongoing control by PFC, and to support the ability to detect (and therefore correct) errors and identify response conflicts more generally (Banich et al., 2000; Botvinick, Braver, Barch, Carter, & Cohen, 2001; Botvinick, Cohen, & Carter, 2004; Erickson et al., 2004; Milham et al., 2001; cf. Fellows & Farah, 2005). Working hand in hand, these two brain systems are thought to support control processes that enable us to keep in mind the information we want to have there and to keep out of mind the information we want left out (Bunge, Ochsner, Desmond, Glover, & Gabrieli, 2001). They do this by modulating activation in subcortical and posterior cortical systems that represent different kinds of visual, auditory, or spatial information and that enable us to remember phone numbers until we dial them, select the right words to say, ignore distracting traffic noise, and the like. In the context of emotion, my colleagues and I hypothesized that lateral PFC and

dACC could modulate brain structures involved in the bottom-up generation of emotion, such as the amygdala or insula.

One other prefrontal system may be important for top-down emotional processing. Guiding and altering our emotional responses on the
basis of stored knowledge, online goals, and delivered strategies requires
not just systems important for implementing control but systems important
for the metacognitive monitoring of their operation. If lateral PFC and
dACC are important for control, then the medial PFC (mPFC) appears to
be important for monitoring (Ochsner, Beer, et al., 2006; Ochsner, Knierim,
et al., 2004). MPFC, and especially its dorsal medial portion, is active
when individuals evaluate their own emotional states (Gusnard, Akbudak,
Shulman, & Raichle, 2001; Lane, Fink, Chau, & Dolan, 1997; K. N.
Ochsner, Knierim, et al., 2004; Paradiso et al., 1999) or the emotional
states of others (Ochsner, Knierim, et al., 2004), when we make attributions about the mental states of others more generally (Gallagher & Frith,
2003), and when we draw inferences about our own or another person's
traits and dispositions (Kelley et al., 2002; Mitchell, Heatherton, &
Macrae, 2002; Mitchell, Macrae, & Banaji, 2006; Ochsner et al., in press).
Interestingly, dorsal mPFC is also involved in the delivered retrieval of
context-appropriate emotional associations from memory in tasks that do
not explicitly involve reference to mental states (Cato et al., 2004; Crosson
et al., 1999). These data suggest that mPFC may be important when we
draw inferences about how we feel, why we feel that way, whether we feel
that way in general, and whether and why other people feel that way, as
well. Thus mPFC may come into play as we track our own changing emotional responses and when we reason about emotional implications of
another person's intentions, actions, and beliefs.

Taken together, these studies provide the foundation for our hypothetical model of the cognitive control of emotion. According to this model,
prefrontal and cingulate systems guide the top-down appraisal of emotional stimuli initially encoded in a bottom-up fashion by the amygdala and
related structures. In the following section, I summarize experiments that
further develop and test this initial working model.

TOWARD A MODEL OF THE COGNITIVE CONTROL
OF EMOTION

The far-reaching aim of our research is to develop a model of the cognitive
control of emotion that makes reference to multiple levels of analysis
(social, cognitive, and neural) and that can provide an account of both
healthy normal and maladaptively abnormal emotional responding. The
development of any such model is, of course, an iterative process in which
theories generate hypotheses that turn into experiments that produce
results, which in turn inform theories, and so on.

The Social Cognitive Neuroscience Approach

The essence of this *social cognitive neuroscience approach* is to use neuro-science data to constrain thinking about the psychological processes that give rise to a specific kind of experience or behavior. Neuroscience data can be said to constrain psychological theorizing insofar as it provides empirical observations that theories must take into account. Robust theories speak to multiple types of data at multiple levels of analysis. By collecting multiple types of data using different methods, we can converge on robust theories of this kind (Ochsner & Kosslyn, 1999).

Note that this way of thinking about neuroscience data as a kind of constraint does not afford them privileged status. Neuroscience data provide dependent variables (DVs) that are neither "better" nor "worse" than many other kinds of DVs that might be collected by any experimental psychologist. Indeed, psychologists use all types of DVs—including choice response times (RTs), self-reports, speed of walking down a hallway, or any other measure—to constrain theory in the sense described here. Data constrain theory by providing observations for which theories must account. In this sense, neuroscience data constrain theory.

This is not to say that all kinds of DVs provide the same kinds of constraints. RTs and the effects of hippocampal damage do tell us different things, as do self-reports of emotional experience and patterns of activation in the amygdala and insula. Our job, as always, is to figure out how to map these different kinds of DVs onto one another and to build theories that explain the relationships among DVs and theoretical constructs couched at different levels of analysis.

That being said, it is important to recognize that information transfer between neuroscience data and psychological theory is bidirectional. Without psychological theory, the hippocampus, for example, is just a bunch of neurons that fire away without rhyme or reason. And without neuroscience data, we might not have developed the notion that there are multiple memory systems, one of which depends critically on the integrity of the hippocampus and many of which do not (Davachi, in press; Schacter, 1997). The mutual constraints between psychological, cognitive, and neural levels of analysis provide the foundation for drawing strong inferences about the validity of psychological theories (Sarter, Berntson, & Cacioppo, 1996).

In this regard, social cognitive neuroscience experiments can be thought of as having two simultaneous goals: (1) to use careful, theory-guided, behavioral experiments to inform our knowledge of brain function and (2) to use knowledge about brain function to inform psychological theory (Ochsner, in press; Ochsner & Lieberman, 2001; Sarter et al., 1996). Cognitive neuroscience tends to emphasize the former, and social psychology the latter mode of investigation, but most every experiment is at least capable of doing both at once.

Although some neuroscientists might reify neuroscience data as perhaps better or more "true" than other types of data, neuroscience methods and the data they produce are better seen as valuable tools in the toolbox of techniques that psychologists can employ to address their questions of interest. The questions you may want to address may not directly benefit from the application or incorporation of neuroscience data, of course. But whatever type of data you collect may constrain theorizing in a similar way. One could ask: Do RT data just speak to the speed with which we can do things? Are accuracy data only about how accurately we can do things? In a literal sense, yes, but in a scientific sense, no. For psychologists of any stripe, DVs are there to tell us something about underlying processing mechanisms. And in that sense, imaging data, electroencephalographic and event-related potential data, neuropsychological data, and so forth, tell us something about processing mechanisms. It is up to our theories to explain what that something is, and multiple kinds of data can inform the construction of those theories.

Two Kinds of Cognitive Control over Emotion

With this approach as a guide, in this section I present the current state of our model by describing experiments that examine two ways in which top-down cognitive processes can be used to regulate bottom-up emotion-generative processes (Ochsner, 2005; Ochsner & Gross, 2005). The first involves the controlled use of attention, and the second, the use of reappraisal to cognitively change the meaning of arousing inputs.

Controlled Attention

Attention is often called the selective aspect of information processing, by which is meant that attention enables us to gate the flow of informational inputs so that only selected stimuli receive further processing. When facing numerous stimuli that each can elicit a different emotional response, we can use selective attention to control the impact the stimuli have on us. By selectively attending to stimuli that generate desired responses and ignoring stimuli that generate undesired responses, we can control what we feel by resolving emotional conflicts.

My colleagues and I have examined the neural bases of this ability using variants of a classic interference paradigm known as the flanker task (Ochsner, Robertson, Cooper, & Gabrieli, 2006). In our affective version of the flanker task, participants viewed three words presented vertically in the center of the screen (see Figure 6.1, top). The participant's job was to judge whether the central target word was positive or negative and to ignore the distracting words that flanked it above and below. On congruent trials these words had the same valence (i.e. positive or negative) as the tar-

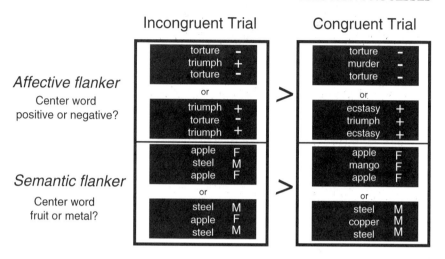

FIGURE 6.1. The structure of trials in the affective and semantic flanker tasks. For both tasks participants were instructed to attend to a central target word and to ignore distracting flanking words presented above and below it. They provided simple binary key-press responses to indicate either its valence (affective flanker) or its semantic category (semantic flanker). On incongruent trials flanking words had the opposite valence or were drawn from a different semantic category, and on congruent trials, words had the same valence or were drawn from the same semantic category. + and - symbols indicate the valence of words on the affective flanker task. M and F indicate the metal or fruit category of words on the semantic flanker task. The symbols were not present on the display during task completion and are provided solely for illustrative purposes.

get, and on incongruent trials these words had the opposite valence. By comparing patterns of brain activation on congruent, as compared with incongruent, trials for this task, we would be able to identify brain systems involved in resulting affective conflicts.

To determine whether the brain systems that support affective conflict resolution are similar to those involved in resolving cognitive conflicts, my colleagues and I compared activation during the affective flanker to activation during a semantic flanker task (see Figure 6.1, bottom). In this task participants again viewed an array of three vertically presented words that in this case were drawn from one of two emotionally neutral semantic categories—metals or fruit. Participants judged the category of the central target word as a metal or a fruit and ignored flanking words that were either from the same or the different category. In keeping with a large prior literature showing that response interference of various kinds slows reaction time, we found that responses were slower on incongruent than on congruent trials for both the affective and semantic flanker tasks.

The critical question was whether the use of selective attention to control affective conflict would involve neural systems similar to or different from those used to resolve cognitive conflict. As the preceding literature review suggests, we had good reason to believe that cognitive conflict should recruit dACC and dorsal lateral PFC regions. Furthermore, there had been suggestions that rostral regions of ACC and adjacent mPFC generally are involved in emotion (e.g., Bush, Luu, & Posner, 2000), in contrast to the cognitive functions of dACC. There were thus two competing hypotheses: Affective conflict could depend on rostral ACC and mPFC, whereas cognitive conflict would depend on dACC; or both types of conflict could recruit dACC regions sensitive to any type of response conflict, and there would be additional response-type-specific regions recruited, which could include mPFC.

The results clearly supported the latter hypothesis. As illustrated schematically in Figure 6.2, incongruent as compared with congruent trials for both the affective and semantic flanker tasks activated common regions of dACC and bilateral dorsal lateral PFC, in keeping with recruitment of these regions in numerous tasks involving cognitive control and response conflict of other kinds (e.g., Banich et al., 2000; Botvinick et al., 2004; Milham et al., 2001; Wager, Jonides, & Reading, 2004; Wager & Smith, 2003).

Interestingly, at the group level, rostral ACC/mPFC was not more active for affective as compared with cognitive conflict. In some cases failures to observe activation of brain systems in overall group contrasts can be attributable to individual differences in the extent to which specific pro-

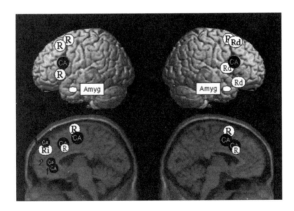

FIGURE 6.2. Lateral (top panels) and medial (bottom panels) cortical regions involved in attentional control (designated by CA), reappraisal in general (designated by R), reappraisal to increase negative emotion (designated by Ri) or reappraisal to decrease negative emotion (designated by Rd). The location of the amygdala, whose activation can be modulated up or down by reappraisal, is indicated by the white circle labeled Amyg. The amygdala is a subcortical structure located on the medial wall of the temporal lobe, and its approximate location beneath the surface of the lateral temporal cortex is indicated here. See text for details of functional interpretations for activated regions.

cesses are engaged. To account for the possibility that individual differences in the tendency to generate and experience emotion could influence activations, this experiment included questionnaires indexing individual differences in trait anxiety (Spielberger, Gorsuch, Lushemne, Vagg, & Jacobs, 1983) and alexithymia (Bagby, Parker, & Taylor, 1994). "Alexithymia" refers to the inability to understand and represent in awareness one's emotional states. Normal individuals differ in the extent to which they are able to recognize their own feelings, although severe emotion recognition deficits may warrant clinical intervention (Lane, Ahern, Schwartz, & Kaszniak, 1997; Lane, Sechrest, Riedel, Shapiro, & Kaszniak, 2000; Sifneos, 1996). We found that both individual difference measures predicted activation during affective conflict. Individuals with high trait anxiety tended to activate dorsal mPFC regions associated with thinking about emotional implications of words and reasoning about affective states (Cato et al., 2004; Ochsner et al., 2005), as well as ventral mPFC regions associated with using affective associations to guide behavior (Ochsner & Gross, 2005). Highly alexithymic individuals *failed* to activate rostral ACC/mPFC regions associated with self-awareness of emotional states. These findings are consistent with the idea that what is special about emotional conflict is not a special mechanism for resolving competing affective responses per se but rather the fact that emotional conflicts elicit awareness of the emotional qualities of conflict-arousing stimuli. Whereas individuals who are highly anxious elaborate and represent in awareness the affective properties of stimuli, alexithymic individuals fail to do so.

The results of this experiment thus support the working model of the cognitive control of emotion by demonstrating that PFC and dACC systems implement domain-general control processes that can be applied to regulating affective or cognitive conflicts and that the extent to which one engages medial systems involved in appraising the emotional value of a stimulus can depend on individual differences in one's ability and tendency to engage specific evaluative processes. These results are also consistent with other studies that have investigated conflicts between competing emotional and cognitive responses (but not affective conflicts per se) that have associated rostral ACC and mPFC with processing the affective connotations of words despite the fact that one is trying to ignore them (Compton et al., 2003; Mohanty et al., 2005; Shin et al., 2001; Whalen, Bush, et al., 1998) and with individual differences in trait anxiety (Bishop, Duncan, Brett, & Lawrence, 2004).

Controlled Appraisal

Although we may possess the capacity to ignore stimuli that elicit undesirable emotional responses, it is neither always possible nor always desirable to do so. For example, one cannot (or at least should not!) ignore a failing grade on an exam, and it might be perilous to ignore critical remarks made by one's relationship partner. To cope with such trying times, one can use cognition to control how one appraises the meaning of aversive stimuli. Thus that failing grade can be construed as a useful wake-up call and reminder to promote good study habits, and apparently critical remarks can be construed appropriately as unintended by-products of your partner's bad day at work (rather than as intentional barbs).

The controlled appraisal of stimuli isn't used only to turn off aversive feelings, however. In some cases, we may turn up the aversive volume by focusing on and elaborating negative appraisals of an event. This may be our conscious goal, as when we try to quell giddiness before an event in which is important to be serious or when we enhance our aggressive impulses before participating in a sporting event. But it may also be the unintended consequence of our conscious thoughts that involve worry, rumination, and anxiety.

To investigate the use of cognitive control to both generate and regulate negative emotion in these ways, we have conducted a series of studies using a simple laboratory paradigm meant to model everyday uses of controlled appraisal. Participants are exposed to a series of emotionally evocative photographs drawn from Peter Lang's International Affective Picture System (IAPS; Lang, Greenwald, Bradley, & Hamm, 1993). The high-arousal negative photographs used in the studies described here typically elicit feelings of disgust, shock, anxiety, and occasionally sadness. As illustrated in Figure 6.3, each photograph is presented in a multipart trial that begins with an instruction word in the center of the screen. This instruction word indicates that participants should either (one baseline trial) simply Look at a stimulus and let themselves respond naturally or reappraise the stimulus in a specified way. Across studies, the means and ends of reappraisal are systematically manipulated, as described subsequently. While

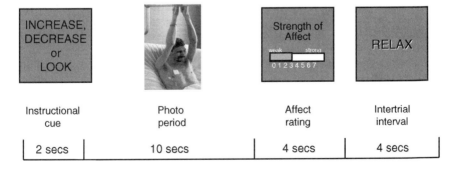

FIGURE 6.3. The structure of trials in a standard reappraisal task. An instructional cue indicates whether participants are to simply look at a stimulus and let themselves respond naturally (baseline trials) or to use some type of reappraisal (described in the text) to either increase or decrease their negative emotion.

the photograph is on the screen, for approximately 8–10 seconds, participants follow the instruction specified by the cue. After the photograph disappears, participants have an opportunity to rate the strength of their current negative affect, from weak to strong, using a scale that appears at the screen's center. Finally, there is an intertrial interval during which participants can relax before the next trial begins.

Contrasting Bottom-Up versus Top-Down Routes to Emotion Generation. To examine the generation of negative emotion, we used this paradigm to contrast bottom-up and top-down routes to emotional appraisal (Ochsner et al., 2006). A bottom-up route to emotional appraisal was modeled using baseline "Look" trials with aversive, as compared with neutral, photographs. By asking participants to respond naturally to photos with intrinsic or culturally learned aversive properties (such as a gunshot wound or a Ku Klux Klan member) as compared with neutral properties (e.g., a neutral facial expression or an office setting), we hypothesized that systems involved in the bottom-up generation of an emotion should be engaged. A top-down route to emotional appraisal was modeled by asking participants to "Increase" their negative responses to neutral photographs. By asking participants to think in negative ways about the context, affects, and outcomes depicted in each photo, we hypothesized that systems involved in a top-down generation of an emotion should be engaged.

The results generally supported the working model (see Figure 6.3). "Look" trials using aversive as compared with neutral photos activated the amygdala bilaterally, as well as a right lateral PFC region associated with sustained attention (Wager, Jonides, & Reading, 2004) and extrastriate visual areas associated with heightened attention to visual inputs (Lane, Chua, & Dolan, 1999). By contrast, "Increase" trials with aversive photos, as compared with "Look" trials with aversive photos, activated the left amygdala, left lateral PFC, and bilateral dACC and mPFC. These results are consistent with the idea that bottom-up and top-down routes to emotional appraisal both depend on amygdala-mediated processes that presumably identify and encode arousing stimuli. In the bottom-up case, the arousal signal comes from properties of the stimulus, whereas in the top-down case the arousal signal comes from one's controlled appraisal of what the stimulus means in the absence of any intrinsically aversive perceptual cues.

These results fit with those from other studies that examine how other ways of manipulating top-down appraisals can modulate processing in bottom-up emotion systems (for a review, see Ochsner & Gross, 2005). For example, anticipation of pleasant or aversive stimuli (e.g., Knutson, Adams, Fong, & Hommer, 2001; O'Doherty et al., 2002; Phelps et al., 2001; Ploghaus et al., 1999; Wager, Rilling, et al., 2004) and placebo-induced beliefs (Lieberman et al., 2004; Petrovic, Kalso, Petersson, & Ingvar, 2002; Wager, Rilling, et al., 2004) have been shown to involve recruitment of lateral and medial PFC systems in combination with modulation of amygdala, insula, and ventral striatum.

Contrasting the Up- and Down-Regulation of Negative Emotion. The basic paradigm illustrated in Figure 6.2 also has been used to ask questions about the neural systems engaged when we use reappraisal to cognitively turn up or turn down our negative emotions (Ochsner, Bunge, Gross, & Gabrieli, 2002; Ochsner, Ray, et al., 2004). Two important questions concern the relationship between the up- and down-regulation of emotion: Are similar top-down control systems engaged? And do they modulate the same bottom-up appraisal systems, albeit in different ways? One hypothesis is that both types of reappraisal rely on a common core set of control systems, including dACC and PFC, used to generate and maintain reappraisal strategies of whatever kind. These control systems could be flexibly deployed to modulate processing in the amygdala in accordance with the goal of reappraisal—turning it up or down as need be. An alternative hypothesis is that each type of reappraisal involves different types of cognitive operations and, as a result, should recruit different top-down control systems. Up-regulation may involve the elaboration and retrieval of emotional associations, which has been associated with dorsal mPFC, whereas down-regulation may involve response inhibitory mechanisms associated with right lateral PFC. To discriminate between these alternative hypotheses, we asked participants to complete three types of trials with aversive photos: baseline Look trials similar to those described previously and Increase and Decrease trials, in which participants appraised the context, affects, and outcomes depicted in photos in either increasingly negative or neutralizing ways.

Imaging results suggested that both hypotheses were correct (Ochsner, Ray, et al., 2004; see also Ochsner et al., 2002). As illustrated schematically in Figure 6.3, both Increase and Decrease (as compared to Look) trials activated left lateral PFC, dACC, and dorsal mPFC regions associated with controlled appraisal of the meaning of a stimulus. Of particular interest is the common reliance of reappraisal and—in the experiment described previously—top-down appraisal on left inferior prefrontal regions known to be important for retrieving information from semantic memory and rehearsing it in verbal working memory (Smith, Jonides, Marshuetz, & Koeppe, 1998; Wagner et al., 2001). This finding is consistent with an account of reappraisal as a deliberately constructed internal narrative that re-represents the meaning of stimuli in goal-congruent ways. In addition, both Increase and Decrease trials modulated the left amygdala, with activity enhanced during photo presentation on Increase trials and diminished during photo presentation on Decrease trials. These data suggest that there is a common functional architecture supporting different types of reappraisal.

Direct comparisons of activity on Increase and Decrease trials revealed neural systems differentially associated with each type of reappraisal.

Increase trials differentially recruited a region of left dorsal mPFC associated with accessing the affective connotations of words and reasoning about one's own or other people's affective mental states (Cato et al., 2004; Ochsner, Knierim, et al., 2004). Decrease trials differentially recruited right dorsolateral and orbitofrontal regions associated with response inhibition (Konishi et al., 1999) and with updating the motivational value of stimuli (O'Doherty, Critchley, Deichmann, & Dolan, 2003).

Converging evidence supporting these findings comes from a growing number of studies that have also begun to investigate related forms of cognitive reappraisal. In general, these studies have found that interactions between top-down control and bottom-up appraisal systems are involved when individuals maintain responses to aversive stimuli after the stimuli disappear (Schaefer et al., 2002); or when they are instructed to "suppress" sexual arousal (Beauregard, Levesque, & Bourgouin, 2001), sadness (Levesque et al., 2003; Levesque et al., 2004), or negative emotion (Phan et al., 2005) or to distance themselves from painful inputs (Kalisch et al., 2005).

Contrasting Self- and Other-Focused Emotional Appraisal. Although studies of cognitive reappraisal generally support the idea that the top-down control of emotion involves prefrontal and cingulate control systems, the precise systems recruited across studies have varied. One reason for this inconsistency could be variability in the specific kinds of reappraisal that participants have been asked to employ. If different types of reappraisal strategies involve qualitatively different types of processing about qualitatively different types of information, it might be expected that different reappraisal strategies would depend on related but distinct control systems. This possibility is consistent with results of the experiments described earlier and also is consistent with the literature on content and process specificity in PFC for different varieties of working memory (D'Esposito et al., 1999; Smith & Jonides, 1998) or episodic memory (Cabeza & Nyberg, 2000; Tulving, 2002).

To investigate this possibility, participants in the Increase/Decrease experiments described earlier were divided into two groups that achieved their emotion regulatory goals using one of two qualitatively distinct reappraisal strategies. Participants assigned to the self-focus group were asked to modulate their negative feelings by either increasing their sense of personal connection to the image (e.g., by imagining it could be a loved one or themselves depicted in the photo) or decreasing their sense of personal connection to the image by adopting a distant, detached, and clinical third-person perspective while viewing it. Participants assigned to the situation-focus group were asked to modulate their negative feelings by reinterpreting the context, affects, and outcomes of pictured persons in increasingly or decreasingly negative ways. We hypothesized that a self-focused strategy might differentially depend on mPFC systems involved in monitoring the extent to which a stimulus is relevant to the self (e.g., Kelley et al., 2002; Ochsner et al., 2006). By contrast, a situation-focused strategy might differentially depend on lateral PFC systems involved in maintaining and manipulating perceptual information (Smith & Jonides, 1998) and in retrieving information about emotion-eliciting contexts from semantic memory (Wagner et al., 2001).

Imaging results provided mixed support for these hypotheses. On the one hand, when negative emotion was increased, there were no differences in activation between the two groups. In retrospect, a lack of difference might be expected, given the way in which my colleagues and I allowed participants to increase their negative emotion in the self-focus group. Participants in this group were asked to reinterpret the outcomes and affects that they themselves or another person could experience, which is very similar to what participants in the situation-focus group were instructed to do. On the other hand, when negative emotion was decreased, our hypotheses were supported: Self-focus participants differentially recruited mPFC, whereas situation-focus participants differentially recruited left lateral PFC.

Although other studies have yet to directly compare and contrast neural systems recruited by qualitatively different kinds of reappraisal strategies, converging evidence is emerging that generally supports the association of mPFC with self-focused (or "me"-focused) processing and lateral PFC with perceptually focused processing. For example, my colleagues and I have shown that when participants view emotionally evocative photographs, mPFC is recruited both when they are asked to appraise their own emotional reactions to the photos and when they appraise emotional states of the central characters depicted in the photos. However, greater mPFC activity is observed for self-focused appraisals, whereas greater left PFC activity is observed for other-focused appraisals. Additional support for this medial–lateral distinction comes from a study of "cold" cognitive control over working memory showing that during task performance individuals high in self-consciousness tend to differentially recruit dorsal mPFC, whereas individuals who are extroverted tend to differentially recruit lateral PFC (Eisenberger, Lieberman, & Satpute, 2005). In a broader context, although this distinction is consistent with a general role for mPFC in metacognitive processing, which by definition involves a high degree of self-awareness, it remains for future work to directly compare appraisal modes that involve internally as compared with externally focused processing.

EXTENSIONS AND FUTURE DIRECTIONS

A primary goal of this chapter is to illustrate the benefits of a social cognitive neuroscience approach by describing the ways in which it has been employed in studying the use of cognition to control the ways in which emotionally evocative stimuli are appraised. Toward that end, we built a working model of the cognitive control of emotion whose initial formulation drew on both cognitive neuroscience and social psychological theory and that was subsequently tested using experiments that employed a social cognitive neuroscience approach. With this initial model in place, the goal of this section is to examine its implications for understanding individual differences in emotion regulatory capacities, to discuss broader questions about the relationships between emotion generation and regulation, and to consider some important questions on the research horizon.

Individual Differences: From Basic Processes to Normal and Abnormal Variation

A comprehensive model of emotion regulation should be able to account for both normal and abnormal variability. The structure of our model suggests a simple way in which such variability could be taken into account: Individuals could vary in the extent to which bottom-up processes tend to generate emotional responses and experiences, the extent to which they possess a repertoire of control strategies and effective top-down processes that can be used to implement them, or some combination of the two. By characterizing bottom-up and top-down emotion processing both psychologically and neurally, we may ultimately be able to account for the normal development of regulatory ability and its breakdown in psychiatric disorders such as depression.

Development

Consider, for example, that between the ages of 8 and 12, working memory and inhibitory capacity undergo a tremendous developmental growth spurt (Bunge, Dudukovic, Thomason, Vaidya, & Gabrieli, 2002; Nelson et al., 2000) and that at about this same time, myelination of the prefrontal cortex increases rapidly as well (Luna et al., 2001). To the extent that the control systems that support response inhibition and working memory are similar to the systems underlying the use of controlled attention or appraisal to regulate emotion, we might expect the interdependence of cognitive control and prefrontal integrity to be mirrored in the emotional domain, as well. My colleagues and I have begun investigating this issue, using the reappraisal task described in the previous section to investigate the capacity to regulate emotion in children ages 8–12, adolescents ages 13–17, and young adults ages 18–22. Initial behavioral results suggest that children have difficulty decreasing their negative emotion using situation-focused reappraisal strategies, whereas the performance of adolescents matches the effective regulation demonstrated by young adults (Ochsner et al., 2006). It remains to be seen whether children recruit different brain systems in an effort to achieve successful regulation. The results of another study examining the attempted "suppression" of sadness in 8- to 10-year-old girls may offer a preliminary answer to this question. When told to "suppress" emotional responses to sad or neutral film clips, children engaged lateral and medial PFC, dACC, and lateral orbitofrontal cortex (Levesque et al., 2004). Although this study did not include an adult comparison group, the authors note that in a previously reported study using adults in the same paradigm they observed fewer regions of prefrontal activation. This suggests that children may need to recruit additional regions to support emotion regulatory strategies.

Dysregulation

The development of cognitive neuroscience applications to psychiatric disorders has proceeded rapidly in the past 15–20 years. For numerous disorders, PET and fMRI studies have been used to identify an underlying "pathophysiology." Initial studies simply compared resting activation in patients with resting activation in controls and identified, for example, relative hyperactivation of the amygdala and hypoactivation of left PFC in depression (Drevets, Gadde, & Krishman, 1997). A problem with such studies, however, is that they do not control the psychological processes engaged by participants, and so it is not clear exactly why resting differences are obtained in between-groups comparisons. Is the scanned environment simply more aversive for a depressed person? Are they attempting to regulate but failing to do so? It is not clear. A second generation of studies constrained the experimental setting by contrasting activation to symptom-provoking stimuli—such as negative trait words in the case of depression, or contamination-related stimuli in the case of obsessive–compulsive disorder—to activation to neutral stimuli of the same type that did not have strong affective associations. By and large, these studies have identified activations in so-called "limbic" structures involved in emotion, including the amygdala, striatum, insula, and orbitofrontal cortex, among others (Breiter et al., 1996; Liberzon et al., 1999; Rauch, Savage, Alpert, Fischman, & Jenike, 1997). Although these studies can directly relate patterns of brain activation to the presence of specific stimuli, they do not control the nature of the appraisal processes participants engage in. As a consequence, results are ambiguous with respect to whether activations do or do not reflect attempts to control the way stimuli are appraised. A third generation of studies has borrowed paradigms from the cognitive neuroscience literature that are known to isolate specific computational processes associated with specific brain systems. These paradigms have begun to identify disorder-specific dysfunction in specific types of recognition, memory, attention, inhibitory, and emotional functions (Bremner et al., 1999; Mohanty et al., 2005; Perlstein, Dixit, Carter, Noll, & Cohen, 2003; Phillips, Drevets, Rauch, & Lane, 2003a, 2003b; Russell et al., 2000).

To date, however, few published studies have investigated the use of cognition to regulate emotional responses. Given that problems with emotion regulation characterize almost every mood, personality, and anxiety disorder listed in the *Diagnostic and Statistical Manual of Mental Disorders* (DSM-IV-TR; American Psychiatric Association, 2000), the importance of understanding the neural bases of emotion regulation is clear. In our own work, my colleagues and I have begun to address this question in the context of depression. Using the reappraisal paradigm described numerous times earlier, we have sought to determine whether depression involves a tendency to generate abnormally strong negative responses, a failure to generate normal positive responses, diminished ability to down-regulate negative responses, or diminished ability to up-regulate positive responses. Initial behavioral results suggest that depressed individuals may be able to cognitively reappraise negative and aversive photographs just as well as controls when using a situation-focused reappraisal strategy.

If this result holds, it raises an intriguing question: If individuals with depression are able to down-regulate their negative and up-regulate their positive emotional responses in a laboratory paradigm, then why do they experience a preponderance of negative affect in everyday life? One might speculate that there are at least two important differences between the lab and the real world. First, our typical reappraisal paradigm elicits feelings of disgust, shock, and anxiety using stimuli that are not highly self relevant and that could be expected to elicit normative negative reactions in all viewers. It is possible, therefore, that depression-relevant, and perhaps idiosyncratically selected, stimuli would pose a greater regulatory challenge for individuals with depression. Second, it is possible that a situation-focused reappraisal strategy draws on processes unimpaired by depression. A self-focused strategy that asks participants to either engage with or disengage from emotional stimuli may be more related to the kinds of self-referential thought that are hallmarks of depressive thinking (Nolen-Hoeksema, 2000; Teasdale et al., 2002). It remains for future research to directly compare individuals with depression and controls in their ability to regulate responses to self-relevant and normatively negative stimuli using self-focused or situation-focused reappraisal strategies.

That being said, it is important to note that individuals with depression are able to benefit from cognitive-behavioral therapies (Teasdale et al., 2002; Teasdale et al., 2001), which suggests that the ability to reappraise— even in negative self-referential contexts—may be intact in depression. An individual-differences analysis of data from our Increase–Decrease study suggests that this may be the case (Ray et al., 2006). In that study we asked participants to complete various measures of the tendency to ruminate, which has been associated with risk for and problems with depression (Nolen-Hoeksema, 2000). Rumination refers to the turning over in one's mind of typically aversive events with the hope of gaining some insight into them. Interestingly, the tendency to ruminate predicted greater increases in amygdala activity on Increase trials and greater decreases in amygdala activity on Decrease trials. Furthermore, when participants decreased negative emotion, the tendency to ruminate was associated with decreases in activation of mPFC regions associated with self-referential processing (e.g., Ray et al., 2005), which suggests that ruminators tended to engage in self-referential processing during the baseline Look condition. These results rather intriguingly suggest that if depression is associated with rumination and if rumination is associated with greater ability to modulate amygdala activation via reappraisal, then individuals with depression might, paradoxically, possess greater capacity to regulate emotion than do controls; their problem may be that they typically are using this capacity to make themselves feel worse rather than better.

Boundary Conditions:
What Do We Mean by Emotion Regulation?

The reader may have noticed that the terms "appraisal" and "reappraisal" have been used somewhat interchangeably throughout this chapter. This flexible usage of terms has both theoretical and empirical motivations. The theoretical motivation stems from the fact that the original definition of reappraisal was meant to convey that a stimulus has been appraised a second time, thereby redirecting an emotional response that already had been generated (Lazarus, 1991). Thus reappraisal is nothing more than appraisal "done over again" in a particular context. The empirical motivation stems from the repeated finding—both in my and my colleagues' work and in that of others—that similar systems are involved in the controlled appraisal of a stimulus to generate emotion and the controlled reappraisal of a stimulus to alter an ongoing emotion. The implication of this similarity is that the differential usage of the terms "appraisal" and "reappraisal" is somewhat artificial, although it still may be useful. What is important is to realize that the typical uses of the terms are limited. In common usage, "appraisal" is used to refer to the bottom-up generation of an emotional response, whereas "reappraisal" is used to refer to the top-down regulation of that response. This chapter suggests that the conflation of bottom-up and top-down processing with appraisal and reappraisal is neither theoretically nor empirically supported and, instead, that one can think of controlled appraisal processes as serving both generative and regulatory functions.

Future Directions

Although there appears to be some support for our initial formulation of a model—or functional architecture—for the cognitive control of emotion, the questions that remain to be answered far outnumber those that already have been addressed. At least three kinds of issues are salient. First, the great majority of research on use of cognition to control emotion has used negative stimuli. Whether it involves experiencing pain, viewing an aversive photograph, or expecting that one of the two soon will occur, there has been a decidedly sinister bent to extant research. Future work should address the relationship between the neural dynamics underlying the control of negative responses and those underlying the control of positive responses. Second, although work is beginning to investigate the ways in which types of control may fractionate into qualitatively different subtypes of control, little work has addressed this issue. It is possible, for example, that some strategies will differ in terms of the kinds of processing that are engaged in (e.g., those involving a self as compared with situation/perceptual/external focus), whereas others will differ because of the mental operations needed to transform responses to distinct kinds of stimuli (e.g., physically painful shock as compared with an aversive sound, odor, or visual image). Third, it will be important for future work to extend basic models to understanding both normal and abnormal individual differences in emotion and emotion control. Only by doing that will we be able to understand how it is that we can remove our "black masks" and see the world through the optimistic eyes of those whose appraisals permit effective emotion control.

ACKNOWLEDGMENTS

The completion of this chapter was supported in part by National Science Foundation Grant No. BCS-93679 and National Institutes of Health Grant No. MH58147.

REFERENCES

Adolphs, R. (2003). Cognitive neuroscience of human social behaviour. *Nature Review Neuroscience, 4*(3), 165–178.
Adolphs, R., Gosselin, F., Buchanan, T. W., Tranel, D., Schyns, P., & Damasio, A. R. (2005). A mechanism for impaired fear recognition after amygdala damage. *Nature, 433*(7021), 68–72.
Adolphs, R., Sears, L., & Piven, J. (2001). Abnormal processing of social information from faces in autism. *Journal of Cognitive Neuroscience, 13*(2), 232–240.
Adolphs, R., Tranel, D., & Damasio, A. R. (1998). The human amygdala in social judgment. *Nature, 393*(6684), 470–474.
American Psychiatric Association. (2000). *Diagnostic and statistical manual of mental disorders* (4th ed., text rev.). Washington, DC: Author.
Anderson, A. K., & Phelps, E. A. (2000). Expression without recognition: Contributions of the human amygdala to emotional communication. *Psychological Science, 11*(2), 106–111.
Anderson, A. K., & Phelps, E. A. (2001). Lesions of the human amygdala impair enhanced perception of emotionally salient events. *Nature, 411*(6835), 305–309.
Anderson, A. K., & Phelps, E. A. (2002). Is the human amygdala critical for the subjective experience of emotion? Evidence of intact dispositional affect in patients with amygdala lesions. *Journal of Cognitive Neuroscience, 14*(5), 709–720.

Bagby, R. M., Parker, J. D., & Taylor, G. J. (1994). The twenty-item Toronto Alexithymia Scale-I: Item selection and cross-validation of the factor structure. *Journal of Psychosomatic Research, 38*(1), 23–32.

Banich, M. T., Milham, M. P., Atchley, R. A., Cohen, N. J., Webb, A., Wszalek, T., et al. (2000). Prefrontal regions play a predominant role in imposing an attentional 'set': Evidence from fMRI. *Brain Research Cognitive Brain Research. 10*(1–2), 1–9.

Beauregard, M., Levesque, J., & Bourgouin, P. (2001). Neural correlates of conscious self-regulation of emotion. *Journal of Neuroscience, 21*(18), RC165.

Bechara, A., Damasio, H., & Damasio, A. R. (2000). Emotion, decision making and the orbitofrontal cortex. *Cerebral Cortex, 10*(3), 295–307.

Beer, J. S., Heerey, E. A., Keltner, D., Scabini, D., & Knight, R. T. (2003). The regulatory function of self-conscious emotion: Insights from patients with orbitofrontal damage. *Journal of Personality and Social Psychology, 85*(4), 594–604.

Beer, J. S., Shimamura, A. P., & Knight, R. T. (2004). Frontal lobe contributions to executive control of cognitive and social behavior. In M. S. Gazzaniga (Ed.), *Cognitive neurosciences* (Vol. 3, pp. 1091–1104). Cambridge, MA: MIT Press.

Bishop, S., Duncan, J., Brett, M., & Lawrence, A. D. (2004). Prefrontal cortical function and anxiety: Controlling attention to threat-related stimuli. *Nature Neuroscience, 7*(2), 184–188.

Botvinick, M. M., Braver, T. S., Barch, D. M., Carter, C. S., & Cohen, J. D. (2001). Conflict monitoring and cognitive control. *Psychological Review, 108*(3), 624–652.

Botvinick, M. M., Cohen, J. D., & Carter, C. S. (2004). Conflict monitoring and anterior cingulate cortex: An update. *Trends in Cognitive Sciences, 8*(12), 539–546.

Breiter, H. C., Rauch, S. L., Kwong, K. K., Baker, J. R., Weisskoff, R. M., Kennedy, D. N., et al. (1996). Functional magnetic resonance imaging of symptom provocation in obsessive–compulsive disorder. *Archives of General Psychiatry, 53*(7), 595–606.

Bremner, J. D., Narayan, M., Staib, L. H., Southwick, S. M., McGlashan, T., & Charney, D. S. (1999). Neural correlates of memories of childhood sexual abuse in women with and without posttraumatic stress disorder. *American Journal of Psychiatry, 156*(11), 1787–1795.

Buchel, C., & Dolan, R. J. (2000). Classical fear conditioning in functional neuroimaging. *Current Opinion in Neurobiology, 10*(2), 219–223.

Bunge, S. A., Dudukovic, N. M., Thomason, M. E., Vaidya, C. J., & Gabrieli, J. D. (2002). Immature frontal lobe contributions to cognitive control in children: Evidence from fMRI. *Neuron, 33*(2), 301–311.

Bunge, S. A., Ochsner, K. N., Desmond, J. E., Glover, G. H., & Gabrieli, J. D. (2001). Prefrontal regions involved in keeping information in and out of mind. *Brain, 124*(Pt. 10), 2074–2086.

Bush, G., Luu, P., & Posner, M. I. (2000). Cognitive and emotional influences in anterior cingulate cortex. *Trends in Cognitive Sciences, 4*(6), 215–222.

Cabeza, R., & Nyberg, L. (2000). Neural bases of learning and memory: Functional neuroimaging evidence. *Current Opinion in Neurology, 13*(4), 415–421.

Calder, A. J., Lawrence, A. D., & Young, A. W. (2001). Neuropsychology of fear and loathing. *Nature Reviews. Neuroscience, 2*(5), 352–363.

Cato, M. A., Crosson, B., Gokcay, D., Soltysik, D., Wierenga, C., Gopinath, K., et al. (2004). Processing words with emotional connotation: An fMRI study of time course and laterality in rostral frontal and retrosplenial cortices. *Journal of Cognitive Neuroscience, 16*(2), 167–177.

Compton, R. J., Banich, M. T., Mohanty, A., Milham, M. P., Herrington, J., Miller, G. A., et al. (2003). Paying attention to emotion: An fMRI investigation of cognitive and emotional stroop tasks. *Cognitive, Affective, and Behavioral Neuroscience, 3*(2), 81–96.

Critchley, H. D., Wiens, S., Rotshtein, P., Ohman, A., & Dolan, R. J. (2004). Neural systems supporting interoceptive awareness. *Nature Neuroscience, 7*(2), 189–195.

Crosson, B., Radonovich, K., Sadek, J. R., Gokcay, D., Bauer, R. M., Fischler, I. S., et al. (1999). Left-hemisphere processing of emotional connotation during word generation. *Neuroreport, 10*(12), 2449–2455.

Davis, M. (1998). Are different parts of the extended amygdala involved in fear versus anxiety? *Biological Psychiatry, 44*(12), 1239–1247.

Delgado, M. R., Nystrom, L. E., Fissell, C., Noll, D. C., & Fiez, J. A. (2000). Tracking the hemodynamic responses to reward and punishment in the striatum. *Journal of Neurophysiology, 84*(6), 3072–3077.

D'Esposito, M., Postle, B. R., Ballard, D., & Lease, J. (1999). Maintenance versus manipulation of information held in working memory: An event-related fMRI study. *Brain Cognitive, 41*(1), 66–86.

Drevets, W. C., Gadde, K., & Krishman, R. (1997). Neuroimaging studies of depression. In D. S. Charney, E. J. Nestler, & B. J. Bunney (Eds.), *Neurobiology of mental illness* (pp. 394–418). New York: Oxford University Press.

Eisenberger, N. I., Lieberman, M. D., & Satpute, A. B. (2005). Personality from a controlled processing perspective: An MRI study of neuroticism, extraversion, and self-consciousness. *Cognitive, Affective, and Behavioral Neuroscience 5*(2), 169196181.

Erickson, K. I., Milham, M. P., Colcombe, S. J., Kramer, A. F., Banich, M. T., Webb, A., et al. (2004). Behavioral conflict, anterior cingulate cortex, and experiment duration: Implications of diverging data. *Human Brain Mapping, 21*(2), 98–107.

Feldman Barrett, L., Ochsner, K. N., & Gross, J. J. (in press). Automaticity and emotion. In J. A. Bargh (Ed.), *Automatic processes in social thinking and behavior.* New York: Psychology Press.

Fellows, L. K., & Farah, M. J. (2004). Different underlying impairments in decision-making following ventromedial and dorsolateral frontal lobe damage in humans. *Cerebral Cortex.*

Fellows, L. K., & Farah, M. J. (2005). Is anterior cingulate cortex necessary for cognitive control? *Brain, 128*(Pt. 4), 788–796.

Gallagher, H. L., & Frith, C. D. (2003). Functional imaging of "theory of mind." *Trends in Cognitive Science, 7*(2), 77–83.

Gusnard, D. A., Akbudak, E., Shulman, G. L., & Raichle, M. E. (2001). Medial prefrontal cortex and self-referential mental activity: Relation to a default mode of brain function. *Proceedings of the National Academy of Sciences of the USA, 98*(7), 4259–4264.

Hamann, S. (2001). Cognitive and neural mechanisms of emotional memory. *Trends in Cognitive Science, 5*(9), 394–400.

Hornak, J., O'Doherty, J., Bramham, J., Rolls, E. T., Morris, R. G., Bullock, P. R., et al. (2004). Reward-related reversal learning after surgical excisions in orbito-frontal or dorsolateral prefrontal cortex in humans. *Journal of Cognitive Neuroscience, 16*(3), 463–478.

Jonides, J., Smith, E. E., Marshuetz, C., Koeppe, R. A., & Reuter-Lorenz, P. A. (1998). Inhibition in verbal working memory revealed by brain activation. *Proceedings of the National Academy of Sciences of the USA, 95*(14), 8410–8413.

Kalisch, R., Wiech, K., Critchley, H. D., Seymour, B., O'Doherty, J. P., Oakley, D. A., Allen, P., & Dolan, R. J. (2005). Anxiety reduction through detachment: Subjective, physiological, and neural effects. *Journal of Cognitive Neuroscience, 17*(6), 874–883.

Kelley, W. M., Macrae, C. N., Wyland, C. L., Caglar, S., Inati, S., & Heatherton, T. F. (2002). Finding the self? An event-related fMRI study. *Journal of Cognitive Neuroscience, 14*(5), 785–794.

Knutson, B., Adams, C. M., Fong, G. W., & Hommer, D. (2001). Anticipation of increasing monetary reward selectively recruits nucleus accumbens. *Journal of Neuroscience, 21*(16), RC159.

Knutson, B., Fong, G. W., Adams, C. M., Varner, J. L., & Hommer, D. (2001). Dissociation of reward anticipation and outcome with event-related fMRI. *Neuroreport, 12*(17), 3683–3687.

Konishi, S., Nakajima, K., Uchida, I., Kikyo, H., Kameyama, M., & Miyashita, Y. (1999). Common inhibitory mechanism in human inferior prefrontal cortex revealed by event-related functional MRI. *Brain, 122*(Pt. 5), 981–991.

LaBar, K. S., & LeDoux, J. E. (1996). Partial disruption of fear conditioning in rats with unilateral amygdala damage: Correspondence with unilateral temporal lobectomy in humans. *Behavioral Neuroscience, 110*(5), 991–997.

Lane, R. D., Ahern, G. L., Schwartz, G. E., & Kaszniak, A. W. (1997). Is alexithymia the emotional equivalent of blindsight? *Biological Psychiatry, 42*(9), 834–844.

Lane, R. D., Chua, P. M., & Dolan, R. J. (1999). Common effects of emotional valence, arousal and attention on neural activation during visual processing of pictures. *Neuropsychologia, 37*(9), 989–997.

Lane, R. D., Fink, G. R., Chau, P. M., & Dolan, R. J. (1997). Neural activation during selective attention to subjective emotional responses. *Neuroreport, 8*(18), 3969–3972.

Lane, R. D., Sechrest, L., Riedel, R., Shapiro, D. E., & Kasszniak, A. W. (2000). Pervasive emotion recognition deficit common to alexithymia and the repressive coping style. *Psychosomatic Medicine, 62*(4), 492–501.

Lang, P. J., Greenwald, M. K., Bradley, M. M., & Hamm, A. O. (1993). Looking at pictures: Affective, facial, visceral, and behavioral reactions. *Psychophysiology, 30*(3), 261–273.

Lazarus, R. S. (1991). *Emotion and adaptation.* Oxford, UK: Oxford University Press.

Lazarus, R. S., & Alfert, E. (1964). Short-circuiting of threat by experimentally altering cognitive appraisal. *Journal of Abnormal and Social Psychology, 69*, 195–205.

LeDoux, J. E. (2000). Emotion circuits in the brain. *Annual Review of Neuroscience, 23*, 155–184.

Levesque, J., Joanette, Y., Mensour, B., Beaudoin, G., Leroux, J. M., Bourgouin, P. & Beauregard, M. (2004). Neural basis of emotional self-regulation in childhood. *Neuroscience, 129*(2), 361–369.

Levesque, J., Eugene, F., Joanette, Y., Paquette, V., Mensour, B., Beaudoin, G., et al. (2003). Neural circuitry underlying voluntary suppression of sadness. *Biological Psychiatry, 53*(6), 502–510.

Levesque, J., Joanette, Y., Mensour, B., Beaudoin, G., Leroux, J. M., Bourgouin, P., et al. (2004). Neural basis of emotional self-regulation in childhood. *Neuroscience, 129*(2), 361–369.

Liberzon, I., Taylor, S. F., Amdur, R., Jung, T. D., Chamberlain, K. R., Minoshima, S., et al. (1999). Brain activation in PTSD in response to trauma-related stimuli. *Biological Psychiatry, 45*(7), 817–826.

Lieberman, M. D. (2000). Intuition: A social cognitive neuroscience approach. *Psychological Bulletin, 126*(1), 109–137.

Lieberman, M. D., Jarcho, J. M., Berman, S., Naliboff, B. D., Suyenobu, B. Y., Mandelkern, M., et al. (2004). The neural correlates of placebo effects: A disruption account. *NeuroImage, 22*(1), 447–455.

Luna, B., Thulborn, K. R., Munoz, D. P., Merriam, E. P., Garver, K. E., Minshew, N. J., et al. (2001). Maturation of widely distributed brain function subserves cognitive development. *NeuroImage, 13*(5), 786–793.

Milham, M. P., Banich, M. T., Webb, A., Barad, V., Cohen, N. J., Wszalek, T., et al. (2001). The relative involvement of anterior cingulate and prefrontal cortex in attentional control depends on nature of conflict. *Brain Research. Cognitive Brain Research, 12*(3), 467–473.

Miller, E. K., & Cohen, J. D. (2001). An integrative theory of prefrontal cortex function. *Annual Review of Neuroscience, 24,* 167–202.

Mitchell, J. P., Heatherton, T. F., & Macrae, C. N. (2002). Distinct neural systems subserve person and object knowledge. *Proceedings of the National Academy of Sciences of the USA, 99*(23), 15238–15243.

Mitchell, J. P., Macrae, C. N., & Banaji, M. R. (In press). The link between social cognition and the self-referential thought in the medial prefrontal cortex. *Journal of Cognitive Neuroscience.*

Mohanty, A., Herrington, J. D., Koven, N. S., Fisher, J. E., Wenzel, E. A., Webb, A. G., et al. (2005). Neural mechanisms of affective interference in schizotypy. *Journal of Abnormal Psychology, 114*(1), 16–27.

Morris, J. S., & Dolan, R. J. (2004). Dissociable amygdala and orbitofrontal responses during reversal fear conditioning. *NeuroImage, 22*(1), 372–380.

Morris, J. S., Ohman, A., & Dolan, R. J. (1999). A subcortical pathway to the right amygdala mediating "unseen" fear. *Proceedings of the National Academy of Sciences of the USA, 96*(4), 1680–1685.

Nelson, C. A., Monk, C. S., Lin, J., Carver, L. J., Thomas, K. M., & Truwit, C. L. (2000). Functional neuroanatomy of spatial working memory in children. *Developmental Psychology, 36*(1), 109–116.

Nolen-Hoeksema, S. (2000). The role of rumination in depressive disorders and mixed anxiety/depressive symptoms. *Journal of Abnormal Psychology, 109*(3), 504–511.

Ochsner, K. N. (2004). Current directions in social cognitive neuroscience. *Current Opinion in Neurobiology, 14*(2), 254–258.

Ochsner, K. N. (2005). Characterizing the functional architecture of affect regulation: Emerging answers and outstanding questions. In J. T. Cacioppo (Ed.), *Social Neuroscience: People thinking about people* (pp. 245–268). Cambridge, MA: MIT Press.

Ochsner, K. N., McRae, K., Ray, R. D., Cooper, J. C., Robertson, E. R., Gross, J. J., et al. (2006). *Neural systems supporting the development of cognitive emotion regulation from adolescence through adulthood.* Unpublished manuscript, Columbia University, New York.

Ochsner, K. N., Beer, J. S., Robertson, E., Cooper, J., Gabrieli, J. D. E., Kihlstrom, J. F., et al. (2005). The neural correlates of direct and reflected self-knowledge. *NeuroImage, 28*(4), 797–814.

Ochsner, K. N., Bunge, S. A., Gross, J. J., & Gabrieli, J. D. (2002). Rethinking feelings: An FMRI study of the cognitive regulation of emotion. *Journal of Cognitive Neuroscience, 14*(8), 1215–1229.

Ochsner, K. N., & Feldman Barrett, L. (2001). A multiprocess perspective on the neuroscience of emotion. In T. J. Mayne & G. A. Bonanno (Eds.), *Emotions: Current issues and future directions* (pp. 38–81). New York: Guilford Press.

Ochsner, K. N., & Gross, J. J. (2005). The cognitive control of emotion. *Trends in Cognitive Sciences, 9*(5), 242–249.

Ochsner, K. N., Knierim, K., Ludlow, D., Hanelin, J., Ramachandran, T., & Mackey, S. (2004). Reflecting upon feelings: An fMRI study of neural systems supporting the attribution of emotion to self and other. *Journal of Cognitive Neuroscience, 16*(10), 1746–1772.

Ochsner, K. N., & Kosslyn, S. M. (1999). The cognitive neuroscience approach. In B. M. Bly & D. E. Rumelhart (Eds.), *Cognitive science* (pp. 319–365). San Diego, CA: Academic Press.

Ochsner, K. N., & Lieberman, M. D. (2001). The emergence of social cognitive neuroscience. *Ameerican Psychologist, 56*(9), 717–734.

Ochsner, K. N., Ray, R. D., Cooper, J. C., Robertson, E. R., Chopra, S., Gabrieli, J. D. E., et al. (2004). For better or for worse: Neural systems supporting the cognitive down- and up-regulation of negative emotion. *NeuroImage, 23*(2), 483–499.

O'Doherty, J., Critchley, H., Deichmann, R., & Dolan, R. J. (2003). Dissociating valence of outcome from behavioral control in human orbital and ventral prefrontal cortices. *Journal of Neuroscience, 23*(21), 7931–7939.

O'Doherty, J. P., Deichmann, R., Critchley, H. D., & Dolan, R. J. (2002). Neural responses during anticipation of a primary taste reward. *Neuron, 33*(5), 815–826.

Paradiso, S., Johnson, D. L., Andreasen, N. C., O'Leary, D. S., Watkins, G. L., Ponto, L. L., et al. (1999). Cerebral blood flow changes associated with attribution of emotional valence to pleasant, unpleasant, and neutral visual stimuli in a PET study of normal subjects. *American Journal of Psychiatry, 156*(10), 1618–1629.

Perlstein, W. M., Dixit, N. K., Carter, C. S., Noll, D. C., & Cohen, J. D. (2003). Prefrontal cortex dysfunction mediates deficits in working memory and prepotent responding in schizophrenia. *Biological Psychiatry, 53*(1), 25–38.

Petrovic, P., Kalso, E., Petersson, K. M., & Ingvar, M. (2002). Placebo and opioid analgesia: Imaging a shared neuronal network. *Science, 295*(5560), 1737-1740.

Phan, K. L., Fitzgerald, D. A., Nathan, P. J., Moore, G. J., Uhde, T. W., & Tancer,

M. E. (2005). Neural substrates for voluntary suppression of negative affect: A functional magnetic resonance imaging study. *Biological Psychiatry, 57*(3), 210–219.

Phelps, E. A., LaBar, K. S., Anderson, A. K., O'Connor, K. J., Fulbright, R. K., & Spencer, D. D. (1998). Specifying the contributions of the human amygdala to emotional memory: A case study. *Neurocase, 4*(6), 527–540.

Phelps, E. A., O'Connor, K. J., Gatenby, J. C., Gore, J. C., Grillon, C., & Davis, M. (2001). Activation of the left amygdala to a cognitive representation of fear. *Nature Neuroscience, 4*(4), 437–441.

Phillips, M. L., Drevets, W. C., Rauch, S. L., & Lane, R. (2003a). Neurobiology of emotion perception: I. The neural basis of normal emotion perception. *Biological Psychiatry, 54*(5), 504–514.

Phillips, M. L., Drevets, W. C., Rauch, S. L., & Lane, R. (2003b). Neurobiology of emotion perception: II. Implications for major psychiatric disorders. *Biological Psychiatry, 54*(5), 515–528.

Ploghaus, A., Tracey, I., Gati, J. S., Clare, S., Menon, R. S., Matthews, P. M., et al. (1999). Dissociating pain from its anticipation in the human brain. *Science, 284*(5422), 1979–1981.

Rauch, S. L., Savage, C. R., Alpert, N. M., Fischman, A. J., & Jenike, M. A. (1997). The functional neuroanatomy of anxiety: A study of three disorders using positron emission tomography and symptom provocation. *Biological Psychiatry, 42*(6), 446–452.

Ray, R. D., Ochsner, K. N., Cooper, J. C., Robertson, E. R., Gabrieli, J. D. E., & Gross, J. J. (2005). Individual differences in trait rumination modulate neural systems supporting the cognitive regulation of emotion. *Cognitive, Affective, and Behavioral Neuroscience 5*(2), 156–168.

Russell, T. A., Rubia, K., Bullmore, E. T., Soni, W., Suckling, J., Brammer, M. J., et al. (2000). Exploring the social brain in schizophrenia: Left prefrontal underactivation during mental state attribution. *American Journal of Psychiatry, 157*(12), 2040–2042.

Sarter, M., Berntson, G. G., & Cacioppo, J. T. (1996). Brain imaging and cognitive neuroscience: Toward strong inference in attributing function to structure. *American Psychologist, 51*(1), 13–21.

Schacter, D. L. (1997). The cognitive neuroscience of memory: perspectives from neuroimaging research. *Philosophical Transactions of the Royal Society of London: Series B. Biological Sciences, 352*(1362), 1689–1695.

Schaefer, S. M., Jackson, D. C., Davidson, R. J., Aguirre, G. K., Kimberg, D. Y., & Thompson-Schill, S. L. (2002). Modulation of amygdalar activity by the conscious regulation of negative emotion. *Journal of Cognitive Neuroscience, 14*(6), 913–921.

Scherer, K. R. (1984). On the nature and function of emotion: A component process approach. In K. R. Scherer & P. Ekman (Eds.), *Approaches to emotion* (pp. 293–317). Hillsdale, NJ: Erlbaum.

Scherer, K. R., Schorr, A., & Johnstone, T. (Eds.). (2001). *Appraisal processes in emotion: Theory, methods, research.* New York: Oxford University Press.

Shin, L. M., Whalen, P. J., Pitman, R. K., Bush, G., Macklin, M. L., Lasko, N. B., et al. (2001). An fMRI study of anterior cingulate function in posttraumatic stress disorder. *Biological Psychiatry, 50*(12), 932–942.

Sifneos, P. E. (1996). Alexithymia: Past and present. *American Journal of Psychiatry, 153*(7, Suppl.), 137–142.

Smith, C. A., & Ellsworth, P. C. (1985). Patterns of cognitive appraisal in emotion. *Journal of Personality and Social Psychology, 48*, 813–838.

Smith, E. E., & Jonides, J. (1998). Neuroimaging analyses of human working memory. *Proceedings of the National Academy of Sciences of the USA, 95*(20), 12061–12068.

Smith, E. E., Jonides, J., Marshuetz, C., & Koeppe, R. A. (1998). Components of verbal working memory: Evidence from neuroimaging. *Proceedings of the National Academy of Sciences of the USA, 95*(3), 876–882.

Spielberger, C. D., Gorsuch, R. L., Lushemne, R., Vagg, P. R., & Jacobs, G. A. (1983). *Manual for the State–Trait Anxiety Inventory (Form Y)*. Palo Alto, CA: Consulting Psychologists Press.

Teasdale, J. D., Moore, R. G., Hayhurst, H., Pope, M., Williams, S., & Segal, Z. V. (2002). Metacognitive awareness and prevention of relapse in depression: Empirical evidence. *Journal of Consulting and Clinical Psychology, 70*(2), 275–287.

Teasdale, J. D., Scott, J., Moore, R. G., Hayhurst, H., Pope, M., & Paykel, E. S. (2001). How does cognitive therapy prevent relapse in residual depression? Evidence from a controlled trial. *Journal of Consulting and Clinical Psychology, 69*(3), 347–357.

Tulving, E. (2002). Episodic memory: From mind to brain. *Annual Review of Psychology, 53*, 1–25.

Wager, T. D., Jonides, J., & Reading, S. (2004). Neuroimaging studies of shifting attention: A meta-analysis. *Neuroimage, 22*(4), 1679–1693.

Wager, T. D., Rilling, J. K., Smith, E. E., Sokolik, A., Casey, K. L., Davidson, R. J., et al. (2004). Placebo-induced changes in FMRI in the anticipation and experience of pain. *Science, 303*(5661), 1162–1167.

Wager, T. D., & Smith, E. E. (2003). Neuroimaging studies of working memory: A meta-analysis. *Cognitive, Affective, and Behavioral Neuroscience, 3*(4), 255–274.

Wagner, A. D., Pare-Blagoev, E. J., Clark, J., & Poldrack, R. A. (2001). Recovering meaning: Left prefrontal cortex guides controlled semantic retrieval. *Neuron, 31*(2), 329–338.

Whalen, P. J., Bush, G., McNally, R. J., Wilhelm, S., McInerney, S. C., Jenike, M. A., et al. (1998). The emotional counting Stroop paradigm: A functional magnetic resonance imaging probe of the anterior cingulate affective division. *Biological Psychiatry, 44*(12), 1219–1228.

Whalen, P. J., Rauch, S. L., Etcoff, N. L., McInerney, S. C., Lee, M. B., & Jenike, M. A. (1998). Masked presentations of emotional facial expressions modulate amygdala activity without explicit knowledge. *Journal of Neuroscience, 18*(1), 411–418.

Winston, J. S., Strange, B. A., O'Doherty, J., & Dolan, R. J. (2002). Automatic and intentional brain responses during evaluation of trustworthiness of faces. *Nature Neuroscience, 5*(3), 277–283.

Winkielman, P. & Berridge, K. C. (2004). Unconscious emotion. Current Directions in Psychological Science, 13, 120-123

III

MOTIVATION PROCESSES

7

Asymmetrical Frontal Cortical Activity, Affective Valence, and Motivational Direction

Eddie Harmon-Jones

In the past decade, there has been a renewed interest in the constructs of approach and withdrawal motivation and how they affect social-psychological processes and behaviors. At the same time, several models of emotion have considered the pleasant-to-unpleasant dimension of emotion an important organizing principle, and several conceptual models have suggested that approach motivation is always related to pleasant emotions and that withdrawal motivation is always related to unpleasant emotions (Watson, 2000). The research I review in this chapter will bear on these issues and on whether these widely held assumptions are indeed valid. But before getting to these issues, I explain how my neuroscience research became involved with social psychological theories and methods.

My interest in approach and withdrawal motivation was sparked by a conceptual question in affective neuroscience that had not been addressed in the mid-1990s—that is, whether high left frontal cortical activation reflects approach motivation or positive affect. Because approach motivation and positive affect often co-occur, these had been confounded in all previous research. The conceptual thinking behind the past research often assumed that approach motivation and positive valence always occurred together. Using social-psychological methods and theories, my colleagues and I were able to disentangle the constructs of affective valence and motivational direction and provide evidence that demonstrated that approach motivation, not positive affect per se, was associated with activation of the left frontal cortex. In addition, our work in affective neuroscience benefited social-psychological theorizing, particularly in relation to anger and aggression processes. In this chapter, I discuss these contributions and demonstrate how integrating neuroscience with social psychology benefits both fields.

Much of the research on asymmetrical frontal brain activity has assessed the activity using alpha frequency band activity derived from the electroencephalograph (EEG). Research has revealed that alpha power is inversely related to other measures of brain activity, such as positron emission tomography (PET; Cook, O'Hara, Uijtdehaage, Mandelkern, & Leuchter, 1998) and functional magnetic resonance imaging (fMRI; Goldman, Stern, Engel, & Cohen, 2002). Additional data from individuals with brain damage supports the research reviewed in this article (e.g., Robinson & Downhill, 1995). Although EEG alpha power is inversely correlated with PET and fMRI measures, it may assess different aspects of brain activity (e.g., pre- vs. postsynaptic potentials).

Because of the recent increase in the use of PET, fMRI, and EEG measurements in social neuroscience, it is important to discuss how these measures differ and the pros and cons of using each one. Ultimately, both PET and fMRI rely on blood flow to brain areas recently involved in neuronal activity, though other changes also affect fMRI, such as oxygen consumption and blood volume changes. Because both PET and fMRI measure blood flow rather than neuronal activity, the activations are not simultaneous with neuronal activations but are blood responses to neuronal responses. Thus there is a biological limit on the time resolution of the response such that, even in the best measurement systems, the peak blood flow response occurs 6–9 seconds after stimulus onset (Reiman, Lane, Van Petten, & Bandettini, 2000). However, there are suggestions that experimental methods can be designed to detect stimulus condition differences as early as 2 seconds after stimulus onset (Bellgowan, Saad, & Bandettini, 2003). Because the brain functions through electrical impulses, and because fMRI and PET measure blood flow in the brain rather than electrical activation, the temporal limitations of the measures are biological. In contrast, EEG measures electrical activations almost instantaneously, at millisecond resolution.

The spatial resolution of EEG, the ability to locate which specific areas of the brain generate the signals recorded, is currently not as good as spatial resolution with PET and fMRI. Much work is being conducted to achieve mathematical solutions to this problem, allowing EEG to achieve better spatial resolution (e.g., Dien, Spencer, & Donchin, 2003; Pascual-Marqui et al., 1999). EEG research is also much less costly than fMRI and PET research. Finally, PET and EEG permit measurement of tonic (e.g., resting, baseline) activity, as well as phasic (e.g., in response to a state manipulation) activity, whereas fMRI permits measurement of phasic but not tonic activity.

Because the majority of research on the frontal asymmetry has used EEG alpha power, I review this research. In this review, I use the term "brain activity" to refer to the inverse of alpha power, as is commonly done in this literature. Moreover, I reserve the use of the term "activation" to refer to state-induced changes in EEG, whereas "activity" can refer to state or trait (baseline) EEG. Finally, the term "relative left frontal activity (or activation)" is used to describe greater left than right frontal activity—a difference or asymmetry score.

Scalp-recorded electrical activity is the result of activity of populations of neurons. The activity can be recorded on the scalp surface because the tissue between the neurons and the scalp acts as a volume conductor. Because the activity generated by one neuron is small, it is thought that the activity recorded at the scalp is the integrated activity of numerous neurons that are active synchronously. Moreover, for activity to be recorded at the scalp, the electric fields generated by each neuron must be oriented in such a way that their effects cumulate. That is, the neurons must be arranged in an open as opposed to closed field. In an open field, the neurons' dendrites are all oriented on one side of the structure, whereas their axons all depart from the other side. Open fields are present where neurons are organized in layers, as in most of the cortex, parts of the thalamus, the cerebellum, and other structures. Because of the need for summation of electrical potentials, the EEG activity is most likely the result of postsynaptic potentials, which have a slower time course and are more likely to be synchronous and summate than presynaptic potentials.

ASYMMETRICAL FRONTAL BRAIN ACTIVITY AND EMOTION

A variety of research approaches have pointed to the importance of the left and right frontal brain regions in emotion and motivation. Initially, research suggested that left frontal brain activity is associated with positive emotions and approach behavior and right frontal brain activity is associated with negative emotions and withdrawal behavior. This research has created an impression that high levels of left frontal activity are more psychologically and physically healthy than low levels of left frontal activity (e.g., Fox, Henderson, Rubin, Calkins, & Schmidt, 2001; Davidson, 1998). Indeed, the past findings have led therapists to create treatment strategies for psychological disorders aimed at increasing left frontal activity (e.g., Baehr, Rosenfeld, & Baehr, 1997; Rosenfeld, Cha, Blair, & Gotlib, 1995).

Relationship between Indices of Trait Affect/Motivation and Resting EEG

A number of studies have examined the relationship between asymmetrical frontal cortical activity recorded during resting baseline and other measures of trait affect and motivation. This research is based on the idea that baseline asymmetrical frontal cortical activity reflects a trait (e.g., Tomarken, Davidson, Wheeler, & Kinney, 1992).

Depression has been found to relate to resting frontal asymmetrical activity, with individuals with depression showing relatively less left than right frontal brain activity. This relationship between depression and asymmetrical frontal activity has been found in individuals identified by self-report indices of depression (Jacobs & Snyder, 1996; Schaffer, Davidson, & Saron, 1983) and in individuals identified through clinical interviews (Allen, Depue, Iacono, & Arbisi, 1993). Moreover, relatively less left frontal activity has been found in individuals who were previously clinically depressed but were in remission status compared with individuals who had never experienced clinical depression (Henriques & Davidson, 1990).

Other research has revealed that trait-positive affect is associated with greater left than right frontal brain activity, whereas trait-negative affect is associated with greater right than left frontal brain activity (e.g., Tomarken, Davidson, Wheeler, & Doss, 1992). In this past research, trait-positive and trait-negative affect were assessed using the Positive and Negative Affect Schedule (PANAS; Watson, Clark, & Tellegen, 1988). Watson et al. have recently stated that they consider this scale a measure of activated positive affect and activated negative affect (Watson, Wiese, Vaidya, & Tellegen, 1999), because the items on the scales assess activated or aroused positive and negative affects (e.g., active, interested, afraid, distressed), not ones lower in arousal (e.g., happy, sad).

Other research has found that trait behavioral activation sensitivity (BAS) relates to greater left than right frontal brain activity (Coan & Allen, 2003; Harmon-Jones & Allen, 1997; Sutton & Davidson, 1997). In this research, BAS was measured by Carver and White's (1994) BIS/BAS questionnaire, which includes items such as "When I want something, I usually go all-out to get it."

Studies have produced inconsistent results regarding the relationship of behavioral inhibition sensitivity (BIS; "I worry about making mistakes") and frontal brain asymmetry. One study found a significant relationship between BIS and greater right than left frontal activity (Sutton & Davidson, 1997), whereas two others found a nonsignificant relationship (Coan & Allen, 2003; Harmon-Jones & Allen, 1997). Although researchers have hypothesized that right frontal brain activity is increased during withdrawal, BIS may not be equivalent to withdrawal motivation (Harmon-Jones & Allen, 1997).

Relationship between Resting EEG and Responses to Emotion-Eliciting Stimuli

Resting baseline frontal asymmetrical activity also predicts emotional responses to emotion-eliciting stimuli. Individuals with relatively greater right than left frontal activity exhibit larger negative affective responses to negative-emotion-inducing films (fear and disgust) and smaller positive affective responses to positive-emotion-inducing films (happiness; Tomarken, Davidson, & Henriques, 1990; Wheeler, Davidson, & Tomarken, 1993). In a related vein, research has found that resting baseline frontal asymmetrical activity predicted evaluative responses to merely exposed stimuli (Harmon-Jones & Allen, 2001). According to Zajonc's (1968) theory, exposing individuals to novel stimuli without reward or punishment (mere exposure) signals safety. Individuals with greater relative right frontal activity reported more favorable attitudes toward familiarized stimuli than did individuals with relative left frontal activity. Other research has found that relative right frontal activity at baseline predicts crying in response to maternal separation in 10-month-old infants (Davidson & Fox, 1989).

Although these effects are based on correlational evidence and hence subject to alternative explanations, a recent study has more strongly suggested that the frontal asymmetry is causally involved in the production of these emotional responses. In this experiment, neurofeedback training was used to manipulate the frontal asymmetry (Allen, Harmon-Jones, & Cavender, 2001). Participants were randomly assigned to receive neurofeedback training designed to increase right frontal relative to left frontal activity or to receive training in the opposite direction. Systematic alterations of frontal asymmetry were observed as a function of neurofeedback training. Moreover, subsequent self-reported affect in response to emotionally evocative film clips was significantly influenced by the direction of neurofeedback training. Individuals trained to increase left frontal activity reported more positive affect in response to the happy film clip than individuals trained to increase right frontal activity.

EEG Activity during Exposure to Emotionally Evocative Situations

Research has also demonstrated that asymmetrical frontal brain activity is associated with state emotional responses. For instance, 10-month-old infants exhibited increased left frontal activation in response to a film clip of an actress generating a happy facial expression as compared with a clip of an actress generating a sad facial expression (Davidson & Fox, 1982). Newborn infants (2–3 days old) evidenced greater relative left-sided activation in frontal regions to sucrose than to water (Fox & Davidson, 1986). Frontal brain activity has been found to relate to facial expressions of positive and negative emotions, as well. For example, Ekman and Davidson (1993) found increased left frontal activation during voluntary facial expressions of smiles of enjoyment (i.e., activation of zygomatic major with concurrent activation of orbicularis oculi, pars lateralis) as compared with voluntary facial expressions of smiles not associated with enjoyment (i.e., activation of zygomatic major without orbicularis oculi, pars lateralis).

More recently, Coan, Allen, and Harmon-Jones (2001) found that voluntary contractions of the facial musculature to form a happy facial expression produced relatively greater left frontal activity and that voluntary contractions of the facial musculature to form a fearful facial expression produced relatively less left frontal activity.

Explanations of the Relationship between Asymmetrical Frontal Brain Activity and Emotion

Primarily, three conceptual models have been designed to explain the observed results. The first view, the *valence model*, has posited that the left frontal brain region is involved in the experience and expression of positive emotion and that the right frontal brain region is involved in the expression and experience of negative emotion (e.g., Ahern & Schwartz, 1985; Gotlib, Ranganath, & Rosenfeld, 1998; Heller, 1990; Heller & Nitschke, 1998; Silberman & Weingartner, 1986). A second view, the *motivation direction model*, has posited that the left frontal brain region is involved in expression of approach-related emotions and that the right frontal brain region is involved in expression of withdrawal-related emotions (Davidson, 1995; Fox, 1991; Harmon-Jones & Allen, 1997; Sutton & Davidson, 1997). A third view, the *valenced motivation model*, has posited that the left frontal brain region is involved in the expression and experience of positive, approach-related emotions and that the right frontal brain region is involved in the expression and experience of negative, withdrawal-related emotions (Davidson, 1998; Tomarken & Keener, 1998).

Because the previously conducted research confounded the valence of emotion with the direction of motivation, it is unable to address whether the frontal asymmetry reflects the valence of the emotion, the direction of the motivation, or a combination of valence and motivation. Often, positive emotion is associated with approach-related motivation, whereas negative emotion is associated with withdrawal-related motivation. Indeed, most contemporary theories of emotion posit that positive emotion is always associated with approach motivation and that negative emotion is always associated with withdrawal motivation (e.g., Watson, 2000; for a different point of view, see Carver, 2001). However, not all emotions behave in accordance with this presumed relationship between the valence of emotion and the direction of motivation. Anger is one of the best examples of a violation of the relationship, because anger is negative in valence (e.g., Lazarus, 1991; Watson et al., 1999), but it often evokes approach motivation (e.g., Berkowitz, 1999; Darwin, 1872/1965; Plutchik, 1980; Young, 1943).

To address the primary emotional/motivation functions of asymmetrical frontal brain activity, my colleagues and I have been examining the emotion of anger. Because anger is a negative emotion that evokes approach motivational tendencies, anger provides the means to unconfound valence from motivational direction. By examining the emotion of anger, we are in a position to answer precisely what the emotional/motivational functions of asymmetrical frontal brain activity are.

ANGER AND APPROACH MOTIVATION

Before reviewing the research on anger and asymmetrical frontal activity, we must consider whether anger is indeed associated with approach motivation. Several lines of research suggest that anger elicits behavioral approach or approach motivation tendencies. In the animal behavior literature, a distinction has been made between offensive or irritable aggression and defensive aggression (Flynn, Vanegas, Foote, & Edwards, 1970; Moyer, 1976). It has been posited that irritable aggression results from anger and that pure irritable aggression "involves attack without attempts to escape from the object being attacked" (Moyer, 1976, p. 187). A number of aggression researchers have suggested that offensive aggression is associated with anger, attack, and no attempts to escape, whereas defensive aggression is associated with fear, attempts to escape, and attack only if escape is impossible (Blanchard & Blanchard, 1984; Lagerspetz, 1969; Moyer, 1976).

In research on humans, Lewis, Sullivan, Ramsay, and Alessandri (1992) found that infants who expressed anger during extinction maintained interest during subsequent relearning, whereas infants who expressed sadness during extinction evidenced decreased interest during relearning. Thus, subsequent to frustrating events, anger may maintain and increase task engagement and approach motivation.

Additional support for the idea that anger is associated with approach motivation comes from tests of the conceptual model that integrated reactance theory with learned helplessness theory (Wortman & Brehm, 1975). According to this model, how individuals respond to uncontrollable outcomes depends on their expectation of being able to control the outcome and the importance of the outcome. Reactance is a state characterized by the emotion of anger and by intensified attempts to achieve the goal. When an individual expects to be able to control outcomes that are important and those outcomes are found to be uncontrollable, psychological reactance is aroused. Thus, for individuals who initially expect control, the first few bouts of uncontrollable outcomes arouse reactance, a motivational state aimed at restoring control. After several exposures to uncontrollable outcomes, these individuals become convinced that they cannot control the outcomes, and they experience decreased motivation (i.e., learned helplessness). In one study testing this model, individuals who exhibited angry feelings in response to one unsolvable problem showed better performance on a subsequent cognitive task than did participants who exhibited less anger (Mikulincer, 1988). The improved performance was presumably due to the associated approach motivational state.

Other research has revealed that state anger relates to high levels of self-assurance, physical strength, and bravery (Harmon-Jones et al., 2006; Izard, 1991), inclinations associated with approach motivation. Additionally, Lerner and Keltner (2001) found that anger and happiness (both trait and state) are associated with optimistic expectations, whereas fear is associated with pessimistic expectations.

Further evidence supporting the conceptualization of anger as involving approach and not withdrawal comes from research on testosterone. Testosterone levels are positively associated with anger and aggression in humans (e.g., Olweus, 1986), and administration of testosterone decreases withdrawal responses in a number of species (e.g., Boissy & Bouissou, 1994; Vandenheede & Bouissou, 1993).

Recently, two additional individual-differences studies were conducted to test the hypothesis that trait anger is related to trait approach motivation (Harmon-Jones, 2003). In both studies, trait BAS, or approach motivation, as assessed by Carver and White's (1994) scale, was positively related to trait anger at the simple correlation level, as assessed by the Buss and Perry (1992) aggression questionnaire. In a second study, BAS was positively correlated with physical aggression. Simultaneously regressing aggression onto BAS, BIS, and general negative affect revealed that physical aggression was positively related to BAS, negatively related to BIS, and positively related to negative affect. These results support the hypothesis that anger is related to approach motivation and strongly challenge theoretical models that assume that approach motivation is associated only with positive affect.

ANGER AND ASYMMETRICAL FRONTAL BRAIN ACTIVITY

Because of the large body of evidence suggesting that anger is associated with approach motivation, anger provided an excellent opportunity to unconfound positive emotional valence from approach motivational direction. We examined the relationship between anger and relative left frontal activation to test whether the frontal asymmetry is due to emotional valence, motivational direction, or a combination of emotional valence and motivational direction.

Asymmetrical Frontal Activity and Trait Anger

In the first study examining the relationship between anger and asymmetrical frontal brain activity (Harmon-Jones & Allen, 1998), EEGs of young adolescents were recorded as they sat quietly for 6 minutes. Trait anger was measured using the Buss and Perry (1992) aggression questionnaire. Results indicated that trait anger was positively related to relatively greater left than right frontal brain activity. Moreover, additional analyses revealed that high levels of trait anger were associated with both increased left frontal activity and decreased right frontal activity. These results suggest that the frontal asymmetry is associated with motivational direction (approach vs. withdrawal) rather than emotional valence.

A second study was conducted to address whether the relationship of anger with increased left frontal activation could be explained by the fact that individuals with high levels of trait anger enjoy the experience of anger more than do individuals with low levels of trait anger. We created a reliable and valid scale that assessed attitude toward anger (Harmon-Jones, 2004). We then examined the relationship between the resting frontal asymmetry, this scale, and trait anger. Results indicated that trait anger related positively to relative left frontal activity. Moreover, although trait anger was directly associated with a more positive attitude toward anger, attitude toward anger did not relate to relative left frontal activity. In addition, statistically controlling for attitude toward anger did not alter the magnitude of the relationship between trait anger and relative left frontal activity. This study suggested that the relationship between trait anger and relative left frontal activity was not due to relative left frontal activity being associated with a more positive feeling toward anger.

Asymmetrical Frontal Activity and State Anger

The trait anger–relative left frontal evidence is correlational and subject to the interpretational difficulties associated with correlational results. Thus it was important to examine whether manipulated anger increases relative left frontal activity. To address this question, participants were randomly assigned to a condition in which they were given insulting or neutral feedback by a confederate. Immediately after the feedback manipulation, EEG was recorded (Harmon-Jones & Sigelman, 2001). Participants were then given the opportunity to aggress against the confederate. In the guise of a second, taste perception, study, participants were asked to give the confederate one of six types of beverages, which ranged from being very pleasant to being very unpleasant. Aggression was measured by the degree of unpleasantness of the beverage that they chose for the confederate to drink.

Results indicated that participants in the insult condition reported feeling more angry and that they behaved more aggressively than participants in the no-insult condition. More important, participants in the insult condition evidenced greater relative left frontal activity than participants in the no-insult condition. Finally, within the insult condition, participants who evidenced greater relative left frontal activity in response to the insult reported feeling more angry and behaved more aggressively.

In addition to the reviewed evidence, other research is consistent with the hypothesis that anger is associated with left frontal activity. For example, as reviewed by van Honk and Schutter (Chapter 10, this volume), research has found that a manipulated increase in left prefrontal activity led participants to attentionally approach angry faces. In contrast, an increase in right prefrontal activity led participants to attentionally avoid angry faces.

Manipulating the Intensity of Approach Motivation in an Anger-Evoking Situation

According to the motivational-direction model of asymmetrical frontal activity, approach motivation is related to left frontal activity, and withdrawal motivation is related to right frontal activity. Thus increased left frontal activation occurs in response to anger-inducing situations because the increase in relative left frontal activity increases approach motivational tendencies that would assist in behavior that may rectify the anger-inducing situation. From this perspective, it follows that if no approach behavior could be taken in response to an anger-provoking situation, then this increase in relative left frontal activation should be less pronounced. If approach and withdrawal motivational tendencies underlie asymmetrical frontal activity, then alterations in motivational intensity should affect the degree of activation in the frontal brain regions.

Several motivational theories posit that the expectancy of success or perceived task difficulty affect motivational intensity (for reviews, see Brehm & Self, 1989; Wright & Kirby, 2001). For the emotion of anger, if a situation creates anger and the individual believes that she can successfully act to alter the situation, then motivational intensity should be relatively high. If the individual believes that no action can be taken, then motivational intensity should be relatively low. Based on the integration of ideas from the motivational model of asymmetrical frontal activity with theories of motivational intensity, we predicted that greater left frontal activation would occur in response to an anger-producing event when persons believe that action can be taken to resolve the situation rather than when persons believe that no action can be taken to resolve the situation.

To test these predictions, university students who paid a sizable portion of their tuition and who were opposed to a tuition increase heard an editorial in which the speaker argued forcefully for a tuition increase. Immediately prior to hearing the editorial, participants were informed that the tuition increase might occur in the future and that petitions were being circulated to attempt to prevent the increase (action-possible condition), or they were informed that the tuition increase would definitely occur (action-impossible condition). Immediately after listening to the editorial, EEGs were recorded, and then participants completed a self-report emotion questionnaire. Finally, participants in the action-possible condition were given the opportunity to sign a petition and take as many petitions as they wanted to have others sign.

Results revealed that participants in the action-possible condition evidenced greater relative left frontal activity than did participants in the action-impossible condition. Moreover, within the action-possible condition, this increase in relative left frontal activity directly related to self-reported anger and behaviors aimed at rectifying the anger-producing event (i.e., whether or not they signed the petition and the number of petitions they took). Interestingly, self-reported anger did not differ between the action-possible and action-impossible conditions. Both conditions reported a large increase in anger after hearing the editorial.

These effects have been conceptually replicated (Harmon-Jones, Lueck, Fearn, & Harmon-Jones, 2006). In this experiment, participants low in racial prejudice were shown neutral, positive, and fear/disgust pictures and pictures intended to provoke anger that depicted instances of racism and hatred (e.g., neo-Nazis, Ku Klux Klan). Prior to viewing the pictures, half of the participants were informed that they would write an essay on why racism is immoral, unjust, and unfair and that this essay would be given to others in order to reduce racism. This manipulation was intended to increase anger-related approach motivation. In addition, personal relevance was manipulated by having half of the participants complete a racial attitudes questionnaire prior to viewing the pictures, whereas the other half completed an attitudes questionnaire about a neutral topic. Results revealed that participants showed greater relative left frontal activity to anger pictures than other picture types only when personal relevance was high and when they expected to engage in approach-related behavior.

The previous two experiments may suggest that relatively greater left frontal activity will occur in response to an angering situation only when there is an explicit approach opportunity. However, it is possible that an explicit approach opportunity is only one feature of an angering situation that intensifies left frontal activity. Other features of the situation or individual might increase approach motivational tendencies and activity in the left frontal cortical region, such as the personality characteristic of anger. That is, individuals who are chronically high in anger may evidence increased left frontal activity (and approach motivational tendencies) in response to angering situations that would not necessarily cause such responses in individuals who are not as chronically angry. This prediction is predicated on the idea that, compared with less angry individuals, angrier individuals have more extensive representations of anger-related information in their associative networks and that, therefore, anger-evoking stimuli should activate parts of their network more readily (Berkowitz, 1990, 1993; Bower, 1981). Among individuals high in trait anger, even mild anger cues might activate parts of the anger network and, through established associations, lead to angry expressive motor responses, physiological reactions, feelings, thoughts, and memories. Indeed, recent studies have shown that individuals high in trait anger respond with greater relative left frontal cortical activity to anger-inducing pictures even when there are no explicit manipulations of personal relevance or approach action expectancy, whereas individuals low in trait anger do not (Harmon-Jones, in press).

On the Reduction of Anger-Related Left Frontal Activity

Past research has suggested that experiencing sympathy for another individual can reduce aggression toward that individual (e.g., see review by Miller & Eisenberg, 1988). We hypothesized that sympathy may reduce aggression by reducing the relative left frontal activity associated with anger. To test this hypothesis, participants were told that they and another student would be writing essays and evaluating each other based on the essays. Participants then wrote a persuasive essay. Afterward, they were instructed in writing to remain completely objective (low sympathy) or to try to imagine how the other person must feel (high sympathy; Batson, 1991; Harmon-Jones, Peterson, & Vaughn, 2003) while they read the other participant's essay. The other participant described his or her difficulties with having multiple sclerosis. Following the reading of the essay, the participant received an evaluation ostensibly written by the other participant. The evaluation contained either neutral ratings and comments (no insult) or negative ratings and comments (insult). Immediately after the evaluation, EEG data were collected. Participants then completed an anger scale and rated the confederate. Results indicated that the low sympathy/insult condition produced greater relative left frontal activity than every other condition. In addition, the low sympathy/insult condition evoked greater left frontal activity and lesser right frontal activity than every other condition when separate estimates of left and right frontal activity were examined. Thus, when participants experienced sympathy for the target person, they did not evidence increased left frontal activity when insulted. Moreover, they expressed less hostile attitudes toward the insulting person than did participants who did not experience sympathy for the insulter. The experiment thus suggested that the alteration of relative left frontal activity via sympathy can reduce angry aggression.

DISCUSSION

The reviewed research provides strong support for the motivational direction model of asymmetrical frontal activity and directly contradicts the valence model and valenced motivation model that have been offered to explain the relationship between emotions and the frontal asymmetry. That the results of the reviewed studies were significantly opposite to the prediction derived from emotional valence models provides particularly strong support for the motivational direction model.

On the Relationship of Angry Feelings and Relative Left Frontal Activity

The research examining the relationship between asymmetrical frontal brain activity and anger began with the assumption that anger is often associated with approach motivation. Indeed, as indicated earlier, much past research has revealed that anger is associated with approach motivation and behavior. However, it is important to note that angry feelings are not inevitably associated with approach motivation and left frontal activity. For instance, in the study in which we examined the relationship between coping potential and left frontal activity (Harmon-Jones, Sigelman, Bohlig, & Harmon-Jones, 2003), we found that regardless of whether individuals expected to be able to resolve the anger-producing event, equally intense feelings of anger were produced by the aversive event. However, relative left frontal activity was increased only when individuals expected to be able to potentially rectify the anger-producing event. In addition, feelings of anger were associated with left frontal activity only in this latter experimental condition. Thus feelings of anger are often, but not inevitably, associated with approach motivation and left frontal activity.

Results from another study are consistent with this interpretation. In this study, results revealed a dissociation between angry feelings and left frontal activity when high levels of sympathy were first aroused for the insulting person (Harmon-Jones, Vaughn-Scott, Mohr, Sigelman, & Harmon-Jones, 2004). In this case, angry feelings were equally high whether or not sympathy was aroused for the insulting person. In contrast, left frontal activity differed between these two conditions, such that left frontal activity was increased following an insult by a person for whom sympathy had not previously been aroused, whereas left frontal activity was not increased when participants first empathized with the insulting person. In fact, in this latter condition, feelings of anger were directly associated with right frontal activity, suggesting that the anger experienced while empathizing with the other person was associated with withdrawal motivation. Future research is needed to assess the experiential and behavioral characteristics of anger that evokes withdrawal and right frontal activity.

Defining Emotional Valence

Consistent with current theories of emotion, the perspective advanced in this chapter assumes that anger is a negative emotion. However, if anger is instead a positive emotion, the valence model of the frontal asymmetry could explain the evidence linking anger to increased left frontal activity. Most perspectives on emotion do not define what is meant by the valence of emotion. Most scientists, like most laypersons, *know* that joy and enthusiasm are positive emotions and that anger and fear are negative emotions. On the rare occasions when valence is discussed, emotions are defined as positive or negative (1) because of the cause of the emotion; (2) because of the emotion's adaptive consequences; (3) or because of the emotion's subjective feeling. Lazarus (1991) noted that the first definition—whether the person–environment relationship is beneficial or harmful—is "the most common, implicit, use of the terms" for positive and negative emotion

(p. 6). By this definition, anger is indeed negative. Anger is evoked by frustrating, painful, or unpleasant circumstances. Thus the reviewed research demonstrates that a negative emotion with approach tendencies is associated with increased left frontal activity.

However, it is still possible that the frontal asymmetry is a function of emotional valence when emotional valence is defined in an alternative manner. In our research, we sought to test whether the valence model of asymmetrical frontal brain activity could explain the relationship of anger and left frontal activity when emotional valence was defined using the *subjective feeling* definition. In the research, we first created a trait questionnaire that demonstrated that there were reliable individual differences in persons' subjective feelings about anger or attitudes toward anger. The questionnaire included 11 items. Example items are: "I like the feeling of power I get from expressing my anger" and "I like how it feels when I am furious." Then we examined the relationship between the subjective feeling of anger and resting baseline left frontal activity. We found that, although trait anger related to both left frontal activity and a more positive subjective feeling about anger, the subjective feeling of anger did not relate to left frontal activity (Harmon-Jones, 2004). Thus, even when using a more arcane definition of emotion, we were unable to find a relationship between positivity of anger and left frontal activity.

Given the difficulties inherent in defining adaptational consequences, we have yet to examine relationships between the adaptational consequences of anger and asymmetrical frontal brain activity. It does appear that anger is associated with increased left frontal activity regardless of whether anger is associated with constructive action (e.g., working to prevent an injustice; Harmon-Jones, Sigelman, et al., 2003) or destructive action (e.g., behavioral aggression; Harmon-Jones & Sigelman, 2001). In sum, the evidence strongly suggests that anger is a negatively valenced emotion that is related to relative left frontal activity because of its association with approach motivation.

Evoking Emotions

Of the emotions examined in the research on brain mechanisms involved in emotions, anger has received less attention than emotions such as fear, sadness, and disgust, which can be induced using established stimuli (e.g., pictures, films). Part of the reason for this relative neglect of anger may be that fear, sadness, and disgust are easier to evoke in the laboratory because active, involving situations are not necessarily required to elicit the emotions. Because the evocation of anger often requires the use of more active and involving situations, the study of anger may require the assistance of social psychologists who are familiar with creating such high-impact settings (see, e.g, Harmon-Jones, Amodio, & Zinner, in press).

On a related note, examinations of emotions other than anger should consider implementing more active and involving situations, as the more active and involving situations may elicit vastly different brain responses than the ones obtained in more passive situations. Indeed, our research has revealed that the manipulation of coping potential (i.e., the belief that one can take action to resolve the anger-producing situation) affects the activation of asymmetrical frontal brain activity but not the experience of anger (Harmon-Jones, Sigelman, et al., 2003). That is, the belief that one can take action to resolve the anger-producing situation produced an increase in left frontal activity and self-reported anger, whereas the belief that one could not act to resolve the anger-producing situation produced an increase in self-reported anger but not an increase in left frontal activity. Given that one of the primary functions of emotions is the motivation of behavior (Brehm, 1999; Frijda, 1986), it is all the more important for emotion researchers to consider the behavioral context in which emotions are evoked.

CONCLUSION

The point of this review is not to suggest that anger is inevitably associated with increased left frontal activity or that left frontal activity is inevitably associated with negative outcomes. Our research has indicated that anger is not inevitably associated with left frontal activity. Instead, the contribution of our research using anger is to suggest that approach motivation, which can involve negative, as well as positive, affective states, is associated with left frontal activity. Moreover, it suggests that a valence model explanation of asymmetrical frontal cortical activity is no longer viable.

For the past few decades, several models of emotion have considered the pleasant-to-unpleasant dimension of emotion an important organizing principle—one that assists in understanding trait mood and situational reactions to significant stimuli at both subjective and physiological levels of analysis. However, recent developments have suggested that this focus on the valence dimension may not adequately capture emotional space. Consideration of motivational direction in the analysis of emotion, particularly as it relates to asymmetrical frontal brain activity, seems especially important. In addition, as psychological science focuses more attention on the empirically neglected positive aspects of psychological life, it is important to keep in mind that approach motivations are not inevitably associated with positive subjective feelings or positive outcomes. The integration of social-psychological theories and methods, mostly developed around the study of anger, with neuroscience led to these discoveries and, as such, benefit both social psychology and neuroscience.

ACKNOWLEDGMENTS

The research presented in this article was funded by grants from the National Institute of Mental Health (Nos. MH60747-01 and MH52662), the National Science Foundation (Nos. BCS-9910702 and BCS 0350435), and the Wisconsin/Hilldale Undergraduate/Faculty Research Fund. Thanks to Cindy Harmon-Jones and Piotr Winkielman for many helpful comments on this chapter.

REFERENCES

Ahern, G. L., & Schwartz, G. E. (1985). Differential lateralization for positive and negative emotion in the human brain: EEG spectral analysis. *Neuropsychologia, 23,* 745–755.

Allen, J. J., Iacono, W. G., Depue, R. A., & Arbisi, P. (1993). Regional EEG asymmetries in bipolar seasonal affective disorder before and after phototherapy. *Biological Psychiatry, 33,* 642–646.

Allen, J. J. B., Harmon-Jones, E., & Cavender, J. (2001). Manipulation of frontal EEG asymmetry through biofeedback alters self-reported emotional responses and facial EMG. *Psychophysiology, 38,* 685–693.

Baehr, E., Rosenfeld, J.P., & Baehr, R. (1997). The clinical use of an alpha asymmetry protocol in the neurofeedback treatment of depression: Two case studies. *Journal of Neurotherapy, 2,* 10–23.

Batson, C. D. (1991). *The altruism question: Toward a social-psychological answer.* Hillsdale, NJ: Erlbaum.

Bellgowan, P. S., Saad, Z. S., & Bandettini, P. A. (2003). Understanding neural system dynamics through task modulation and measurement of functional MRI amplitude, latency, and width. *Proceedings of the National Academy of Sciences of the USA, 100,* 1415–1419.

Berkowitz, L. (1990). On the formation and regulation of anger and aggression: A cognitive–neoassociationistic analysis. *American Psychologist, 45,* 494–503.

Berkowitz, L. (1993). Towards a general theory of anger and emotional aggression: Implications of the cognitive–neoassociationistic perspective for the analysis of anger and other emotions. In R. S. Wyer, Jr., & T. K. Srull (Eds). *Advances in social cognition: Vol. 6. Perspectives on anger and emotion* (pp. 1–46). Hillsdale, NJ: Erlbaum.

Berkowitz, L. (1999). Anger. In T. Dalgleish & M. J. Power (Eds.), *Handbook of cognition and emotion* (pp. 411–428). Chichester, UK: Wiley.

Blanchard, D. C., & Blanchard, R. J. (1984). Affect and aggression: An animal model applied to human behavior. *Advances in the Study of Aggression, 1,* 1–62.

Boissy, A., & Bouissou, M. F. (1994). Effects of androgen treatment on behavioral and physiological responses of heifers to fear-eliciting situations. *Hormones and Behavior, 28,* 66–83.

Bower, G. H. (1981). Mood and memory. *American Psychologist, 36,* 129–148.

Brehm, J. W. (1999). The intensity of emotion. *Personality and Social Psychology Review, 3,* 2–22.

Brehm, J. W., & Self, E. (1989). The intensity of motivation. *Annual Review of Psychology, 40,* 109–131.

Buss, A. H., & Perry, M. (1992). The aggression questionnaire. *Journal of Personality and Social Psychology, 63*, 452–459.

Carver, C. S. (2001). Affect and the functional bases of behavior: On the dimensional structure of affective experience. *Personality and Social Psychology Review, 5*, 345–356.

Carver, C. S., & White, T. L. (1994). Behavioral inhibition, behavioral activation, and affective responses to impending reward and punishment: The BIS/BAS scales. *Journal of Personality and Social Psychology, 67*, 319–333.

Coan, J. A., & Allen, J. J. B. (2003). Frontal EEG asymmetry and the behavioral activation and inhibition systems. *Psychophysiology, 40*, 106–114.

Coan, J. A., Allen, J. J. B., & Harmon-Jones, E. (2001). Voluntary facial expression and hemispheric asymmetry over the frontal cortex. *Psychophysiology, 38*, 912–925.

Cook, I. A., O'Hara, R., Uijtdehaage, S. H. J., Mandelkern, M., & Leuchter, A. F. (1998). Assessing the accuracy of topographic EEG mapping for determining local brain function. *Electroencephalography and Clinical Neurophysiology, 107*, 408–414.

Darwin, C. (1965). *The expression of the emotions in man and animals.* Chicago: University of Chicago Press. (Original work published 1872)

Davidson, R. J. (1995). Cerebral asymmetry, emotion, and affective style. In R. J. Davidson & K. Hugdahl (Eds.), *Brain asymmetry* (pp. 361–387). Cambridge, MA: MIT Press.

Davidson, R. J. (1998). Anterior electrophysiological asymmetries, emotion, and depression: Conceptual and methodological conundrums. *Psychophysiology, 35*, 607–614.

Davidson, R. J., & Fox, N. A. (1982). Asymmetrical brain activity discriminates between positive and negative affective stimuli in human infants. *Science, 218*, 1235–1236.

Davidson, R. J., & Fox, N. A. (1989). Frontal brain asymmetry predicts infants' response to maternal separation. *Journal of Abnormal Psychology, 98*, 127–131.

Dien, J., Spencer, K. M., & Donchin, E. (2003). Localization of the event-related potential novelty response as defined by principal components analysis. *Cognitive Brain Research, 17*(3), 637–650.

Ekman, P., & Davidson, R. J. (1993). Voluntary smiling changes regional brain activity. *Psychological Science, 4*, 342–345.

Flynn, J., Vanegas, H., Foote, W., & Edwards, S. B. (1970). Neural mechanisms involved in a cat's attack on a rat. In R. Whalen, R. F. Thompson, M. Verzeano, & N. Weinberger (Eds.), *The neural control of behavior* (pp. 135–173). New York: Academic Press.

Fox, N. A. (1991). If it's not left, it's right. *American Psychologist, 46*, 863–872.

Fox, N. A., & Davidson, R. J. (1986). Taste-elicited changes in facial signs of emotion and the asymmetry of brain electrical activity in human newborns. *Neuropsychologia, 24*, 417–422.

Fox, N. A., Henderson, H. A., Rubin, K. H., Calkins, S. D., & Schmidt, L. A. (2001). Continuity and discontinuity of behavioral inhibition and exuberance: Psychophysiological and behavioral influences across the first four years of life. *Child Development, 72*, 1–21.

Frijda, N. H. (1986). *The emotions.* Cambridge, UK: Cambridge University Press.

Goldman, R. I., Stern, J. M., Engel, J., Jr., & Cohen, M. S. (2002). Simultaneous EEG and fMRI of the alpha rhythm. *Neuroreport, 13*, 2487–2492.

Gotlib, I. H., Ranganath, C., & Rosenfeld, J. P. (1998). Frontal EEG alpha asymmetry, depression, and cognitive functioning. *Cognition and Emotion, 12*, 449–478.

Harmon-Jones, E. (2003). Anger and the behavioural approach system. *Personality and Individual Differences, 35*, 995–1005.

Harmon-Jones, E. (2004). On the relationship of anterior brain activity and anger: Examining the role of attitude toward anger. *Cognition and Emotion, 18*, 337–361.

Harmon-Jones, E. (in press). Trait anger predicts relative left frontal cortical activation to anger-inducing stimuli. *International Journal of Psychophysiology*.

Harmon-Jones, E., & Allen, J. J. B. (1997). Behavioral activation sensitivity and resting frontal EEG asymmetry: Covariation of putative indicators related to risk for mood disorders. *Journal of Abnormal Psychology, 106*, 159–163.

Harmon-Jones, E., & Allen, J. J. B. (1998). Anger and frontal brain activity: EEG asymmetry consistent with approach motivation despite negative affective valence. *Journal of Personality and Social Psychology, 74*, 1310–1316.

Harmon-Jones, E., & Allen, J. J. B. (2001). The role of affect in the mere exposure effect: Evidence from psychophysiological and individual-differences approaches. *Personality and Social Psychology Bulletin, 27*, 889–898.

Harmon-Jones, E., Amodio, D. M., & Zinner, L. (in press). Social-psychological methods of emotion elicitation. In J. A. Coan & J. J. B. Allen (Eds.), *Handbook of emotion elicitation and assessment*. New York: Oxford University Press.

Harmon-Jones, E., Harmon-Jones, C., Abramson, L., Nelson, B., Rupsis, M. M., Burck, A. L., et al. (2006). *PANAS positive affect is associated with state and trait anger*. Manuscript submitted for publication.

Harmon-Jones, E., Lueck, L., Fearn, M., & Harmon-Jones, C. (2006). The effect of personal relevance and approach-related action expectation on relative left frontal cortical activity. *Psychological Science, 17*, 434–440.

Harmon-Jones, E., Peterson, H., & Vaughn, K. (2003). The dissonance-inducing effects of an inconsistency between experienced empathy and knowledge of past failures to help: Support for the action-based model of dissonance. *Basic and Applied Social Psychology, 25*, 69–78.

Harmon-Jones, E., & Sigelman, J. (2001). State anger and frontal brain activity: Evidence that insult-related relative left prefrontal activation is associated with experienced anger and aggression. *Journal of Personality and Social Psychology, 80*, 797–803.

Harmon-Jones, E., Sigelman, J. D., Bohlig, A., & Harmon-Jones, C. (2003). Anger, coping, and frontal cortical activity: The effect of coping potential on anger-induced left frontal activity. *Cognition and Emotion, 17*, 1–24.

Harmon-Jones, E., Vaughn-Scott, K., Mohr, S., Sigelman, J., & Harmon-Jones, C. (2004). The effect of manipulated sympathy and anger on left and right frontal cortical activity. *Emotion, 4*, 95–101.

Heller, W. (1990). The neuropsychology of emotion: Developmental patterns and implications for psychopathology. In N. L. Stein, B. Leventhal, & T. Trabasso (Eds.), *Psychological and biological approaches to emotion* (pp. 167–211). Hillsdale, NJ: Erlbaum.

Heller, W., & Nitschke, J. B. (1998). The puzzle of regional brain activity in depression and anxiety: The importance of subtypes and comorbidity. *Cognition and Emotion, 12*, 421–447.

Henriques, J. B., & Davidson, R. J. (1990). Regional brain electrical asymmetries discriminate between previously depressed and healthy control subjects. *Journal of Abnormal Psychology, 99*, 22–31.

Izard, C. E. (1991). *The psychology of emotions*. New York: Plenum Press.

Jacobs, G. D., & Snyder, D. (1996). Frontal brain asymmetry predicts affective style in men. *Behavioral Neuroscience, 110*, 3–6.

Lagerspetz, K. M. J. (1969). Aggression and aggressiveness in laboratory mice. In S. Garattini & E. B. Sigg (Eds.), *Aggressive behavior* (pp. 77–85). New York: Wiley.

Lazarus, R. S. (1991). *Emotion and adaptation*. New York: Oxford University Press.

Lerner, J. S., & Keltner, D. (2001). Fear, anger, and risk. *Journal of Personality and Social Psychology, 81*, 146–159.

Lewis, M., Sullivan, M. W., Ramsay, D. S., & Alessandri, S. M. (1992). Individual differences in anger and sad expressions during extinction: Antecedents and consequences. *Infant Behavior and Development, 15*, 443–452.

Mikulincer, M. (1988). Reactance and helplessness following exposure to unsolvable problems: The effects of attributional style. *Journal of Personality and Social Psychology, 54*, 679–686.

Miller, P. A., & Eisenberg, N. (1988). The relation of empathy to aggressive and externalizing/antisocial behavior. *Psychological Bulletin, 103*, 324–344.

Moyer, K. E. (1976). *The psychobiology of aggression*. New York: Harper & Row.

Olweus, D. (1986). Aggression and hormones: Behavioral relationship with testosterone and adrenaline. In D. Olweus, J. Block, & M. Radke-Yarrow (Eds.), *Development of antisocial and prosocial behavior: Research, theories, and issues* (pp. 51–72). Orlando, FL: Academic Press.

Pascual-Marqui, R. D., Lehmann, D., Koenig, T., Kochi, K., Merlo, M. C., Hell, D. et al. (1999). Low resolution brain electromagnetic tomography (LORETA) functional imaging in acute, neuroleptic-naive, first-episode, productive schizophrenia. *Psychiatry Research: Neuroimaging, 90*, 169–179.

Plutchik, R. (1980). *Emotion: A psychoevolutionary synthesis*. New York: Harper & Row.

Reiman, E. M., Lane, R. D., Van Patten, C., & Bandettini, P. A. (2000). Positron emission tomography and functional magnetic resonance imaging. New York: Cambridge University Press.

Robinson, R. G., & Downhill, J. E. (1995). Lateralization of psychopathology in response to focal brain injury. In R. J. Davidson & K. Hugdahl (Eds.), *Brain asymmetry* (pp. 693–711). Cambridge, MA: MIT Press.

Rosenfeld, J.P., Cha, G., Blair, T., & Gotlib, I. H. (1995). Operant (biofeedback) control of left–right frontal alpha power differences: Potential neurotherapy for affective disorders. *Biofeedback and Self-Regulation, 20*, 241–258.

Schaffer, C. E., Davidson, R. J., & Saron, C. (1983). Frontal and parietal electroencephalogram asymmetry in depressed and nondepressed subjects. *Biological Psychiatry, 18*, 753–762.

Silberman, E. K., & Weingartner, H. (1986). Hemispheric lateralization of functions related to emotion. *Brain and Cognition, 5*, 322–353.

Sutton, S. K., & Davidson, R. J. (1997). Prefrontal brain asymmetry: A biological substrate of the behavioral approach and inhibition systems. *Psychological Science, 8,* 204–210.

Tomarken, A. J., Davidson, R. J., & Henriques, J. B. (1990). Resting frontal brain asymmetry predicts affective responses to films. *Journal of Personality and Social Psychology, 59,* 791–801.

Tomarken, A. J., Davidson, R. J., Wheeler, R. E., & Doss, R. (1992). Individual differences in anterior brain asymmetry and fundamental dimensions of emotion. *Journal of Personality and Social Psychology, 62,* 676–687.

Tomarken, A. J., Davidson, R. J., Wheeler, R. E., & Kinney, L. (1992). Psychometric properties of resting anterior EEG asymmetry: Temporal stability and internal consistency. *Psychophysiology, 29,* 576–592.

Tomarken, A. J., & Keener, A. D. (1998). Frontal brain asymmetry and depression: A self-regulatory perspective. *Cognition and Emotion, 12,* 387–420.

Vandenheede, M., & Bouissou, M. F. (1993). Effect of androgen treatment on fear reactions in ewes. *Hormones and Behavior, 27,* 435–448.

Watson, D. (2000). *Mood and temperament.* New York: Guilford Press.

Watson, D., Clark, L. A., & Tellegen, A. (1988). Development and validation of brief measures of positive and negative affect: The PANAS scales. *Journal of Personality and Social Psychology, 54,* 1063–1070.

Watson, D., Wiese, D., Vaidya, J., & Tellegen, A. (1999). The two general activation systems of affect: Structural findings, evolutionary considerations, and psychobiological evidence. *Journal of Personality and Social Psychology, 76,* 820–838.

Wheeler, R. E., Davidson, R. J., & Tomarken, A. J. (1993). Frontal brain asymmetry and emotional reactivity: A biological substrate of affective style. *Psychophysiology, 30,* 82–89.

Wortman, C. B., & Brehm, J. W. (1975). Responses to uncontrollable outcomes: An integration of reactance theory and the learned helplessness model. In L. Berkowitz (Ed.), *Advances in experimental social psychology* (Vol. 8, pp. 278–336). New York: Academic Press.

Wright, R. A., & Kirby, L. D. (2001). Effort determination of cardiovascular response: An integrative analysis with applications in social psychology. In M. P. Zanna (Ed.), *Advances in experimental social psychology,* (Vol. 33, pp. 255–307). San Diego: Academic Press.

Young, P. T. (1943). *Emotion in man and animal: Its nature and relation to attitude and motive.* New York: Wiley.

Zajonc, R. B. (1968). Attitudinal effects of mere exposure. Journal of Personality and Social Psychology, 9(2, Part 2), 1–27.

8

Reward

NEURAL CIRCUITRY FOR SOCIAL VALUATION

Brian Knutson and G. Elliott Wimmer

During an Enlightenment-era correspondence with Pierre de Fermat, Blaise Pascal proposed that individuals compute "expected value" (EV) as the product of the expected magnitude and probability of a potentially favorable gamble. Since then, the notion of EV has played a pivotal role in both psychological (Bandura, 1977; Rotter, 1972) and economic theory (von Neumann & Morgenstern, 1944). Although theorists sometimes assume that people will behave in ways that will maximize EV, empirical research has documented exceptions (Kahneman & Tversky, 1979). Nonetheless, anticipated gain magnitude and probability provide useful anchors for attempts to understand how people process rewards. If the brain computes EV prior to a potentially rewarding outcome, then scientists can elicit and study the representation of EV. In this overview, we describe neuroimaging research designed to elucidate how the brain represents EV and then consider emerging evidence that neural representation of EV extends to, pervades, and may even influence social exchange.

BACKGROUND

If the amount of effort an animal expends to obtain a stimulus indexes value, then self-stimulation represents one of the most extreme examples of valuation. Social psychologist James Olds and physicist Peter Milner serendipitously discovered self-stimulation in 1954, while attempting to electrically stimulate arousal centers in the midbrain of rats (Olds &

Milner, 1954). Olds and Milner noticed that a rat that had had an electrode erroneously implanted near the nucleus accumbens (NAcc) rather than in arousal centers of the midbrain not only showed energized behavior when stimulated but also spontaneously returned to the corner of a table where it had been stimulated the day before. After devising an apparatus that allowed the rat to self-administer stimulation by pressing a bar, Olds and Milner found that the rat worked vigorously to do so, to the point of exhaustion and the exclusion of all other activities (e.g., eating, drinking, sex, and sleep). Since its discovery, self-stimulation behavior has been demonstrated in all other mammalian species studied (Olds & Fobes, 1981), including humans (Bishop, Elder, & Heath, 1963).

Brain sites that support self-stimulation ascend from deep in the midbrain to higher subcortical regions (i.e., lateral hypothalamus, medial amygdala, and ventral striatum). Some cortical regions also support self-stimulation but do so less robustly (i.e., orbitofrontal cortex and mesial prefrontal cortex). Subsequent innovations in histochemical mapping indicated that the neurotransmitter dopamine could be found in many of these regions (Falck & Hillarp, 1959). Regions deep in the midbrain appeared to house the bodies of dopamine neurons, which projected to the subcortical and cortical regions. Microinjection studies later indicated that rats would expend similar effort to self-administer dopamine-like chemicals to many of these sites (McBride, Murphy, & Ikemoto, 1999). Methods for visualizing synaptic activity on a subsecond time scale revealed dopamine release in subcortical and cortical projection areas as rats anticipated rewards ranging from food to sex to commonly abused drugs (Wightman & Robinson, 2002). Finally, electrophysiological recording of midbrain dopamine neurons in monkeys indicated that even after learning had stabilized, dopamine neurons continued to fire during anticipation of rewards but transiently ceased firing when anticipated rewards were not delivered (Schultz, Dayan, & Montague, 1997). Together, this remarkable progression of findings implicates mesolimbic dopamine projections in both self-stimulation behavior and reward anticipation and, by extension, in the computation of EV.

Most self-stimulation studies have been conducted with nonhuman subjects due to the invasiveness of implanting electrodes in the brain. However, technology for visualizing human brain activity became available near the end of the 20th century. For instance, positron emission tomography (PET) enabled visualization of local neural utilization of oxygen, glucose, and even certain neurotransmitters. In addition to demonstrating that dopamine is released in the ventral striatum when people play engaging games (Koepp et al., 1998; Pappata et al., 2002; Zald et al., 2004), PET researchers have demonstrated that dopamine release in the ventral striatum caused by amphetamine injection correlates with self-reported positive arousal (or euphoria) but not with negative arousal (or fear; Drevets et al., 2001; Mawlawi et al., 2001; Volkow et al., 1999). However, although PET can give researchers clues about what neurotransmitters are released, its temporal resolution (i.e., approximately 120 seconds per brain scan) limits inferences about when release occurs. On the other hand, although event-related functional magnetic resonance imaging (fMRI) provides information only about local changes in oxygenation (hereafter "activation"), it does provide adequate temporal resolution (i.e., about 1–2 seconds per brain scan) for researchers to infer when activation occurs. Thus the remainder of this overview focuses primarily on rapidly emerging findings from event-related fMRI.

MONETARY REWARD

Determination of the neural basis of valuation in humans constitutes one of the most basic challenges presently confronting affective neuroscience (Davidson & Sutton, 1995; Panksepp, 1991). Thus our laboratory initially used event-related fMRI to attempt to identify brain regions that represent components of EV (i.e., the magnitude and probability of expected gains). As exemplified by rapid advances in vision research (Engel et al., 1994), programmatic functional brain mapping research often progresses through stages that include (1) visualization of relevant brain regions; (2) parametric manipulation of activation in those regions; and (3) exploration of alternative functional hypotheses for activation in those regions. Thus an initial challenge was to visualize activation in the mesolimbic pathway in general and in the ventral striatum in particular. Although event-related fMRI provides adequate spatiotemporal resolution for visualizing second-to-second activation changes in small subcortical regions, we faced the additional challenge of identifying compelling incentives. We adopted monetary incentives because they are widely valued (i.e., most people will work for money), can carry either positive or negative value (i.e., can be gained or lost), and can be scaled to different magnitudes (and thus parameterized). Inspired by the early research of Pavlov with dogs (Pavlov, 1927) and more recent work of Schultz with monkeys (Schultz et al., 1997), we designed a "monetary incentive delay" (MID) task for use in humans undergoing fMRI (Knutson, Westdorp, Kaiser, & Hommer, 2000).

Honoring a traditional ethological distinction between appetitive and consummatory behavior (Craig, 1918), the MID task is designed to evoke both anticipation of and reactions to monetary gain and loss (see Figure 8.1). A typical MID task trial includes four components: (1) viewing a cue (cue; 250–2,000 milliseconds); (2) waiting (anticipation; 2,000–3,000 milliseconds); (3) responding to a rapidly presented target with a button press (target; 160–350 milliseconds); (4) receipt of trial-based and cumulative feedback about gain or loss (outcome; 2,000 milliseconds; Knutson, Fong, Bennett, Adams, & Hommer, 2003). On all trials, participants are instructed to respond as rapidly as possible when targets appear, with the

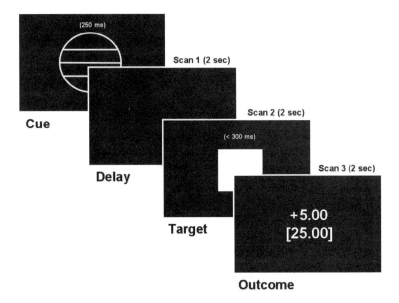

FIGURE 8.1. Monetary incentive delay task trial structure. Adapted from Knutson, Fong, Bennett, Adams, and Hommer (2003). Copyright 2003 by Elsevier. Adapted by permission.

goal of pressing the button before targets disappear. Cue features (e.g., shape, horizontal or vertical lines) indicate whether participants can acquire gains or avoid losses by responding to the subsequently presented targets. Because of the separation of anticipation and outcome periods in the task, investigators can infer which brain regions were recruited by different stages of incentive processing.

The MID task is designed to change affect rather than overt behavior. Behavioral performance can be controlled across incentive conditions by varying the range of target speeds, which are typically set to a challenging but not impossible level of difficulty (e.g., to elicit a hit rate of 66%). However, different conditions reliably elicit distinct affective experiences. Specifically, presentation of gain cues primarily elicits positive arousal (e.g., "excitement"), whereas presentation of loss cues primarily elicits negative arousal (e.g., "anxiety") proportional to cue magnitude (Knutson et al., 2003). Changes in anticipatory affect have been verified using both retrospective and online ratings (Knutson, Nielsen, Larkin, & Carstensen, 2005). Interestingly, both gain and loss anticipation and outcomes elicit changes in valence, but whereas anticipation also elicits increased arousal, outcomes do not.

Combined with event-related fMRI, the MID task has yielded novel insights about the dynamics of human reward processing. In the first published fMRI study to manipulate monetary incentives, we observed striatal and mesial frontal activation when participants engaged in incentive trials (both gain and loss) versus nonincentive trials over the course of the entire trial (Knutson et al., 2000). However, these activations occurred in regions that were located more dorsal than the mesolimbic pathway, suggesting that whole-trial comparisons did not afford adequate temporal resolution for resolving more rapid anticipatory changes in activation. Indeed, in a second study that utilized several different magnitudes of incentives in which modeling focused on anticipation only, the more ventral NAcc was preferentially activated by gain anticipation but not loss anticipation (Knutson, Adams, Fong, & Hommer, 2001). A third study in which anticipation and outcome were analyzed separately replicated this finding and further indicated that gain outcomes instead activated the mesial prefrontal cortex (MPFC; Knutson, Fong, Adams, Varner, & Hommer, 2001). Whereas the magnitude of anticipated gain was manipulated in these studies, the probability of anticipated gain was held constant (i.e., approximately 66% probability of obtaining gain or avoiding loss in a given trial).

In a subsequent study, we manipulated the probability, as well as the magnitude, of anticipated gain, thus independently altering both components of EV. Whereas NAcc activation was proportional to the magnitude of anticipated gains as in prior studies, MPFC activation was sensitive to the probability of anticipated gains (Knutson, Taylor, Kaufman, Peterson, & Glover, 2005). Together, these results not only verify the involvement of mesolimbic circuitry in the computation of both components of EV (see Figure 8.2) but also further imply that whereas NAcc activation increases with anticipated gain magnitude, MPFC activation increases with anticipated gain probability. Theoretically, the findings suggest a possible mechanism for peoples' insensitivity to probability during risk assessment (Kahneman & Tversky, 1979), as cortical representation of probability may require more effortful processing than subcortical representation of magnitude. Clinically, the findings suggest that patients with cortical lesions of the MPFC (e.g., the historic case of Phineas Gage) may be able to anticipate gain magnitude but may be less able to adjust expectations according to gain probability (Camille et al., 2004; Knutson & Cooper, 2005).

Together, these findings demonstrate NAcc activation during gain anticipation and verify that this activation increases proportional to anticipated gain magnitude. Comparison of the gain anticipation hypothesis with alternative accounts of NAcc activation is ongoing but presently incomplete. The design of the MID task can address some prominent alternative hypotheses. According to one account, the NAcc activates in response to surprising or unpredicted stimuli (Berns, McClure, Pagnoni, & Montague, 2001), which implies that activation should occur in response to all incentive outcomes. However, in the MID task, the most robust NAcc activation occurs during gain anticipation rather than in response to gain outcomes. A

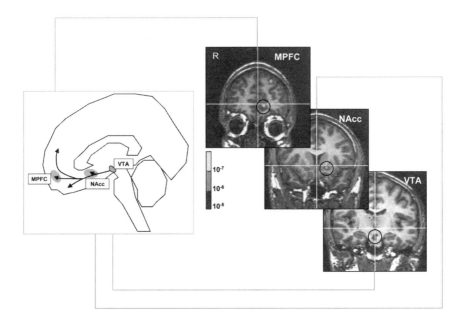

FIGURE 8.2. Activation in mesolimbic volumes of interest correlate with a linear model of expected value (i.e., anticipated gain magnitude X probability. MPFC; mesial prefrontal cortex; NAcc, nucleus accumbens; VTA, ventral tegmental area; Adapted from Knutson, Taylor, Kaufman, Peterson, and Glover (2005). Copyright 2005 by the Society for Neuroscience. Adapted by permission.

second account posits that the NAcc activates during anticipation of any arousing or salient event (positive or negative; Berridge & Robinson, 1998), which implies that the NAcc should show similar increases in activation during gain or loss anticipation, as subjects report experiencing similar levels of arousal when anticipating gains and losses. However, we have repeatedly and consistently observed greater NAcc activation during anticipation of gains than losses. A third account posits that NAcc activation facilitates motor preparation (Mogenson, Jones, & Yim, 1980), which again implies that the NAcc should show similar activation during anticipation of gains and losses, as participants respond to obtain gains and avoid losses with similar speed. However, again, the NAcc shows greater activation during anticipation of gains than during anticipation of losses. A fourth account might posit that NAcc activation should occur in the context of learning and thus should show less activation after learning has stabilized (Dickinson, 1994). However, even after implicit and explicit learning have stabilized, we continue to observe prominent NAcc activation during anticipation of gains. Various combinations of these hypotheses remain to be tested, but at present, the gain anticipation hypothesis best fits the pattern of NAcc activation observed in several experiments. But it may be associated positive arousal rather than goal representation that best correlates with NAcc activation, as individual differences in positive arousal correlate with individual differences in NAcc activation to large potential gains of the same magnitude (Bjork et al., 2004; Knutson, Adams, et al., 2001; Knutson, Taylor, et al., 2005).

Although the preceding overview focuses on the work of our laboratory, many other investigators have successfully used monetary rewards to elicit mesolimbic activation with fMRI, starting with initial demonstrations (Delgado, Nystrom, Fissell, Noll, & Fiez, 2000; Elliott, Friston, & Dolan, 2000) and followed by increasingly sophisticated paradigms that have been well summarized elsewhere (Knutson & Cooper, 2005; McClure, York, & Montague, 2004; O'Doherty, 2004). Other researchers have independently replicated the finding that anticipation of gains elicits greater mesolimbic activation than anticipation of losses (Breiter, Aharon, Kahneman, Dale, & Shizgal, 2001) and that anticipation of gains elicits increased activation in the NAcc whereas gain outcomes elicit activation of the MPFC (Wittmann et al., 2005), even in noncontingent tasks that do not require a motor response (Ramnani, Elliott, Athwal, & Passingham, 2004).

OTHER REWARDS

fMRI researchers have also discovered that other rewards elicit activity in mesolimbic circuits, including pleasant tastes (Berns et al., 2001; O'Doherty, Rolls, Francis, Bowtell, & McGlone, 2001), pleasant smells (Anderson et al., 2003; Gottfried, O'Doherty, & Dolan, 2003), pleasant touch (Rolls et al., 2003), and pleasant sounds (such as music; Menon & Levitin, 2005). Importantly, all of these researchers empirically demonstrated that participants judged stimuli to be pleasant relative to neutral or unpleasant stimuli. However, most of these studies focused on brain responses to stimulus delivery and did not control for anticipation. One study distinguished anticipation from outcome in the case of cued delivery of pleasant, neutral, and unpleasant tastes (O'Doherty, Deichmann, Critchley, & Dolan, 2002). The investigators reported activation of midbrain, ventral striatum, and orbitofrontal cortex (OFC) during anticipation of pleasant taste but only of OFC in response to pleasant taste receipt or outcome. Though more work remains to be done, these findings are consistent with the notion that NAcc activation during gain anticipation generalizes to nonmonetary rewards. Notably, although rewarding stimuli elicit mesolimbic activation, these activations do not critically appear to depend on whether rewards are unlearned (a.k.a. "primary"), such as pleasant taste, or learned (a.k.a. "secondary"), such as money.

If NAcc activation occurs during gain anticipation, then it might bias subsequent cognition and behavior in ways that can promote the seeking of gains (Ikemoto & Panksepp, 1999). With respect to cognition, we have recently demonstrated that monetary reward cues can enhance memory for subsequently presented scenes and that this memory enhancement effect depends on the extent to which cues elicit NAcc and midbrain activation in individual participants (Adcock, Thangavel, Whitfield-Gabrieli, Knutson, & Gabrieli, 2006). With respect to behavior, because risk involves weighing potential gains against potential losses, one might hypothesize that an increase in gain anticipation would promote risky choices, whereas an increase in loss anticipation would instead promote riskless choices. Using a financial trading task in combination with fMRI, we recently demonstrated that anticipatory NAcc activation predicts switching to a risk-seeking strategy (i.e., choosing stocks rather than bonds), whereas anterior insula activation predicts the opposite switch to a risk-avoidant strategy (i.e., choosing bonds rather than stocks; Kuhnen & Knutson, 2005). Thus emerging evidence is beginning to suggest that anticipatory NAcc activation may modulate subsequent cognition and behavior in ways that promote gain seeking.

Up to this point, we have implicated mesolimbic circuitry in general, and the NAcc in particular, in anticipation of various rewards and also possibly in modulating subsequent behavior. Many questions still remain to be answered. For instance, fMRI visualization of neural activation related to gain anticipation raises the question of whether a distinct circuit related to loss anticipation can be visualized (e.g., the anterior insula; Kuhnen & Knutson, 2005). Another set of questions regards whether these findings will generalize to the realm of social interaction. Specifically, can socially rewarding stimuli also activate mesolimbic circuitry, and can activation of these regions also influence subsequent social behavior?

SOCIAL REWARD

As with the broader spectrum of rewards, social rewards can be specifically defined as attributes or behavior of others that an organism will expend effort to obtain and that can either be unlearned or learned. Even in the case of novel social stimuli such as faces, people prefer symmetrical to asymmetrical structures and smiling to frowning expressions (Grammer & Thornhill, 1994; Knutson, 1996). However, people can also rapidly and flexibly learn to assign reward value to novel social stimuli, with lasting consequences. In this section, we examine whether unlearned and learned socially rewarding stimuli elicit mesolimbic activation and whether mesolimbic activation can influence subsequent social behavior (Adolphs, 2001).

Following initial reports of amygdalar activation to fearful faces (Breiter et al., 1996), some of the first fMRI studies to focus on social incentives utilized facial stimuli. An initial study reported ventral striatal activation to forward-gazing faces that participants rated as attractive

(Kampe, Frith, Dolan, & Frith, 2001). However, as noted in a later correction (Kampe, Frith, Dolan, & Frith, 2002), activation foci were located in the thalamus rather than the ventral striatum, as initially reported. A subsequent study reported mesolimbic activation in general and NAcc activation in particular in male participants exposed to female faces (Aharon et al., 2001). NAcc activation correlated both with rated attractiveness and with the number of button presses participants made to continue viewing the female faces in a separate behavioral experiment. Both of these studies had block designs and so may have included activation that occurred during both anticipation and outcome. To control for anticipatory confounds, a third study used an event-related design and reported that both male and female participants showed increased activation of the mPFC and OFC as a function of the face's participant-rated attractiveness and whether the face was judged as happy or not (O'Doherty et al., 2003). Together, these findings suggest that both the attractiveness and the happiness of novel faces can activate the MPFC, and they further raise the possibility that anticipation of viewing attractive faces may activate the NAcc, though the last implication has not been directly tested.

For some, other novel social rewards may include erotic stimuli (Lang, Greenwald, Bradley, & Hamm, 1993). A number of fMRI studies have investigated neural correlates of exposure to erotic visual stimuli. Initial studies primarily contrasted erotic films with nonerotic films among heterosexual males and reported widespread activations of subcortical and cortical regions, including but not limited to mesolimbic regions (Arnow et al., 2002; Garavan et al., 2000; Karama et al., 2002; Mouras et al., 2003; Park et al., 2001). Unlike studies of other rewarding social stimuli (e.g., faces), studies of erotic films may produce more widespread activation because investigators have modeled responses to lengthy and dynamic stimuli rather than to discrete static images. Accordingly, when investigators concurrently measured online affective indices such as penile tumescence during viewing of erotic films and correlated these with brain activation, they found more focused mesolimbic and mesial cortical patterns of activation (Arnow et al., 2002; Ferretti et al., 2005). Further, subsequent studies of more temporally constrained erotic pictures clearly demonstrate ventral striatal activation, as well as increased activation of visual processing pathways, in both male and female participants, who reported similar levels of sexual motivation (Hamann, Herman, Nolan, & Wallen, 2004).

Social reward can also be learned, as in the case of bonding. Prototypical examples include the nurturing attachment that develops between mother and infant, as well as the romantic attachment that develops between lovers. Accordingly, fMRI experiments have begun to investigate neural responses to infants and lovers. With respect to infants, one study reported lateral OFC activation when mothers viewed their own versus other infants, and this activation was correlated with positive mood when viewing the pictures (Nitschke et al., 2004). However, this study suffered from signal loss in the MPFC and the striatum. A second study without signal loss in these regions similarly reported activation of lateral OFC but also of the striatum (including ventral striatum) when mothers viewed pictures of their own versus other infants (Bartels & Zeki, 2004). These studies suggest that viewing one's own infant can activate mesolimbic circuitry. fMRI researchers have also investigated exposure to pictures of lovers. An initial study reported that viewing pictures of lovers versus friends activated striatal regions, as well as the anterior insula and anterior cingulate (Bartels & Zeki, 2000), and these results were replicated in a follow-up study (Bartels & Zeki, 2004). A third study of recent lovers (i.e., relationships begun less than 3 months prior to the study) also found that viewing lovers versus acquaintances activated striatal regions and midbrain nuclei, but not the other cortical regions (Aron et al., 2005). Thus studies suggest that viewing pictures of lovers can activate striatal and midbrain regions of the mesolimbic circuit.

In addition to innate bonding mechanisms, social reward can be learned over the course of repeated interactions. For instance, all human cultures value reciprocity, and repeated reciprocity represents an evolutionarily stable strategy that can sustain cooperation, even among strangers (Trivers, 1971). Behavioral economists have devised ingenious games to elicit reciprocity (or not), such as the prisoner's dilemma game (Axelrod & Hamilton, 1981). In an iterated version of the prisoner's dilemma, two players repeatedly and independently choose either to cooperate or defect. If they mutually cooperate, both win, and if they mutually defect, both lose. However, if one player defects and the other cooperates, the defector wins more than if he or she had cooperated, whereas the cooperator loses more than if he or she had defected. The standard in behavioral economics is for partners to play with actual money, and all of the studies described here adhere to this standard.

In an initial fMRI study of the prisoner's dilemma game, investigators found that mutually cooperative outcomes (rated as most desirable by the female participants) elicited more mesolimbic activation (specifically, in the NAcc, caudate, MPFC, and anterior cingulate) than did outcomes elicited by other strategies. Further, peak activation in the NAcc, but not other regions, correlated with a tendency to engage in repeated mutual cooperation (Rilling et al., 2002). Similar but less robust patterns of mesolimbic activation were observed when participants played against a computer. These researchers replicated the same pattern of findings in a follow-up study that utilized a one-shot version of the prisoner's dilemma game with both male and female participants. After participants chose to cooperate, activation in NAcc and MPFC increased when partners also cooperated but decreased when partners chose to defect. In another study, participants first played a prisoner's dilemma game outside the scanner with partners (identified by pictures) who consistently responded to the participant's cooperation with either cooperation or defection (Singer, Kiebel, Winston, Dolan,

& Frith, 2004). In a subsequent fMRI session, participants showed increased medial amygdala, putamen/NAcc, and left insula activation while viewing pictures of intentional cooperators versus nonplayers. Thus social stimuli arbitrarily associated with prior cooperation also can elicit mesolimbic activation.

Another game that elicits social reciprocity is the trust game, in which an investor receives money and then decides how much to either invest in a trustee or retain. The invested amount then triples, and the trustee must decide how much to pay back the investor or retain (Berg, Dickhaut, & McCabe, 1995). In an fMRI study, pairs of participants were scanned simultaneously while playing repeated trust games (King-Casas et al., 2005). When trustees learned that the investor had increased their investment relative to previous investments, activation increased in the head of the caudate/NAcc. As the task progressed and investments increased, the onset of this activation in the trustees' brain began earlier, until it preceded revelation of increased investments.

However, social reciprocation need not always involve cooperation. In some cases, people will expend inordinate amounts of effort and time to reciprocate defection, even at the risk of substantial personal loss (e.g., the case of revenge). Using PET imaging rather than fMRI, researchers investigated brain activation associated with anticipation of revenge in the context of a trust game with male participants (de Quervain et al., 2004). The researchers gave money to participants, who then invested in trustees. After the investment tripled, trustees then either cooperated by returning part of the investment or defected by returning nothing. Investors could then decide whether or not to punish defectors (by taking away their money), during which time their brains were scanned with PET. Participants who chose to punish defectors showed activation of the head of the caudate (just above the NAcc). The investigators inferred that this activation was related to the desire to punish defectors, as activation in the head of the caudate predicted how much money participants were willing to spend to punish defectors in a separate condition.

Other researchers scanned participants with fMRI as they played a more complicated matrix game for money, in which participants attempted to coordinate choices with a partner outside the scanner to maximize earnings. Some choices maximized only the participant's earnings or only the partner's earnings, whereas others maximized the pair's joint earnings. Participants had to take the perspectives of their partners and imagine their partners taking their own perspectives in order to identify "equilibrium" solutions that would maximally benefit both partners. While undergoing fMRI, participants either simultaneously chose with the partner or simply guessed their partner's strategy. The only brain area that showed significant activation when participants coordinated to choose equilibrium solutions versus merely identifying partners' strategies was the NAcc (Bhatt & Camerer, 2005).

As with research utilizing other types of rewards, the collective findings of these social game studies are consistent with the notion that NAcc activation indexes gain anticipation (Knutson, Adams, et al., 2001). Gain anticipation may occur in the context of reciprocated cooperation, but it also may occur prior to reciprocated defection (e.g., in the case of anticipated revenge; Knutson, 2004), and it seems related to social coordination in all cases. Although the findings suggest that social rewards activate qualitatively similar regions to other types of rewards, they also raise the possibility that social rewards may have a more pronounced quantitative effect on mesolimbic activation than monetarily equivalent nonsocial rewards. Of course, social coordination may additionally engage qualitatively distinct brain areas associated with other functions (not reviewed here), such as regions implicated in perspective taking, which lie along the mesial wall of the prefrontal cortex (Gallagher & Frith, 2003; McCabe, Houser, Ryan, Smith, & Trouard, 2001).

In addition to converging with literature on other rewards, neuroimaging research on social rewards brings new light to bear on how neuroscience methods can inform the study of social behavior. Although social behavior is complex, prediction of complex phenomena does not necessarily require complex theory. The dynamic interplay of simple mechanisms might also generate complex behavior (Braitenberg, 1984). For example, neuroimaging evidence suggests that a process as simple as reward anticipation (and accompanying affect) may underlie a diverse range of social phenomena, including cooperation, revenge, moral attribution, and strategic coordination. Thus neuroimaging may inform an understanding of social behavior by helping researchers to deconstruct complex processes and to winnow out unnecessarily complex theories based on questionable assumptions. Social behavior can be studied empirically, incrementally, hierarchically, and systematically from a neuroscience perspective.

IMPLICATIONS

Humans are not just information processors. Humans are also value processors. In fact, value may take precedence over other types of information (Zajonc, 1980), because organisms that cannot efficiently assess value may not survive long enough to represent their genes in future generations (Panksepp, Knutson, & Burgdorf, 2002). Because they cannot survive or reproduce alone, social connections are among the most highly valued of incentives for mammals (MacLean, 1990). Thus mammalian value computation should not only reside deep in the processing hierarchy but should also be especially attuned to social incentives. To survive and procreate, mammals should not only be able to assess value reactively but also proactively. Indeed, one reason for the expansion of the forebrain in primates (Semendeferi, Lu, Schenker, & Damasio, 2002) may involve enhancing the ability to assign value to future events, particularly those related to social interaction.

Emerging techniques that allow researchers to visualize neural activity at the speed of phenomenology will revolutionize psychology. Part of this revolution will be methodological. Researchers can now track second-to-second changes in small and deep brain regions long implicated in affect in other mammals (e.g., rats). Technical development is still rapidly advancing, and many investigators have yet to avail themselves of the spatial and temporal resolution afforded by event-related fMRI. Accumulating evidence suggests that excessive averaging over either time or space can obscure meaningful fluctuations in subcortical activity. A parallel methodological challenge involves developing tools that can track ongoing changes in psychological phenomena, such as affect, with adequate temporal resolution, which could then be directly correlated with changes in brain activation. Hopefully in the future, not only will psychology inform neuroimaging, but neuroimaging will also reciprocally inform psychology. For instance, we have repeatedly observed that NAcc activation correlates with increases in positive arousal. Based on this association, one might predict that people will experience more positive arousal at any point in a given task when NAcc activation increases. This prediction has been confirmed in the case of the MID task, in which online affect probes have revealed that positive arousal increases most markedly during gain anticipation, rather than in response to gain outcomes (Knutson, Nielsen, et al., 2005). Additionally, linking brain activity to function may help drive predictions about how current brain activity could influence subsequent behavior. For instance, emerging evidence suggests that NAcc activation may promote gain-seeking financial behavior, as well as cooperation with friends and punishment of enemies. Of course, the difficult work of testing alternative functional accounts of brain activation must also proceed. In the case of affect, this endeavor will require designs that utilize subjectively compelling stimuli while controlling for sensorimotor demands, valence, arousal, and anticipation.

Another part of the coming revolution will be theoretical. Neuroimaging has revealed a beautiful and elegant confluence of results. The NAcc is activated not only by anticipation of nonsocial rewards such as money, food, or pleasant sensations but also by anticipation of social rewards, such as interacting with one's child or lover, rewarding a friend, or punishing an enemy. Thus neuroimaging findings may bring together previously disparate domains of inquiry and reveal surprising and useful connections between them. The current data suggest that social interaction is a multilayered process that powerfully involves affect. By implication, theories that attempt to describe and predict social interaction should strive to assign a central role for affect.

Although surprisingly coherent, the existing findings raise more questions than they answer. If a mechanism for gain anticipation responds to social incentives and modulates subsequent social behavior, what other motivational circuits also play a role, how many are there, and how do they dynamically interact? At minimum, based both on brain stimulation data (Panksepp, 1998) and the statistical independence of self-reported positive arousal and negative arousal (Watson & Tellegen, 1985), one might postulate a loss anticipation system (Kuhnen & Knutson, 2005). Candidate regions might include those involved in the anticipation of pain, such as the periaqueductal gray, ventromedial hypothalamus, lateral amygdala, anterior insula, and anterior cingulate (Panksepp, 1998). Different neurochemicals might modulate activity of these distinct circuits (Depue & Collins, 1999; Knutson et al., 1998). Further, what kinds of control systems govern or modulate the activity of these deep motivational systems, how many are there, and how do they dynamically interact? For instance, our findings suggest that in the case of gain anticipation, the MPFC may modulate activity in the NAcc and enable people to correct their expectations of reward when violated or to keep probabilistic concerns in mind (Knutson, Taylor, et al., 2005). Finally, do social incentives recruit these systems differently than nonsocial incentives, and what additional circuitry promotes social interaction?

The goal of this overview is not to provide an exhaustive survey but, rather, to highlight a hypothesis that may prove useful to social neuroscientists. The hypothesis that NAcc activation indexes gain anticipation (and thereby generates an appetitive signal) provides a simple but powerful unifying framework both for consolidating diverse findings and also for generating predictions about future cognition and behavior. The hypothesis generalizes to both nonsocial and social rewards. It not only predicts where in the brain and when in time activation will occur but also how brain activation might influence subsequent behavior. At present, we know something, but not much. By applying neuroscience tools to the study of social behavior, we feel certain in predicting that we have much to gain.

ACKNOWLEDGMENTS

Brian Knutson was supported by a National Alliance on Schizophrenia and Depression Young Investigator Award and National Institute of Aging Seed Grant No. AG024957 during manuscript preparation. We thank Meghana Bhatt, Jeffrey Cooper, and Jeanne L. Tsai for helpful comments on previous drafts.

REFERENCES

Adcock, R. A., Thangavel, A., Whitfield-Gabrieli, S., Knutson, B., & Gabrieli, J. D. E. (2006). Reward-motivated learning: Mesolimbic activation precedes memory formation. *Neuron, 50,* 507–517.

Adolphs, R. (2001). The neurobiology of social cognition. *Current Opinion in Neurobiology, 11,* 231–239.

Aharon, I., Etcoff, N. L., Ariely, D., Chabris, C. F., O'Connor, E., & Breiter, H. C. (2001). Beautiful faces have variable reward value: fMRI and behavioral evidence. *Neuron, 32*, 537–551.

Anderson, A. K., Christoff, K., Stappen, I., Panitz, D., Ghahremani, D. G., Glover, G. H., et al. (2003). Dissociated neural representations of intensity and valence in human olfaction. *Nature Neuroscience, 6*, 196–202.

Arnow, B., Desmond, J. E., Banner, L. L., Glover, G. H., Solomon, A., Polan, M. L., et al. (2002). Brain activation and sexual arousal in healthy, heterosexual males. *Brain, 125*, 1–10.

Aron, A., Fisher, H. E., Mashek, D. J., Strong, G., Li, H. F., & Brown, L. L. (2005). Reward, motivation, and emotion systems associated with early-stage intense romantic love. *Journal of Neurophysiology, 94*, 327–337.

Axelrod, R., & Hamilton, W. D. (1981). The evolution of cooperation. *Science, 211*, 1390–1396.

Bandura, A. (1977). *Social learning theory.* Englewood Clifs, NJ: Prentice Hall.

Bartels, A., & Zeki, S. (2000). The neural basis of romantic love. *NeuroReport, 11*, 3829–3834.

Bartels, A., & Zeki, S. (2004). The neural correlates of maternal and romantic love. *NeuroImage, 21*, 1155–1166.

Berg, J., Dickhaut, J., & McCabe, K. (1995). Trust, reciprocity, and social history. *Games and Economic Behavior, 10*, 122–142.

Berns, G. S., McClure, S. M., Pagnoni, G., & Montague, P. R. (2001). Predictability modulates human brain response to reward. *Journal of Neuroscience, 21*, 2793–2798.

Berridge, K. C., & Robinson, T. E. (1998). What is the role of dopamine in reward: Hedonic impact, reward learning, or incentive salience? *Brain Research Reviews, 28*, 309–369.

Bhatt, M., & Camerer, C. F. (2005). Self-referential thinking and equilibrium as states of mind in games: fMRI evidence. *Games and Economic Behavior, 25*, 424–459.

Bishop, M. P., Elder, S. T., & Heath, R. G. (1963). Intracranial self-stimulation in man. *Science, 140*, 394–396.

Bjork, J. M., Knutson, B., Fong, G. W., Caggiano, D. M., Bennett, S. M., & Hommer, D. W. (2004). Incentive-elicited brain activation in adolescents: Similarities and differences from young adults. *Journal of Neuroscience, 24*, 1793–1802.

Braitenberg, V. (1984). *Vehicles: Experiments in synthetic psychology.* Cambridge, MA: MIT Press.

Breiter, H. C., Aharon, I., Kahneman, D., Dale, A., & Shizgal, P. (2001). Functional imaging of neural responses to expectancy and experience of monetary gains and losses. *Neuron, 30*, 619–639.

Breiter, H. C., Etcoff, N. L., Whalen, P. J., Kennedy, W. A., Rauch, S. L., Buckner, R. L., et al. (1996). Response and habituation of the human amygdala during visual processing of facial expression. *Neuron, 17*, 875–887.

Camille, N., Coricelli, G., Sallet, J., Pradat-Diehl, P., Duhamel, J. R., & Sirigu, A. (2004). The involvement of the orbitofrontal cortex in the experience of regret. *Science, 304*, 1167–1170.

Craig, W. (1918). Appetites and aversions as constituents of instincts. *Biological Bulletin, 34*, 91–107.

Davidson, R., & Sutton, S. (1995). Affective neuroscience: The emergence of a discipline. *Current Opinions in Neurobiology, 5*(2), 217–224.

de Quervain, D. J., Fischbacher, U., Treyer, V., Schellhammer, M., Schnyder, U., Buck, A., et al. (2004). The neural basis of altruistic punishment. *Science, 305*, 1254–1258.

Delgado, M. R., Nystrom, L. E., Fissell, C., Noll, D. C., & Fiez, J. A. (2000). Tracking the hemodynamic response to reward and punishment in the striatum. *Journal of Neurophysiology, 84*, 3072–3077.

Depue, R. A., & Collins, P. F. (1999). Neurobiology of the structure of personality: Dopamine, facilitation of incentive motivation, and extraversion. *Behavioral and Brain Sciences, 22*, 491–517.

Dickinson, A. (1994). Instrumental conditioning. In N. J. Mackintosh (Ed.), *Animal learning and cognition* (pp. 45–79). New York: Academic Press.

Drevets, W. C., Gautier, C., Price, J. C., Kupfer, D. J., Kinahan, P. E., Grace, A. A., et al. (2001). Amphetamine-induced dopamine release in human ventral striatum correlates with euphoria. *Biological Psychiatry, 49*, 81–96.

Elliott, R., Friston, K. J., & Dolan, R. J. (2000). Dissociable neural responses in human reward systems. *Journal of Neuroscience, 20*, 6159–6165.

Engel, S. A., Rumelhart, D. E., Wandell, B. A., Lee, A. T., Glover, G. H., Chichilnisky, E. J., et al. (1994). fMRI of human visual cortex. *Nature, 369*, 525.

Falck, B., & Hillarp, N. A. (1959). On the cellular localization of catecholamines in the brain. *Acta Anatomica, 38*, 277–279.

Ferretti, A., Caulo, M., Del Gratta, C., Di Matteo, R., Merla, A., Montorsi, F., et al. (2005). Dynamics of male sexual arousal: Distinct components of brain activation revealed by fMRI. *NeuroImage, 26*, 1086–1096.

Gallagher, H., & Frith, C. (2003). Functional imaging of "theory of mind." *Trends in Cognitive Science, 7*, 77–83.

Garavan, H., Pankiewicz, J., Bloom, A., Cho, J. K., Sperry, L., Ross, T. J., et al. (2000). Cue-induced cocaine craving: Neuroanatomical specificity for drug users and drug stimuli. *American Journal of Psychiatry, 157*, 1789–1798.

Gottfried, J. A., O'Doherty, J., & Dolan, R. J. (2003). Appetitive and aversive olfactory learning in humans studied using event-related functional magnetic resonance imaging. *Journal of Neuroscience, 22*, 10829–10837.

Grammer, K., & Thornhill, R. (1994). Human (*Homo sapiens*) facial attractiveness and sexual selection: The role of symmetry and averageness. *Journal of Comparative Psychology, 108*, 233–242.

Hamann, S. B., Herman, R. A., Nolan, C. L., & Wallen, K. (2004). Men and women differ in amygdala response to visual sexual stimuli. *Nature Neuroscience, 7*, 411–416.

Ikemoto, S., & Panksepp, J. (1999). The role of nucleus accumbens dopamine in motivated behavior: A unifying interpretation with special reference to reward-seeking. *Brain Research Reviews, 31*, 6–41.

Kahneman, D., & Tversky, A. (1979). Prospect theory: An analysis of decision under risk. *Econometrica, 47*, 263–291.

Kampe, K. K., Frith, C. D., Dolan, R. J., & Frith, U. (2001). Reward value of attractiveness and gaze. *Nature, 413*, 589.

Kampe, K. K., Frith, C. D., Dolan, R. J., & Frith, U. (2002). Correction. *Nature, 416*, 602.

Karama, S., Lecours, A. R., Leroux, J. M., Bourgouin, P., Beaudoin, G., Joubert, S., et al. (2002). Areas of brain activation in males and females during viewing of erotic film excerpts. *Human Brain Mapping, 16*, 1–13.

King-Casas, B., Tomlin, D., Anen, C., Camerer, C. F., Quartz, S. R., & Montague, P. R. (2005). Getting to know you: Reputation and trust in a two-person economic exchange. *Science, 308*, 78–83.

Knutson, B. (1996). Facial expressions of emotion influence interpersonal trait inferences. *Journal of Nonverbal Behavior, 20*, 165–182.

Knutson, B. (2004). Sweet revenge? *Science, 305*, 1246–1247.

Knutson, B., Adams, C. M., Fong, G. W., & Hommer, D. (2001). Anticipation of increasing monetary reward selectively recruits nucleus accumbens. *Journal of Neuroscience, 21*, RC159.

Knutson, B., & Cooper, J. C. (2005). Functional magnetic resonance imaging of reward prediction. *Current Opinion in Neurobiology, 18*, 411–417.

Knutson, B., Fong, G. W., Adams, C. M., Varner, J. L., & Hommer, D. (2001). Dissociation of reward anticipation and outcome with event-related FMRI. *NeuroReport, 12*, 3683–3687.

Knutson, B., Fong, G. W., Bennett, S. M., Adams, C. M., & Hommer, D. (2003). A region of mesial prefrontal cortex tracks monetarily rewarding outcomes: Characterization with rapid event-related FMRI. *NeuroImage, 18*, 263–272.

Knutson, B., Nielsen, L., Larkin, G., & Carstensen, L. L. (2006). *Affect dynamics: Tracking trajectories through affect space.* Manuscript submitted for publication.

Knutson, B., Taylor, J., Kaufman, M. T., Peterson, R., & Glover, G. (2005). Distributed neural representation of expected value. *Journal of Neuroscience, 25*, 4806–4812.

Knutson, B., Westdorp, A., Kaiser, E., & Hommer, D. (2000). FMRI visualization of brain activity during a monetary incentive delay task. *NeuroImage, 12*, 20–27.

Knutson, B., Wolkowitz, O. M., Cole, S. W., Chan, T., Moore, E. A., Johnson, R. C., et al. (1998). Selective alteration of personality and social behavior by serotonergic intervention. *American Journal of Psychiatry, 155*, 373–379.

Koepp, M. J., Gunn, R. N., Lawrence, A. D., Cunningham, V. J., Dagher, A., Jones, T., et al. (1998). Evidence for striatal dopamine release during a video game. *Nature, 393*(6682), 266–268.

Kuhnen, C. M., & Knutson, B. (2005). The neural basis of financial risk-taking. *Neuron, 47*, 620–628.

Lang, P. J., Greenwald, M. K., Bradley, M. M., & Hamm, A. O. (1993). Looking at pictures: Affective, facial, visceral and behavioral reactions. *Psychophysiology, 30*, 261–273.

MacLean, P. D. (1990). *The triune brain in evolution.* New York: Plenum Press.

Mawlawi, O., Martinez, D., Slifstein, M., Broft, A., Chatterjee, R., Hwang, D., et al. (2001). Imaging human mesolimbic dopamine transmission with positron emission tomography: I. Accuracy and precision of D2 receptor parameter measurements in ventral striatum. *Journal of Cerebral Blood Flow and Metabolism, 21*, 1034–1057.

McBride, W. J., Murphy, J. M., & Ikemoto, S. (1999). Localization of brain reinforcement mechanisms: Intracranial self-administration and intracranial place-conditioning studies. *Behavioral Brain Research, 101*, 129–152.

McCabe, K., Houser, D., Ryan, L., Smith, V., & Trouard, T. (2001). A functional imaging study of cooperation in two-person reciprocal exchange. *Proceedings of the National Academy of Sciences of the USA, 98,* 11832–11835.

McClure, S. M., York, M. K., & Montague, P. R. (2004). The neural substrates of reward processing in humans: The modern role of fMRI. *Neuroscientist, 10,* 260–268.

Menon, V., & Levitin, D. J. (2005). The rewards of music listening: Response and physiological connectivity of the mesolimbic system. *NeuroImage, 28,* 175–184.

Mogenson, G. M., Jones, D. L., & Yim, C. Y. (1980). From motivation to action: Functional interface between the limbic system and the motor system. *Progress in Neurobiology, 14,* 69–97.

Mouras, H., Stoleru, S., Bittoun, J., Glutron, D., Pelegrini-Issac, M., Paradis, A., et al. (2003). Brain processing of visual sexual stimuli in healthy men: A functional magnetic resonance imaging study. *NeuroImage, 20,* 855–869.

Nitschke, J. B., Nelson, E. E., Rusch, B. D., Fox, A. S., Oakes, T. R., & Davidson, R. J. (2004). Orbitofrontal cortex tracks positive mood in mothers viewing pictures of their newborn infants. *NeuroImage, 21,* 583–592.

O'Doherty, J., Rolls, E. T., Francis, S., Bowtell, R., & McGlone, F. (2001). Representation of pleasant and aversive taste in the human brain. *Journal of Neurophysiology, 85,* 1315–1321.

O'Doherty, J. P. (2004). Reward representations and reward-related learning in the human brain: Insights from neuroimaging. *Current Opinion in Neurobiology, 14,* 769–776.

O'Doherty, J. P., Deichmann, R., Critchley, H. D., & Dolan, R. J. (2002). Neural responses during anticipation of a primary taste reward. *Neuron, 33,* 815–826.

O'Doherty, J. P., Winston, J. S., Critchley, H. D., Perrett, D., Burt, D. M., & Dolan, R. J. (2003). Beauty in a smile: The role of medial orbitofrontal cortex in facial attractiveness. *Neuropsychologia, 41,* 147–155.

Olds, J., & Milner, P. (1954). Positive reinforcement produced by electrical stimulation of septal area and other regions of rat brain. *Journal of Comparative and Physiological Psychology, 47,* 419–427.

Olds, M. E., & Fobes, J. L. (1981). The central basis of motivation: Intracranial self-stimulation studies. *Annual Review of Psychology, 32,* 523–574.

Panksepp, J. (1991). Affective neuroscience: A conceptual framework for the study of emotions. In K. Strongman (Ed.), *International reviews of studies in emotions* (Vol. 1, pp. 59–99). Chichester, UK: Wiley.

Panksepp, J. (1998). *Affective neuroscience: The foundations of human and animal emotions.* New York: Oxford University Press.

Panksepp, J., Knutson, B., & Burgdorf, J. (2002). The role of emotional brain systems in addictions: A neuro-evolutionary perspective. *Addiction, 97,* 459–469.

Pappata, S., Dehaene, S., Poline, J. B., Gregoire, M. C., Jobert, A., Delforge, J., et al. (2002). In vivo detection of striatal dopamine release during reward: A PET study with [(11)C]raclopride and a single dynamic scan approach. *NeuroImage, 16,* 1015–1027.

Park, K., Seo, J. J., Kang, H. K., Ryu, S. B., Kim, H. J., & Jeong, G. W. (2001). A new potential of blood oxygenation level dependent (BOLD) functional MRI for evaluating cerebral centers of penile erection. *International Journal of Impotence Research, 13,* 73–81.

Pavlov, I. P. (1927). *Conditioned reflexes: An investigation of the physiological activity of the cerebral cortex.* Oxford, UK: Oxford University Press.

Ramnani, N., Elliott, R., Athwal, B. S., & Passingham, R. E. (2004). Prediction error for free monetary reward in the human prefrontal cortex. *NeuroImage, 23*(3), 777–786.

Rilling, J. K., Gutman, D. A., Zeh, T. R., Pagnoni, G., Berns, G. S., & Kilts, C. D. (2002). A neural basis for social cooperation. *Neuron, 35,* 395–405.

Rolls, E. T., O'Doherty, J., Kringelbach, M. L., Francis, S., Bowtell, R., & McGlone, F. (2003). Representations of pleasant and painful touch in the human orbitofrontal and cingulate cortices. *Cerebral Cortex, 13,* 308–317.

Rotter, J. B. (1972). *Applications of a social learning theory of personality.* New York: Holt.

Schultz, W., Dayan, P., & Montague, P. R. (1997). A neural substrate of prediction and reward. *Science, 275,* 1593–1599.

Semendeferi, K., Lu, A., Schenker, N., & Damasio, H. (2002). Humans and great apes share a large frontal cortex. *Nature Neuroscience, 5,* 272–276.

Singer, T., Kiebel, S. J., Winston, J. S., Dolan, R. J., & Frith, C. D. (2004). Brain responses to the acquired moral status of faces. *Neuron, 41,* 653–662.

Trivers, R. L. (1971). The evolution of reciprocal altruism. *Quarterly Review of Biology, 46,* 35–57.

Volkow, N. D., Wang, G., Fowler, J. S., Logan, J., Gatley, S. J., Wong, C., et al. (1999). Reinforcing effects of psychostimulants in humans are associated with increases in brain dopamine and occupancy of D2 receptors. *Journal of Pharmacology and Experimental Therapeutics, 291,* 409–415.

von Neumann, J., & Morgenstern, O. (1944). *Theory of games and economic behavior.* Princeton, NJ: Princeton University Press.

Watson, D., & Tellegen, A. (1985). Toward a consensual structure of mood. *Psychological Bulletin, 98,* 219–235.

Wightman, R. M., & Robinson, D. L. (2002). Transient changes in mesolimbic dopamine and their association with "reward." *Journal of Neurochemistry, 82,* 721–735.

Wittmann, B. C., Schott, B. H., Guderian, S., Frey, J. U., Heinze, H. J., & Duzel, E. (2005). Reward-related fMRI activation of dopaminergic midbrain is associated with enhanced hippocampus-dependent long-term memory formation. *Neuron, 45,* 459–467.

Zajonc, R. B. (1980). Feeling and thinking: Preferences need no inferences. *American Psychologist, 35,* 151–175.

Zald, D. H., Boileau, I., El-Dearedy, W., Gunn, R. N., McGlone, F., Dichter, G. S., et al. (2004). Dopamine transmission in the human striatum during monetary reward tasks. *Journal of Neuroscience, 24,* 4105–4112.

9

A Biobehavioral Model of Implicit Power Motivation Arousal, Reward, and Frustration

Oliver C. Schultheiss

POWER MOTIVATION: DEFINITION, MEASUREMENT, AND VALIDITY

Like members of many other social species, humans show marked individual differences in how much they seek and enjoy power. Some people are driven to become socially visible and dominate their fellow human beings, whereas others do not seem to care much for any kind of self-assertion and feel comfortable keeping a low social profile. Such individual differences in the drive for power have been conceptualized and studied over the past 50 years through the prism of the power motive construct. The power motive (also sometimes labeled *need* Power, or *n* Power) represents an enduring affective preference for having impact on other people or the world at large (Winter, 1973). Individuals with a strong power motive experience the consummation of the impact incentive as pleasurable and rewarding, whereas individuals with a weak power motive do not derive much pleasure from having impact. Accordingly, the former are more motivated than the latter to seek out opportunities to have impact on others.

From the start, research on the power motive was guided by the notion that introspective access to motivational states and traits is limited and that motives should therefore be assessed indirectly—hence the attribute *implicit* (McClelland, 1984). In their groundbreaking research on the achievement motive, David McClelland and John Atkinson had shown that experimentally aroused motivational states alter the content of stories that

176

individuals write about picture cues in specific ways that can be codified into reliable scoring systems (McClelland, Atkinson, Clark, & Lowell, 1953). The McClelland–Atkinson approach was first applied toward the development of a measure of implicit power motivation by Veroff (1957), who compared the stories written by candidates in student elections with stories written by students not running for office, and later by Uleman (1972), who devised a scoring system by comparing stories written by students who acted as powerful experimenters with those written by students assigned to the less powerful role of research participant. Winter (1973) conducted additional studies employing experimental arousal of power motivation and cross-validated and combined the content-coding categories he had derived in his research with those identified earlier by Veroff (1957) and Uleman (1972). According to Winter's (1973) integrated scoring system, power imagery is scored whenever a story character expresses a power concern through strong, forceful actions; provides unsolicited help, support, or advice; tries to control or regulate others' behavior; tries to influence, persuade, bribe, or argue with another person; tries to impress another person or the world at large; arouses strong, nonreciprocal emotions in others; or is concerned with reputation and prestige.

The scoring system is applied to imaginative stories that participants write in response to four to six picture cues showing people in everyday situations that are slightly suggestive of themes of power and dominance (e.g., a ship's captain talking to a passenger, two women working in a laboratory, a couple in a nightclub; see Smith, 1992, for reproductions of these and other commonly used pictures). This procedure of collecting imaginative stories for scoring is called the Picture Story Exercise (PSE) and is derived from Morgan and Murray's (1935) Thematic Apperception Test. Before scorers can code PSE stories for motivational content, they are required to achieve > 85% reliability on scoring materials prescored by an expert (Smith, 1992). This rigorous criterion ensures high interrater reliability: In studies in which two scorers coded the same PSE independently for motivational imagery, interrater agreement is usually 80–100%. Stability of power motive scores across assessments is substantial, too (see Schultheiss & Pang, in press, for an overview of research on the reliability of implicit motive scores). For instance, Winter and Stewart (1977) reported a retest correlation of .61 for a 1-week interval, and Koestner, Franz, and Hellmann (1991; cited in Smith, 1992) obtained a retest correlation of .55 for an 8-month interval.

A large body of literature supports the validity of Winter's power motive measure (reviewed in McClelland, 1987a; Winter, 1996). For instance, consistent with the notion that power motivation should promote social success and visibility, power-motivated individuals have been found to draw others' attention through risky choices and behaviors (e.g., McClelland & Watson, 1973), to be more likely to ascend to higher levels of management in large corporations (e.g., McClelland & Boyatzis, 1982), to pursue more successful careers (McClelland & Franz, 1992), and to be more sexually active than individuals low in power motivation (e.g., Schultheiss, Dargel, & Rohde, 2003a). The darker side of power motivation is represented by findings involving this need in alcohol abuse, relationship violence, and political radicalism (Lichter & Rothman, 1981; Mason & Blankenship, 1987; McClelland, Davis, Kalin, & Wanner, 1972). Strong evidence for the validity of the power motive measure also comes from research on political behavior and between-group processes. Adapting his power motive scoring system for use with any kind of running text, Winter (1991) found that U.S. presidents whose inaugural speeches were more saturated with power motivation imagery were more likely to wage war, to be assassinated, and to be rated as great by historians than U.S. presidents with fewer power images in their inaugural speeches. Increases and decreases of power motivation assessed in political documents have also been shown to be associated with peaceful and violent outcomes of international crises (Winter, 1987; see also Winter, 1993).

Importantly, the power motive and other implicit motives, such as the needs for affiliation and achievement, are more likely to become aroused by and respond to *nonverbal cues* than to verbal stimuli (Schultheiss, 2001). Klinger (1967) showed that individuals respond to watching an affiliation-oriented or achievement-oriented experimenter with increases in affiliation or achievement motivation expressed in PSE stories, even if they cannot hear the experimenter's verbal instructions. In a similar vein, Schultheiss and Brunstein (1999; 2002) demonstrated that experimenters who assigned and described a power-related goal verbally to their participants failed to arouse participants' power motive. Only after participants had an opportunity to translate the verbally assigned goal into an experiential format through a goal imagery exercise did their power motive predict goal commitment and task performance. Recent research indicates that facial expressions of emotion are particularly salient nonverbal cues for the power motive. Power-motivated individuals attend to and condition well in response to expressions signaling another person's low dominance and submission (e.g., surprise) and attend away from and show poor conditioning in response to expressions signaling another person's high dominance (e.g., anger, but also a smiling face; Schultheiss & Hale, in press; Schultheiss, Pang, Torges, Wirth, & Treynor, 2005).

Consistent with their nonverbal-processing bias, implicit motives are particularly likely to show an effect on behavior if *nondeclarative measures* (e.g., measures of behaviors and processes that are not controlled by a person's view of herself or himself or by the person's explicit intentions) are employed, but they have very limited or no effects on declarative measures of motivation (i.e., measures that tap into a person's conscious sense of self and the beliefs, judgments, decisions, and attitudes associated with it). The differential effect of motives on declarative and nondeclarative measures was first observed by deCharms, Morrison, Reitman, and McClelland

(1955), who found that the PSE measure of achievement motivation predicted performance on a scrambled-word test (a nondeclarative measure) but not participants' attribution of achievement-related traits to themselves or others (declarative measures of motivation). Later, Biernat (1989) showed that the PSE achievement motive measure predicted performance on a math task (a nondeclarative measure of motivation) but not participants' decisions to serve as group leaders on another task (a declarative measure of motivation). In a similar vein, Brunstein and Hoyer (2002) found that high-achievement individuals showed superior performance on a vigilance task (nondeclarative measure) but were not more likely than low-achievement individuals to continue on the task if given the choice (declarative measure). Last, Schultheiss and Brunstein (2002) found that the PSE power motivation measure predicts nonverbal (e.g., gesturing, facial expressions) and paraverbal (e.g., speech fluency) behaviors on a persuasion task but not the actual content of the arguments presented, which can be conceived of as a declarative measure.

To summarize, implicit power motivation is assessed through content coding of picture stories and other kinds of verbal material. Motive scores derived in this manner provide an objective, reliable, and valid measure of an individual's need to have impact on others or the world at large. Consistent with the nonconscious, implicit nature of motives assessed per content coding, the power motive is particularly responsive to nonverbal cues but not to verbal–symbolic stimuli and more likely to influence nondeclarative indicators of motivation than declarative ones. There is also considerable evidence for a biological root of implicit power motivation, to which I turn next.

ENDOCRINE AND LEARNING CORRELATES
OF POWER MOTIVATION

Power Motivation Arousal and Sympathetic Catecholamines

Initial evidence for a link between implicit power motivation and individual differences in physiological responses to social stimuli came from a study conducted by Steele (1973; see McClelland, 1987a, for further details of this research). Steele compared participants whose power motive had been aroused through the presentation of inspirational speeches (e.g., Winston Churchill's speech at Dunkirk) with participants from a control condition who had listened to travel tapes and participants who had listened to an achievement-arousing tape. The dependent variables were changes on the PSE measure of power motivation and urinary metabolites of epinephrine (E) and norepinephrine (NE), two catecholamines that are released by the sympathetic nervous system (SNS) under conditions of acute stress. Steele found not only that participants in the power-arousal condition had significantly higher postarousal power motive scores than control-group and achievement-arousal participants but also that postarousal power motive scores were correlated .71 with increases in E and .66 with increases in NE in this group. In contrast, catecholamine changes from before to after the experimental manipulation were not significantly associated with power motive scores in control-group and achievement-arousal participants. These findings suggested that power motivation arousal is uniquely associated with an enhanced response of the SNS, as reflected in sympathetic catecholamine increases.

Further support for a link between power motivation and SNS activation came from a study by McClelland, Floor, Davidson, and Saron (1980). They found that power-motivated male students who experienced frequent power challenges in their daily lives (e.g., being physically threatened or encountering difficulties when dealing with the college administration) and who were unable to spontaneously express power-related impulses (as reflected in high activity inhibition scores on the PSE; cf. Schultheiss & Brunstein, 2002) had significantly higher urinary E levels than all other participants.

In another study, McClelland, Ross, and Patel (1985) assessed salivary NE in students both immediately and 105 minutes after an important midterm examination to measure their acute stress response and also took a baseline measure of salivary NE several days after the exam. The midterm exam was considered to be a challenge for power-motivated individuals because students' status and prestige in college are associated with their academic standing and, hence, how well they do on examinations. Students whose power motive was stronger than their affiliation motive showed a strong and sustained increase in NE after the exam, whereas students whose affiliation motive was stronger than their power motive showed only a slight NE postexam increase relative to baseline levels. These findings provide further evidence for the notion that implicit power motivation, in interaction with specific power-arousing situations and cues, predicts SNS activation and catecholamine release.

McClelland (1987b) speculated that NE, which is released both peripherally and centrally in response to situational challenges, is associated with the experience of having impact and thus represents a biological basis of power motivation reward. A role for NE as the reward substrate of power motivation is unlikely for three reasons, though. First, despite initial speculations about a rewarding role of NE (e.g., Stein, 1975), depriving the brain of NE, either by lesion or chemical depletion, does not impair animals' capacity for intracranial self-stimulation, a classical measure of reward and reinforcement (see Rolls, 1999, for a summary). Second, NE is released in the context not only of power-related challenges but also of other acute stressors (such as jumping from an airplane or escaping a predator), which makes a specific role for NE in power motivation reward even less likely. Third, the studies on power motivation and catecholamine release conducted by McClelland and colleagues were not designed to actually reward or frustrate power-motivated individuals' need for impact nor to examine what happens on incentive consummation. Rather, they can be viewed as evidence for a role for NE (and E) in power motivation arousal and thus in heightened sensitivity to cues predicting, and energization of behavior directed toward attainment of, the impact incentive.

Testosterone's Role in Power Motivation Reward

A hormone with a stronger claim to a specific role in power motivation is the gonadal steroid testosterone (T). In animals and humans, high levels of T have been found to be associated with dominance, social success, enhanced libido, and assertive and violent behavior (e.g., Albert, Jonik, & Walsh, 1992; Carter, 1992; Mazur & Booth, 1998; Monaghan & Glickman, 1992). In many primates, dominant males show transient T increases in response to dominance challenges (Bernstein, Gordon, & Rose, 1983; Mazur, 1985; Sapolsky, 1987). Human males respond with T increases to winning, and with T decreases to losing, dominance contests such as tennis matches, chess tournaments, or even games of chance against another person (reviewed in Mazur & Booth, 1998). The relationship between dominance and T is less well documented for women (Mazur & Booth, 1998), whose free T levels are about one-fourth to one-sixth of those usually observed in healthy men. However, consistent with the notion that T is crucial for female dominance, too, some research shows that elevated T levels in women lead to enhanced physiological and attentional responses to angry faces (van Honk et al., 1999, 2001), that high-T women occupy higher occupational positions than low-T women in various social hierarchies (e.g., Dabbs, Alford, & Fielden, 1998; Purifoy & Koopmans, 1979), and that female prisoners who rank high in the prison hierarchy or who have a history of showing unprovoked aggression are characterized by high T levels (Dabbs & Hargrove, 1997; Dabbs, Ruback, Frady, Hopper, & Sgoutas, 1988).

Subjectively, high T levels are associated with feelings of vigor and activation (Dabbs, Strong, & Milun, 1997; Sherwin, 1988a). T is an effective antidepressant in clinical populations with very low or absent endogenous T production (e.g., Rabkin, Wagner, & Rabkin, 1996), but, at supraphysiological doses, it can also lead to addiction (Pope & Katz, 1994). Consistent with T's addictive properties, animal studies show that T has reinforcing effects. Systemically or locally administered T increases dopamine transmission in the nucleus accumbens (e.g., Packard, Schroeder, & Alexander, 1998), which is at the heart of the brain's incentive motivation system (Cardinal, Parkinson, Hall, & Everitt, 2002). Administration of T has also been shown to reinforce behavior in conditioned place preference paradigms (Alexander, Packard, & Hines, 1994; Wood, Johnson, Chu, Schad, & Self, 2004). T-induced conditioned place preference can be abolished by the concomitant administration of dopamine antagonists

(Packard et al, 1998; Schroeder & Packard, 2000). Accumbens-mediated reinforcing effects of T are particularly pronounced after T has been metabolized to 3α-androstanediol (Frye, Rhodes, Rosellini, & Svare, 2002).

Over the past several years, my laboratory has been dedicated to exploring the link between implicit power motivation and T. In several studies, we have found a slight positive association between basal T levels and the implicit power motive (Schultheiss, Campbell, & McClelland, 1999; Schultheiss, Dargel, & Rohde, 2003b; Schultheiss, Wirth, et al., 2005). However, this association emerges more clearly for men than for women (cf. Schultheiss et al., 2003b). In a study using an experimental arousal design similar to Steele's (1973), we found that relative to a motivationally neutral documentary film, a movie depicting the aggressive pursuit of dominance (*The Godfather: Part II*) elicited increases in power motivation on the PSE in both men and women but T increases only in men with high basal T levels and not in women (Schultheiss, Wirth, & Stanton, 2004). Moreover, in power-arousal-group participants, T changes from before to immediately after the movie correlated substantially with changes in PSE power motive scores among men (bipartial $r = .86$; $p = .001$), whereas T and power motive changes were not significantly associated among women (bipartial $r = -.13$; ns). Although these findings may suggest that the power motive and power motivation arousal are not specifically associated with T in women, it is also conceivable that the relatively higher measurement error for the comparatively low female T levels and the smaller magnitude of situation-induced T changes in women may mask a more substantial positive association between T and power motivation in women.

Going beyond correlational links between T and power motivation or power motivation arousal, my colleagues and I have also explored how the power motive influences individuals' T responses and instrumental learning in response to experimentally varied victory and defeat in dominance contests. In our dominance-contest studies, same-sex dyads competed on several rounds of an implicit-learning task that required participants to repeatedly execute a complex visuomotor pattern. The outcome of this contest was varied such that the designated "winner" won most rounds and the designated "loser" accordingly lost most of the time. Participants' motivational dispositions and personalities were assessed with a PSE and questionnaires at the beginning of the study; their salivary T levels and their mood were assessed several times before and after the contest; and instrumental learning was assessed by determining their learning gains on the implicit-learning task after the contest. Notably, participants had no conscious intention to acquire the visuomotor pattern featured on the implicit learning task, nor did they become aware of the fact that they had learned anything in the first place. Thus learning was implicit in the sense that it happened automatically and was not mediated by declarative processes (e.g., through explicit memory and self-instruction).

Across three studies conducted with young male adults in the United States and Germany, we consistently found that, 15 to 20 minutes after the contest, power motivation predicted T increases after a victory and T decreases after a defeat (Schultheiss et al., 1999; Schultheiss & Rohde, 2002; Schultheiss, Wirth, et al., 2005). However, when we examined the effect of power motivation on women's T responses to the contest outcome, we found a very different pattern of results. In women, power motivation predicted a general sustained postcontest T increase (averaged across assessments at 0, 15 and 30 minutes after the contest; semipartial $r = .29$, $p = .01$), regardless of contest outcome. This increase was particularly strong in power-motivated losers immediately after the contest, whereas power-motivated winners showed only a very slight and nonsignificant T increase at this time.

In contrast to these sex differences in hormonal responses to social victory and defeat, implicit power motivation predicted contest-outcome effects on instrumental learning (sequence execution accuracy) in exactly the same way and magnitude in men and women. In both genders, power motivation was associated with enhanced instrumental learning among winners and impaired instrumental learning among losers. These findings represent a replication of similar results obtained by Schultheiss and Rohde (2002) in a male German sample. Together with that earlier study, they provide straightforward evidence ·for a moderating role of the implicit power motive in instrumental learning of behavior that has impact on others (i.e., beating one's opponent in the contest) and the inhibition of behavior that led to the frustration of the need for impact (i.e., being beaten by one's opponent).

Consistent with the reinforcing effects of T documented in animal experiments, we also found that men's T changes 15 to 20 minutes postcontest were associated with instrumental learning and statistically mediated the effect of power motivation on learning. Schultheiss and Rohde (2002) reported that among power-motivated winners, T increases transmitted the boosting effect of power motivation on implicit learning among winners, and Schultheiss, Wirth, et al. (2005) found that high-power losers' T decreases translated into impaired implicit learning. (That neither study found the mediation effect in both winners and losers can probably be explained by the fact that the effect of power motivation and T changes was smaller among losers than among winners in Schultheiss and Rohde's [2002] study and vice versa in Schultheiss, Wirth, et al.'s [2005] study.) Although Schultheiss and Rohde's (2002) and Schultheiss, Wirth, et al.'s (2005) findings cannot conclusively establish a causal reinforcing role for T in instrumental learning, such a causal effect could, in principle, be documented by administering androgen receptor antagonists such as flutamide to participants before they enter a dominance contest, thus preventing T and its metabolites from boosting dopamine transmission in the brain's reinforcement circuits.

Paralleling the absence of reports on reinforcing effects of T on behavior in female animals, Schultheiss, Wirth, et al. (2005) did not find any evidence for a reinforcing effect of T on implicit learning in women. In fact, higher postcontest T levels even showed a *negative* association with one aspect of implicit learning (speed of visuomotor pattern execution), which is inconsistent with a role of T in reinforcement. The lack of evidence for a reinforcing effect of T on instrumental learning in females does not rule out priming effects of T on power-motivated behaviors. Animal studies show that T lowers the threshold for aggressive behavior in males and females (Albert et al., 1992), and the previously cited research on the effects of T on women's emotional responding to social threats and challenges suggests a priming role of T on female assertiveness in humans, too. Consistent with the hypothesis that T primes self-assertion in women, we found that female losers, who had the strongest T increases immediately after the contest, also showed the greatest increase in power imagery in response to a postcontest PSE picture suggesting aggression (a woman with an angry face and bared teeth; bipartial $r = .34$, $p < .05$) but not to nonaggressive PSE pictures (female judges, women playing basketball; bipartial $r = .11$, *ns*). Thus, although elevated T levels after a social defeat do not reinforce instrumental behavior in women, they are associated with what seems to be a compensatory need to assert oneself forcefully.

Finally, our studies also provide pervasive evidence for a dissociation between declarative and nondeclarative measures of motivation and motivational outcomes. Declarative measures of power motivation (such as the dominance and aggression scales of Jackson's [1984] Personality Research Form [PRF] or the social potency and aggression scales of Tellegen's [1982] Multidimensional Personality Questionnaire) did not show consistent or substantial correlation with the nondeclarative PSE measure of power motivation or predict, conjointly with contest outcome, T changes and instrumental learning in a consistent or meaningful way in any of our studies. For instance, in the male sample studied by Schultheiss, Wirth, et al. (2005), self-reported dominance motivation (from the PRF) correlated .07 (*ns*) with implicit power motivation. The correlation between self-reported dominance motivation and T changes 15 minutes postcontest was −.05 among losers and −.11 among winners (semipartial *r*s, *p*s > .10). Likewise, the correlation between self-reported dominance motivation and implicit learning was −.15 among both losers and winners (*p*s > .10). Conversely, although the implicit power motive, in combination with contest outcome, significantly predicted both T changes and instrumental learning (nondeclarative criterion measures), it failed to predict participants' self-reported affective responses (a declarative criterion measure) to the contest outcome in the Schultheiss and Rohde (1999, 2002) and Schultheiss, Wirth, et al. (2005) studies. The sole strong predictor of participants' postcontest moods in all of these studies was the contest outcome, with winners reporting feeling happy and strong and losers reporting feeling sad and weak after the contest. Notably, self-reported affect after the contest also did not significantly correlate with either T changes or implicit learning gains in any study. This pattern of results led Schultheiss, Wirth, et al. (2005) to conclude that "conscious experience of pleasure or displeasure is not a necessary corollary of reward and reinforcement" (p. 186).

Frustrated Power Motivation and Cortisol Changes

Although T appears to scale the reward value of outcomes of dominance-related social interactions in men and may subserve a general power-motivation-enhancing function in women, recent evidence points to a role for cortisol in frustrated power motivation in both genders. Wirth, Welsh, and Schultheiss (2006) analyzed saliva samples collected in Schultheiss and Rohde's (2002) study and in a dominance-contest study conducted with male and female U.S. college students for cortisol (C) levels. C is released by the adrenals under stress, particularly if the stress is uncontrollable, and induces the body to shunt available energy into coping with the stressor. Although C is not consistently related to declarative measures of negative affect and stress, it increases reliably in stress-induction paradigms (Dickerson & Kemeney, 2004) and is chronically elevated in individuals with depression (Rothschild, 2003). Wirth et al. (2006) found that across both German and U.S. samples, implicit power motivation predicted increased C after the contest in losers and decreased C after the contest in winners. According to this finding, a social defeat was particularly stressful for high-power individuals but not for low-power individuals (who may actually have been comfortable with the defeat; see Schultheiss, Wirth, et al., 2005, for a discussion of this issue).

TOWARD A BIOBEHAVIORAL MODEL OF POWER MOTIVATION

So far, I have reviewed evidence implicating the sympathetic catecholamines in power motivation arousal, the gonadal steroid testosterone in male power motivation reward and power-motivated women's response to dominance challenges in general, and the adrenal steroid cortisol in frustrated or stressed power motivation. In the remainder of this chapter, I review research that suggests that the observed hormonal changes are not independent of each other but represent a coherent, integrated endocrine response to dominance challenges, and I sketch out how power motivation interacts with situational cues and outcomes to affect hormonal changes and behavior in men and women.

Male Power Motivation

In men, the major source of androgens (including T) are the testes, with androgen release being driven by pulses of luteinizing hormone (LH) from the pituitary. These LH pulses and their decline over the course of the day account for the wave-like release of T, with T peaks occurring every 1 to 3 hours, and for the typical circadian profile of T, with high levels in the morning and low levels in the evening; but they are in all likelihood too slow to account for the rapid T changes that Schultheiss and Rohde (2002) and Schultheiss, Wirth, et al. (2005) observed after the contest in men. However, Sapolsky (1986, 1987) has demonstrated in his research on social status and reproductive physiology in baboons that other mechanisms are involved in T secretion besides the LH pathway. He found that the sympathetic catecholamines E and NE have a stimulatory effect on testicular T secretion within minutes, whereas cortisol released from the adrenals inhibits T secretion just as quickly. Thus the balance between sympathetic catecholamines and cortisol determines whether T release is transiently increased or decreased. Sapolsky (1987) observed that dominant baboons showed a comparatively strong catecholamine response and weak cortisol response to stress, leading to a T increase within 30 minutes (the same time window in which Schultheiss and Rohde, 2002, and Schultheiss, Wirth, et al., 2005, observed transient T peaks in power-motivated winners), whereas low-ranking animals showed a comparatively weak catecholamine response and strong cortisol response to stress, leading to a rapid decline of T.

Research on the relationship between stress hormones and T in humans provides results that are consistent with Sapolsky's (1987) stress-hormone balance model of T release. For instance, Gerra et al. (1996) reported a correlation of .62 for plasma T and NE levels in young male adults, which suggests that these hormones, although released by different glands, are functionally related in humans, too. Eubank, Collins, Lovell, Dorling, and Talbot (1997) measured stress hormones and T in marathon canoeists before an important competition and split their participants into two groups: facilitators, who viewed the competition as a positive challenge, and debilitators, who felt distressed in the face of the contest. In the group of facilitators, T and plasma E and NE increased before the competition, whereas C remained low. In contrast, debilitators showed decreased T and catecholamine levels but increased C levels immediately before the competition. Finally, the combined T and C data collected from the same sample of German males by Schultheiss and Rohde (2002) and Wirth et al. (in press; Study 1) reveal that an inhibitory effect of C on T may emerge only after a defeat: C increases 20 minutes postcontest were associated with T decreases in losers (bipartial $r = -.33$, $p = .06$), whereas a positive relationship between changes in both hormones was obtained in winners (bipartial $r = .35$, $p = .05$). Consistent with Sapolsky's (1987) balance model, the lack of an inhibiting effect of C on T increases in winners may have been due to an increased release of catecholamines (not assessed), whose stimulatory effect on T release outweighed the inhibitory effect of C.

Sapolsky's (1987) stress-hormone balance model of T release, in conjunction with the previously reviewed literature on the rewarding properties of T, provide a framework for integrating the endocrine and behavioral changes associated with power motivation arousal and satisfaction/ frustration in men. According to the model outlined in Figure 9.1, in individuals high in power motivation, power-related situational cues and contexts elicit a specific increase in sympathetic catecholamines (as observed by McClelland et al., 1980; McClelland et al., 1985), which prime the individual for asserting him- or herself against others. Physiologically, the increasing levels of sympathetic catecholamines result in increases in cardiovascular tone, oxygen uptake, and availability of energy in the form of glucose and fatty acids (Kaplan, 2000). Psychologically, increased levels of sympathetic catecholamines are associated with enhanced sensory signal-to-noise ratio and vigilance (Robbins, 1997). The overall result of these changes make the power-motivated person more physiologically, psychologically, and behaviorally prepared for dealing with a dominance challenge or for taking advantage of an opportunity to have impact on others.

The described sympathetic nervous system changes occur on the order of seconds and minutes. To the extent that they persist, fanned by feedback from the environment signaling to the individual that the challenge can be effectively countered and controlled (Henry, 1992), they have a stimulatory effect on the testicles, thus inducing the release of T observed in power-motivated contest winners 15 to 20 minutes postcontest in Schultheiss and

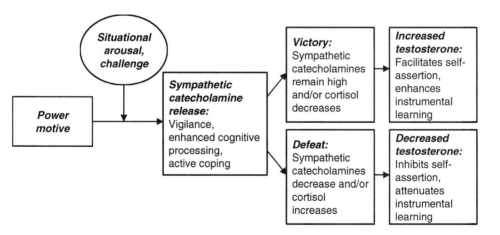

FIGURE 9.1. Biobehavioral model of male power motivation arousal and reward/ frustration.

Rohde's (2002) and Schultheiss, Wirth, et al.'s (2005) studies and the transient T increase observed in dominant primates when their dominance is challenged (Bernstein et al., 1983; Sapolsky, 1987). In males, this T increase has two short-term effects: First, it temporarily lowers the threshold for aggression, thus making the individual more pugnacious and willing to defend or assert his dominance over others (Albert et al., 1992; Sapolsky, 1987). Second, through its anabolic effects, increased T helps to increase muscle strength within minutes to hours, which would provide physiological backup for the individual's increased proneness to engage in dominance conflicts with others (Tsai & Sapolsky, 1996). Victory-induced T increases also have a long-term effect on behavior by their effects on dopamine transmission in the striatum, which accentuate learning of the behaviors that ultimately led to victory (cf. Frye et al., 2002; Packard et al., 1998).

To the extent that a power-motivated individual loses control over the outcome of a contest, however, the stress-hormone balance tilts the other way, toward a net increase of C over sympathetic catecholamines (note that catecholamines may increase under these conditions, too; however, their effect is likely to be offset by the strong C increases). The net effect of this shift in stress hormones is an increased inhibitory action of C on testicular T release that outweighs the stimulatory effect on catecholamines and results in the stagnating or decreasing T levels observed in power-motivated losers by Schultheiss and Rohde (2002), Schultheiss et al. (1999), and Schultheiss, Wirth, et al. (2005). The increased C levels may reflect a switch from dealing with a challenge that can be met to adjusting to an uncontrollable stressor, consistent with the fact that the individual has lost dominance and thus control over his opponent. Psychologically, decreased C levels raise the aggression threshold for the individual through removing inhibition on T release. Thus it will take a stronger stimulus to make him engage in another dominance encounter than previously, and this may protect the individual from further costly defeats (cf. Mazur, 1985). Reduced T may also be causally involved in impaired learning of behavior that was "instrumental" for the defeat by attenuating striatal dopamine transmission and thus the "glue" that would help consolidate goal-directed behavior. However, it is also conceivable that reduced C has a direct attenuating effect on reinforcement through its inhibiting effects on dopamine synthesis and turnover (cf. Pacak et al., 2002). Whatever the precise mechanism, its outcome ensures that behavior that was counterproductive to the power-motivated individual's goal of having impact will not make it into the individual's repertoire of power-related skills.

Female Power Motivation

My tentative biobehavioral model of female power motivation is similar to the male model in most respects (see Figure 9.2). Thus, based on the

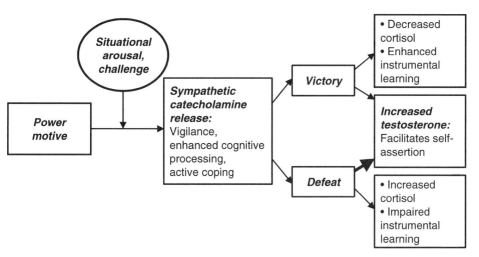

FIGURE 9.2. Biobehavioral model of female power motivation arousal and reward/frustration. The bold arrow reflects Schultheiss, Wirth, et al.'s (2005) finding that for power-motivated women, a social defeat transiently raises testosterone more than does a victory.

research reviewed previously, it is clear that situations and contexts that arouse or challenge a woman's power motivation stimulate the release of sympathetic catecholamines, which induce physiological and psychological changes conducive to active coping with the task at hand. Likewise, in the studies reported by Schultheiss, Wirth, et al. (2005), power-motivated women do not differ from power-motivated men in their learning responses to the contest outcome: Winners show enhanced, losers show impaired, instrumental learning. Finally, power-motivated women, like power-motivated men, respond with a C increase to a social defeat (Wirth et al., in press).

The model of female power motivation differs from the male model in two crucial respects, though. First, there is no evidence that T increases are associated with instrumental learning and reinforcement in women. Schultheiss, Wirth, et al. (2005) failed to find significant positive correlations between women's postcontest T increases and indicators of instrumental learning of behavior that had been involved in winning or losing the contest. As mentioned previously, this finding is in agreement with the animal literature on the reinforcing properties of T, which so far have been documented for male mammals only. Note, however, that this lack of a role of T in reinforcement in females does not preclude such a role for other gonadal steroids, such as estradiol or T precursors and metabolites. Also, because there is considerable evidence for a role of elevated T in female dominance and aggression (discussed earlier), the absence of reinforcing effects of T in women does not seem to diminish T's role as a facilitator of power-motivated behavior.

Second, there is little evidence that Sapolsky's (1987) stress-hormone balance model of T release and inhibition applies to females in the same way that it applies to males. In contrast to their pronounced stimulatory effect on the testes, sympathetic catecholamines do not seem to be capable by themselves of stimulating androgen release from the female ovaries (Dyer & Erickson, 1985). Moreover, whatever stimulatory or inhibitory effects stress hormones may exert on T release from the ovaries would not have a strong influence on circulating levels of T in women, because the relative contribution of the gonads to overall T levels is comparatively much smaller in women than in men—hence the substantially lower total T levels in women. In contrast, the adrenal glands represent a more significant source of circulating androgens in women than in men (Ojeda, 2000). Schultheiss, Wirth, et al. (2005) therefore proposed that the rise in T observed in power-motivated women (and particularly in losers) after a contest may be the result of increased androgen release from the adrenal cortex, possibly triggered by increased stress-axis activation. Because women may be more sensitive to even slight changes in T (Sherwin, 1988b), the T-increasing effect of (lost) dominance challenges may make power-motivated women more likely to seek and engage in further opportunities to assert themselves.

Clearly, the biobehavioral model of female power motivation is much more speculative and in need of empirical corroboration than the model of male power motivation, for which numerous converging lines of evidence exist in the animal and human literatures. It is notable that the lack of research in the hormonal correlates and mechanisms of female dominance behavior, deplored by Sapolsky in 1987, persisted more than 10 years later, when Mazur and Booth (1998) concluded that the empirical literature on the role of T in female dominance is scant and disparate, and continues until this day. To the extent that the unequal allocation of research efforts to the endocrine correlates of dominance in men and women is due to researchers' implicit or explicit assumption that issues of dominance are more salient or important among men, consultation of the literature on implicit power motivation may provide a healthy corrective. In their review of gender differences in implicit motives, Stewart and Chester (1982) concluded that women and men do not substantially differ in their average level of power motivation, in the cues and stimuli that arouse their need for power, or in the behaviors that they employ to have impact on others (see also Pang & Schultheiss, 2005; Schultheiss & Brunstein, 2001; Schultheiss et al., 2004). Given the strong links between implicit power motivation and physiological processes, the power motive construct may therefore represent a particularly suitable vantage point from which to study the hormonal correlates of dominance and self-assertion in women.

ACKNOWLEDGMENTS

This chapter is dedicated to the memory of James McBride Dabbs, a pioneer of endocrinological methods in personality and social psychology.

The research reported in this chapter was supported by Deutsche Forschungsmeinschaft Grant Nos. SCHU 1210/1-2, 1-3, and 2-2 and National Institute of Mental Health Grant No. 1 R03 MH63069-01. This research would not have been possible without the help and generous contributions of my colleagues and collaborators Joachim Brunstein, Kenneth Campbell, Anja Dargel, David McClelland, Joyce Pang, Wolfgang Rohde, Steven Stanton, Cynthia Torges, Kathryn Welsh, and Michelle Wirth.

REFERENCES

Albert, D. J., Jonik, R. H., & Walsh, M. L. (1992). Hormone-dependent aggression in male and female rats: Experiential, hormonal, and neural foundations. *Neuroscience and Biobehavioral Reviews, 16*(2), 177–192.

Alexander, G. M., Packard, M. G., & Hines, M. (1994). Testosterone has rewarding affective properties in male rats: Implications for the biological basis of sexual motivation. *Behavioral Neuroscience, 108*, 424–428.

Bernstein, I. S., Gordon, T. P., & Rose, R. M. (1983). The interaction of hormones, behavior, and social context in nonhuman primates. In B. B. Svare (Ed.), *Hormones and aggressive behavior* (pp. 535–561). New York: Plenum Press.

Biernat, M. (1989). Motives and values to achieve: Different constructs with different effects. *Journal of Personality, 57*, 69–95.

Brunstein, J. C., & Hoyer, S. (2002). Implizites und explizites Leistungsstreben: Befunde zur Unabhängigkeit zweier Motivationssysteme [Implicit versus explicit achievement strivings: Empirical evidence of the independence of two motivational systems]. *Zeitschrift für Pädagogische Psychologie, 16*, 51–62.

Cardinal, R. N., Parkinson, J. A., Hall, J., & Everitt, B. J. (2002). Emotion and motivation: The role of the amygdala, ventral striatum, and prefrontal cortex. *Neuroscience and Biobehavioral Reviews, 26*, 321–352.

Carter, C. S. (1992). Hormonal influences on human sexual behavior. In J. B. Becker, S. M. Breedlove, & D. Crews (Eds.), *Behavioral endocrinology* (pp. 131–142). Cambridge MA: MIT Press.

Dabbs, J. M., Alford, E. C., & Fielden, J. A. (1998). Trial lawyers and testosterone: Blue-collar talent in a white-collar world. *Journal of Applied Social Psychology, 28*, 84–94.

Dabbs, J. M., & Hargrove, M. F. (1997). Age, testosterone, and behavior among female prison inmates. *Psychosomatic Medicine, 59*, 477–480.

Dabbs, J. M., Ruback, R. B., Frady, R. L., Hopper, C. H., & Sgoutas, D. S. (1988). Saliva testosterone and criminal violence among women. *Personality and Individual Differences, 9*, 269–275.

Dabbs, J. M., Strong, R., & Milun, R. (1997). Exploring the mind of testosterone: A beeper study. *Journal of Research in Personality, 31*, 577–587.

deCharms, R., Morrison, H. W., Reitman, W., & McClelland, D. C. (1955). Behavioral correlates of directly and indirectly measured achievement motivation. In

D. C. McClelland (Ed.), *Studies in motivation* (pp. 414–423). New York: Appleton-Century-Crofts.

Dickerson, S. S., & Kemeny, M. E. (2004). Acute stressors and cortisol responses: A theoretical integration and synthesis of laboratory research. *Psychological Bulletin, 130*(3), 355–391.

Dyer, C. A., & Erickson, G. F. (1985). Norepinephrine amplifies human chorionic gonadotropin-stimulated androgen biosynthesis by ovarian theca-interstitial cells. *Endocrinology, 116*(4), 1645–1652.

Eubank, M., Collins, D., Lovell, G., Dorling, D., & Talbot, S. (1997). Individual temporal differences in pre-competition anxiety and hormonal concentration. *Personality and Individual Differences, 23*, 1031–1039.

Frye, C. A., Rhodes, M. E., Rosellini, R., & Svare, B. (2002). The nucleus accumbens as a site of action for rewarding properties of testosterone and its 5a-reduced metabolites. *Pharmacology, Biochemistry and Behavior, 74*, 119–127.

Gerra, G., Avanzini, P., Zaimovic, A., Fertonani, G., Caccavari, R., Delsignore, R., et al. (1996). Neurotransmitter and endocrine modulation of aggressive behavior and its components in normal humans. *Behavioural Brain Research, 81*, 19–24.

Henry, J. P. (1992). Biological basis of the stress response. *Integrative Physiological and Behavioral Science, 27*(1), 66–83.

Jackson, D. N. (1984). *Personality Research Form* (3rd ed.). Port Huron, MI: Sigma Assessment Systems.

Kaplan, N. M. (2000). The adrenal glands. In J. E. Griffin & S. R. Ojeda (Eds.), *Textbook of endocrine physiology* (4th ed., pp. 328–356). New York: Oxford University Press.

Klinger, E. (1967). Modeling effects on achievement imagery. *Journal of Personality and Social Psychology, 7*, 49–62.

Lichter, S. R., & Rothman, S. (1981). Jewish ethnicity and radical culture: A social psychological study of political activists. *Political Psychology, 3*, 116–157.

Mason, A., & Blankenship, V. (1987). Power and affiliation motivation, stress, and abuse in intimate relationships. *Journal of Personality and Social Psychology, 52*, 203–210.

Mazur, A. (1985). A biosocial model of status in face-to-face primate groups. *Social Forces, 64*, 377–402.

Mazur, A., & Booth, A. (1998). Testosterone and dominance in men. *Behavioral and Brain Sciences, 21*, 353–397.

McClelland, D. C. (1984). *Motives, personality, and society: Selected papers*. New York: Praeger.

McClelland, D. C. (1987a). *Human motivation*. New York: Cambridge University Press.

McClelland, D. C. (1987b). Biological aspects of human motivation. In F. Halisch & J. Kuhl (Eds.), *Motivation, intention, and volition* (pp. 11–19). Berlin: Springer.

McClelland, D. C., Atkinson, J. W., Clark, R. A., & Lowell, E. L. (1953). *The achievement motive*. New York: Appleton-Century-Crofts.

McClelland, D. C., & Boyatzis, R. E. (1982). Leadership motive pattern and long-term success in management. *Journal of Applied Psychology, 67*, 737–743.

McClelland, D. C., Davis, W. N., Kalin, R., & Wanner, E. (1972). *The drinking man*. New York: Free Press.

McClelland, D. C., Floor, E., Davidson, R. J., & Saron, C. (1980). Stressed power motivation, sympathetic activation, immune function, and illness. *Journal of Human Stress, 6*, 11–19.

McClelland, D. C., & Franz, C. E. (1992). Motivational and other sources of work accomplishments in mid-life: A longitudinal study. *Journal of Personality, 60*, 679–707.

McClelland, D. C., Ross, G., & Patel, V. (1985). The effect of an academic examination on salivary norepinephrine and immunoglobulin levels. *Journal of Human Stress, 11*, 52–59.

McClelland, D. C., & Watson, R. I. (1973). Power motivation and risk-taking behavior. *Journal of Personality, 41*, 121–139.

Monaghan, E. P., & Glickman, S. E. (1992). Hormones and aggressive behavior. In J. B. Becker, S. M. Breedlove, & D. Crews (Eds.), *Behavioral endocrinology* (pp. 261–285). Cambridge MA: MIT Press.

Morgan, C., & Murray, H. A. (1935). A method for investigating fantasies: The Thematic Apperception Test. *Archives of Neurology and Psychiatry, 34*, 289–306.

Ojeda, S. R. (2000). Female reproductive function. In J. E. Griffin & S. R. Ojeda (Eds.), *Textbook of endocrine physiology* (4th ed., pp. 202–242). New York: Oxford University Press.

Pacak, K., Tjurmina, O., Palkovits, M., Goldstein, D. S., Koch, C. A., Hoff, T., et al. (2002). Chronic hypercortisolemia inhibits dopamine synthesis and turnover in the nucleus accumbens: An in vivo microdialysis study. *Neuroendocrinology, 76*(3), 148–157.

Packard, M. G., Schroeder, J. P., & Alexander, G. M. (1998). Expression of testosterone conditioned place preference is blocked by peripheral or intra-accumbens injection of alpha-flupenthixol. *Hormones and Behavior, 34*(1), 39–47.

Pang, J. S., & Schultheiss, O. C. (2005). Assessing implicit motives in U. S. college students: Effects of picture type and position, gender and ethnicity, and cross-cultural comparisons. *Journal of Personality Assessment, 85*(3), 280–294.

Pope, H. G., & Katz, D. L. (1994). Psychiatric and medical effects of anabolic-androgenic steroid use. *Archives of General Psychiatry, 51*, 375–382.

Purifoy, F. E., & Koopmans, L. H. (1979). Androstenione, testosterone, and free testosterone concentration in women of various occupations. *Social Biology, 26*, 179–188.

Rabkin, J. G., Wagner, G., & Rabkin, R. (1996). Testosterone replacement therapy in HIV illness. *General Hospital Psychiatry, 17*, 37–42.

Robbins, T. W. (1997). Arousal systems and attentional processes. *Biological Psychology, 45*(1–3), 57–71.

Rolls, E. T. (1999). *The brain and emotion*. Oxford, UK: Oxford University Press.

Rothschild, A. J. (2003). The hypothalamic–pituitary–adrenal axis and psychiatric illness. In O. M. Wolkowitz & A. J. Rothschild (Eds.), *Psychoneuroendocrinology: The scientific basis of clinical practice* (pp. 139–163). Arlington, VA: American Psychiatric.

Sapolsky, R. M. (1986). Stress-induced elevation of testosterone concentration in high ranking baboons: Role of catecholamines. *Endocrinology, 118*(4), 1630–1635.

Sapolsky, R. M. (1987). Stress, social status, and reproductive physiology in free-living baboons. In D. Crews (Ed.), *Psychobiology and reproductive behavior: An evolutionary perspective* (pp. 291–322). Englewood Cliffs, NJ: Prentice Hall.

Schroeder, J. P., & Packard, M. G. (2000). Role of dopamine receptor subtypes in the acquisition of a testosterone conditioned place preference in rats. *Neuroscience Letters, 282*(1–2), 17–20.

Schultheiss, O. C. (2001). An information processing account of implicit motive arousal. In M. L. Maehr & P. Pintrich (Eds.), *Advances in motivation and achievement: Vol. 12. New directions in measures and methods* (pp. 1–41). Greenwich, CT: JAI Press.

Schultheiss, O. C., & Brunstein, J. C. (1999). Goal imagery: Bridging the gap between implicit motives and explicit goals. *Journal of Personality, 67*, 1–38.

Schultheiss, O. C., & Brunstein, J. C. (2001). Assessing implicit motives with a research version of the TAT: Picture profiles, gender differences, and relations to other personality measures. *Journal of Personality Assessment, 77*(1), 71–86.

Schultheiss, O. C., & Brunstein, J. C. (2002). Inhibited power motivation and persuasive communication: A lens model analysis. *Journal of Personality, 70*, 553–582.

Schultheiss, O. C., Campbell, K. L., & McClelland, D. C. (1999). Implicit power motivation moderates men's testosterone responses to imagined and real dominance success. *Hormones and Behavior, 36*(3), 234–241.

Schultheiss, O. C., Dargel, A., & Rohde, W. (2003a). Implicit motives and sexual motivation and behavior. *Journal of Research in Personality, 37*, 224–230.

Schultheiss, O. C., Dargel, A., & Rohde, W. (2003b). Implicit motives and gonadal steroid hormones: Effects of menstrual cycle phase, oral contraceptive use, and relationship status. *Hormones and Behavior, 43*, 293–301.

Schultheiss, O. C., & Hale, J. A. (in press). Implicit motives modulate attentional orienting to perceived facial expressions of emotion. *Motivation and Emotion.*

Schultheiss, O. C., & Pang, J. S. (in press). Measuring implicit motives. In R. W. Robins, R. C. Fraley, & R. F. Krueger (Eds.), *Handbook of research methods in personality psychology.* New York: Guilford Press.

Schultheiss, O. C., Pang, J. S., Torges, C. M., Wirth, M. M., & Treynor, W. (2005). Perceived facial expressions of emotion as motivational incentives: Evidence from a differential implicit learning paradigm. *Emotion, 5*(1), 41–54.

Schultheiss, O. C., & Rohde, W. (1999). *Relationship between implicit power motivation and self-reported mood after winning or losing a dominance contest.* Unpublished raw data.

Schultheiss, O. C., & Rohde, W. (2002). Implicit power motivation predicts men's testosterone changes and implicit learning in a contest situation. *Hormones and Behavior, 41*, 195–202.

Schultheiss, O. C., Wirth, M. M., & Stanton, S. J. (2004). Effects of affiliation and power motivation arousal on salivary progesterone and testosterone. *Hormones and Behavior, 46*(5), 592–599.

Schultheiss, O. C., Wirth, M. M., Torges, C. M., Pang, J. S., Villacorta, M. A., & Welsh, K. M. (2005). Effects of implicit power motivation on men's and women's implicit learning and testosterone changes after social victory or defeat. *Journal of Personality and Social Psychology, 88*(1), 174–188.

Sherwin, B. B. (1988a). Affective changes with estrogen and androgen replacement therapy in surgically menopausal women. *Journal of Affective Disorders, 14*(2), 177–187.

Sherwin, B. B. (1988b). A comparative analysis of the role of androgen in human male and female sexual behavior: Behavioral specificity, critical thresholds, and sensitivity. *Psychobiology, 16*, 416–425.

Smith, C. P. (Ed.). (1992). *Motivation and personality: Handbook of thematic content analysis.* New York: Cambridge University Press.

Steele, R. S. (1973). *The physiological concomitants of psychogenic motive arousal in college males.* Unpublished doctoral dissertation, Harvard University.

Stein, L. (1975). Norepinephrine reward pathways: Role in self-stimulation, memory consolidation, and schizophrenia. *Nebraska Symposium on Motivation, 22*, 113–159.

Stewart, A. J., & Chester, N. L. (1982). Sex differences in human social motives: Achievement, affiliation, and power. In A. J. Stewart (Ed.), *Motivation and society: A volume in honor of David C. McClelland* (pp. 172–218). San Francisco: Jossey-Bass.

Tellegen, A. (1982). *Multidimensional Personality Questionnaire.* Unpublished manuscript.

Tsai, L. W., & Sapolsky, R. M. (1996). Rapid stimulatory effects of testosterone upon myotubule metabolism and sugar transport, as assessed by silicon microphysiometry. *Aggressive Behavior, 22*, 357–364.

Uleman, J. S. (1972). The need for influence: Development and validation of a measure, in comparison with need for power. *Genetic Psychology Monographs, 85*, 157–214.

van Honk, J., Tuiten, A., Hermans, E., Putman, P., Koppeschaar, H., Thijssen, J., et al. (2001). A single administration of testosterone induces cardiac accelerative responses to angry faces in healthy young women. *Behavioral Neuroscience, 115*(1), 238–242.

van Honk, J., Tuiten, A., Verbaten, R., van den Hout, M., Koppeschaar, H., Thijssen, J., et al. (1999). Correlations among salivary testosterone, mood, and selective attention to threat in humans. *Hormones and Behavior, 36*(1), 17–24.

Veroff, J. (1957). Development and validation of a projective measure of power motivation. *Journal of Abnormal and Social Psychology, 54*, 1–8.

Winter, D. G. (1973). *The power motive.* New York: Free Press.

Winter, D. G. (1987). Enhancement of an enemy's power motivation as a dynamic of conflict escalation. *Journal of Personality and Social Psychology, 52*, 41–46.

Winter, D. G. (1991). Measuring personality at a distance: Development of an integrated system for scoring motives in running text. In D. J. Ozer, J. M. Healy, & A. J. Stewart (Eds.), *Perspectives in personality* (Vol. 3, pp. 59–89). London: Kingsley.

Winter, D. G. (1993). Power, affiliation, and war: Three tests of a motivational model. *Journal of Personality and Social Psychology, 65,* 532–545.

Winter, D. G. (1996). *Personality: Analysis and interpretation of lives.* New York: McGraw-Hill.

Winter, D. G., & Stewart, A. J. (1977). Power motive reliability as a function of retest instructions. *Journal of Consulting and Clinical Psychology, 45,* 436–440.

Wirth, M. M., Welsh, K., & Schultheiss, O. C. (2006). Salivary cortisol changes in humans after winning or losing a dominance contest depend on implicit power motivation. *Hormones and Behavior, 49,* 346–352.

Wood, R. I., Johnson, L. R., Chu, L., Schad, C., & Self, D. W. (2004). Testosterone reinforcement: Intravenous and intracerebroventricular self-administration in male rats and hamsters. *Psychopharmacology, 171*(3), 298–305.

10

Vigilant and Avoidant Responses to Angry Facial Expressions
DOMINANCE AND SUBMISSION MOTIVES

Jack van Honk and Dennis J. L. G. Schutter

In primitive animals, approach- and withdrawal-related emotion is initiated in limbic affective circuits and is observed as the fight-or-flight response. In humans, these primordial forms of approach and withdrawal were the building blocks for the development of the cortically controlled emotions anger and anxiety in the left and the right prefrontal cortices, respectively. Beneficial socioemotional human behavior in the end, however, importantly depends on effective communication between the lower, subcortical, and the higher, cortical, regions of the brain. Hypothesizing from this simple psychobiological framework that borrows from several theories of emotion, we have in recent years been investigating approach- and withdrawal-related emotion in terms of attentional and physiological responses to angry facial expressions. We researched relations with personality characteristics assessed by self-report and investigated the roles of the hormones cortisol and testosterone, of the left and the right prefrontal cortex (PFC), and of the left and the right parietal cortex. To find more direct evidence and to scrutinize involved brain mechanisms, controlled hormone administrations and repetitive transcranial magnetic stimulation (rTMS) were applied, and autonomic measures, electroencephalography (EEG), and functional magnetic resonance imaging (fMRI) were employed.

Findings led to a more specified psychobiological model wherein the avoidant submissive response to the angry face is mediated by anxiety, cortisol, and the right hemisphere, whereas anger, testosterone, and the left hemisphere process the approach-related dominant response to the facial expression. Finally, evidence from novel analytic EEG applications demonstrated the importance of subcorticocortical communication in the model.

THE EVOLUTIONARY NEUROBIOLOGY OF APPROACH- AND WITHDRAWAL-RELATED EMOTION

The emotions of approach and withdrawal evolved 350 million years ago as fight or flight when the first reptiles wandered the earth. It was only then that this bipolar affective reactivity became optional because the sympathetic nervous system became attached to the cardiovascular and respiratory systems (Campbell, Wood & McBride, 1997). Hundreds of millions of years passed wherein animals largely depended on affective reflexive forms of approach and withdrawal. Just 10 million years ago in the human primate, during the enormous expansion of the cortical structures, primordial emotion migrated into the prefrontal cortex. Ten thousand years ago, the basic motivations became manifest as the cortically controlled emotions anger and anxiety in modern humans (Berridge, 2003). To reduce conflict among the antagonistic action tendencies, this implementation seems to have taken place in a lateralized fashion (Davidson, 2004). The approach-related emotion anger is processed by the left prefrontal cortex, whereas the withdrawal emotion anxiety is processed by the right prefrontal cortex (Harmon-Jones, 2003, 2004). This recent evolutionary system possesses cognitive control that enables flexible, less predictable responses to modern social-emotional environments.

In psychological laboratories, attentional mechanisms are often studied using artificial stimuli such as meaningless probes. Attention in the real world is, however, determined by motivation, and our attentional systems are specifically tuned to perceptual cues associated with threat. Depending on the individual's motivational stance, attention is unconsciously directed toward—or away from—an emotionally threatening stimulus. When consciously detected as a result of higher level cortical processing, the attentional response can undergo cognitive control and can be modulated in terms of inhibition or excitation. In this heuristic framework, the subcortical structures are predominantly involved in unconscious rudimentary forms of motivated attention, whereas cortical structures perform conscious control. It should, however, be noted that the use of the term "consciousness" in this respect must be distinguished from the affective forms of consciousness discussed in recent philosophical-evolutionary models (Panksepp, 2003). Nevertheless, a heuristic division between conscious and unconscious aspects of motivated attention can serve as a valuable framework in the investigation of different features of approach- and withdrawal-related human emotion (van Honk & de Haan, 2001). The most successful paradigm in investigating these conscious and unconscious aspects of motivated attention is the emotional Stroop task (Williams, Matthews, & MacLead, 1996).

THE EMOTIONAL STROOP TASK

Fifteen hundred years ago, Augustine of Hippo already predicted that emotionally charged stimuli would involuntarily attract attention, especially during emotional states and disturbances. The ancient hypothesis was recently repeatedly confirmed using the emotional Stroop task (Williams et al., 1996), which showed that, in particular, participants with anxiety selectively attend threatening words. In the emotional Stroop task, the colors in which threatening and neutral words are printed have to be named as fast as possible, and the meaning of the words must be ignored. The mean color-naming latencies for emotional stimuli minus the mean color-naming latencies for neutral stimuli provide so-called attentional-bias scores. Positive attentional-bias scores indicate that attention is allocated toward the emotional stimulus (i.e., vigilance), whereas negative attentional-bias scores indicate that attention is allocated away from the emotional stimulus (i.e., avoidance). Attentional biases for threat are, according to Mathews and MacLeod (1994), emotional responses of evolutionary origin—affectively driven changes in information processing when fight or flight may be required in potentially threatening situations. In the human world, however, part of their adaptive value is lost because the flight-or-fight response is far less often executed. As a result, they may have lost some of their adaptiveness, and they now play a role in the etiology and maintenance of the disorders of fear and anxiety (McEwen, 1994).

Interestingly, the slowdown in color naming of threatening compared with neutral words has been demonstrated not only in supraliminal, or unmasked, conditions but also in subliminal, or masked, conditions. In the subliminal, or masked, emotional Stroop task, conscious recognition of the words is precluded by short presentation of the words and immediate replacement by a pattern mask (e.g., meaningless, reversed, and rotated letter-string in the same color). Participants with both clinical and nonclinical anxiety selectively attend to masked threatening words, whereas only the groups with clinical anxiety tend to show vigilant attention to unmasked threatening words (Williams et al., 1996). It has been argued that the difference between the groups indicates defective conscious countercontrol in the clinical groups, as conscious countercontrol would serve as mood protection and logically depends on access to consciousness (Reiman, 1997).

A problem in the previously discussed research is the use of linguistic material: Not only is the threat value of words limited, but also the evolutionary necessity of fast responses to verbal information seems questionable at least (McNally, 1995). Evolutionary explanations in emotion research warrant the use of stimuli having significance in ancestral environments (Tooby & Cosmides, 1995). Biologically relevant pictures should permit more direct access to our primordial motivational emotional system (Panksepp, 2003), and their crucial features may even travel an ancient thalamic–amygdala shortcut to the limbic system (LeDoux, 1996). Angry facial expressions are candidates for processing in rapid fashions, with their perceptual characteristics reaching subcortical feature detectors and speeding up the activation of the arousal system (Öhman, 1993). Though the crude perceptual analysis increases the chance of a false-alarm response, it speeds up fight-or-flight preparation and diminishes the chance of a crucial miss.

In an extensive line of aversive conditioning experiments, Öhman and colleagues (see Öhman, 1993) demonstrated conditioning superiority for masked angry faces (compared with happy faces) and suggested that individuals are "biologically prepared" to associate fear with angry faces. The more biologically prepared responses to the masked angry faces would have been evoked because they skipped the longer cortical route and merely traveled the thalamic–amygdala pathway. Crucial evidence was found during an aversive conditioning paradigm in a positron emission tomography (PET) study. Morris, Öhman, and Dolan (1999) demonstrated that a subcortical pathway is predominantly involved in the processing of masked angry faces, whereas a cortical route predominantly processes the unmasked angry face. It should, however, be noted that amygdala-driven affective responses to threatening angry faces do not necessarily promote flight (Öhman, 1993; Whalen, 1998); they may promote fight as well. The amygdala is strongly implicated in aggression and plays an essential role in the social response to the angry facial expression (Kling & Brothers, 1992). When confronted with such social threat, the individual does not necessarily show fearful submission; those high in the dominance hierarchy may choose to aggress to defend status. The findings of Öhman (1993) during aversive conditioning may indicate that angry faces are easily attached to fear, but this does not tell us everything about evolved properties of the angry face in the social system. These dual-sided properties may well provide insights into the antagonism between fear and aggression on the subcortical level and between anger and anxiety on the cortical level.

DOMINANCE AND SUBORDINATION

It has been argued that within species, the emotion fear antagonizes aggressive motivation (DeCantanzara, 1999). In the early primate's social systems, within the boundaries of this antagonism it is decided who is going to take the aggressive dominant stance and who is more to likely to be fearful and submissive. In humans, however, it is conceivable that more complex environments required elaborated coordination and execution of action plans, causing the "cognitively controlled" emotions anger and anxiety to evolve. A workable distinction between fear and anxiety is given by Mathews and Mackintosh (1998). They regard fear as the basic emotion arising from the operation of a phylogenetically older limbic system subserving detection and reactions to danger, whereas "human" anxiety entails more complex cognitive processing and symbolic representations of potential danger wherein the prefrontal cortex is implicated. Fear is defined as a response to present danger, whereas anxiety involves the anticipation of potential danger (Lang, Davis, & Öhman, 2000). In a threatening social encounter, when an individual is confronted with an angry threat, the affective reaction of a person who is fearful or anxious would be to show diminished eye contact and to gaze away from the direction of threat (Hock, 1993). Fear and anxiety carry the submissive motivation to orient away from social threat, which reduces the possibility of encountering aggression (Van Honk et al., 2000). The aforementioned subcorticocortical emotional processing can also be applied to anger and aggression, although it is somewhat more problematic because aggression refers to the action itself, whereas anger entails the disposition for aggressive action that should orient attention toward social threat. This relates to the adaptation that allows anger-prone individuals to protect themselves from injury or status loss by readiness for fight (Lemerise & Dodge, 1993).

Interestingly, rodents seem to dominate in aggressive ways exclusively, likely because in their social systems symbolic rituals did not evolve to nonaggressively establish and maintain social hierarchies (Brothers, 1990). In primates, the angry facial expression evolved to function as a threat signal in dominance encounters (Öhman, 1993), with vigilant responses in terms of an enduring threatening angry gaze signaling dominance and avoidant responses in terms of eye or gaze aversion symbolizing submission and preventing aggression (Mazur & Booth, 1998). The ability to adaptively react to the facial expression of anger is thus crucial for efficient social-emotional functioning. By forewarning of the possibility of punishment, the angry face curtails the behaviors of those involved in social misconduct (Blair, 2003). The threat of anger in itself is often sufficient; socially deviant behavior is terminated, and hierarchical relations are established and maintained by submissive behavior toward the dominant animal displaying anger (Öhman, 1993). However, depending on the social relation between sender and receiver, angry faces can be responded to with both fearful submission and aggressive dominance (Dimberg & Öhman, 1996), action patterns that are in humans controlled by the emotions anger and anxiety (van Honk, Tuiten, van den Hout, et al., 2001). Working within the boundaries of this heuristic, we constructed an emotional Stroop task employing angry and neutral faces that attempts to mimic the real-life face-to-face dominant–submissive interaction under both supraliminal and subliminal conditions.

THE FACE-TO-FACE PARADIGM

This emotional Stroop task compares color-naming latencies of neutral and angry faces from Ekman and Friesen's (1976) pictures of facial affect. Multiple duplications of each model are made and colored by placing a red, green, blue, or yellow transparent folio in front of the picture in the slide frame. The stimuli are back-projected through a milk-colored glass screen into the experimental room using a tachistoscope. In the supraliminal, or unmasked, task, one trial consists of a fixation cross shown for 750 milliseconds, followed by the target slide (the colored, neutral, or angry face). A microphone connected to a voice-level detector is placed in front of the participant. Initiation of vocal response is registered by the computer's clock and subsequently terminates the target presentation. Neutral faces and threat faces are presented in random order. The subliminal, or masked, version of the Stroop task uses target slides identical to the supraliminal version. As masking stimuli we use cut, randomly reassembled, and rephotographed pictures of faces displayed in the same color as the targets. In the task, after a short (30-millisecond) presentation, the target stimulus is immediately replaced by a masking stimulus to block conscious awareness of the target. Again participants are instructed to name the color as fast as possible. Figure 10.1 gives an impression of the task characteristics in both conditions. Finally, a forced-choice awareness check was used to control for conscious recognition. As noted earlier, the mean color-naming laten-

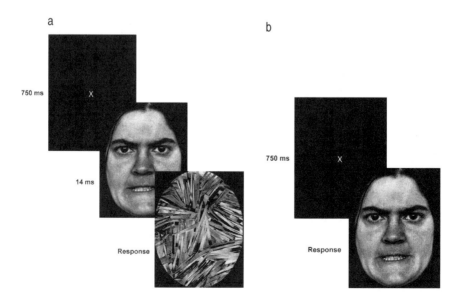

FIGURE 10.1. Masked (a) and unmasked (b) emotional Stroop task.

cies for emotional stimuli minus the mean color-naming latencies for neutral stimuli are the crucial attentional bias scores.

PERSONALITY CHARACTERISTICS

Two experiments were performed that investigated the relationship between trait anger, trait anxiety, and the attentional response to the masked and unmasked angry facial expressions (van Honk, Tuiten, van den Hout, et al., 2001). In the first experiment, participants were selected on high and low trait anger by means of the State–Trait Anger Scale (STAS; Spielberger et al., 1983) from a large pool of students and only an unmasked version of the Stroop task was used. Selected groups were subsequently reallocated to low and high trait anxiety scores by way of a median split on basis of the State–Trait Anxiety Inventory (STAI; Spielberger, Gorsuch, & Lushene, 1970). However, no relation between trait anxiety and the attentional response to the angry face was found, whereas individuals scoring high on trait anger diverged from those scoring low on trait anger by showing attentional vigilance toward angry faces (van Honk, Tuiten, van den Hout, et al., 2001). It should, however, be noted that the preselection had been based on trait anger scores. In a follow-up experiment, therefore, not only were an unmasked and a masked version of the Stroop task used but also selection was based on high and low trait anxiety scores involving a large population of students. Strikingly, again no effects on anxiety were found, whereas medium split reallocation of participants based on trait anger scores indicated that participants high in trait anger selectively attended *toward* angry faces in the unmasked task and the masked task (see Figure 10.2).

The effects on trait anger are in line with our suggestion that vigilant responses to angry facial expressions are driven by dominance motives. But what about the submission motives, given the absence of effects on anxiety? A recent study by Putman, Hermans, and van Honk (2004) throws light on this issue. These authors used self-reports of *social* anxiety and demonstrated that individuals with relatively higher levels of social anxiety selectively attended *away* from the angry facial expression (Putman et al., 2004). Notably, in the latter study, this effect was found in the masked task exclusively (Putman et al., 2004) supporting the suggestion that unconscious emotion processing provides a purer measure of motivated attention, unconfounded by the whims of consciousness (Öhman et al., 1997). Moreover, in a recent study with people with social phobia, this effect was observed again, although now during both masked and unmasked exposure conditions (Hermans, Putman & van Honk, 2006). These findings crucially support the model of Williams et al. (1996), wherein the inability for conscious countercontrol results in attentional biases for threat in both masked and unmasked tasks, which was suggested to be indicative of psychopathology. Furthermore, methodological changes in the social anxiety

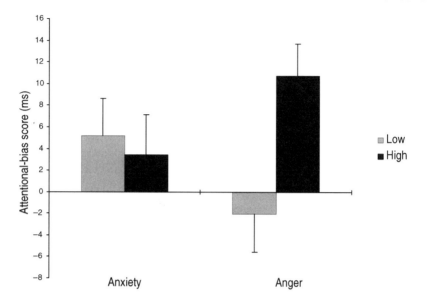

FIGURE 10.2. Mean attentional bias scores and standard deviations in pre-selected anxiety groups and reallocated (median split) anger groups for masked data ($n = 42$).

studies included the use of computer display instead of tachistoscope and the control for emotion per se by adding the happy facial expression (see Putman et al., 2004). Taken together, the findings on anger and social anxiety can be discussed in terms of evolutionary evolved content-specific responses to the facial expression of anger and explained in terms of anger-driven dominance and social anxiety–driven submission motives (van Honk, Schutter, Hermans, & Putnam, 2004). It is therefore interesting to observe that on the endocrine level, end products of the hypothalamic–pituitary–adrenal (HPA) and the hypothalamic–pituitary–gonadal (HPG) axes, the steroid hormones cortisol and testosterone, are associated with a concurring dichotomy in social motives. High basal levels of cortisol relate to socially anxious, avoidant, and submissive behavior (Kagan, Reznick, & Snidman, 1988; Schulkin, Gold, & McEwen, 1998; Sapolsky, 1990), whereas high basal levels of testosterone have been related to anger, social aggression, and interpersonal dominance (Perski, Smith, & Bassu, 1971; Mazur & Booth, 1998).

STEROID HORMONES

Steroid hormones act on motivation and emotion by way of mediating structural and functional neurochemical changes in the limbic system that influence the way individuals react to internal events and external stimuli (Schulkin, 2003). In this way steroid hormones are important in the control of our social-emotional behavior and might be important neuromodulators to research in social neuroscience. With respect to vigilant and avoidant emotional responses to angry faces, clear-cut hypotheses can be postulated for testosterone and cortisol, because—as noted—they are unmistakably involved in dominant and submissive behavior. Hypothesizing from findings reported earlier, high levels of testosterone predict vigilant attention toward angry facial expressions, whereas high levels of cortisol predict the attentionally avoidant response to this socially threatening stimulus.

In an attempt to find support for this notion, we measured salivary testosterone and cortisol levels of participants and indexed the selective response to the angry faces in the Stroop task. Testosterone and cortisol were measured from saliva because this gives a sound reflection of the unbound, free fraction of testosterone that reaches the target tissues of the brain and controls for invasive, stress-inducing confounding influences of blood sampling. In the first study, testosterone was targeted, and only the unmasked emotional Stroop task was applied. It was found that participants with high levels of salivary testosterone selectively attended to angry faces (van Honk et al., 1999). Despite the fact that males have on average multiple times the amount of testosterone that females do, these relations were independent of gender, as can be seen from Figure 10.3.

Next, both masked and unmasked versions of the Stroop task were applied in a follow-up experiment investigating the role of cortisol (van Honk et al., 1998). It is shown in Figure 10.4 that participants with high levels of cortisol selectively attended away from angry faces, but only if these were masked.

In sum, the vigilant attentional response to the angry face seems to be mediated by both anger and testosterone (van Honk et al., 1999; van

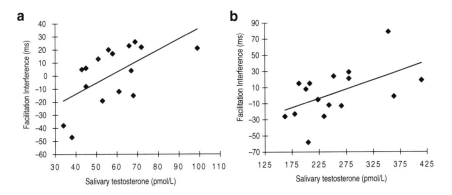

FIGURE 10.3. Scatterplots of testosterone levels (T-6) versus interference scores in women (a) and men (b).

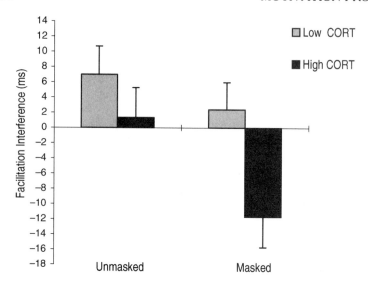

FIGURE 10.4. Bars represent mean interference scores and standard deviations in median split cortisol (CORT) groups in the unmasked and the masked conditions.

Honk, Tuiten, van den Hout, et al., 2001), the steroid associated with social aggression and interpersonal dominance (Dabbs & Hargrove, 1997). On the other hand, individuals with social anxiety and participants with high levels of cortisol selectively attend away from angry faces, though most reliably when these are masked (Putman et al., 2004; van Honk et al., 1998).

Although in line with the hypotheses, the current findings are correlational, making it difficult to draw firm conclusions concerning causality. More definitive evidence for a role of steroid hormones in emotional responses to angry faces might be obtained by hormone administration. Furthermore, for grasping the physiological mechanism involved in the selective response to the angry face, cardiac responses could be used as a dependent measure. For instance, the cardiac defense reflex, an acceleration of the heartbeat within 5 seconds after stimulus presentation, indicates increased preparation for fight or flight (Lang, Bradley, & Cuthbert, 1998). In a double-blind placebo-controlled design, we investigated the effects of a single dose of testosterone (0.5 mg) in healthy young women on cardiac responses to neutral, happy, and angry faces (van Honk, Tuiten, Hermans, et al., 2001). Given the more vigilant response to angry faces observed in women with high baseline levels of testosterone (van Honk et al., 1999), it was hypothesized that the cardiac defense reflex to angry faces would be elevated by testosterone administration. Results can be seen in Figure 10.5, which demonstrates that testosterone elevates cardiac defense reflexes to angry faces but not to happy and neutral faces.

This effect was suggested to be due to the encouragement of dominance behavior, though this explanation might be criticized because the physiological change could be interpreted as enhanced fear (cf. Mogg & Bradley, 1998). However, in a variety of animals, it has been demonstrated that testosterone treatment enhances dominance in social confrontations by *reducing* fearfulness toward threatening conspecifics (Biossy & Bouissou, 1994). The single dose of testosterone administered to women might likewise have reduced fearfulness and enhanced willingness to fight or defend status in social challenges.

It has been suggested that the central effects of steroids on motivation and emotion primarily involve the phylogenetically older brain structures (van Honk & de Haan, 2001). Steroids act by binding to specific steroid responsive neurons that occupy a wide but selective range of nuclei in the limbic system (Wood, 1996). In concert with sensory cues from the external environment, testosterone and cortisol may facilitate or inhibit aggres-

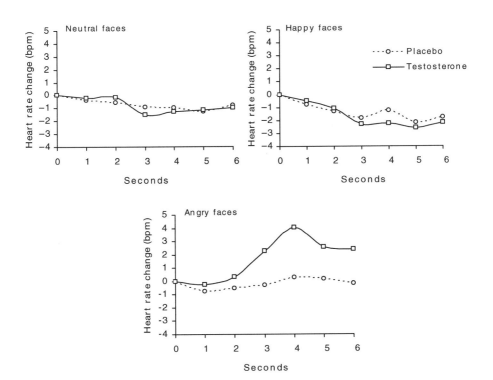

FIGURE 10.5. Mean heart rate changes in beats per minute (bpm) from baseline (1 second prestimulus) during 6 seconds poststimulus for neutral, happy, and angry faces.

sive dominant and fearful submissive behavior by affecting networks of these steroid-receptor-containing neurons, which in turn interact with other integrative neural circuits influencing motivation. In fact, anatomical evidence in rodents indicates that steroid–responsive neuron networks can filter and channel sensory information, leading to selection of specific stimuli, subsequently initiating a cascade of events leading to the behavioral response (Cottingham & Phaff, 1986). A key neuroanatomical component of these neuron networks is the amygdala (Wood, 1996). The central nucleus of the amygdala innervates brainstem centers that control heart rate (Kling & Brothers, 1992), and recent evidence from neuroimaging studies (PET and fMRI) indicate a role for the human amygdala in attentional and autonomic responses to angry facial expressions (Whalen, 1998; Morris et al., 1999). It can thus be expected that the amygdala plays an important role in the elevated cardiac responses to angry faces observed after testosterone administration. To scrutinize this hypothesis, we investigated whether a single administration of testosterone would truly activate the amygdala in response to angry compared with happy faces. A relative increase was indeed observed in the right-sided amygdala (Hermans, Ramsey, & van Honk, in press). These neuroimaging data reveal how the unfortunate choice in human emotion research to concentrate almost exclusively on fear and anxiety may result in faulty reasoning concerning the functions of the amygdala. Exaggerated amygdala activity to emotive stimuli can indicate fear or fearlessness, depending on the nature of the stimulus at hand.

Not only do steroids modulate neuronal communication and brain–social environment communication, but the social environment can also influence the endocrine system. Reciprocal interactions between the steroid hormones cortisol and testosterone and the social system have been abundantly demonstrated. A rise in social status causes an increase in testosterone (Rose, Bernstein, & Gordon, 1975; Rahe, Karson, Howard, Rubin, & Poland, 1990), whereas status loss makes testosterone levels drop (e.g., Kreuz, Rose, & Jennings, 1972; Thompson, Dabbs, & Frady, 1990). Furthermore, the HPA and the HPG axes can work cooperatively. When facing social competition or social threat, individuals show (short term) increases in testosterone, and cortisol often goes up as well (Elias, 1981; Booth, Shelley, Mazur, Tharp, & Kittok, 1989; Gladue, Boechler, & McCaul, 1989). This is especially seen in those who are often victorious (Salvador, Simon, Suay, & Llorens, 1987) or who are inclined to defend their status (Cohen, Nisbett, Bowdle, & Schwarz, 1996). Notably, increases in, at least, testosterone are unlikely to influence motivation and emotion directly, given the rather slow time courses of action in the brain. On the peripheral levels, cortisol and testosterone can, however, prepare the body within seconds for competition by directly mobilizing energy through raising blood glucose levels (Service, 1995) and muscle metabolism (Tsai & Sapolski, 1996).

In another experiment we attempted to evoke cortisol and testosterone responses by means of the "face-to-face competition" inherent in the Stroop task using angry faces and, most important, to see whether possible increases would be related to the emotional response to the angry face. Thus, using masked and unmasked versions the emotional Stroop task, we investigated whether the vigilant attentional response toward the angry face would lead to a bodily preparation for aggression seen as pre- to posttask testosterone and cortisol increases, while the avoidant attentional response toward the angry face would lead to "physiological withdrawal" in terms of testosterone and cortisol declines (van Honk et al., 2000). The different exposure conditions might additionally reveal a role for conscious recognition of facial threat. Participants showing a vigilant response to both the unmasked and the masked angry faces demonstrated significant increases in cortisol, whereas cortisol decreased in both tasks in participants showing an avoidant response. Testosterone significantly increased in participants showing the vigilant response to angry faces and decreased in participants showing avoidance, but these effects occurred only in the masked tasks (see Figure 10.6).

In sum, apart from the dissociation between the masked and the unmasked tasks for testosterone, the relations were observed as hypothesized. With respect to the difference between masked and unmasked findings, it has been argued that during higher order conscious processing, cognitive inhibitory mechanisms are able to put up a defense barrier to control

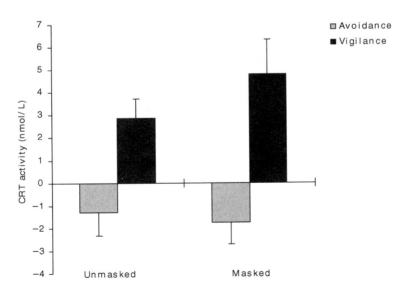

FIGURE 10.6a. Mean (and *SEM*) salivary cortisol (CRT) response for the Avoidance participant groups and the Vigilance participant groups in the unmasked and the masked task.

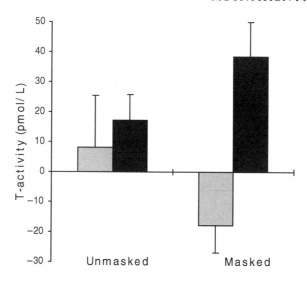

FIGURE 10.6b. Mean (and *SEM*) salivary testosterone (T) response in the Avoidance participant groups and the Vigilance participant-groups in the unmasked and the masked task.

for emotional reactions that might endanger the individual (Plutchik, 1993). A brain structure implicated in this process is the orbitofrontal cortex (OFC), which is known to modulate both physiological and attentional responses to consciously recognized emotionally laden stimuli (Reiman, 1997). Putting the consciousness issue aside for a moment, the findings from the Stroop task on steroid hormones fit observations of behavior and physiology in the primate social system. During social confrontations—that is, when individuals are confronted with dominant figures displaying anger, the adaptive regulatory function of those low in the dominance hierarchy is to avoid injury and energy loss through inhibited behavioral and physiological responses (Sapolsky, 1990; Nesse, 2000). Those high in the hierarchy must, however, prepare their bodies for vigorous action to defend status aggressively if necessary (van Honk et al., 2000; van Honk, Hermans, et al., 2002).

Our data from the masked and unmasked tasks, combined with the fMRI data, indicate that subcortical unconscious affective processing properties are strongly implicated in the relations between steroid hormones and the emotional responses to the angry faces. These results may well find their cortical and conscious manifestations when one applies single sessions of rTMS over the left and the right PFC to influence the *emotional states* of anger and anxiety. RTMS is a technique capable of changing emotional processing by targeting cortical primary sites (Wassermann & Lisanby, 2001). Transient changes in affective processing after a single trial of rTMS over left or right PFC should particularly be observed in conscious instead of unconscious indices of motivation and emotion.

THE PREFRONTAL CORTEX

Multiple hypotheses have been postulated regarding the asymmetrical involvement of the cerebral cortex in emotional processing. The right-hemisphere hypothesis, a prevalent view for more than a century, argues that emotional processing is a function of the right hemisphere (Borod et al., 1998). This hypothesis has, however, been falsified by the work of Davidson and colleagues, who recorded electrical brain activity and repeatedly found evidence for the valence hypothesis wherein it is proposed that the left PFC is involved in approach-related positive affect and the right PFC in withdrawal-related negative affect (Davidson, 1988, 1998, 2004). Deriving the alpha (8–12 Hz) power (μV^2) from resting state EEG has been claimed to index cortical inactivity ("idling"). Positive mood has been linked to relatively reduced left to right PFC alpha activity (i.e., increased neural activity), whereas negative mood has been associated with lowered right to left PFC alpha activity as indexed by the PFC asymmetry (log transformed right PFC alpha power – log transformed left PFC alpha power).

The link between approach- and withdrawal-related affect and frontal asymmetry has proven to be highly reliable over the years, but the positive–negative distinction is problematic, because the negative emotion anger has also been shown to be lateralized to the left (Harmon-Jones, 2004). This is not so strange, because anger is the prototypical emotion of approach: an energizer driven by motives of reward with aggressive tendencies (Harmon-Jones 2004, van Honk & Schutter, 2006). Findings and theoretical elaborations by Harmon-Jones (2003, 2004) have provided a revision in theorizing on approach- and reward-related emotional processing. On the basis of an extensive line of evidence demonstrating links between the left PFC, anger, and aggression, he proposed a model of motivational direction that drops the "positive–negative" valence dimensions and simply suggests that the approach-related emotions are processed by the left PFC and the withdrawal-related emotions by the right PFC. To summarize some existing data, anxious behavior and the expression of the emotion fear is associated with relatively more right-sided EEG alpha power (Harmon-Jones & Allen, 1997; Kalin, Larson, Shelton, & Davidson, 1998), whereas, for anger proneness and the expression of anger, evidence points at relatively more left prefrontal activity (Coan, Allen, & Harmon-Jones, 1999; Harmon-Jones & Allen, 1998).

Interestingly, asymmetrical prefrontal brain activation can be changed by rTMS. TMS is a technique capable of temporarily changing the excitability of specific regions of the cortex, depending on stimulation parameters. TMS is based on Faraday's law of electromagnetic induction and can be utilized to investigate brain function more directly by applying brief magnetic pulses to either disrupt or facilitate cortical information processing (Grafman & Wassermann, 1999). TMS is a noninvasive method in which an electrical current is conveyed into the brain through a brief but strong magnetic field. Near conducting nerve tissue that is radially oriented to the TMS pulse (Bohning, 2000), the magnetic field is subsequently transformed back into an electrical current that causes a transmembrane potential that, when strong enough, induces neural depolarization and an action potential. The effect of a single TMS pulse on the brain is normally short-lasting (i.e., milliseconds). However, when TMS pulses are applied in trains, called repetitive TMS, the effect can outlast the actual stimulation time. Schutter, van Honk, d'Alfonso, Postma, and de Haan (2001), for instance, found significant changes in electrical brain activity 1 hour after applying 20 minutes of slow-frequency rTMS over the dorsolateral PFC. Because the magnetic field decays exponentially with distance, current TMS technology allows scientists to target only cortical tissue directly. However, distant transsynaptic effects demonstrating effective connectivity have been shown as well (Paus, Castro-Alamancos, & Petrides, 2001). Stimulation frequencies around 1Hz, called slow frequency or inhibitory TMS, is argued to reduce cortical excitability, whereas frequencies exceeding 5Hz, called fast frequency or excitatory rTMS, increase cortical excitability (Pascual-Leone, Walsh, & Rothwell, 2000).

Recently, we performed an rTMS experiment in which we sought to influence the frontal asymmetry of emotion. Inhibitory rTMS was applied to the left and the right PFC of human participants on separate occasions, and selective attention for angry faces was indexed using unmasked and masked versions of the emotional Stroop task (d'Alfonso, van Honk, Hermans, Postma, & de Haan, 2000). It was hypothesized that right PFC stimulation would result in the left PFC becoming relatively more active, leading to a more vigilant response to the angry face, whereas left PFC stimulation would make the right PFC more active, leading to an avoidant response. Emotionally vigilant responses after right PFC rTMS and emotionally avoidant responses after left PFC rTMS were observed and, as might be expected, this time only in the unmasked task (van Honk & De Haan, 2001). These findings, displayed in Figure 10.7, not only provide support for Harmon-Jones's model of motivational direction but also show that emotional processing on the level of the PFC is of a conscious nature. A rTMS study using fearful faces provides further support for these notions (van Honk, Schutter, et al., 2002).

For the d'Alfonso et al. (2000) study, additional analyses were performed on sympathetic and parasympathetic activity of the heart that have been monitored during the motivational task after the rTMS experiment. Increases in selective attention to angry facial expressions after right compared with left PFC rTMS were accompanied by right compared with left PFC rTMS elevations in sympathetic activity (see Figure 10.8). On the basis

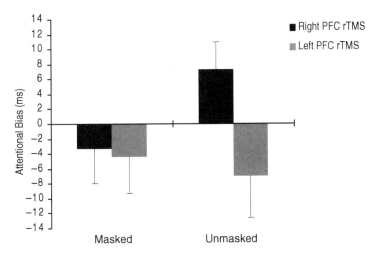

FIGURE 10.7. Mean attentional bias scores (+ *SEM*) for angry faces after slow inhibitory rTMS over the right and left prefrontal cortext.

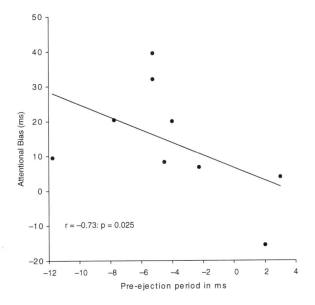

FIGURE 10.8. Scatterplot represents right relative to left rTMS-induced changes in pre-ejection period (PEP) during the Stroop task versus right relative to left rTMS induced changes in attentional-bias scores.

of this evidence and given the inhibitory parameter settings applied, it can be argued that a left-PFC lateralized, sympathetic mechanism directed attention toward the angry facial expression (van Honk, Hermans, et al., 2002). This refutes the suggestion that right prefrontal lateralized parasympathetic mechanisms would be involved in the attentive processing of anger (Hughdahl & Johnsen, 1991). The latter notion is based on evidence from aversive conditioning paradigms wherein angry faces seem easily associated with fear or anxiety. However, our data show that aversive conditioning paradigms tell us little about the evolutionary evolved unconditioned emotional properties of the facial expression of anger (van Honk, Tuiten, & Van den Hout, et al., 2001).

THE PARIETAL CORTEX

Research into emotion and the cerebral cortex has been concentrating on the prefrontal regions. There is, however, also evidence for the involvement of the parietal cortex in emotion and emotional disorders (Davidson, 1984; Davidson & Henriques, 2000). To find evidence for a role of the parietal cortex in approach- and withdrawal-related emotion, we performed a study in which participants underwent EEG baseline recordings from prefrontal and parietal electrode sites that were followed by a modified dot probe task using neutral, happy, and angry faces. The dot probe task is a spatially oriented motivated attention task, which therefore should be particularly sensitive to the spatial properties of the parietal cortex. As in the Stroop task, a central fixation cross remains visible for 750 milliseconds. The faces are now, however, presented for 500 milliseconds, a few degrees to the periphery. They are immediately followed by a probe (the capital character A or O) on either the left or the right side; that is, in a location at which a neutral or emotional face had been presented. Presentation of the probe is terminated by computer registration of the vocal response of the participant. Participants were instructed to focus on the fixation cross at the start of each new trial and to identify as fast and accurately as possible the capital character A or O. Bias scores were calculated by subtracting the average latencies to probes replacing an neutral face from the probes replacing an emotional face. Negative difference scores indicate more time needed to identify the probes, that is, avoidance of the emotional faces, whereas positive scores reflect more vigilant attention to emotional faces. The relationships between prefrontal and parietal brain EEG asymmetries in the alpha and beta frequency range and selective attention to angry and happy faces were investigated by means of correlational analyses (Schutter et al., 2002). Data revealed that relatively increased right-sided resting-state baseline beta activity over the parietal cortex exclusively predicted an attentionally more avoidant response to the angry facial expression, as can be seen in Figure 10.9. Thus the dimensions of approach and withdrawal

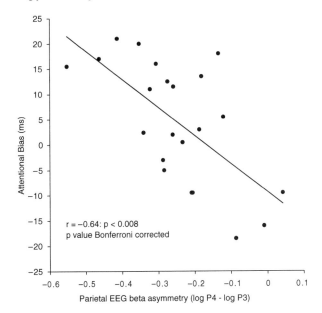

FIGURE 10.9. Averaged brain asymmetries from the P3 and P4 electrode sites and mean attentional bias for angry facial expressions in milliseconds (ms). Increased relative right EEG beta asymmetry is associated with avoidant responses to the angry facial expression.

over the parietal cortex indexed by the dot probe task were in concordance with those found over the PFC on basis of the Stroop task using rTMS (d'Alfonso et al., 2000). The dominant motivational stance can be linked to the left hemisphere and the submissive stance to the right hemisphere.

In an attempt to gather stronger evidence, an rTMS study was performed over the right parietal cortex in a placebo-controlled design, using locally inhibitory frequency parameter settings. Dependent measures were again attentional biases for angry faces, measured by the dot probe task, this time together with indices of autonomic activity (skin conductance and heart rate; van Honk et al., 2003). It was hypothesized that right parietal rTMS should induce more vigilant attentional responses to the angry faces, accompanied by an increase of cardiac activity (van Honk et al., 2002) during the performance of the dot probe task. The effect on the dot probe task was observed, but only when the faces appeared in the left-hemisphere field, indicating that rTMS induced specific right-hemispheric changes seen as a significant reduction in the avoidant response to the angry face that was observed after placebo (see Figure 10.10a). Furthermore, this reduction in avoidance—or enhanced vigilance—to the angry face was accompanied by a task-dependent elevation in heart rate (see Figure 10.10b). When these are taken together with the data from the emotional Stroop task using

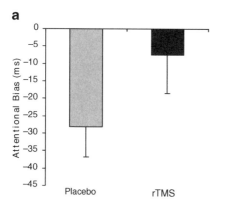
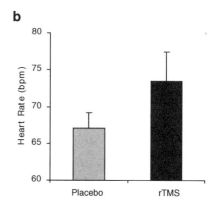

FIGURE 10.10. Mean (*SEM*) attentional biases for angry facial expressions in milliseconds (ms) in the left hemifield and mean (*SEM*) heart rate in beats per minute (bpm) during performance of the motivated attention task after placebo and rTMS.

rTMS and the EEG, it seems justifiable to assume that for both the PFC and the parietal cortex, the right hemisphere more strongly carries the motives of submission, whereas the left hemisphere seems to carry dominant motivation when one encounters social threat.

Until now, unconscious and conscious forms of approach- and withdrawal-related emotion were treated in relative isolation, as were the brain regions involved. Steroid-hormone mediated unconscious affective processing was argued to be mainly mediated on the subcortical level of the brain, whereas specific properties of the PFC and the parietal cortex were predominantly involved in conscious emotion. An important question for social neuroscience is what brings the different cortical and subcortical aspects of emotional approach- and withdrawal-related emotion together, because these systems rarely act in isolation. How do the evolutionary older and newer brain regions communicate during the social-emotional incidents described earlier, and which neurochemical processes might be involved? Interestingly, most of the answers bring us back to the steroid hormones, as they regulate not only brain communication but also the communication between the brain and the social environment.

THE COMMUNICATING SOCIAL EMOTIONAL BRAIN

Social-emotional behavior concerns meaningful conspecific communication and depends on brain communication and the communication between the brain and the social environment. Steroids are importantly involved in brain communication and are in constant interaction with the social environment. Methods capable of estimating the communication between different brain regions, not only on the corticocortical level (Nunez et al., 1997), but also on the subcortical–cortical level, are EEG coherence analyses computed within or across frequency bands (Knyazev & Slobodskaya, 2003). Both are important because appropriate social-emotional functioning depends not only on corticocortical or "horizontal" brain communication but also, in particular, on effective communication between the subcortical and the cortical affective brain (Mayberg et al., 1999)—so-called "vertical" brain communication. This is of interest because, apart from influencing cortical and subcortical processing (Schutter, Peper, Kahn, & van Honk, 2005; Tops et al., 2005; Schulkin, 2003), steroids seem to bridge phylogeny by influencing the communication between the older subcortical and the newer cortical layers of the brain. Evidence builds on an evolutionary-oriented brain theory wherein the phylogenetically different subcortical and cortical brain systems relate to oscillations in slow-frequency and fast-frequency EEG bands (Robinson, 1999). Relative increases or decreases in subcortical–cortical communication are computed by correlating the change in power between these bands, and it has repeatedly been demonstrated that elevated subcortical–cortical cross-talk, as indexed by EEG, is accompanied by the behaviorally avoidant, fearful stance, whereas reduced cross-talk was linked to reward-driven, approach-related behaviors (Knyazev & Slobodskaya, 2003; Knyazev, Savostyanov, & Levin, 2004). In agreement with the affective properties of the steroid hormones, it was found that cortisol increases subcortical–cortical communication (Schutter & van Honk, 2005) and shifts the frontal asymmetry of emotion to the right (Tops et al., 2005) while decreasing the communication between the prefrontal and the parietal structures of the cortex (Schutter, van Honk, Koppeschaar, & Kahn, 2002). On the basis of the preceding, these effects can be interpreted as increases in the fearful-submissive motivational stance. Enhanced communication between the left PFC and the right parietal cortex was, on the other hand, observed after testosterone administration (Schutter et al., 2005), an effect that seems to be preceded by a reduction in subcorticocortical communication (Schutter & van Honk, 2004) and that is accompanied by increases in approach-related motivation and emotion. Given the inherent antagonism between cortisol and testosterone on the physiological and psychological levels (Viau, 2002; van Honk, Peper, & Schutter, 2005) this evidence provides initial insights into how these steroid hormones influence brain communication and thereby set the motivational stance for dominance or submission.

REFERENCES

Berridge, K. C. (2003). Comparing the emotional brains of humans and other animals. In R. J. Davidson & Scherer (Eds.), *Handbook of affective sciences* (pp. 25–51). New York: Oxford University Press.

Blair, R. J. (2003). Facial expressions, their communicatory functions and neurocognitive substrates. *Philosophical Transactions of the Royal Society of London (B) Biological Sciences, 358,* 561–572.

Bohning, D. E. (2000). Introduction and overview of TMS physics, in M. S. George & R. H. Belmaker (Eds.), *Transcranial magnetic stimulation in neuropsychiatry* (pp. 3–44). Washington: American Psychiatric Press.

Boissy, A., and Bouissou, M. F. (1994). Effects of androgen treatment on behavioral and physiological responses of heifers to fear-eliciting situations. *Hormones and Behavior, 28,* 66–83.

Booth, A., Shelley, G., Mazur, A., Tharp, G., & Kittok, R. (1989). Testosterone and winning and losing in human competition. *Hormones and Behavior, 23,* 556–571.

Borod, J. C., Cicero, B. A., Obler, L. K., Welkowitz, J., Erhan, H. M., Santschi, C., et al. (1998). Right hemisphere emotional perception: Evidence across multiple channels. *Neuropsychology, 12,* 446–458.

Brothers, L. (1990). The neural basis of primate social communication. *Motivation and Emotion, 14,* 81–91.

Cambell, B. A., Wood, G., & McBride, T. (1997). Origins of orienting and defensive response: An evolutionary perspective. In P. J. Lang & M. T. Balaban (Eds.), *Attention and orienting: Sensory and motivational processes* (pp. 41–68). Hillsdale, NJ: Erlbaum.

Coan, J. A., Allen, J. J. B., & Harmon-Jones, E. (1999). Approach/withdraw motivational states, emotion, and facial feedback. *Psychophysiology, 36,* S41.

Cohen, D., Nisbett, R. E., Bowdle, B. F., & Schwarz, N. (1996). Insult, aggression, and the southern culture of honor: An "experimental ethnography." *Journal of Personality and Social Psychology, 70,* 945–960.

Cottingham, S. L., & Phaff, D. (1986). Interconnectedness of steroid hormone-binding neurons: Existence and implications. *Current Topics in Neuroendocrinology, 7,* 223–249.

Dabbs, J. M., Jr., & Hargrove, M. F. (1997). Age, testosterone, and behavior among female prison inmates. *Psychosomatic Medicine, 59,* 477–480.

d'Alfonso, A., van Honk, J., Hermans, E. J., Postma, A., & De Haan, E. (2000). Laterality effects in selective attention to threat after rTMS at the prefrontal cortex. *Neuroscience Letters, 280,* 195–198.

Davidson, R. J. (1984). Affect: Cognition and hemispheric lateralization. In C. E. Izard, J. Kagan, & R. B. Zajonc (Eds.), *Emotions, cognition and behavior* (pp. 320–365). Cambridge, UK: Cambridge University Press.

Davidson, R. J. (1988). EEG measures of cerebral asymmetry: Conceptual and methodological issues. *International Journal of Neuroscience, 39,* 71–89.

Davidson, R. J. (1998). Affective style and affective disorders: Perspectives from affective neuroscience. *Cognition and Emotion, 12,* 307–330.

Davidson, R. J., & Henriques, J. (2000). Regional brain function in sadness and depression. In J. C. Borod (Ed.), *The neuropsychology of emotion* (pp. 269–297). New York: Oxford University Press.

Davidson, R. J. (2004). What does the prefrontal cortex "do" in affect? Perspectives on frontal EEG asymmetry research. *Biological Psychology, 67,* 219–233.

DeCantanzara, D. A. (1999). *Motivation and emotion.* Upper Saddle River, NJ: Prentice Hall.

Dimberg, U., & Öhman, A. (1996). Behold the wrath: Psychophysiological responses to facial stimuli. *Motivation and Emotion, 20,* 149–182.

Elias, M. (1981). Serum cortisol, testosterone, and testosterone binding glubolin responses to competitive fighting in human males. *Aggressive Behavior, 7,* 215–224.

Ferin, M. (1993). Neuropeptides, the stress response, and the hypothamalo–pituitary–gonadal axis in the female rhesus monkey. *Annals of the New York Academy of Sciences, 679,* 106–116.

Gladue, B. A., Boechler, M., & McCaul, K. D. (1989). Hormonal response to competition in human males. *Aggressive Behavior, 15,* 409–422.

Grafman, J., & Wassermann, E. M. (1999). Transcranial magnetic stimulation can measure and modulate learning and memory. *Neuropsychologia, 37,* 159–167.

Harmon-Jones, E. (2003). Early career award: Clarifying the emotive functions of asymmetrical frontal cortical activity. *Psychophysiology, 40,* 838–848.

Harmon-Jones, E. (2004). Contributions from research on anger and cognitive dissonance to understanding the motivational functions of asymmetrical frontal brain activity. *Biological Psychology, 67,* 51–76.

Harmon-Jones, E., & Allen, J. J. B. (1997). Behavioral activation sensitivity and resting frontal EEG asymmetry: Covariation of putative indicators related to risk of mood disorders. *Journal of Abnormal Psychology, 106,* 159–163.

Harmon-Jones, E., & Allen, J. J. B. (1998). Anger and frontal brain activity: EEG asymmetry consistent with approach motivation despite negative affective valence. *Journal of Personality and Social Psychology, 74,* 1310–1316.

Hermans, E. J., Putnam, P., & van Honk, J. (2006). *Reduced processing of angry threat in social phobia.* Unpublished raw data.

Hermans, E., Ramsey, N. F., & van Honk, J. (in press). Testosterone increases neural activiation in a primordial aggression circuit during the processing of anger. *Biological Psychiatry.*

Hock, M. (1993). Coping dispositions, attentional directions, and anxiety states. In H. W. Krohne (Ed.); *Attention and avoidance* (pp. 139–169). Bern, Switzerland: Hogrefe & Huber.

Hugdahl, K.,& Johnsen, B. H. (1991). Brain asymmetry and human electrodermal conditioning. *Integrative Physiology and Behavior Science, 26,* 39–44.

Kagan, J., Reznick, S., & Snidman, N. (1988) Biological bases of childhood shyness. *Science, 24,* 169–171.

Kalin, N. H., Larson, C., Shelton, C. E., & Davidson, R. J. (1998). Asymmetric frontal brain activity, cortisol, and behavior associated with fearful temperament in rhesus monkeys. *Behavioral Neuroscience, 112,* 286–292.

Kling, A. S., & Brothers, L. A. (1992). The amygdala and social behavior. In J. P. Aggleton (Ed.), *The amygdala* (pp. 353–377). New York: Wiley-Liss.

Knyazev, G. G., Savostyanov, A. N., & Levin, E. A. (2004). Alpha oscillations as a correlate of trait anxiety. *International Journal of Psychophysiology, 53,* 147–160.

Knyazev, G. G., & Slobodskaya, H. R. (2003). Personality trait of behavioral inhibition is associated with oscillatory systems reciprocal relationships. *International Journal of Psychophysiology, 48,* 247–261.

Kreuz, L., Rose, R., & Jennings, J. (1972). Suppression of plasma testosterone levels and psychological stress. *Archives of General Psychiatry, 26,* 479–482.

Lang, P. J., Davis, M., & Öhman, A. (2000). Fear and anxiety: Animal models and human cognitive psychophysiology. D*Journal of Affective Disorders, 61,* 137–159.

Lang, P. J., Bradley, M. M., & Cuthbert, B. N. (1998). Motivated attention: Affect, activation and action. In P. J. Lang, R. F. Simons, & M. Balaban (Eds.), *Attention and orienting* (pp. 97–135). Mahwah, NJ: Erlbaum.

LeDoux, J. E. (1996). *The emotional brain.* New York: Simon & Schuster.

Lemerise, E. A., & Dodge, K. A. (1993). The development of anger and hostile interventions. In M. Lewis & J. M. Haviland-Jones (Eds.), *Handbook of emotions* (pp. 537–546). New York: Guilford Press.

Mathews, A., & Mackintosh, B. (1998). A cognitive model of selective processing in anxiety. *Cognitive Therapy and Research, 22,* 539–560.

Mathews, A., & MacLeod, C. (1994). Cognitive approaches to emotion and emotional disorders. *Annual Review of Psychology, 45,* 25–50.

Mayberg, H. S., Liotti, M., Brannan, S. K., McGinnis, S., Mahurin, R. K., Jarebec, P. A., et al. (1999). Reciprocal limbic-cortical function and negative mood: Converging PET findings in depression and normal sadness. *American Journal of Psychiatry, 156,* 675–682.

Mazur, A., & Booth, A. (1998). Testosterone and dominance. *Behavioral and Brain Sciences, 21,* 353–397.

McEwen, B. S. (1994). Stressful experience, brain, and emotions: Developmental, genetic, and hormonal influences. In M. S Gazzaniga (Ed.), *The cognitive neurosciences* (pp. 1117–1135). New York: MIT Press.

McNally, R. J. (1995). Automaticity and anxiety disorders. *Behaviour Research and Therapy, 33,* 747–754.

Mogg, K., & Bradley, B. P. (1998). A cognitive-motivational analysis of anxiety. *Behavior Research and Therapy, 36,* 809–848.

Morris, J. S., Öhman, A., and Dolan, R. J. (1999). A subcortical pathway to the amygdala mediating "unseen" fear. *Proceedings of the National Academy of Sciences of the USA, 96,* 1680–1685.

Nesse, R. M. (2000). Is depression an adaptation. *Archives of General Psychiatry, 57,* 14–20.

Nunez, P. L., Srinivasan, R., Westdorp, A. F., Wijesinghe, R. S., Tucker, D. M., Silberstein, R. B., et al. (1997). EEG coherency: I. Statistics, reference electrode, volume conduction, Laplacians, cortical imaging, and interpretation at multiple scales. *Electroencephalography and Clinical Neurophysiology, 103,* 499–515.

Öhman, A. (1993). Fear and anxiety as emotional phenomena: Clinical phenomenology, evolutionary perspectives, and information processing mechanisms. In M. Lewis & J. M. Haviland-Jones (Eds.), *Handbook of emotions* (pp. 511–536). New York: Guilford Press.

Öhman, A (1997). A fast blink of the eye: Evolutionary preparedness for pre-attentive processing of threat. In P. J. Lang, R. F. Simons, and M. T. Balaban (Eds.), *Attention and orienting: Sensory and motivational processing* (pp. 165–184). Hillsdale, NJ: Earlbaum.

Panksepp, J. (2003). At the interface of the affective, behavioral, and cognitive neurosciences: Decoding the emotional feelings of the brain. *Brain and Cognition, 52,* 4–14.

Pascual-Leone, A., Walsh, V., & Rothwell, J. (2000). Transcranial magnetic stimulation in cognitive neuroscience: Virtual lesion, chronometry, and functional connectivity. *Current Opinion in Neurobiology, 10,* 232–237.

Paus, T., Castro-Alamancos, M. A., & Petrides, M. (2001). Cortico-cortical connectivity of the human mid-dorsolateral frontal cortex and its modulation by repetitive transcranial magnetic stimulation. *European Journal of Neuroscience, 14,* 1405–1411.

Perski, H., Smith, K., & Bassu, G. K. (1971). Relation of psychologic measures of aggression and hostility to testosterone production in man. *Psychosomatic Medicine, 33,* 265–277.

Plutchik, R. (1993). Emotions and their vicissitudes: Emotions and psychopathology. In M. Lewis & J. M. Haviland (Eds.), *Handbook of emotions* (pp. 53–66). New York: Guilford Press.

Putman, P., Hermans, E. & van Honk, J. (2004) Selective attention to threatening faces in an emotional Stroop task: It's BAS, not BIS. *Emotion, 4,* 305–311.

Rahe, R., Karson, S., Howard, N., Rubin, R., & Poland, R. (1990). Psychological and physiological assessments on American hostages freed from captivity in Iran. *Psychosomatic Medicine, 52,* 1–16.

Reiman, E. M. (1997). The application of positron emission tomography to the study of normal and pathologic emotions. *Journal of Clinical Psychiatry, 58,* 4–12.

Robinson, D. L. (1999). The technical, neurological, and psychological significance of "alpha," "delta," and "theta" waves confounded on EEG evoked potentials: A study of peak latencies. *Clinical Neuropsychology, 110,* 1427–1434.

Rose, R. M., Bernstein, I. S., & Gordon, T. (1975). Consequences of social conflict on testosterone levels in rhesus monkeys. *Psychosomatic Medicine,* 37, 50–61.

Sapolsky, R. (1990). Adrenocortical function, social rank, and personality among wild baboons. *Biological Psychiatry, 28,* 862–878.

Salvador, A., Simon, V., Suay, F., & Llorens, L. (1987). Testosterone and cortisol responses to competitive fighting in human males. *Aggressive Behavior, 13,* 9–13.

Schulkin, J. (2003). *Rethinking homeostasis: Allostatic regulation in physiology and pathophysiology.* Cambridge, MA: MIT Press.

Schulkin, J., Gold, P. W., & McEwen B. S. (1998). Induction of corticotropin-releasing hormone gene expression by glucocorticoids: Implications for understanding the states of fear and anxiety and allostatic load. *Psychoneuroendocrinology, 23,* 219–243.

Schutter, D. J. L. G., Peper, J. S., Kahn, R. S., & van Honk, J (in press). Administration of testosterone increases functional connectivity in a cortico-cortical depression circuit. *Journal of Neuropsychiatry and Clinical Neurosciences.*

Schutter, D. J. L. G., van Honk, J., d'Alfonso, A., Postma, A., & de Haan, E. H. F. (2001). Effects of slow rTMS as the right dorsolateral prefrontal cortex on EEG asymmetry and mood. *Neuroreport, 12,* 345–347.

Schutter, D. J. L. G., van Honk, J., d'Alfonso, A. A. L., Postma, A., & de Haan, E. H. F. (2001). Effects of slow rTMS at the right dorsolateral prefrontal cortex on EEG asymmetry and mood. *Neuroreport, 12,* 445–447.

Schutter, D. J. L. G., van Honk, J., Koppeschaar, H. P. F., & Kahn, R. S. (2002) Cortisol and reduced interhemispheric coupling between the left prefrontal and the right parietal cortex. *Journal of Neuropsychiatry and Clinical Neurosciences, 14,* 89–90.

Schutter, D. J. L. G., & van Honk, J. (in press). Salivary cortisol levels and the coupling of midfrontal delta-beta oscillations. *International Journal of Psychophysiology*.

Service, F. J. (1995). Hypoglycemic disorders. *The New England Journal of Medicine*, *332*, 1144–1152.

Spielberger, C. D., Gorsuch, R. L., & Lushene, R. D. (1970). *Manual for the State–Trait Anxiety Inventory*. Palo Alto, CA: Consulting Psychologists Press.

Thompson, W., Dabbs, J., Jr., & Frady, R. (1990). Changes in saliva testosterone during a 90-day shock incarceration program. *Criminal Justice and Behavior*, *17*, 246–252.

Tooby, J., & Cosmides, L. (1995). Mapping the evolved functional organisation of mind and brain. In M. S. Gazzaniga (Ed.), *The cognitive neurosciences* (pp. 1185–1197). New York: MIT Press.

Tops, M., Wijers, A. A., van Staveren, A. S., Bruin, K. J., Den Boer, J. A., Meijman, T. F., et al. (2005). Acute cortisol administration modulates EEG alpha asymmetry in volunteers. *Biological Psychology*, *69*, 181–193.

Tsai, L. W., & Sapolski, R. M. (1996). Rapid stimulatory effects of testosterone upon myotubule metabolism and sugar transport, as assessed by silicon microphysiometry. *Aggressive Behavior*, *22*, 357–364.

van Honk, J., & de Haan, E. (2001). Cortical and subcortical routes for conscious and unconscious processing of emotional faces. In B. De Gelder, C. A. Heywood, & E. de Haan (Eds.), *Varieties of unconscious processing* (pp. 222–237). Oxford, UK: Oxford University Press.

van Honk, J., Hermans, E. J., d'Alfonso, A. A. L., Schutter, D. J. L. G., van Doornen, L., & de Haan, E. H. F. (2002). A left-prefrontal lateralized, sympathetic mechanism directs attention towards social threat: Evidence from rTMS. *Neuroscience Letters*, *319*, 99–102.

van Honk, J., Peper, J. S., & Schutter, D. J. L. G. (2005). Testosterone reduces unconscious fear but not consciously experienced anxiety. *Biological Psychiatry*, *58*, 218–225.

van Honk, J., & Schutter, D. J. L. G. (2006). Unmasking feigned sanity: A neurobiological model of emotion processing in primary psychopathy. *Cognitive Neuropsychiatry*, *11*, 285–306.

van Honk, J., Schutter, D. J. L. G, d'Alfonso, A. A. L., Kessels, R. P. C., &, de Haan E. H. F. (2002). 1Hz rTMS over the right prefrontal cortex reduces vigilant attention to unmasked but not to masked fearful faces. *Biological Psychiatry*, *52*, 312–317.

van Honk, J., Schutter, D. J. L. G., Hermans, E. J., & Putman, P. (2004). Testosterone, cortisol, dominance, and submission: Biologically prepared motivation, no psychological mechanisms involved. *Behavioral Brain Sciences*, *27*, 1–2.

van Honk, J., Schutter, D. J. L. G., Putman, P., De Haan, E. H. F., & D'Alfonso, A. A. L. (2003). Reductions in phenomenological, physiological and attentional indices of depression after 2Hz rTMS over the right parietal cortex. *Psychiatry Research*, *120*, 95–101.

van Honk, J., Tuiten, A., Hermans, E., Putman, P., Koppeschaar, H. F., & Verbaten, R. (2001). A single administration of testosterone induces cardiac accelerative responses to angry faces in healthy young women. *Behavioral Neuroscience*, *115*, 238–242.

van Honk J., Tuiten, A., van den Hout, M., de Haan, E., & Stam H. (2001).

Attentional biases for angry faces: Relationships to trait anger and anxiety. *Cognition and Emotion, 15,* 279–297.

van Honk, J., Tuiten, A., van den Hout, M., Koppeschaar, H., Thijssen, J., de Haan, E., et al. (1998). Baseline salivary cortisol levels and preconscious selective attention for threat. *Psychoneuroendocrinology, 23,* 741–747.

van Honk J., Tuiten, A, van den Hout M., Koppeschaar, H., Thijssen, J., de Haan, E., et al. (2000). Conscious and preconscious selective attention to social threat: Different neuroendocrine response patterns. *Psychoneuroendocrinology, 25,* 577–591.

van Honk, J., Tuiten, A., Verbaten, R., van den Hout, M., Koppeschaar, H., Thijssen, J., et al. (1999). Correlations among salivary testosterone, mood, and selective attention to threat in humans. *Hormones and Behavior, 36,* 17–24.

Viau, V. (2002). Functional cross-talk between the hypothalamic–pituitary–gonadal and adrenal axes. *Journal of Neuroendocrinology, 14,* 506–513.

Wassermann, E. M., & Lisanby, S.H. (2001). Therapeutic application of repetitive transcranial magnetic stimulation: A review. *Clinical Neurophysiology, 112,* 1367–1377.

Whalen, P. J. (1998). Fear, vigilance, and ambiguity: Initial neuroimaging studies of the human amygdala. *Current Directions in Psychological Science, 7,* 177–188.

Williams, J. M. G., Mathews, A., & MacLeod, C. (1996). The emotional Stroop task and psychopathology. *Psychological Bulletin, 120,* 3–24.

Wood, R. I. (1996). Functions of the steroid-responsive neural network in the control of male hamster sexual behavior. *Trends in Endocrinology and Metabolism, 7,* 338–344.

IV

ATTITUDES AND
SOCIAL COGNITION

11

Attitudes and Evaluation

TOWARD A COMPONENT PROCESS FRAMEWORK

William A. Cunningham and Marcia K. Johnson

One of the most exciting developments in social psychology is the recent increase in interest in integrating theories and methods of social psychology, cognitive psychology, and cognitive neuroscience. Just as the social-cognitive revolution that began in the 1980s provided new insights into social processes, an additional level of analysis—identifying the neural correlates of these processes—promises a more complete understanding of important constructs such as attitudes, prejudice, and emotional regulation.

In this chapter we review social neuroscience research, examining the evaluative processes that underlie attitudes. It is difficult to think of a social-psychological concept more central than attitudes (Eagly & Chaiken, 1993). The sense that something is good or bad, positive or negative, pleasant or unpleasant, or to be approached or avoided is critical to almost any behavior. Indeed, the processes of evaluation and associated behavioral choice are ubiquitous though often invisible in daily life. Yet, as is increasingly clear, even simple evaluations are often the integrated outcome of multiple affective and cognitive component processes.

EVALUATIVE PROCESSES AND ATTITUDES

Attitudes, most simply put, are our likes and dislikes (Bem, 1970). Although such a definition can conjure images of valence tags (the equivalent of little pluses and minuses) associated with representations of objects, events, concepts, and so forth, Allport (1935) highlighted the importance of not defining attitudes as rigid, tightly bound responses to a particular stimulus. That is, attitudes are not simple if–then rules that operate as an S–R association between the perception of a stimulus and a specific feeling, opinion, or behavior. Rather, he suggested that the concept of attitude must include the idea of flexibility, and he defined an attitude as "a mental and neural state of readiness, organized through experience, exerting a directive or dynamic influence upon the individual's response to all objects and situations with which it is related" (p. 810). Allport (1935) additionally suggested that the way to achieve dynamic, flexible attitudes that may include ambivalence was by "reducing attitudes to small enough components" (p. 820). Following this line of thinking, by making representations of attitudes small enough (e.g., breaking a representation–attitude association [R–A] into R_1–A_1, R_2–A_2, R_3–A_3, etc.), a simple concept of attitude might be retained, and combinations of attitude representations would permit levels of attitude complexity.

We take a similar approach in this chapter, suggesting that attitude *processes* can be reduced to more elemental units. That is, we suggest that attitudes are the outcome of multiple affective and cognitive processes, variously recruited and/or tuned to meet situational and motivational constraints. Although few attitude theorists would deny the flexible nature of the processes that underlie attitudes, there has been a (perhaps only implicit) representation focus in most of social psychology. Attitudes tend to be treated as representations directly retrieved from memory in response to perceptual cues. Admittedly, the distinction between representation and process may be somewhat artificial, but we want to shift the emphasis from attitudes as retrieved to attitudes as constructed dynamically within particular contexts (e.g., situational, cognitive, motivational). Thus attitudes and evaluations, and especially the subjective experience associated with attitudes, comes from a cognitive–affective system that likely operates in a dynamic and integrated fashion (see Schwarz & Bohner, 2001; Wilson & Hodges, 1992).

An analogy can be made between the concept of an attitude and the concept of a memory. According to the source monitoring framework (Johnson, Hashtroudi, & Lindsay, 1993; Johnson & Raye, 1981), remembering is not simply retrieval of a trace but rather an attribution about the nature of a mental experience (see also Jacoby, Kelley, & Dywan, 1989). Mental experiences result from a combination of associative and more constructive processes, and attributions or judgments about them are based on a weighted average of various features or types of information, including additional information that may be retrieved in the service of monitoring the origin of the mental experience (e.g., imagination or perception). Furthermore, the weights associated with different features or other types of evidence are affected by current context (e.g., motivational state, hypotheses). The activation of information can occur relatively automatically or via more reflective processes, and the activated information can be evaluated relatively automatically or by more reflective processes (i.e., although information that arises relatively automatically is often evaluated relatively automatically and information that arises more reflectively is evaluated more reflectively, this is not necessarily the case). Similarly, attitudes can be viewed as the result of a weighting of the affective qualities associated with currently activated information. Some evaluative qualities arise more automatically and some with more reflective effort (e.g., Johnson & Multhaup, 1992), and some contribute to the attitude more automatically and some with more reflection.

THE ATTITUDE SYSTEM

As in the social cognitive tradition that underlies much social neuroscience research, we assume that in order to understand attitudes, one needs to understand the cognitive architecture that underlies perception and thought. However, even before fully specifying the component cognitive processes that give rise to our mental experiences, we can move toward a component process framework by considering two general ways that components could be defined—in terms of types of information processed or in terms of the type of operation engaged. With respect to type of information, historically in the attitude–emotion domain, stimuli have been assumed to include two key attributes—valence and intensity. With respect to type of process, as in cognition in general, in the attitude–emotion domain, the distinction between implicit and explicit processes has been important. Here we consider recent evidence that either or both of these two simple ways of conceptualizing components of attitudes are reflected in identifiable neural areas or circuits. In addition, we also briefly consider the relation between attitudes and emotion, whether there are separate neural correlates of positively and negatively valenced stimuli, the possibility that the same neural systems flexibly process positive and negative stimuli depending on motivational goals, and how ambivalence is reflected in brain activity. In this chapter, we focus primarily on affectively based attitudes. That is, for the purposes of this chapter, attitudes are evaluations infused by emotion.

Attitudes and Emotion

The psychological study of attitudes has been naturally linked to the study of affect and emotional processing. Thurstone (1931) provided a parsimonious definition of attitudes as simply "the affect for or against a psychological object" (p. 261). Research spanning almost a century has indicated that our self-perceived bodily states are linked to our evaluative judgments (Bem, 1972; Damasio, 1994; James, 1884). For example, in extending findings that electrodermal activity (e.g., the skin's ability to conduct electricity) varied as a function of the emotionality of presented stimuli (Smith,

1922), electrodermal activity has been found to vary with attitude extremity (Dysinger, 1931) and agreement with presented attitude statements (Dickson & McGinnies, 1966). In addition, other psychophysiological methods have been developed that are sensitive to attitude valence and extremity, such as facial electromyography (EMG; e.g., changes in electrical potentials over particular muscles in the face; Cacioppo, Petty, Losch, & Kim, 1986). More recently, research using event-related potentials (ERP) and functional magnetic resonance imaging (fMRI) has demonstrated links between neural activity in regions associated with emotion and attitudes (e.g., Cunningham et al., 2003; Cunningham, Raye, & Johnson, 2004).

Arousal and Valence

For some time, emotion researchers have found that apparently discrete emotional experiences can be characterized along two orthogonal dimensions. Although the names of these dimensions vary from theory to theory, they typically involve a dimension of positivity and negativity (valence) and a dimension of intensity (arousal; Russell, 1979). This distinction between valence and arousal has had a long history in social psychology. In their two-factor theory of emotion, Schacter and Singer (1962) suggested that emotions are derived from a combination of arousal and cognitions used to explain the arousal. In several studies, participants who were experimentally aroused (e.g., given a dose of epinephrine) reported experiencing greater emotional responses consistent with their situations, but only when they were unaware of the effects of the arousal manipulations. Such findings suggest that one first experiences a visceral autonomic response to a stimulus or situation that is devoid of valence, and then one cognitively interprets this bodily state and generates a specific positive or negative emotion (see also Cannon, 1929; James, 1884).

In this conception, arousal is associated with an experienced bodily state and valence with a cognitive appraisal. Of course, these autonomic and cognitive responses could overlap in time rather than being serial, and they could interact in producing specific emotions and attitudes. Converging evidence for the distinction between arousal and valence has been provided by recent functional neuroimaging studies. In three fMRI studies that manipulated or parametrically analyzed both valence and arousal such that the two could be examined orthogonally, different brain areas were associated with valence and arousal (Anderson et al., 2003; Cunningham, Raye, & Johnson, 2004; Small et al., 2003). In each of these studies, arousal was associated with amygdala activation, and negative valence was associated with right prefrontal activation. In addition, Adolphs, Russell, and Tranel (1999) asked both a patient with bilateral amygdala damage and controls to rate the valence and arousal of various stimuli. The patient with amygdala damage rated stimuli to have the same valences as controls did but rated the emotional intensity of stimuli differently.

Positive and Negative Substrates?

In addition to evidence dissociating valence and arousal, other evidence suggests that positive and negative components of valence may also be processed distinctly (Cacioppo & Berntson, 1994). For example, Davidson and colleagues have found, using EEG, that there appear to be separate systems for approach- and avoidance-related behavior (Davidson & Irwin, 1999). Viewing or thinking about negative information results in greater right-sided EEG activity than viewing or thinking about something positive (Cunningham, Espinet, DeYoung, & Zelazo, 2005; Davidson, Ekman, Saron, Senalis, & Friesen, 1990, Jones & Fox, 1992). Interestingly, anger, which is a negative but approach-related emotion, is associated with greater left than right EEG activity (Harmon-Jones & Allen, 1998). Thus laterality does not appear to be synonymous with positivity or negativity per se but rather behavioral tendencies associated with evaluative processing.

In the imaging domain, Sutton, Davidson, Donzella, Irwin, and Dottl (1997) found using PET that viewing negatively valenced pictures was associated with activation in the right orbital frontal cortex and the right inferior frontal cortex, whereas viewing positively valenced pictures was associated with activation in the left pre- and postcentral gyri. More recently, evidence for right lateralized processing of negative information has been found using fMRI (Anderson et al., 2003; Cunningham et al., 2003; Cunningham, Raye, & Johnson, 2004). Specifically, areas of the right inferior frontal cortex and anterior insula consistently appear to be involved more in processing negative than positive valenced stimuli. Other studies have found that areas of the orbitofrontal cortex (OFC; Anderson et al., 2003; Nitschke et al., 2003; Kringelbach, O'Doherty, Rolls, & Andrew, 2003) and basal ganglia (Delgado, Nystrom, Fissell, Noll, & Fiez, 2000) are involved primarily in the processing of positive affect, with the OFC being involved in the first-order association between a stimulus and its reinforcement value and the ventral striatum system being involved in the processing of rewards (Knutson & Cooper, 2005; see Wager, Phan, Liberzon, & Taylor, 2003, for a meta-analysis). Although such findings do not necessarily imply that the processing of positive and negative information is fully dissociated, this suggests that they may involve at least partially separable circuits.

To the extent that the processing of positive and negative information relies on different brain regions, an important question to resolve regards the different processing time associated with each. Predictions based on the idea of a negativity bias propose that negative information takes priority in processing, both in terms of more rapid responses and greater overall influence (Cacioppo & Berntson, 1994; Cacioppo & Gardner, 1999; Ito, Larsen, Smith, & Cacioppo, 1998). Thus one might expect negative stimuli to be processed more quickly than positive stimuli in terms of brain activity. Although several studies have investigated potential differences in response time to negative and positive stimuli, the answer to this question remains unclear.

Several studies have found that the processing of negative information may occur quite rapidly in the processing stream. For example, Kawasaki et al. (2001) found that the processing of negative, but not neutral or positive, stimuli occurred 120–160 milliseconds after stimulus presentation in single-cell recordings of the human OFC. In addition, negative stimuli appear to be differentiated from positive stimuli in posterior perception areas, as indexed by the early P1 component (Smith, Cacioppo, Larsen, & Chartrand, 2003). Some have suggested that negative information is privileged such that it is processed more quickly than positive information—a temporal negativity bias (Cacioppo & Gardner, 1999). Providing support for this idea, Carretie, Martin-Loeches, Hinojosa, & Mercado (2001), using magnetoencephalography (MEG), found that negative stimuli were processed 200 milliseconds more quickly than positive stimuli in the OFC. Similarly, some ERP components, such as the P200, appear to occur more rapidly to negative than positive stimuli (Carretie, Mercado, Tapia, & Hinojosa, 2001). Yet other studies have suggested a primacy for positive stimuli. In a study using faces with various expressions, Batty and Taylor (2003) found that the N170 component occurred more quickly to faces with pleasant emotional expressions than negative emotional expressions.

There are several potential explanations for these discrepancies. First, if positive and negative information are processed by different brain areas, these separable aspects of information may be processed at different rates for different processes. Thus for some processes negative information may be processed more quickly, and for others positive information may be processed more quickly (Cunningham, Espinet, et al., 2005). Second, we might expect motivational goals to affect the time courses of the processing of valence. In other words, it may not be that positive or negative information is processed more quickly per se, but rather that motivation and attention may determine whether positive or negative information is processed more quickly depending on situational and motivational factors. Third, valence may be confounded with some other variable, such as emotional intensity or motivational significance, and differences may reflect this other variable.

Flexible Tuning of Arousal and/or Valence Components?

Presumably, increased states of arousal direct attention toward motivationally salient stimuli in complex environments and prepare an organism for behavior. Because different stimuli may be deemed "important" at different times, a general arousal or vigilance system that is itself independent of valence might function most efficiently. This system presumably is involved in monitoring the environment, detecting potentially relevant changes, and redirecting attention, such that significant emotional stimuli can receive enhanced processing. Either after attention has been directed, or perhaps in parallel, whether a stimulus is positive or negative is computed. Consistent with the idea of a functional connection between arousal and attention, studies have demonstrated similar effects for both positive and negative stimuli in brain areas associated with attention, such as the anterior cingulate gyrus and visual sensory areas (Schupp, Junghofer, Weike, & Hamm, 2003).

Recent evidence suggests that chronic differences in tuning for valenced information (positivity vs. negativity bias), as well as situational variables, may direct attention and the perception of emotional intensity. We (Cunningham, Raye, & Johnson, 2005) presented participants with positively and negatively valenced stimuli during fMRI scanning. After scanning, participants completed an individual-differences measure of their prevention and promotion focus orientation (i.e., participants indicated whether they were more motivated by positive or negative stimuli; e.g., see Higgins, 1997). As participants were more promotion focused, greater activation was observed in the amygdala, anterior cingulate gyrus, and extrastriate cortex for positive stimuli. As participants were more prevention-focused, greater activation was observed in these same regions for negative stimuli. Thus the amygdala and attentional brain regions were tuned not toward a particular valence but rather toward stimuli that were motivationally important. Similarly, Canli, Sivers, Whitfield, Gotlib, and Gabrieli (2002) found that amygdala activation for happy faces was correlated with extraversion, and Mather et al. (2004) found that, whereas amygdala activation was greater for negative stimuli for young adults, it was greater for positive stimuli for older adults. Presumably, happy faces signal an important environmental cue for extraverts (more so than for introverts), and positive stimuli are more important for older adults than for younger adults, consistent with other evidence of an age shift in the relative salience of negative and positive stimuli (Charles, Mather, & Carstensen, 2003). Thus, although the motivational significance of stimuli may differ between people, similar structures are involved in processing these stimuli.

Implicit and Explicit Processes in Attitudes

Most current social cognitive theories of attitude propose that two sets of processes/systems underlie evaluation (see Chaiken & Trope, 1999). Although these models use different names for the processes and seek to explain different aspects of attitudes (e.g., structure, function, persuasion, etc.), they typically propose one system that operates relatively automatically and effortlessly and another that requires more cognitive attention or effort (Chaiken, 1980; Gilbert, Pelham, & Krull, 1988; Fazio, 1990; Greenwald & Banaji, 1995; Petty & Cacioppo, 1984). Often the second, more effortful, system is proposed to play a corrective role in attitudinal processing by updating or modifying an initial response or judgment deemed to be inappropriate or suboptimal given current motivational and situational constraints (Devine, 1989; Fazio, 1990; Petty & Wegener, 1993). Following this logic, dominant models of attitude have suggested that attitudes reflect dissociated memory representations (Greenwald & Banaji, 1995). That is, automatic processes activate implicit attitudes, and controlled processes activate explicit attitudes.

We suggest that thinking about attitudes as having both implicit and explicit components is useful as a heuristic, but attitudes very likely do not break down into a simple implicit–explicit dichotomy. At a coarse-grained level of analysis, some processes can be thought of as being relatively automatic, reflexive, and not initiated consciously. Others involve more conscious deliberation and usually require more time to initiate. But some "implicit" processes are more automatic than others, and some "explicit" processes require more deliberation than others. Thus we suggest that implicit–explicit or automatic–controlled are not dichotomous categories and that they likely do not operate in an all-or-none fashion. Different explicit (or implicit) evaluations may recruit different processes and brain systems. Moreover, we suggest that these implicit and explicit processes begin to interact or become integrated throughout the processing stream. For example, as time increases between the initiation of evaluative processing and the response we measure, additional component processes can be engaged that may provide a richer and more elaborate attitude. In fact, some researchers suggest that at least some attentional processing is necessary for emotional processing to initiate (Pessoa & Ungerleider, 2005). Thus, although we refer to the relative automaticity of processes for the purposes of description, we endorse neither a rigid dichotomy nor a single-factor continuum.

Early/Unaware Emotional Processing

Given the importance of arousal in directing attention, it is not surprising that these computations occur at a very early stage of information processing. In a study of face perception, Asley, Vuilleumier, and Swick (2004) found that ERP signals differed between emotional and nonemotional faces as early as 120 to 160 milliseconds after stimulus presentation (see also Pizzagalli et al., 2002; Eimer & Holmes, 2002). In fact, ERP differences to emotional stimuli compared with neutral stimuli have been observed as early as 94 milliseconds after stimulus presentation in occipital regions (Batty & Taylor, 2003). What is particularly interesting about this rapid emotional processing is that structural processing and identification of facial features is thought not to occur until 170 milliseconds after stimulus presentation (Sagiv & Bentin, 2001), suggesting that the processing of emotional expression, a signal that can denote safety or danger, may occur in parallel with facial structural encoding processes. In other words, emotional significance may be processed before a stimulus has been fully identified (e.g., see Niedenthal & Kitayama, 1994; Zajonc, 1980).

Moreover, not only are these early emotional processes relatively automatic, but they also may occur in the absence of conscious awareness. Several studies have now demonstrated psychological signs of emotional processing to stimuli that participants do not report even having seen. For example, skin conductance and ERP signals have been detected to the subliminal presentation of emotional faces as rapidly as 100 milliseconds after stimulus presentation (Öhman & Soares, 1996; Williams et al., 2004). Functional MRI studies have found amygdala activation to subliminal presentations of fearful faces (Whalen et al., 1998) and angry faces that have been previously associated with an aversive stimulus (Morris, Öhman, & Dolan, 1998).

More Complex Emotional Processing

Because the processing of *some* aspects of emotional intensity can occur relatively automatically does not mean that *all* of emotional processing is automatic, unconscious, or inevitable. As more time is available for evaluation, additional processing components can be brought to bear. Explicit evaluation may induce both more cognitively complex attitudes and more affectively complex attitudes. For example, simple emotions (e.g., fear, joy) can arise from relatively automatic processing of a stimulus, whereas more complex emotions (e.g., remorse, jealously, empathy) typically involve more reflective processing (e.g., Johnson & Multhaup, 1992). Cunningham, Raye, and Johnson (2004) found that some brain regions (e.g., an area of the OFC and the temporal pole) were associated with emotional intensity only when participants were making a reflective evaluation. Thus the emotional qualities accompanying an evaluative judgment made with or without reflection may be qualitatively distinct. For example, for some people, the term "affirmative action" may elicit relatively simple feelings of fear or anger arising from automatic processing and guilt, jealousy, hope, or other complex emotions arising with reflective processing.

Additional evidence for differences in the functional roles of emotional processes (e.g., gut responses vs. more cognitive aspects) in evaluation comes from work by Bechara and colleagues using the Iowa Gambling Task (see Bechara, 2004, for a review). In this task, participants select cards from different decks of cards with different reward contingencies. Some decks provide high immediate gains but are disadvantageous overall (providing, on average, fewer rewards), whereas others provide small rewards but are advantageous overall (on average providing higher rewards). Although patients with OFC damage showed normal skin conductance responses (SCRs) when receiving rewards and punishments, they did not show anticipatory SCR prior to their decisions. This dissociation suggests that some emotional processes are involved in the planning and simulation of emotional experience to make a decision and others are involved in the processing of current rewards and punishments.

Ambivalence and Control

Explicit evaluation involves monitoring, manipulating, inhibiting, controlling, or differentially weighting evaluative information to reach an evaluative judgment. When contrasting tasks that require evaluative and nonevaluative judgments, we find greater activation in medial areas of the prefrontal cortex (PFC) when participants make evaluative judgments and in lateral areas of the PFC when participants make nonevaluative judgments (Cunningham et al., 2003; Cunningham, Raye, & Johnson, 2004). More important, several of the prefrontal regions were associated with the processing of attitude complexity (having simultaneous positive and negative responses) or with control of an initial response. The functional role of more reflective/controlled evaluative processes may be to respond to and mitigate evaluative complexity by withholding responses until more information is available, by integrating multiple sources of information, and/or by deliberately retrieving additional memory representations.

Such processes are particularly important when stimuli are more complex; for example, when both positive and negative aspects are activated simultaneously (perhaps by different subsystems). This simultaneous state of feeling both positively and negatively, or ambivalence, has been shown behaviorally when people win or lose at a task but do not win or lose as much as they might have; for example, winning only $5 when it was possible to win $9 (Larsen, McGraw, Mellers, & Cacioppo, 2004). At the neural level, an area of right OFC (BA47) shows greater activation when participants make good–bad judgments about ambivalent compared with nonambivalent (e.g., neutral, clearly positive, or clearly negative) stimuli (Cunningham et al., 2003; Cunningham, Raye, & Johnson, 2004).

In such cases of attitude conflict, it is necessary to engage in control processes to reduce the cognitive or affective inconsistency that ambivalence brings (Festinger, 1954; Heider, 1946). As in monitoring memories (e.g., Johnson et al., 1993), the functional role of more reflective or controlled processes in evaluation may be to withhold responding until more information is available, to integrate multiple sources or dimensions of information, and/or to retrieve additional information. Through these additional control processes, evaluations can be brought into line with personal values, motivational goals, or situational constraints.

Brain regions that are involved in the regulation of affective states, including areas of the anterior PFC and anterior cingulate gyrus (Cunningham, Raye, & Johnson, 2004; Ochsner, Bunge, Gross, & Gabrieli, 2002), are similar to those involved in cognitive control more generally (Cohen, Botvinick, & Carter, 2000; MacDonald, Cohen, Stenger, & Carter, 2000; Johnson, Raye, Mitchell et al., 2005). Interestingly, several of these regions are involved in control, whether one is down-regulating (dampening) or up-regulating (enhancing) emotional experience (Ochsner et al., 2004). Furthermore, the degree of prefrontal EEG asymmetry is correlated with a decreased startle response to evocative stimuli, suggesting a direct role of the lateral PFC in the control of emotional states (Jackson et al., 2003).

As in processes associated with arousal or valence, the processes associated with ambivalence and control are likely to occur with different temporal dynamics or at different points in the processing stream, with at least two sets of processes involved in the processing of attitudinal ambivalence. With respect to cognitive conflict and control, Botvinick, Braver, Barch, Carter, and Cohen (2001) propose that there are separable conflict-detection and regulatory systems. Whereas the conflict-detection system is proposed to operate relatively automatically, the regulation system requires or is associated with more controlled processing. Providing support for this proposed distinction in the domain of evaluation, Cunningham, Raye, and Johnson (2004) presented participants with concepts and asked participants to either make an evaluative judgment about the concept (is it good or bad?) or a nonevaluative judgment about the concept (is it abstract or concrete?). Following scanning, participants rated each of the concepts presented during the fMRI part of the study for valence (how good or bad was it?), emotional intensity, and the degree to which they tried to control their initial response to the concept. In this study, we found that some brain areas, such as ventrolateral PFC, correlated with self-reported ratings of control to particular stimuli, even when making nonevaluative judgments. Although this may suggest that these processes are automatic, when participants made explicitly evaluative good–bad judgments, these regions were significantly more active. In addition, other brain regions were active only when participants had an agenda to evaluate, such as areas in anterior PFC. This suggests that ambivalence, and the control induced by ambivalence, may be hierarchically organized such that different degrees of reflection are necessary for different processes of control. Consistent with this idea, Amodio and colleagues (2004) found ERP signals associated with control that occurred less than 200 milliseconds after the presentation of black and white faces. Yet, despite signals that control was engaged, participants on average still showed evidence of prejudice in that they were more likely to misperceive a tool as a gun when it was preceded by a black than by a white face, suggesting that more time or additional processes are necessary for more complete control.

APPLICATIONS FOR PREJUDICE RESEARCH

An early focus for the social neuroscience study of attitudes has been the important domain of prejudice. Initial studies demonstrated a role for the amygdala in the processing of other-race faces. Hart et al. (2000) demonstrated that, for white participants, amygdala activation to supraliminal black faces habituated more slowly than to white faces, and that the reverse pattern was found for black participants. They concluded that all faces are processed immediately for their threat value, but that in-group faces are deemed safe more quickly than out-group faces. The role of the amygdala in intergroup perception was further demonstrated by Phelps et al. (2000), who showed that greater amygdala activation to Black than to White faces was correlated with an indirect measure of race bias that reflects the extent to which black is associated with bad and white with good, the race Implicit Association Test (IAT). Interestingly, neither of these studies showed overall greater amygdala activation to black faces relative to white faces for white participants.

One potential explanation for not finding the expected greater amygdala activation to black than to white faces is that control processes may inhibit or reconstrue an activated emotional response. That is, rather than automatic attitude being separate from controlled aspects of attitude, the two systems may be more dynamically linked. Thus, for participants viewing long blocks of black or white faces (as in Hart et al., 2000, and Phelps et al., 2000), control processes may dampen any automatic effects that would otherwise be observed. Consistent with this hypothesis, Cunningham, Johnson, et al. (2004) found that 12 out of 13 white participants showed greater activation to black than to white faces (which were randomly intermixed), but only when the faces were presented briefly and masked such that participants did not report seeing the faces. As one might expect given our control hypothesis, for faces that could be clearly seen, the decreased activation to black relative to white faces was accompanied by activation in areas of the PFC and the anterior cingulate gyrus—areas that are associated with cognitive control.

Interestingly, it appears that mental activities that counteract prejudiced thoughts may diminish control in other situations. According to Baumeister, Bratslavsky, Muraven, and Tice (1998), regulation is a limited resource, and any act of control uses up resources not only at the time of control but also for some time afterward while the system recuperates. Richeson and Shelton (2003) found that after nonprejudiced white participants interacted with a black individual, they subsequently performed worse at the Stroop task, a task that requires cognitive control for incompatible trials (e.g., reporting that the word *green* is in a red print color). In a followup fMRI study, Richeson, Baird, et al. (2003) used fMRI to scan white participants while they viewed black and white faces. Afterward, participants performed the Stroop task. As in Cunningham, Johnson, et al. (2004), greater activation was observed in the right lateral PFC while participants viewed black compared with white faces. Furthermore, the degree of right PFC activity while viewing black faces during the fMRI task predicted subsequent Stroop performance, with those with the most right PFC activity performing the worst later. Presumably, the cognitive cost of control was manifested in the subsequent cognitive task.

We note that the amygdala should not be considered *the* source of prejudice but rather one component that may contribute to biased responses in the context of a larger attitude system. For example, Phelps, Cannistraci, and Cunningham (2003) reported on a patient who, despite bilateral amygdala damage, still showed evidence of automatic race biases on an indirect measure of automatic associations, suggesting that automatic evaluative responses are possible without an amygdala. This should not necessarily be surprising, as amygdala activation seems now to be better characterized as processing emotionally significant stimuli rather than simply negative, fearful, or threatening stimuli (Canli, Silvers, Whitfield, Gotlib, & Gabrieli, 2004; Cunningham, Johnson, et al., 2004; Mather et al., 2004). In the processing of social groups and people or objects in general, other areas are associated with processing emotional intensity and valence; notably, right PFC and OFC. Additional patient work examining which aspects of evaluative processing are impaired with particular forms of damage would be informative.

CONCLUSIONS

Evaluations arise from multiple component cognitive and affective processes that work in concert to make judgments about the world. Any given process does not typically work alone in an all-or-none fashion, but rather various combinations of processes generate qualitatively different evaluative outcomes. Different situational and motivational constraints, including whether or not an explicit evaluation is required, activate different component processes, resulting in different overall evaluations of a stimulus. Thus the same stimulus can produce quite different subjective evaluative experiences (e.g., a positive attitude in one circumstance and a negative in one another). Attitudes can be thought of as the constructed output of combinations of currently active component processes.

Already, neuroimaging results suggest that different patterns of brain activity are associated with emotional intensity, positivity, negativity, ambivalence, and control and that activity in different areas may have different temporal signatures. Furthermore, compared with implicit expression of attitudes, having a goal to explicitly evaluate a stimulus that activates additional brain areas associated with the processing of each of these aspects. Our evolving component-process framework assumes that implicit and explicit evaluation are not wholly independent; common processes may be involved in the formation of both quick-and-crude automatic judgments and more systematically derived reflective judgments. Future research is needed to understand how these basic processes work in more dynamic and integrated ways to construct attitudinal states.

A challenge for future research is to understand how disparate elements or processes become unified to give rise to phenomenal experience and behavior. It is likely that prefrontal regions, such as areas in medial PFC that receive inputs from throughout the brain, function as polymodal integration centers. To the extent that different processes unfold at different rates, this means that evaluations may vary from second to second (or millisecond to millisecond) as new information is processed. For example, if a judgment is required early in the processing stream, an evaluation can be based only on relatively automatic processing of simple emotional responses (initial arousal and/or valence). More reflective processing of these aspects typically requires time to initiate, as does regulation and control. Interestingly, with practice, regulation and control can be accomplished via more automatic processes (e.g., Moskowitz, Gollwitzer, Wasel, & Schaal, 1999). Attitudes, in this framework, reflect the current processing of an integrated information processing system at any given time. At some point, a judgment may be required, and this state is the person's attitude at that given moment. The particular ways in which information is constrained, weighed, and integrated as attitudes are constructed online is a challenging problem. Also of particular interest are the conditions under which the result is not a unified evaluation—the conditions under which ambivalence persists.

Although understanding attitudes presents a considerable challenge for analysis, there is a rich history of relevant theoretical ideas and findings from social and cognitive psychology and intriguing new findings from social cognitive neuroscience. Variability in an individual's attitudes toward the nominally same stimulus may mean that there is more than one "true" attitude—that different attitudes reflect particular combinations of elements at different times to satisfy different constraints. As social neuroscience investigations of attitude and evaluation continue, it is likely that a clearer picture of this dynamic system will emerge, yielding better understanding of how important aspects of attitudes arise from the intersection of emotional and cognitive processes. Attitudes are evaluative outcomes, reflecting the way that aspects of experience that are typically labeled as emotional (valence, intensity, ambivalence) arise from processes that are typically labeled as cognitive (perceptual and reflective). In other words, just as emotion and cognition (e.g., Johnson & Multhaup, 1992) and motivation and cognition (e.g., Johnson & Sherman, 1990), are interactively linked, attitudes are not something apart from the cognitive, affective, and behavioral processes that contribute to them and that they in turn contribute to. In this dynamic, integrated system, attitudes and emotions in turn influence cognitive processes (including in ways that we sometimes label as motivational).

ACKNOWLEDGMENTS

Preparation of this chapter and some of the research described was supported by a grant from the National Institutes of Health (No. MH 62196). We thank Carol Raye, Philip Zelazo, Kris Preacher, Norman Farb, and Jay Van Bavel for helpful comments on an early version of this chapter.

REFERENCES

Adolphs, R., Russell, J. A, & Tranel, D. (1999). A role for the human amygdala in recognizing emotional arousal from unpleasant stimuli. *Psychological Science, 10,* 167–171.

Allport, G. W. (1935). Attitudes. In C. Murchison (Ed.), *Handbook of social psychology* (pp. 798–844). Worcester, MA: Clark University Press.

Amodio, D. M., Harmon-Jones, E., Devine, P. G., Curtin, J. J., Hartley, S. L., & Covert, A. E. (2004). Neural signals for the detection of unintentional race bias. *Psychological Science, 15,* 88–93.

Anderson, A. K., Christoff, K., Stappen I., Panitz, D., Ghahremani, D. G., Glover, G., et al. (2003). Dissociated neural representations of intensity and valence in human olfaction. *Nature Neuroscience, 6,* 196–202.

Asley, V., Vuilleumier, P., & Swick, D. (2004). Time course and specificity of event-related potentials to emotional expressions. *NeuroReport, 15,* 211–216.

Batty, M., & Taylor, M. J. (2003). Early processing of the six basic facial emotional expressions. *Cognitive Brain Research, 17,* 613–620.

Baumeister, R. F., Bratslavsky, E., Muraven, M., & Tice, D. M. (1998). Ego depletion: Is the active self a limited resource? *Journal of Personality and Social Psychology, 74,* 1252–1265.

Bechara, A. (2004). The role of emotion in decision making: Evidence from neurological patients with orbitofrontal damage. *Brain and Cognition, 55,* 30–40.

Bem, D. J. (1970). Beliefs, attitudes, and human affairs. Belmont, CA: Brooks/Cole.

Bem, D. J. (1972). Self-perception theory. In L. Berkowitz (Ed.), *Advances in experimental social psychology* (Vol. 6, pp. 1–62). New York: Academic Press.

Botvinick, M. M., Braver, T. S., Barch, D. M., Carter, C. S., & Cohen, J. D. (2001). Conflict monitoring and cognitive control. *Psychological Review, 108,* 624–652.

Cacioppo, J. T., & Bernston, G. (1994). Relationship between attitudes and evaluative space: A critical review, with emphasis on the separability of positive and negative substrates. *Psychological Bulletin, 115,* 401–423.

Cacioppo, J. T., & Gardner, W. L. (1999). Emotion. *Annual Review of Psychology, 50,* 191–214.

Cacioppo, J. T., Petty, R. E., Losch, M. E., & Kim, H. S. (1986). Electromyographic activity over facial muscle regions can differentiate the valence and intensity of affective reactions. *Journal of Personality and Social Psychology, 50,* 260–268.

Canli, T., Sivers, H., Whitfield, S. L., Gotlib, I. H., & Gabrieli, J. D. (2002). Amygdala response to happy faces as a function of extraversion. *Science, 296,* 2191.

Cannon, W. (1929). *Bodily changes in pain, hunger, fear and rage.* New York: Appleton.

Carretie, L., Martin-Loeches, M., Hinojosa, J. A., & Mercado, F. (2001). Emotion and attention studies through event-related potentials. *Journal of Cognitive Neuroscience, 13,* 1109–1128.

Carretie, L., Mercado, F., Tapia, M., & Hinojosa, J. A. (2001). Emotion, attention, and the "negativity bias," studied through event-related potentials. *International Journal of Psychophysiology, 41,* 7–85.

Chaiken, S. (1980). Heuristic versus systematic information processing and the use of source versus message cues in persuasion. *Journal of Personality and Social Psychology, 39*, 752–766.

Chaiken, S., & Trope, Y. (Eds.). (1999). *Dual-process theories in social psychology*. New York: Guilford Press.

Charles, S. T., Mather, M., & Carstensen, L. L. (2003). Aging and emotional memory: The forgettable nature of negative images for older adults. *Journal of Experimental Psychology: General, 132*, 310–324.

Cohen, J. D., Botvinick, M., & Carter, C. S. (2000). Anterior cingulate and prefrontal cortex: Who's in control? *Nature Neuroscience, 3*, 421–423.

Cunningham, W. A., Espinet, S. D., DeYoung, C. G., & Zelazo, P. D. (2005). Attitudes to the right—and left: Frontal ERP asymmetries associated with stimulus valence and processing goal. *NeuroImage, 28*, 827–834.

Cunningham, W. A, Johnson, M. K., Gatenby, J. C., Gore, J. C., & Banaji, M. R. (2003). Component processes of social evaluation. *Journal of Personality and Social Psychology, 85*, 639–649.

Cunningham, W. A., Johnson, M. K., Raye, C. L., Gatenby, J. C., Gore, J. C., & Banaji, M. R. (2004). Separable neural components in the processing of black and white faces. *Psychological Science, 15*, 806–813.

Cunningham, W. A., Raye, C. L., & Johnson, M. K. (2004). Implicit and explicit evaluation: fMRI correlates of valence, emotional intensity, and control in the processing of attitudes. *Journal of Cognitive Neuroscience, 16*, 1717–1729.

Cunningham, W. A., Raye, C. L., & Johnson, M. K. (2005). Neural correlates of evaluation associated with promotion and prevention regulatory focus. *Cognitive, Affective, and Behavioral Neuroscience, 5*, 202–211

Damasio, A. R. (1994). *Descartes' error: Emotion, reason, and the human brain*. New York: Putnam.

Davidson, R. J., Ekman, P., Saron, C. D., Senulis, J. A., & Friesen, W. V. (1990). Approach–withdrawal and cerebral asymmetry: emotional expression and brain physiology: I. *Journal of Personality and Social Psychology, 58*, 330–341.

Davidson, R. J., & Irwin, W. (1999). The functional neuroanatomy of emotion and affective style. *Trends in Cognitive Science, 3*, 11–21.

Delgado, M. R., Nystrom, L. E., Fissel, C., Noll, D. C., & Fiez, J. A. (2000). Tracking the hemodynamic responses to reward and punishment in the striatum. *Journal of Neurophysiology, 84*, 3072–3077.

Devine, P. G. (1989). Stereotypes and prejudice: Their automatic and controlled components. *Journal of Personality and Social Psychology, 56*, 5–18.

Dickson, H. W., & McGinnies, E. (1966). Affectivity in the arousal of attitudes as measured by galvanic skin response. *American Journal of Psychology, 79*, 584–587.

Dysinger, D. W. (1931). A comparative study of affective responses by means of the impressive and expressive methods. *Psychological Monographs, 41*, 14–31.

Eagly, A. H., & Chaiken, S. (1993). *The psychology of attitudes*. Forth Worth, TX: Harcourt Brace Jovanovich.

Eimer, M., & Holmes, A. (2002). An ERP study on the time course of emotional face processing. *Neuroreport, 13*, 427–431.

Fazio, R. H. (1990). Multiple processes by which attitudes guide behavior: The MODE model as an integrative framework. In M. P. Zanna (Ed.), *Advances in experimental social psychology* (Vol. 23, pp. 75–109). New York: Academic Press.

Festinger, L. (1954). A theory of social comparison processes. *Human Relations, 7,* 117–140.

Gilbert, D. T., Pelham, B. W., & Krull, D. S. (1988). On cognitive busyness: When person perceivers meet persons perceived. *Journal of Personality and Social Psychology, 54,* 733–740.

Greenwald, A. G., & Banaji, M. R. (1995). Implicit social cognition: Attitudes, self-esteem, and stereotypes. *Psychological Review, 102,* 4–27.

Harmon-Jones, E., & Allen, J. J. B. (1998). Anger and frontal brain activity: EEG asymmetry consistent with approach motivation despite negative affective valence. *Journal of Personality and Social Psychology, 74,* 1310–1316.

Hart, A. J., Whalen, P. J., Shin, L. M., McInerney, S. C., Fischer, H., & Rauch, S. L. (2000). Differential response in the human amygdala to racial outgroup vs. ingroup face stimuli. *NeuroReport, 11,* 2351–2355.

Heider, F. (1946). Attitudes and cognitive organization. *Journal of Psychology, 21,* 107–112.

Higgins, E. T. (1997). Beyond pleasure and pain. *American Psychologist, 52,* 1280–1300.

Ito, T. A., Larsen, J. T., Smith, N. K., & Cacioppo, J. T. (1998). Negative information weighs more heavily on the brain: The negativity bias in evaluative categorizations. *Journal of Personality and Social Psychology, 75,* 887–900.

Jackson, D. C., Mueller, C. J., Dolski, I., Dalton, K. M., Nitschke, J. B., Urry, H. L., et al. (2003). Now you feel it, now you don't: Frontal brain electrical asymmetry and individual differences in emotion regulation. *Psychological Science, 14,* 612–617.

Jacoby, L. L., Kelley, C. M., & Dywan, J. (1989). Memory attributions. In H. L. Roediger & F. I. M. Craik (Eds.), *Varieties of memory and consciousness: Essays in honor of Endel Tulving* (pp. 391–422). Hillsdale, NJ: Erlbaum.

James, W. (1884). What is an emotion? *Mind, 9,* 188–205.

Johnson, M. K., Hashtroudi, S., & Lindsay, D. S. (1993). Source monitoring. *Psychological Bulletin, 114,* 3–28.

Johnson, M. K., & Multhaup, K. S. (1992). Emotion and MEM. In S. Christianson (Ed.), *Handbook of emotion and memory: Research and theory* (pp. 33–66). Hillsdale, NJ: Erlbaum.

Johnson, M. K., & Raye, C. L. (1981). Reality monitoring. *Psychological Review, 88,* 67–85.

Johnson, M. K., Raye, C. L., Mitchell, K. J., Greene, E. J., Cunningham, W. A., & Sanislow, C. A. (2005). Using fMRI to investigate a component process of reflection: Prefrontal correlates of refreshing a just activated representation. *Cognitive, Affective, and Behavioral Neuroscience, 5,* 339–361.

Johnson, M. K., & Sherman, S. J. (1990). Constructing and reconstructing the past and the future in the present. In E. T. Higgins & R. M. Sorrentino (Eds.), *Handbook of motivation and cognition: Vol. 2. Foundations of social behavior* (pp. 482–526). New York: Guilford Press.

Jones, N. A., & Fox, N. A. (1992). Electroencephalogram asymmetry during emotionally evocative films and its relation to positive and negative affectivity. *Brain and Cognition, 20,* 280–299.

Kawasaki, H., Kaufman, O., Damasio, H., Damasio, A. R., Granner, M., Bakken, H., et al. (2001). Single-neuron responses to emotional visual stimuli recorded in human ventral prefrontal cortex. *Nature Neuroscience, 4,*15–16.

Knutson, B., & Cooper, J. C. (2005). Functional magnetic resonance imaging of reward prediction. *Current Opinion in Neurology, 18,* 411–417.

Kringelbach, M. L., O'Doherty, J. O., Rolls, E. T., & Andrew, C. (2003). Activation of the human orbitofrontal cortex to a liquid food stimulus is correlated with its subjective pleasantness. *Cerebral Cortex, 13,* 1064–1071.

Larsen, J. T., McGraw, A. P., Mellers, B. A., & Cacioppo, J. T. (2004). The agony of victory and the thrill of defeat: Mixed emotional reactions to disappointing wins and relieving losses. *Psychological Science, 15,* 325–330.

MacDonald, A. W., Cohen, J. D., Stenger, V. A., & Carter, C. S. (2000). Dissociating the role of dorsolateral prefrontal cortex and anterior cingulate cortex in cognitive control. *Science, 288,* 1835–1837.

Mather, M., Canli, T., English, T., Whitfield, S., Wais, P., Ochsner, K., et al. (2004). Amygdala responses to emotionally valenced stimuli in older and younger adults. *Psychological Science, 15,* 259–263.

Morris, J. S., Öhman, A., & Dolan, R. J. (1998). Conscious and unconscious emotional learning in the human amygdala. *Nature, 393,* 467–470.

Moskowitz, G. B., Gollwitzer, P. M., Wasel, W., & Schaal, B. (1999). Preconscious control of stereotype activation through chronic egalitarian goals. *Journal of Personality and Social Psychology, 77,* 176–184.

Niedenthal, P. M., & Kitayama, S. (1994). *The hearts' eye: Emotional influences in perception and attention.* San Diego: Academic Press.

Nitschke, J. B., Nelson, E. E., Rusch, B. D., Fox, A. S., Oakes, T. R., & Davidson, R. J. (2003). Orbitofrontal cortex tracks positive mood in mothers viewing pictures of their newborn infants. *NeuroImage, 21,* 583–592.

Ochsner, K. N., Bunge, S. A., Gross, J. J., & Gabrieli, J. D. E. (2002). Rethinking feelings: An fMRI study of the cognitive regulation of emotion. *Journal of Cognitive Neuroscience, 14,* 1215–1229.

Ochsner, K. N., Ray, R., Cooper, J., Robertson, E., Chopra, S., Gabrieli, J. D. E., et al. (2004). For better or for worse: Neural systems supporting the cognitive up- and down-regulation of negative emotion. *NeuroImage, 23,* 483–499.

Öhman, A., & Soares, J. J. F. (1996). Emotional conditioning to masked stimuli: Expectancies for aversive outcomes following nonrecognized fear-relevant stimuli. *Journal of Experimental Psychology: General, 127,* 69–82.

Pessoa, L., & Ungerleider, L.G. (2005). Visual attention and emotional perception. In L. Itti, G. Rees, & J. K. Tsotsos (Eds.), *Neurobiology of attention* (pp. 160–166). San Diego, CA: Elsevier.

Petty, R. E., & Cacioppo, J. T. (1984). The effects of involvement on responses to argument quantity and quality: Central and peripheral routes to persuasion. *Journal of Personality and Social Psychology, 46,* 69–81.

Petty, R. E., & Wegener, D. T. (1993). Flexible correction processes in social judgment: Correcting for context-induced contrast. *Journal of Experimental Social Psychology, 29,* 137–165.

Phelps, E. A., Cannistraci, C. J., & Cunningham, W. A. (2003). Intact performance on an indirect measure of face bias following amygdala damage. *Neuropsychologia, 41,* 203–208.

Phelps, E. A., O'Connor, K. J., Cunningham, W. A., Funayama, E. S., Gatenby, J. C., Gore, J. C., et al. (2000). Performance on indirect measures of race evaluation predicts amygdala activation. *Journal of Cognitive Neuroscience, 12,* 729–738.

Pizzagalli, D. A., Lehmann, D., Hendrick, A. M., Regard, M., Pascual-Marqui, R. D., & Davidson, R. J. (2002). Affective judgments of faces modulate early activity (~160 ms) within the fusiform gyri, *NeuroImage, 16*, 663–677.

Richeson, J. A., Baird, A. A., Gordon, H. L., Heatherton, T. F., Wyland, C. L., Trawalter, S., et al. (2003). An fMRI investigation of the impact of interracial contact on executive function. *Nature Neuroscience, 6*, 1323–1328.

Richeson, J. A., & Shelton, J. N. (2003). When prejudice does not pay: Effects of interracial contact on executive function. *Psychological Science, 14*, 287–290.

Russell, J. A. (1979). Affective space is bipolar. *Journal of Personality and Social Psychology, 37*, 345–356.

Sagiv, N., & Bentin, S. (2001). Structural encoding of human and schematic faces: Holistic and part-based processes. *Journal of Cognitive Neuroscience, 13*, 937–951.

Schachter, S., & Singer, J. (1962). Cognitive, social and physiological determinants of emotional state. *Psychological Review, 69*, 379–399.

Schupp, H. T., Junghofer, M., Weike, A. I., & Hamm, A. O. (2003). Attention and emotion: An ERP analysis of facilitated emotional stimulus processing. *Neuroreport, 14*, 1107–1110.

Schwarz, N., & Bohner, G. (2001). The construction of attitudes. In A. Tesser & N. Schwarz (Eds.), *Blackwell handbook of social psychology: Intraindividual processes* (Vol. 1, pp. 413–435). Oxford, UK: Blackwell.

Small, D. M., Gregory, M. D., Mak, Y. E., Gitelman, D., Mesulam, M. M., & Parrish, T. (2003). Dissociation of neural representation of intensity and affective valuation in human gustation. *Neuron, 39*, 701–711.

Smith, N. K., Cacioppo, J. T., Larsen, J. T., & Chartrand, T. L. (2003). May I have your attention please: Electrocortical responses to positive and negative stimuli. *Neuropsychologia, 41*, 171–183.

Smith, W. (1922). *The measurement of emotion*. London: Paul.

Sutton, S. K., Davidson, R. J., Donzella, B., Irwin, W., & Dottl, D. A. (1997). Manipulating affective state using extended picture presentations. *Psychophysiology, 34*, 217–226.

Thurstone, L. L. (1931). Measurement of social attitudes. *Journal of Abnormal and Social Psychology, 26*, 249–269.

Wager, T. D., Phan, K. L., Liberzon, I., & Taylor, S. F. (2003). Valence, gender, and lateralization of functional brain anatomy in emotion: A meta-analysis of findings from neuroimaging. *NeuroImage, 19*, 513–531.

Whalen, P. J., Rauch, S. L., Etcoff, N. L., McInerney, S. C., Lee, M. B., & Jenike, M. A. (1998). Masked presentations of emotional facial expressions modulate amygdala activity without explicit knowledge. *Journal of Neuroscience, 18*, 411–418.

Williams, L. M., Liddell, B. J., Rathjen, J., Brown, K. J., Gray, J., Phillips, M., et al. (2004). Mapping the time course of nonconscious and conscious perception of fear: An integration of central and peripheral measures. *Human Brain Mapping, 21*, 64–74.

Wilson, T. D., & Hodges, S. (1992). Attitudes as temporary constructions. In L. Martin & A. Tesser (Eds.), *The construction of social judgments* (pp. 37–66). Hillsdale, NJ: Erlbaum.

Zajonc, R. B. (1980). Feeling and thinking: Preferences need no inferences. *American Psychologist, 35*, 151–175.

12

A Social Cognitive Neuroscience Model of Human Empathy

Jean Decety

The construct of empathy denotes, at a phenomenological level of description, a sense of similarity between the feelings one person experiences and those expressed by others. It can be conceived of as an interaction between any two individuals, with one experiencing and sharing the feeling of the other. This sharing of feelings does not necessarily imply that one will act or even feel impelled to act in a supportive or sympathetic way (empathy's paradox is that this ability may be used for both helpful and hurtful purposes). Moreover, the social and emotional situations that elicit empathy can become quite complex depending on the feelings experienced by the observed and the relationship of the target to the observer (Feshbach, 1997). This capacity to understand others and experience their feelings in relation to oneself illustrates the social nature of the self, its inherent intersubjectivity. Humans are indeed an intrinsically social and gregarious species. And virtually all of their actions (including their thoughts, desires, and feelings) are directed toward or are produced in response to others (Batson, 1990).

The goal of this chapter is to provide a model of empathy that articulates data from social psychology and neuroscience (including neuropsychology). The former discipline has an extensive history of research in the domain of empathy, whereas the latter has only recently begun to investigate its neural bases. Bridging social psychology and cognitive neuroscience provides important guidelines for investigating the neural processes underlying empathy. On the other hand, cognitive neuroscience may help disambiguate competing social theories. To that end, instead of addressing each of these research domains separately, I marshal theoretical notions and findings from these different approaches with the guidance of an overarching conceptual framework. This framework considers that empathy involves parallel and distributed processing in a number of dissociable computational mechanisms. Shared neural representations, self-awareness, mental flexibility, and emotion regulation constitute the basic macro-components of empathy, which are mediated by specific neural systems. Consequently, damage to each of these components may lead to an alteration of empathic behavior and produce selective social disorders, depending on which aspect is disrupted.

It seems evident from the descriptions of comparative psychologists and ethologists that some behaviors homologous to empathy can be observed in other species (e.g., Plutchik, 1987). For de Waal (1996) empathy is not an all-or-nothing phenomenon, and many forms of empathy exist between the extremes of mere agitation at the distress of another and full understanding of their predicament. Many other comparative psychologists, however, view empathy as a kind of induction process by which emotions, both positive and negative, are shared and by which the probabilities of similar behavior are increased in the participants. In the view developed in this chapter, this is not a sufficient mechanism to account for the full-blown ability of human empathy. This does not mean that some aspects of empathy are not present in other species, such as motor mimicry and emotion contagion (see de Waal & Thompson, 2005). Emotions and feelings may indeed be shared between individuals, but humans are also able to intentionally "feel for" and act on behalf of other people whose experiences may differ greatly from their own (Batson, 1991; Decety & Hodges, 2006; Davis, 1994). Empathic concern is often associated with prosocial behaviors such as helping kin and has been considered as a chief enabling process for altruism (Batson, 1991). Wilson (1998) suggested that empathic helping behavior has evolved because of its contribution to genetic fitness (kin selection). In humans and other mammals, an impulse to care for offspring is almost certainly genetically hardwired. It is far less clear that an impulse to care for siblings, more remote kin, and similar nonkin is genetically hardwired (Batson, 2006). The emergence of altruism, of empathizing with and caring for those who are not kin, is thus not easily explained within the framework of neo-Darwinian theories of natural selection. Social learning explanations of kinship patterns in human helping behavior are thus highly plausible. However, one of the most striking aspects of human empathy is that it can be felt for virtually any target—even targets of a different species. In addition, as emphasized by Harris (2000), humans, unlike other primates, can put their emotions into words, allowing them not only to express emotion but also to report on current, as well as past, emotions. These reports provide an opportunity to share, explain, and regulate emotional experience with others that is not found in other species. Conversation helps to develop empathy, for it is often here that one learns of shared experiences and feelings. Moreover, this self-reflexive capability (which includes emotion regulation) may be an important difference between humans and other animals (Povinelli, 2001).

Overall, this evolutionary conceptual view is compatible with the hypothesis that advanced levels of social cognition may have arisen as an emergent property of powerful executive functioning assisted by the representational properties of language (Barrett, Henzi, & Dunbar, 2003). However, these higher levels operate on previous levels of organization and should not be seen as independent of or conflicting with one another. Evolution has constructed layers of increasing complexity, from nonrepresentational to representational and metarepresentational mechanisms, which need to be taken into account for a full understanding of human empathy.

BREAKING DOWN EMPATHY
INTO ITS CONSTITUTIVE COMPONENTS

For many psychologists, empathy implies at least three different processes: feeling what another person is feeling; knowing what another person is feeling; and having the intention to respond compassionately to another person's distress (Thompson, 2001). Yet, regardless of the particular terminology that is used, there is broad agreement among scholars on three primary aspects: (1) an affective response to another person, which often, but not always, entails sharing that person's emotional state; (2) a cognitive capacity to take the perspective of the other person; and (3) some self-regulatory and monitoring mechanisms that modulate inner states (e.g., Batson, 1991; Davis, 1996; Decety & Hodges, 2006; Eisenberg, 2000; Hodges & Wegner, 1997; Preston & de Waal, 2002). According to Ickes (1997), empathy is a complex form of psychological inference in which observation, memory, knowledge, and reasoning are combined to yield insights into the thoughts and feelings of others. As such, empathy involves not only the affective experience of the other person's actual or inferred emotional state but also some minimal recognition and understanding of another's emotional state (or most likely emotional state). This definition captures the multidimensional nature of empathy and makes explicit reference to some minimal mentalizing capacity. This latter concept refers to the broad social cognitive ability used by humans to explain and predict their own behavior and that of others by attributing to them independent mental states, such as belief, desires, emotions, or intentions (Flavell, 1999).

Of all the sources from which one can draw insight as to the constituents of human empathy, psychotherapeutic schools provide the most interesting experience-related knowledge. Indeed, empathy plays a central role in psychotherapies, as almost all of them involve intersubjective communication between individuals in order for the clinician to understand his or her client sufficiently to proceed along a treatment path (Bohart & Greenberg, 1997). Although it is not a major construct in psychoanalysis, Freud (1921/1955) wrote that empathy was indispensable when it came to taking a position regarding another person's mental life and considered it as the process that plays the largest part in our understanding of what is inherently foreign to our ego in other people. A number of analysts have pointed out that empathy involves resonating with the other's unconscious affect and experiencing his or her experience with him or her while the empathizer maintains the integrity of his or her own person intact. For instance, Basch (1983) speculated that, because their respective autonomic nervous systems are genetically programmed to respond in like fashion, a given affective expression by a member of a particular species tends to recruit a similar response in other members of that species.

> This is done through the promotion of an unconscious autonomic imitation of the sender's bodily state and facial expression by the receiver. It generates in the receiver the autonomic response associated with that bodily state and facial expression, which is to say, the receiver experiences an affect identical with that of the sender. (p. 108)

Such a view subsequently received direct empirical validation by a series of studies conducted by Levenson and Ruef (1992). They found evidence that a perceiver's accuracy in inferring a target's negative emotional states was related to the degree of physiological synchrony between the perceiver and the target. In other words, when two people feel similar emotions, they more accurately perceive each other's intentions and motivations.

The model proposed here suggests that four major functional components dynamically interact to produce the experience of empathy:

1. Affective sharing between the self and the other, based on the automatic perception–action coupling and resulting shared representations.
2. Self-awareness. Even when there is some temporary identification between the observer and its target, there is no confusion between self and other.
3. Mental flexibility to adopt the subjective perspective of the other.
4. Regulatory processes, including emotion regulation.

In this view, none of these components can account solely for the potential of human empathy. The four components are intertwined and interact with one another to produce the subjective experience of human empathy. For instance, sharing emotion without self-awareness corresponds to the phenomenon of emotional contagion, which takes the form of "total identification without discrimination between one's feelings and those of the other" (de Waal, 1996). This model of empathy combines both representational aspects—that is, memories that are localized in distributed neural networks that encode information and that, when temporarily activated, enable access to this stored information—and processes, that is, computational procedures that are localized and are independent of the nature or modality of the stimulus that is being processed (see Figure 12.1).

Like many emotion-related processes, some components involved in empathy occur implicitly, without awareness, in a bottom-up fashion. This is the case with the emotion-sharing and motor-mimicry aspect. Other components require explicit top-down processing, such as perspective taking, representing our own thoughts and feelings as well as those of others, and also some aspects of emotion regulation.

AFFECTIVE SHARING BETWEEN SELF AND OTHER

Emotional expression and perception are an integral part of social interaction (Schulkin, 2004). Bodily expressions constitute an external, perceivable indication of people's intentions and emotions. At one level, emotional expressions are governed by rules and can be elicited by simple stimuli, as in the example of disgust in the presence of bitter taste. However, humans and other animals also use bodily expressions to communicate various type of information to members of their own species. Understanding other people's emotional signals has clear adaptive advantages and is especially important in the formation and maintenance of social relationships.

Social psychological research shows that humans mimic unintentionally and unconsciously a wide range of behaviors, such as accents, tone of voice, rate of speech, and posture and mannerisms, as well as moods (e.g., Chartrand & Bargh, 1999). This tendency to automatically mimic and synchronize one's own emotional behavior with that of others, also known as the phenomenon of emotion contagion, facilitate the smoothness of social interaction and may even foster empathy (Hatfield, Cacioppo, & Rapson, 1994). For instance, a study demonstrated that participants who had been mimicked by the experimenter were more helpful and generous toward other people than nonmimicked participants (Van Baaren, Holland, Kawakami, & Van Knippenberg, 2004). They also found that these beneficial consequences of mimicry were not restricted to behavior directed toward the mimicker but included behavior directed toward people not directly involved in the mimicry situation. Interestingly, individuals with autism who are profoundly impaired in social and emotional abilities do not show spontaneous mimicry, but they can perform voluntary mimicry well (McIntosh, Reichmann-Decker, Winkielman & Wilbarger, 2006). Such a core deficit in involuntary motor resonance may be the seed for their profound impairment in basic emotional connectedness.

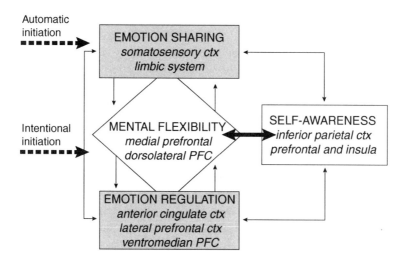

FIGURE 12.1. Schematic overview of the major processes involved in empathy. This model contends that empathy depends on bottom-up and top-down processes. It combines both representational aspects (i.e., memories that are localized in distributed neural networks that encode information and, when temporarily activated, enable access to this stored information, e.g., shared affective representations) and processes (i.e., computational procedures that are neurally localized and are independent of the nature or modality of the stimulus that is being processed—e.g., decoupling mechanism between self and other). Motor resonance that leads to emotion sharing is mediated by the perception–action mechanism (Preston & de Waal, 2002). The medial prefrontal cortex/paracingulate sulcus has a key role in decoupling between first-person and third-person information (Gallagher & Frith, 2003). The right inferior parietal cortex, at the junction with temporoparietal cortex, plays a critical role in the distinction between self-produced actions and emotions and those generated by others (Decety & Grèzes, 2006). This heteromodal association cortex, which receives input from the lateral and posterior thalamus, as well as visual, auditory, somaesthetic, and limbic areas, has reciprocal connections to the prefrontal cortex and to the temporal lobes. Because of these anatomical characteristics, this region is a key neural locus for self-processing that is involved in multisensory body-related information processing, as well as in the processing of phenomenological and cognitive aspects of the self. The ventromedial prefrontal cortex has been described as a convergence zone in which information from the amygdala, hippocampus, and sensory regions interacts to influence social behavior (Damasio, 1994). The insular cortex is the main cortical target of interoceptive afferents and mediates the interoceptive state of the body (Craig, 2002). The lateral prefrontal cortex and the anterior cingulate are part of a circuit that regulates emotion and cognition (Davidson et al., 2000). Note the bidirectional links between the (widely distributed) areas in which representation of emotions are temporarily activated (including autonomic and somatic responses) during empathic experience and the areas involved in emotion regulation. Each area has unique patterns of corticocortical connections, which determine its function, and differences in neural activity during the experience of empathy are produced by distributed subsystems of brain regions. Even though there is massive parallel processing, the dynamic of activation in these regions is also an important aspect to be investigated further.

This automatic mapping between self and other is supported by considerable empirical literature in the domain of perception and action, which has been marshaled under the common-coding theory (Prinz, 1997). Its core assumption is that actions are coded in terms of the perceivable effects (i.e., the distal perceptual events) they should generate. This theory also states that perception of an action activates action representations to the degree that the perceived and the represented action are similar (Wilson & Knoblich, 2005). Furthermore, these representations may be shared between individuals. Indeed, the meaning of a given object, action, or social situation may be common to several people and may activate corresponding distributed patterns of neural activation in their respective brains (Decety & Sommerville, 2003; Jeannerod, 1999). This sharing explains how we come to understand each other; that is, the isomorphism between action representations allows the individual to implicitly know the goal of others through the use of her or his own action representation system.

In neuroscience, evidence for this perception–action coupling ranges from electrophysiological recordings in monkeys, in which mirror neurons in the ventral premotor and posterior parietal cortices fire during both goal-directed actions and observation of the same actions performed by another individual (Rizzolatti, Fogassi, & Gallese, 2001), to functional neuroimaging experiments in humans that demonstrate that the neural circuit involved in action execution overlaps with that activated when actions are observed (Blakemore & Decety, 2001). This neural network includes the premotor cortex, the parietal lobule, the supplementary motor area, and the cerebellum. In addition, a number of neuroimaging studies have shown that similar brain areas are reliably activated while imagining one's own action, imagining another's action, and imitating actions performed by a model (Decety & Chaminade, 2003a; Decety & Grèzes, 2006).

The perception–action mechanism accounts (at least partly) for emotion sharing, which constitutes the core mechanism for empathy (Preston & de Waal, 2002). This model posits that perception of emotion activates in the observer the neural mechanisms that are responsible for the generation of similar emotion. Such a system prompts the observer to resonate with the emotional state of another individual, with the observer activating the motor representations and associated autonomic and somatic responses that stem from the observed target, that is, a sort of inverse mapping. For example, while watching someone smile, the observer activates the same facial muscles involved in producing a smile at a subthreshold level, and this would create the corresponding feeling of happiness in the observer. There is evidence for such a mechanism in the recognition of emotion from facial expression. For instance, viewing facial expressions triggers expressions on one's own face, even in the absence of conscious recognition of the stimulus (Dimberg, Thunberg, & Elmehed, 2000; Wallbott, 1991). Making a facial expression generates changes in the autonomic nervous system and is associated with feeling the corresponding emotion. In a series of experiments, Levenson, Ekman and Friesen (1990) instructed participants to produce facial configurations for anger, disgust, fear, happiness, sadness, and surprise while heart rate, skin conductance, finger temperature, and somatic activity were monitored. They found that such a voluntary facial activity produced significant levels of subjective experience of the associated emotions, as well as specific and reliable autonomic measures. Recently an fMRI experiment confirmed and extended these findings by showing that, when participants are required to observe or to imitate facial expressions of various emotions, increased neurodynamic activity is detected in the superior temporal sulcus, the anterior insula, and the amygdala, as well as in areas of the premotor cortex corresponding to the facial representation (Carr, Iacoboni, Dubeau, Mazziotta, & Lenzi, 2003).

The finding of paired deficits between emotion production and emotion recognition also provides strong arguments in favor of this model. A lesion study carried out with a large number of neurological patients by Adolphs and colleagues (Adolphs, Damasio, Tranel, Cooper, & Damasio, 2000) found that damage within the right somatosensory-related cortices (including primary and secondary somatosensory cortices, insula, and anterior supramarginal gyrus) impaired patients' ability to judge other people's emotional states from viewing their faces. A study of brain-damaged individuals found that recognizing emotions from prosody draws on the right frontoparietal cortex (Adolphs, Damasio, & Tranel, 2002). This finding is consistent with the hypothesis that the recognition of emotion in others requires the perceiver to reconstruct images of somatic and motoric components that would normally be associated with producing and experiencing the emotion signaled in the stimulus (Adolphs et al., 2002).

Moreover, several dramatic case studies support the idea that the same neural systems are involved both in the recognition and in the expression of specific emotion. Adolphs, Tranel, Damasio, and Damasio (1995) investigated S.M., a 30-year-old patient, whose amygdala was bilaterally destructed by a metabolic disorder. Consistent with the prominent role of the amygdala in mediating certain negatively valenced emotions such as fear, S.M. was found to be impaired in both the recognition of fear from facial expressions and in the phenomenological experience of fear. Another case, N. M., who suffered from bilateral amygdala damage and left thalamic lesion, was found to be impaired in recognizing fear from facial expressions and exhibited an equivalent impairment in fear recognition from body postures and emotional sounds (Sprengelmeyer et al., 1999). The patient also reported reduced anger and fear in his everyday experience of emotion. There is also evidence for paired deficits for the emotion of disgust. Calder, Keane, Manes, Antoun, and Young (2000) described patient N.K., with left insula and putamen damage, who was selectively impaired in recognizing social signals of disgust from multiple modalities (facial expressions, nonverbal sounds, and emotional prosody) and who was less disgusted than controls by disgust-provoking scenarios. Further and direct support for a specific role of the left insula in both the recognition and the experience of disgust was recently provided by an fMRI study in which participants inhaled odorants producing a strong feeling of disgust and, in another condition, watched video clips showing the facial expression of disgust. It was found that observing such facial expressions and feelings of disgust activated the same sites in the anterior insula and anterior cingulate cortex (Wicker et al., 2003).

The expression of pain provides a crucial signal, which can motivate caring behaviors in others. Interestingly, a single-neuron recording study in neurological patients has documented pain-related neurons in the anterior cingulate cortex (ACC) that respond both to actual stimulation (thermal stimuli) and to the observation of the same stimuli delivered to another individual (Hutchison, Davis, & Lozano, 1999). A first fMRI study demonstrated that the ACC, the anterior insula, cerebellum, and brainstem were activated when healthy participants experienced a painful stimulus, as well as when they observed a signal indicating that another person was receiving a similar stimulus, but only the actual experience of pain resulted in activation in the somatosensory cortices and in subcalosal cingulate cortex (Singer et al., 2004). Similar results were also reported by Morrison, Lloyd, di Pellegrino, and Roberts (2004) in a study in which participants were scanned during a condition of feeling a moderately painful pinprick stimulus to the fingertips and another condition in which they witnessed another person's hand undergo similar stimulation. Both conditions resulted in common hemodynamic activity in a pain-related area in the right dorsal ACC. Common activity in response to noxious tactile and visual stimulation was restricted to the right inferior Brodmann's area (BA) 24b. In contrast, the primary somatosensory cortex showed significant activations in response to noxious tactile, but not visual, stimuli. The different response patterns in the two areas are consistent with the ACC's role in coding the motivational–affective dimension of pain, which is associated with the preparation of behavioral responses to aversive events. These findings are supported by an fMRI study conducted by Jackson, Meltzoff, and Decety (2005) in which participants were shown still photographs depicting right hands and feet in painful or neutral everyday-life situations and asked to imagine the level of pain that these situations would produce. Significant activation in regions involved in the affective aspects of pain processing, notably the ACC, the thalamus, and the anterior insula, was detected, but no activity was seen in the somatosensory cortex. Moreover, the level of activity within the ACC was strongly correlated with participants' mean ratings of pain attributed to the different situations. In a follow-up fMRI study, Jackson, Brunet, Meltzoff, and Decety (2006), again using pictures of hands and feet in painful scenarios, instructed the participants to imagine and rate the level of pain perceived from two different perspectives (self vs. other). Results indicated that both the self and other perspectives are associated with activation in the neural network involved in the processing of the affective aspect of pain, including the ACC and the insula. However, the self-perspective yielded higher pain ratings and involved the pain matrix more extensively, including the secondary somatosensory cortex, the mid-insula, and the posterior part of the subcalosal cingulate cortex. Adopting the perspective of the other was associated with increased activation in the right temporoparietal junction. In addition, distinct subregions were activated within the insular cortex for the two perspectives (anterior aspect for others and more posterior for self). These neuroimaging data highlight both similarities and self–other distinctiveness as important aspects of human empathy. The experience of pain in oneself is associated with more caudal activations (within area 24), consistent with spinothalamic nociceptive projections, whereas the perception of pain in others is represented in more rostral (and dorsal) regions (within area 32). A similar rostrocaudal organization is observed in the insula, which is consistent with its anatomical connectivity and electrophysiological properties. For instance, painful sensations are evoked in the posterior part of the insula (and not in the anterior part) by direct electrical stimulation of the insular cortex in neurological patients (Ostrowsky et al., 2002). Altogether, these findings are in agreement with the fact that indirect pain representations (as elicited by the observation of pain in others) are qualitatively different from the actual experiences of pain.

A positron emission tomography (PET) study investigated the neural response to externally (watching emotion-laden film clips) versus internally (autobiographical scripts) generated emotions (Reiman et al., 1997). Both film-generated emotion and recall-generated emotion were associated with symmetrical increases in the medial prefrontal cortex and thalamus. The film condition also resulted in activation of the hypothalamus, the amygdala, the anterior temporal cortex, and the occipito–temporo–parietal junction, whereas the recall condition was specifically associated with activation in the anterior insula and orbitofrontal cortex. Thus there is an overlap between externally and internally produced emotions, but this overlap is partial. It should be noted that the films and recall scripts included three emotions (happiness, sadness, and disgust), which were not analyzed separately.

A more recent neuroimaging study demonstrated the involvement of shared representations (in both emotion-processing areas and fronto-parietal networks) when participants feel sympathy for another individual (Decety & Chaminade, 2003b). In this study, participants were presented with a series of video clips showing individuals telling sad and neutral stories as if they had personally experienced them. At the end of each movie, participants were asked to rate the mood of the actor and also how likable they found that person. Watching sad stories versus neutral stories was associated with increased activity in emotion-processing-related structures (including the amygdala and parietofrontal areas) predominantly in the right hemisphere.

Altogether, shared representations between self and other at the cortical level have been documented for action understanding, emotion recognition, and pain processing. This mechanism offers an interesting foundation
for intersubjectivity because it provides a functional bridge between first-
person information and third-person information (Decety & Sommerville,
2003), which allows an automatic connection between the self and the
other. There is no specific cortical site for shared representations: Their
neural underpinnings are widely distributed, and the pattern of activation
(and also, presumably, deactivation) varies according to the processing
domain, the particular emotion, and the stored information. However,
such a mechanism is necessary but not sufficient for empathic understanding. The awareness that others exist as separate entities is a prerequisite
component of empathy.

SELF–OTHER AWARENESS

Individuals who are self-aware, as evidenced by being able to become the
object of their own attention, experience a sense of psychological continuity over time and space (Gallup, 1998). It has been speculated that any
organisms capable of self-recognition would have an introspective awareness of their own mental states and the ability to ascribe mental states to
others (Humphrey, 1990). A clear sense of self may have evolved to solve at
least two kinds of adaptive problems: (1) the self is the repository of the
social feedback one receives from others, and (2) it allows one to model
and understand the internal, subjective worlds of others, making easier to
infer intentions and causes that lay behind observed behaviors, thus
improving interaction efficacy (Forgas & Williams, 2002). Interestingly,
the development of self- and other mental state understanding is functionally linked to that of executive functions—that is, the processes that serve
to monitor and control thought and actions, including self-regulation, planning, cognitive flexibility, response inhibition, and resistance to interference
(Russell, 1996). There is increasingly clear evidence of a specific developmental link between the development of mentalizing and improved self-
control at around the age of 4 (Carlson & Moses, 2001). The development
of cognitive control is related to the maturation of the prefrontal cortex
(Tamm, Menon, & Reiss, 2002). In addition, there is hard evidence that a
region around the paracingulate sulcus in the medial prefrontal cortex
plays a specific role in mentalizing. This region contains spindle cells, a
class of large projection neurons found only in great apes and humans,
which are thought to be involved in coordinating widely distributed neural activity involving emotion and cognition (Allman, Hakeem, Erwin,
Nimchinsky, & Hof, 2001). This region has been found to be reliably activated by mentalizing tasks of various cognitive difficulty, ranging from
judging the emotion in another person's gaze to detection of intention in

simple dynamic animations, attribution of intention to cartoons characters, story comprehension, detection of social transgression, and appreciation of humor (Gallagher & Frith, 2003).

Self-awareness does not rely on a specific brain region. Rather, it arises from the interaction between processes distributed in the brain, especially the prefrontal cortex and the inferior parietal lobule. Neuropsychological research supports a preeminent role for the right frontal lobe in self-related processing. For instance, Keenan, Nelson, O'Connor, and Pascual-Leone (2001) demonstrated that patients undergoing a Wada test were temporarily desensitized with regard to the recognition of their own faces when the right hemisphere was anesthetized. This was not the case when the left hemisphere was anesthetized. Right hemisphere damage has also been found to be linked with impairments in autobiographical memory and self-evaluation. Furthermore, clinical examination has shown that personal confabulation (akin to the creation of fictitious stories about the self) appears to be associated with damage to the right frontal lobe (Feinburg, 2001).

Based on these numerous studies (and many others not reviewed here), it was argued that the right hemisphere is a key player in self-awareness and mental state attribution (Keenan, Gallup, & Falk, 2003). It is worth noting that Keenan et al.'s definition of consciousness includes awareness of one's own thoughts, as well as awareness of others' thoughts. Similar (but not identical) neural processing for self and other raises the question of how we distinguish between representations activated by the self and those activated by others.

Neuroscience research indicates that the right inferior parietal cortex, in conjunction with prefrontal areas and the insula, may be critical in distinguishing the self from the other and therefore in navigating shared representations. The inferior parietal cortex is a heteromodal association area, which receives input from the lateral and posterior thalamus, as well as visual, auditory, somesthetic, and limbic areas. It has reciprocal connections to the prefrontal cortex and to the temporal lobes (Eidelberg & Galaburda, 1984). These multiple connections confer on this region a role in the elaboration of an image of the body in space and in time (Benton & Silvan, 1993), on which the sense of agency depends. Accumulating empirical evidence indicates that the parietal cortex plays a major role in the sense of agency in distinguishing between self-produced actions and actions generated by others (Blakemore & Frith, 2003; Jackson & Decety, 2004, for reviews). Interestingly, the right inferior parietal cortex–right temporo-parietal junction is also involved when participants mentally simulate the actions from a third-person perspective in comparison with first-person perspective (Ruby & Decety, 2001). There are new findings suggesting that this mechanism is also at play while one is thinking about others. For instance, it has been demonstrated that when participants are asked to adopt another person's perspective to evaluate that person's beliefs (Ruby

& Decety, 2003), imagine his or her feelings (Ruby & Decety, 2004), and imagine his or her pain (Jackson, Brunet, et al., 2005), as compared with their own perspective, the right inferior parietal cortex is strongly involved.

All the aforementioned evidence strongly suggests that the inferior parietal cortex, in conjunction with the prefrontal cortex, plays a pivotal role in the sense of self by comparing the source of sensory signals (whether they originate from the self or from the environment). Such a function is crucial for empathy in order to maintain a minimal distinction between the self and the other and to keep track of the origin of the feelings.

MENTAL FLEXIBILITY TO ADOPT
THE PERSPECTIVE OF THE OTHER

Empathy may be initiated by a variety of situations—for instance, by seeing another person in distress or in discomfort, by imagining someone else's behavior, by reading a narrative in a fiction book, or by seeing a moving TV report. However, in these conditions, empathy requires one to adopt more or less consciously the subjective point of view of the other.

Several social psychologists have suggested and documented through empirical work that our default mode to reasoning about others is biased toward self-perspective and that this constitutes a general feature of human cognition (e.g., Hodges & Wegner, 1997; Keysar, 1994; Royzman, Cassidy, & Baron, 2003). Stated in other words, people are fundamentally egocentric and have difficulty getting beyond their own perspective when anticipating what others are thinking or feeling. Usually people are unaware of this projective tendency, which also applies to goals. This view is consistent with the shared-representations mechanism. One sees others through one's own embodied cognition and uses one's own knowledge (including beliefs, opinions, attitudes, feelings) as the primary basis for understanding others. Self-perspective may thus be considered as the default mode of the human mind. It is a very parsimonious and advantageous mechanism for understanding and predicting the behavior of others. Yet it is far from perfect, as individual differences in people's thoughts and emotions abound. Errors in taking the perspective of others stem from the inability to suppress the self-perspective, and many costly social misunderstandings are rooted in people's failure to recognize the degree to which their construals of a situation may differ from those of others (Decety & Hodges, 2006; Hodges & Wegner, 1997). For successful social interaction, and empathic understanding in particular, an adjustment must operate on these shared representations. Whereas the projection of self-traits onto the other does not necessitate any significant store of knowledge about the other, empathic understanding requires the inclusion of other characteristics within the self. An essential aspect of empathy is to recognize the other person as like the self, while maintaining a clear separation between self and other. Hence, mental flexibility and self-regulation are important components of empathy. One needs to calibrate one's own perspective that has been activated by the interaction with the other, or even by its mere imagination. Such calibration requires prefrontal cortex executive resources, as demonstrated by neuroimaging studies in healthy participants, as well as neuropsychological observations.

A series of three neuroimaging studies with healthy volunteers investigated the neural underpinning of perspective taking in three different modalities (i.e., motoric, conceptual, and emotional) of self–other representations. In a first study, participants were scanned while they were asked to either imagine themselves performing a variety of everyday actions (e.g., winding a watch) or to imagine another individual performing similar actions (Ruby & Decety, 2001). Both conditions were associated with common activation in the supplementary motor area (SMA), premotor cortex, and the occipitotemporal region. This neural network corresponds to the shared motor representations between the self and the other. Taking the perspective of the other to simulate his or her behavior resulted in selective activation of the frontopolar cortex and right inferior parietal lobule. In a second study, medical students were shown a series of affirmative health-related sentences (e.g., "taking antibiotic drugs causes general fatigue") and were asked to judge their truthfulness either according to their own perspective (i.e., as experts in medical knowledge) or according to the perspective of a layperson (Ruby & Decety, 2003). The set of activated regions recruited when the participants put themselves in the shoes of a layperson included the medial prefrontal cortex, the frontopolar cortex, and the right inferior parietal lobule. In a third study, the participants were presented with short written sentences that depicted real-life situations (e.g., "someone opens the toilet door that you have forgotten to lock"), which are likely to induce social emotions (e.g., shame, guilt, pride), or other situations that were emotionally neutral (Ruby & Decety, 2004). In one condition, they were asked to imagine how they would feel if they were experiencing these situations. And in another condition, they were asked to imagine how their mothers would feel in those situations. Reaction times were statistically greater when the participants imagined emotion-laden situations as compared with neutral ones, both from their own perspective and from the perspective of their mothers. Neurodynamic changes were detected in the frontopolar cortex, the ventromedial prefrontal cortex, the medial prefrontal cortex, and the right inferior parietal lobule when the participants adopted the perspective of their mothers, regardless of the affective content of the situations depicted. Cortical regions that are involved in emotional processing, including the amygdala and the temporal poles, were found activated in the conditions that integrated emotion-laden situations. Consistent findings were reported from a MRI study in which participants were asked to make food preference judgments about themselves or about someone else (a person whom they new fairly well).

Self-judgments were associated with increases in the medial prefrontal cortex, the anterior insula, and secondary somatosensory areas. Judgments of the other resulted in activation of the medial prefrontal cortex, the frontopolar cortex, and the posterior cingulate (Seger, Stone, & Keenan, 2004).

One of the most striking findings of these studies that investigated self-versus-others perspective is the systematic involvement of the frontopolar cortex, medial prefrontal cortex, and posterior cingulate when the participants adopt the perspective of another person. Converging evidence from clinical neuropsychology and neuroscience points to the frontopolar cortex as being chiefly involved in inhibitory or regulating processing. Frontal damage may result in impaired perspective-taking ability and a lack of cognitive flexibility (Eslinger, 1998). Anderson, Bechara, Damasio, Tranel, and Damasio (1999) reported the cases of two patients with early damage to the anterior prefrontal cortex (encompassing the frontopolar cortex) who, when tested on moral dilemmas, exhibited an excessively egocentric perspective. A major study of patients with limited focal lesions to the frontal lobe, who were tested for visual perspective taking and detecting deception, revealed a dissociation of performance within the frontal lobes (Stuss, Gallup, & Alexander, 2001). Right frontal lobe lesions were associated with impaired visual perspective taking, whereas medial frontal lesions, particularly right ventral, were associated with impaired detection of deception.

These findings support the hypothesis that an inhibitory component is required to regulate and tone down the self-perspective tendency and allow the cognitive and affective flexibility necessary to the evaluation of the other's perspective. Such a view is compatible with the role of the prefrontal cortex in top-down control of behavior (Miller & Cohen, 2001). An alternative interpretation of the role of the frontopolar cortex in adopting the perspective of another individual is based on the distinction between different psychological operations mediated by distinct subregions of the prefrontal cortex. There is evidence that the frontopolar cortex is involved in the process of evaluating self-generated responses and is recruited when the task requires monitoring and manipulation of information that has been internally represented (Christoff & Gabrieli, 2000). Adopting the subjective perspective of another individual so as to understand his or her feelings is a self-generated process that operates on internally represented information fed by the internal activation of shared representations.

EMOTION REGULATION

Emotion regulation refers to the processes by which individuals influence which emotions they have, when they have them, and how they experience and express these emotions (Gross, 1998). It also applies to the modulation of the behavioral and the physiological dimensions of emotion. It is likely that the emotional state and affective consequences generated in the self from the perception or imagination of the other's affective state require some regulation and control for the experience of empathy. Indeed, without such control, the mere activation of the perception–action mechanism, including the associated autonomic and somatic responses, could lead to emotional contagion or emotional distress. Such regulation is also important in modulating one's own vicarious emotion so that it is not experienced as aversive. Previous research indicates that emotion regulation is positively related to feelings of concern for the other person (Derryberry & Rothbart, 1988; Eisenberg et al., 1994). In contrast, people who experience their emotions intensely, especially negative emotions, are prone to personal distress, that is, an aversive emotional reaction such as anxiety or discomfort based on the recognition of another's emotional state or condition (Eisenberg, Shea, Carlo, & Knight, 1991). Chronic incapacity to suppress negative emotion may be a key factor in anxiety and aggressive and violent behavior (Jackson, Malmstadt, Larson, & Davidson, 2000).

A circuit that includes several interconnected regions of the prefrontal cortex, amygdala, hippocampus, ACC, insular cortex, and ventral striatum has been acknowledged to be implicated in various aspects of emotion regulation (Davidson, Putnam, & Larson, 2000). In neurology, the term "self-regulatory disorder" has been coined for the syndrome exhibited by patients with ventromedial prefrontal cortex damage (particularly on the right). This syndrome is defined as the inability to regulate behavior according to internal goals and constraints (Levine, Freedman, Dawson, Black, & Stuss, 1999). It arises from the inability to hold a mental representation of the self online and to use this self-related information to inhibit inappropriate responses. Interestingly, the orbitofrontal, ventromedial, and dorsolateral cortices have been reported in the neurological literature to be involved in empathy. Notably, damage to the orbitofrontal is associated with a wide range of social-emotional deficits, including impaired social judgment and disinhibited behavior. For instance, Stone, Baron-Cohen, and Knight (1998) found that patients with bilateral lesions of the orbitofrontal cortex are impaired in the "faux pas" task. This task requires both an understanding of false or mistaken belief and an appreciation of the emotional impact of a statement on the listener. A study conducted by Stuss and colleagues (2001) extended this finding by showing that only lesions in the right orbitofrontal produce such a deficit. In addition, a number of clinical studies reported a relationship between the deficit in empathy and performance of cognitive flexibility tasks among patients with lesions in the dorsolateral regions, whereas those with orbitofrontal cortex lesions were more impaired in empathy but not in cognitive flexibility (Grattan, Bloomer, Archambault, & Eslinger, 1994; Shamay-Tsoory, Tomer, Berger, & Aharon-Peretz, 2003). The ventromedial prefrontal cortex, with its reciprocal connections with brain regions involved in emotional processing (amygdala), memory (hippocampus), and executive functions (dorsolateral prefrontal cortex), also plays a major role in emotion regulation. Damasio's (1994) somatic-markers hypothesis, which posits that memories of somatic states that are associated with particular experiences or outcomes are stored in the ventromedial prefrontal cortex, is directly relevant in the process of affective regulation. Recent work by Shamay-Tsoory, Tomer, Berger, Goldsher, and Aharon-Peretz (2005) supports this hypothesis. They tested patients with lesions of the ventromedial prefrontal cortex or dorsolateral prefrontal cortex with three theory-of-mind tasks (second-order beliefs and faux pas) that differed in the level of emotional processing involved. They found that patients with ventromedial lesions were most impaired in the faux pas task but presented normal performance in the second-order-belief tasks. The authors further argued that, in order to detect faux pas, one is required not only to understand the knowledge of the other but also to have empathic understanding of the other's feelings. Finally, the ACC is part of a circuit involved in a form of attention that serves to regulate both cognitive and emotional processing (Bush, Luu, & Posner, 2000). Its lesion produces a host of symptoms, which include apathy, inattention, dysregulation of autonomic functions, and emotional instability.

Neuroimaging research has recently begun to investigate neural mechanisms involved in affective reappraisal, a cognitive strategy used to regulate emotion. For instance, an fMRI experiment on emotion reappraisal has detected coactivation of the lateral prefrontal and medial prefrontal cortices and decreased activity in the medial orbitofrontal cortex and the amygdala (Ochsner, Bunge, Gross, & Gabrieli, 2002). Another study identified a circuit composed of the right orbitofrontal, right dorsolateral prefrontal cortex, and anterior cingulate for voluntary suppression of sadness (Lévesque et al., 2003). One recent fMRI study investigated whether observation of distress in others leads to empathic concern and altruistic motivation or to personal distress and egoistic motivation (Lamm, Batson & Decety, in press). In this experiment behavioral measures and event-related fMRI were used to explore the effect of perspective taking and emotion regulation on empathy processing while participants watched video clips of patients expressing pain resulting from medical treatment. Video clips were presented either with the instruction to imagine the feelings of the patient ("imagine other") or to imagine oneself to be in the patient's situation ("imagine self"). Need for emotion regulation was manipulated by providing information that the medical treatment had or had not been successful. Behavioral measures clearly demonstrated that imagery and reappraisal instructions were effective. Neuroimaging data showed consistent activity in the insular cortex and anterior medial cingulate cortex (aMCC). Graded responses related to the imagery instructions were observed in dorsal insula, aMCC, and left and right parietal cortex. Emotion regulation resulted in hemodynamic changes in anterior paracingulate cortex, subgenual ACC, and orbitofrontal and right temporal cortex. These findings support the view that the response to the pain of others can be modulated by cognitive and motivational processes. These processes influence whether observing a conspecific in need of help will result in empathic concern, an important prerequisite for helping behavior.

EMPATHY AS A SIMULATION OF THE SUBJECTIVITY OF THE OTHER

The way our nervous system is organized and tailored by evolution provides the basic biological mechanism for resonating with others. This shared-representations mechanism, driven by the common coding, between perception and action, provides the default mode to implicitly relate to others and may be responsible for the projective tendency to ascribe one's own characteristics and self-traits to others (Decety & Sommerville, 2004; Decety & Jackson, 2004). However, this tendency needs to be regulated (or calibrated) when sharing emotions or when adopting the perspective of others in order to understand their feelings and behave appropriately (Decety & Hodges, 2006). This requires additional computational mechanisms, including monitoring and manipulation of internal information generated by the activation of the shared representations between the self and the other. In addition, there are limits to the extent to which the experiences are isomorphic, as demonstrated by the nonoverlapping neural areas.

One of the core components of empathy relies on the unconscious neural/mental simulation of the emotional state of others. This idea is far from new (e.g., Damasio, 1994; Gallese & Goldman, 1998; Goldman, 1993). For instance, Ax (1964) suggested that empathy might be thought of as "an autonomic nervous system state which tends to simulate that of another person" (p. 11). This idea fits neatly with the notion of embodiment, which refers both to actual bodily states and to simulations of experience in the brain's modality-specific systems for perception, action, and the introspective systems that underlie conscious experiences of emotion, motivation, and cognitive operations (Niedenthal, Barsalou, Winkielman, Krauth-Gruber, & Ric, 2005). However, this simulation is not exclusively under automatic management and, at least in humans, falls under conscious control. This makes empathy, as described here, an intentional capacity. Without self-awareness and emotion regulation processing, there may be no true empathy. The automatic activation of shared representations would instead be associated with anxiety and discomfort and would lead to responses oriented to the self (e.g., emotional distress). Such a formulation is also consistent with the observation that prosocial behaviors, which stem from empathy, emerge during child development in parallel with self-conscious emotions (Lewis, 1999). These emotions require self-evaluation and comparison with other people, as well as some form of emotion regulation. Forming an explicit representation of another person's feelings, as an intentional agent, thus necessitates additional computational mechanisms beyond the shared-representation level. This requires that second-order representations of the other are available to consciousness (a decoupling mechanism between first-person information and second-person information), for which the anterior paracingulate cortex plays a unique function (Frith & Frith, 2003). Thus human empathy cannot be described only as a simple resonance of affect between the self and other. It involves an explicit representation of the subjectivity of the other and a minimal self–other distinction. Recent neuroimaging investigations of the perception of pain in others support such a view (Jackson, Meltzoff, & Decety, 2005; Jackson, Brunet, et al., 2005; Lamm et al., 2006; Morrison et al., 2004; Singer et al., 2004). Indeed, all these studies have shown that part of the neural network (including the ACC and the anterior insula) mediating self-experienced pain is shared when empathizing or observing the pain in others and also that nonoverlapping aspects within these regions are specifically activated for the self or the other. This supports the idea that personal and vicarious experiences at some level differ physiologically (Craig, 1968) and result in qualitatively distinct responses. Finally, empathy also necessitates emotion regulation, in which the ventral prefrontal cortex, with its strong connections with the limbic system, dorsolateral, and medial prefrontal areas, plays an important role.

To conclude and sum up, empathy refers to an emotional response that is produced by the emotional state of another individual without losing sight of whose feelings belong to whom. This response is contingent on cognitive, as well as emotional, factors and involves parallel and distributed processing in a number of dissociable computational mechanisms. Shared representations, self-awareness, mental flexibility, and emotion regulation constitute the basic macro components of empathy, which are mediated by specific neural systems. These components may comprise more elementary components that future social neuroscience research will elucidate. Moreover, because this model assumes that empathy relies on dissociable information-processing components, it predicts a variety of structural or functional dysfunctions, depending on which aspect is disrupted (see Blair, 2005; Decety & Jackson, 2004).

REFERENCES

Adolphs, R., Damasio, H., & Tranel, D. (2002). Neural systems for recognition of emotional prosody: A 3-D lesion study. *Emotion, 2*, 23–51.

Adolphs, R., Damasio, H., Tranel, D., Cooper, G., & Damasio, A. (2000). A role for the somatosensory cortices in the visual recognition of emotion as revealed by three-dimensional lesion mapping. *Journal of Neuroscience, 20*, 2683–2690.

Adolphs, R., Tranel, D., Damasio, H., & Damasio, A. (1995). Fear and the human amygdala. *Journal of Neuroscience, 15,* 5879–5891.

Allman, J. M., Hakeem, A., Erwin, J. M., Nimchinsky, E., & Hof, P. (2001). The anterior cingulate cortex: The evolution of an interface between cognition and emotion. *Annals of the New York Academy of Sciences, 935,* 107–117.

Anderson, S. W., Bechara, A., Damasio, H., Tranel, D., & Damasio, A. R. (1999). Impairment of social and moral behavior related to early damage in human prefrontal cortex. *Nature Neuroscience, 2,* 1032–1037.

Ax, A. A. (1964). Goals and methods of psychophysiology. *Psychophysiology, 1,* 8–25.

Barrett, L., Henzi, P., & Dunbar, R.I.M. (2003). Primate cognition: From what now to what if. *Trends in Cognitive Science, 7,* 494–497.

Basch, M. F. (1983). Empathic understanding: A review of the concept and some theoretical considerations. *Journal of the American Psychoanalytic Association, 31,* 101–126.

Batson, C. D. (1990). How social an animal? The human capacity for caring. *American Psychologist, 45,* 336–346.

Batson, C. D. (1991). Empathic joy and the empathy–altruism hypothesis. *Journal of Personality and Social Psychology, 61,* 413–426.

Batson, C. D. (2006). Folly bridges. In P. A. M. van Lange (Ed.), *Bridging social psychology* (pp. 59–64). Mahwah, NJ: Erlbaum.

Benton, A., & Silvan, A. B. (1993). Disturbance of body schema. In K. M. Heilman & E. Valenstein (Eds.), *Clinical neuropsychology* (pp. 123–140). Oxford, UK: Oxford University Press.

Blair, R. J. R. (2005). Responding to the emotions of others: Dissociating forms of empathy through the study of typical psychiatric populations. *Consciousness and Cognition, 14,* 698–718.

Blakemore, S.-J., & Decety, J. (2001). From the perception of action to the understanding of intention. *Nature Reviews. Neuroscience, 2,* 561–567.

Blakemore, S.-J., & Frith, C. D. (2003). Self-awareness and action. *Current Opinion in Neurobiology, 13,* 219–224.

Bohart, A., & Greenberg, L. S. (1997). *Empathy reconsidered.* Washington, DC: American Psychological Association.

Bush, G., Luu, P., & Posner, M. I. (2000). Cognitive and emotional influences in anterior cingulate cortex. *Trends in Cognitive Science, 4,* 215–222.

Calder, A. J., Keane, J., Manes, F., Antoun, N., & Young, A. W. (2000). Impaired recognition and experience of disgust following brain injury. *Nature Neuroscience, 3,* 1077–1078.

Carlson, S. M., & Moses, L. J. (2001). Individual differences in inhibitory control and children's theory of mind. *Child Development, 72,* 1032–1053.

Carr, L., Iacoboni, M., Dubeau, M. C., Mazziotta, J. C., & Lenzi, G. L. (2003). Neural mechanisms of empathy in humans: A relay from neural systems for imitation to limbic areas. *Proceedings of the National Academy of Science of the USA, 100,* 5497–5502.

Chartrand, T. L., & Bargh, J. A. (1999). The chameleon effect: The perception–behavior link and social interaction. *Journal of Personality and Social Psychology, 71,* 464–478.

Christoff, K., & Gabrieli, J. D. E. (2000). The frontopolar cortex and human cognition: Evidence for a rostrocaudal hierarchical organization within the human prefrontal cortex. *Psychobiology, 28,* 168–186.

Craig, A. D. (2002). How do you feel? Interoception: The sense of the physiological condition of the body. *Nature Reviews. Neuroscience, 3,* 655–666.

Craig, K. D. (1968). Physiological arousal as a function of imagined, vicarious and direct stress experiences. *Journal of Abnormal Psychology, 73,* 513–520.

Damasio, A. R. (1994). *Descartes' error: Emotion, reason, and the human brain.* New York: Oxford University Press.

Davidson, R. J., Putnam, K. M., & Larson, C. L. (2000). Dysfunction in the neural circuitry of emotion regulation: A possible prelude to violence. *Science, 289,* 591–594.

Davis, M. H. (1996). *Empathy: A social psychological approach.* Boulder, CO: Westview Press.

de Waal, F. B. M. (1996). *Good Natured: The origins of right and wrong in humans and other animals.* Cambridge, MA: Harvard University Press.

de Waal, F. B. M., & Thompson, E. (2005). Primates, monks and the mind: The case of empathy. *Journal of Consciousness Studies, 12,* 38–54.

Decety, J., & Chaminade, T. (2003a). When the self represents the other: A new cognitive neuroscience view of psychological identification. *Consciousness and Cognition, 12,* 577–596.

Decety, J., & Chaminade, T. (2003b). Neural correlates of feeling sympathy. *Neuropsychologia, 41,* 127–138.

Decety, J., & Grèzes, J. (2006). The power of stimulation: Imagining one's own and other's behavior. *Brain Research, 1079,* 4–14.

Decety, J., & Hodges, S. D. (2006). The social neuroscience of empathy. In P. A. M. van Lange (Ed.), *Bridging social psychology* (pp. 103–109). Mahwah, NJ: Erlbaum.

Decety, J., & Jackson, P. L. (2004). The functional architecture of human empathy. *Behavioral and Cognitive Neuroscience Reviews, 3,* 71–100.

Decety, J., & Sommerville, J. A. (2003). Shared representations between self and others: A social cognitive neuroscience view. *Trends in Cognitive Science, 7,* 527–533.

Derryberry, D., & Rothbart, M. K. (1988). Arousal, affect, and attention as components of temperament. *Journal of Personality and Social Psychology, 55,* 958–966.

Dimberg, U., Thunberg, M., & Elmehed, K. (2000). Unconscious facial reactions to emotional facial expressions. *Psychological Science, 11,* 86–89.

Eidelberg, D., & Galaburda, A. M. (1984) Inferior parietal lobule. *Archives of Neurology, 41,* 843–852.

Eisenberg, N. (2000). Emotion, regulation, and moral development. *Annual Review of Psychology, 51,* 665–697.

Eisenberg, N., Fabes, R. A., Murphy, B., Karbon, M., Maszk, P., Smith, M., et al. (1994). The relations of emotionality and regulation to dispositional and situational empathy-related responding. *Journal of Personality and Social Psychology, 66,* 776–797.

Eisenberg, N., Shea, C. L., Carlo, G., & Knight, G. (1991). Empathy-related responding and cognition: A "chicken and the egg" dilemma. In W. Kurtines & J. Gewirtz (Eds.), *Handbook of moral behavior and development: Vol. 2. Research* (pp. 63–68). Hillsdale, NJ: Erlbaum.

Eslinger, P. J. (1998). Neurological and neuropsychological bases of empathy. *European Neurology, 39*, 193–199.

Feinburg, T. E. (2001). *Altered egos: How the brain creates the self.* New York: Oxford University Press.

Feshbach, N. D. (1997). Empathy: The formative years implications for clinical practice. In A.C. Bohart & L.S. Greenberg (Eds.), *Empathy reconsidered* (pp. 33–59). Washington, DC: American Psychological Association.

Flavell, J. H. (1999). Cognitive development: Children's knowledge about the mind. *Annual Review of Psychology, 50*, 21–45.

Forgas, J. P., & Williams, K. D. (2002). *The social self.* New York: Psychology Press.

Freud, S. (1955). Group psychology and the analysis of the ego. In J. Strachey (Ed. & Trans.), *The standard edition of the complete psychological works of Sigmund Freud* (Vol. 18, pp. 67–143). London: Hogarth Press. (Original work published 1921)

Frith, U., & Frith, C. D. (2003). Development and neurophysiology of mentalizing. *Philosophical Transactions of the Royal Society of London: Series B. Biological Sciences, 358*, 459–473.

Gallagher, H. L., & Frith, C. D. (2003). Functional imaging of theory of mind. *Trends in Cognitive Sciences, 7*, 77–83.

Gallese, V., & Goldman, A. I. (1998). Mirror neurons and the simulation theory of mind-reading. *Trends in Cognitive Sciences, 2*, 493–501.

Gallup, G. G. (1998). Self-awareness and the evolution of social intelligence. *Behavioural Processes, 42*, 239–247.

Goldman, A. I. (1993). Ethics and cognitive science. *Ethics, 103*, 337–360.

Grattan, L. M., Bloomer, R. H., Archambault, F. X., & Eslinger, P. J. (1994). Cognitive flexibility and empathy after frontal lobe lesion. *Neuropsychiatry, Neuropsychology, and Behavioral Neurology, 7*, 251–257.

Gross, J. J. (1998). The emerging field of emotion regulation: An integrative review. *Review of General Psychology, 2*, 271–289.

Harris, P. L. (2000). Understanding emotion. In M. Lewis & J. M. Haviland-Jones (Eds.), *Handbook of emotions*, 2nd ed. (pp. 281–292). New York: Guilford Press.

Hatfield, E., Cacioppo, J., & Rapson, R. (1994). *Emotional contagion.* New York: Cambridge University Press.

Hodges, S. D., & Wegner, D. M. (1997). Automatic and controlled empathy. In W. Ickes (Ed.), *Empathic accuracy* (pp. 311–339). New York: Guilford Press.

Humphrey, N. (1990). The uses of consciousness. In J. Brockman (Ed.), *Speculations: The reality club* (pp. 67–84). New York: Prentice-Hall.

Hutchison, W. D., Davis, K. D., & Lozano, A. M. (1999). Pain-related neurons in the human cingulate cortex. *Nature Neuroscience, 2*, 403–405.

Ickes, W. (1997). *Empathic accuracy.* New York: Guilford Press.

Jackson, D. C., Malmstadt, J. R., Larson, C. L., & Davidson, R. J. (2000). Suppression and enhancement of emotional responses to unpleasant pictures. *Psychophysiology, 37*, 512–522.

Jackson, P. L., & Decety, J. (2004). Motor cognition: A new paradigm to study self–other interactions. *Current Opinion in Neurobiology, 14*, 259–263.

Jackson, P. L., Brunet, E., Meltzoff, A. N., & Decety, J. (2006). Empathy examined through the neural mechanisms involved in imagining how I feel versus how you feel pain. *Neuropsychologia, 44,* 752–761.

Jackson, P. L., Meltzoff, A. N., & Decety, J. (2005). How do we perceive the pain of others: A window into the neural processes involved in empathy. *Neuro-Image, 24,* 771–779.

Jeannerod, M. (1999). To act or not to act: Perspective on the representation of actions. *Quarterly Journal of Experimental Psychology, 52A,* 1–29.

Keenan, J. P., Gallup, G. G., & Falk, D. (2003). *The face in the mirror: The search for the origins of consciousness.* New York: HarperCollins.

Keenan, J. P., Nelson, A., O'Connor, M., & Pascual-Leone, A. (2001). Self-recognition and the right hemisphere. *Nature, 409,* 305.

Keysar, B. (1994). The illusory transparency of intention: Linguistic perspective taking in text. *Cognitive Psychology, 26,* 165–208.

Lamm, C., Batson, C. D., & Decety, J. (in press). The neural basis of human empathy—effects of perspective-taking and cognitive appraisal: An event-related fMRI study. *Journal of Cognitive Neuroscience.*

Levenson, R. W., Ekman, P., & Friesen, W. V. (1990). Voluntary facial action generates emotion-specific autonomic nervous system activity. *Psychophysiology, 27,* 363–384.

Levenson, R. W., & Ruef, A. M. (1992). Empathy: A physiological substrate. *Journal of Personality and Social Psychology, 63,* 234–246.

Lévesque, J., Eugène, F., Joanette, Y., Paquette, V., Mensour, B., Beaudoin, G., et al. (2003). Neural circuitry underlying voluntary suppression of sadness. *Biological Psychiatry, 53,* 502–510.

Levine, B., Freedman, M., Dawson, D., Black, S. E., & Stuss, D. T. (1999). Ventral frontal contribution to self-regulation: Convergence of episodic memory and inhibition. *Neurocase, 5,* 263–275.

Lewis, M. (1999). Social cognition and the self. In P. Rochat (Ed.), *Early social cognition* (pp. 81–98). New York: Erlbaum.

McIntosh, D.N., Reichmann-Decker, A., Winkielman, P., & Wilbarger, J.L. (2006). When the social mirror breaks: Deficits in automatic, but not voluntary mimicry of emotional facial expressions in autism. *Developmental Science, 9,* 295–302.

Miller, E. K., & Cohen, J. D. (2001). An integrative theory of prefrontal cortex function. *Annual Review of Neurosciences, 24,* 167–202.

Morrison, I., Lloyd, D., di Pellegrino, G., & Roberts, N. (2004). Vicarious responses to pain in anterior cingulate cortex: Is empathy a multisensory issue? *Cognitive, Affective, and Behavioral Neuroscience, 4,* 270–278.

Niedenthal, P. M., Barsalou, L. W., Winkielman, P., Krauth-Gruber, S., & Ric, F. (2005). Embodiment in attitudes, social perception, and emotion. *Personality and Social Psychology Review, 9,* 184–211.

Ochsner, K. N., Bunge, S. A., Gross, J. J., & Gabrieli, J. D. E. (2002). Rethinking feelings: An fMRI study of the cognitive regulation of emotion. *Journal of Cognitive Neuroscience, 14,* 1215–1229.

Ostrowsky, K., Magnin, M., Ryvlin, P., Isnard, J., Gueno, M., & Maugui re, F. (2002). Representation of pain and somatic sensation in the human insula: A study of responses to direct electrical cortical stimulation. *Cerebral Cortex, 12,* 376–385.

Plutchik, R. (1987). Evolutionary bases of empathy. In N. Eisenberg, & J. Strayer

(Eds.), *Empathy and its development* (pp. 38–46). New York: Cambridge University Press.

Povinelli, D. J. (2001). *Folk physics for apes*. New York: Oxford University Press.

Prinz, W. (1997). Perception and action planning. *European Journal of Cognitive Psychology, 9*, 129–154.

Preston, S. D., & de Waal, F. B. M. (2002). Empathy: Its ultimate and proximate bases. *Behavioral and Brain Sciences, 25*, 1–72.

Reiman, E. M., Lane, R. D., Ahern, G. L., Schwartz, G. E., Davidson, R. J., Friston, K. J., et al. (1997). Neuroanatomical correlates of externally and internally generated emotion. *American Journal of Psychiatry, 154*, 918–925.

Rizzolatti, G., Fogassi, L., & Gallese, V. (2001). Neurophysiological mechanisms underlying the understanding and the imitation of action. *Nature Review Neuroscience, 2*, 661–670.

Royzman, E. B., Cassidy, K. W., & Baron, J. (2003). I know you know: Epistemic egocentrism in children and adults. *Review of General Psychology, 7*, 38–65.

Ruby, P., & Decety, J. (2001). Effect of subjective perspective taking during simulation of action: A PET investigation of agency. *Nature Neuroscience, 4*, 546–550.

Ruby, P., & Decety, J. (2003). What you believe versus what you think they believe: A neuroimaging study of conceptual perspective taking. *European Journal of Neuroscience, 17*, 2475–2480.

Ruby, P., & Decety, J. (2004). How would you feel versus how do you think she would feel? A neuroimaging study of perspective taking with social emotions. *Journal of Cognitive Neuroscience, 16*, 988–999.

Russell, J. (1996). *Agency and its role in mental development*. Hove, UK: Psychology Press.

Schulkin, J. (2004). *Bodily sensibility*. New York: Oxford University Press.

Seger, C. A., Stone, M., & Keenan, J. P. (2004). Cortical activations during judgments about the self and another person. *Neuropsychologia, 42*, 614–629.

Shamay-Tsoory, S. G., Tomer, R., Berger, B. D., & Aharon-Peretz, J. (2003). Characterization of empathy deficits following prefrontal brain damage: The role of right ventromedial prefrontal cortex. *Journal of Cognitive Neuroscience, 15*, 1–14.

Shamay-Tsoory, S. G., Tomer, R., Berger, B. D., Goldsher, D., & Aharon-Peretz, J. (2005). Impaired affective theory of mind is associated with ventromedial prefrontal damage. *Cognitive and Behavioral Neurology, 18*, 55–67.

Singer, T., Seymour, B., O'Doherty, J., Kaube, H., Dolan, R. J., & Frith, C. D. (2004). Empathy for pain involves the affective but not sensory components of pain. *Science, 303*, 1157–1161.

Sprengelmeyer, R., Young, A. W., Schroeder, U., Grossenbacher, P. G., Federlein, J., Buttner, T., et al. (1999). Knowing no fear. *Proceedings of the Royal Society of London: Series B. Biological Sciences, 266*, 2451–2456.

Stone, V. E., Baron-Cohen, S., & Knight, R. T. (1998). Frontal lobe contributions to theory of mind. *Journal of Cognitive Neuroscience, 10*, 640–646.

Stuss, D. T., Gallup, G., & Alexander, M. P. (2001). The frontal lobes are necessary for theory of mind. *Brain, 124*, 279–286.

Tamm, L., Menon, V., & Reiss, A. L. (2002). Maturation of brain function associated with response inhibition. *Journal of American Children and Adolescent Psychiatry, 41*, 1231–1238.

Thompson, E. (2001). Empathy and consciousness. *Journal of Consciousness Studies, 8,* 1–32.

Van Baaren, R. B., Holland, R. W., Kawakami, K., & Van Knippenberg, A. (2004). Mimicry and prosocial behavior. *Psychological Science, 15,* 71–74.

Wallbott, H. G. (1991). Recognition of emotion from facial expression via imitation? Some indirect evidence for an old theory. *British Journal of Social Psychology, 30,* 207–219.

Wicker, B., Keysers, C., Plailly, J., Royet, J. P., Gallese, V., & Rizzolatti, G. (2003). Both of us disgusted in my insula: The common neural basis of seeing and feeling disgust. *Neuron, 40,* 655–664.

Wilson, E. O. (1988). *On human nature.* Cambridge, MA: Harvard University Press.

Wilson, M., & Knoblich, G. (2005). The case for motor involvement in perceiving conspecifics. *Psychological Bulletin, 131,* 460–473.

13

How Dynamics of Thinking Create Affective and Cognitive Feelings
PSYCHOLOGY AND NEUROSCIENCE OF THE CONNECTION BETWEEN FLUENCY, LIKING, AND MEMORY

Tedra Fazendeiro, Troy Chenier, and Piotr Winkielman

The past two decades have witnessed an explosion of research on the interaction between affect and cognition. One stream of this research explores this interaction by studying how affective stimuli and states influence various forms of cognition, including attention, perception, categorization, reasoning, and memory (for overview, see Eich, Kihlstrom, Bower, Forgas, & Niedenthal, 2000). Other research, including ours, focuses on the reverse direction of this interaction and investigates how cognition influences affect. However, we take a unique approach. Typically, research on cognitive influences on affect explores how specific beliefs about the stimulus and its context (i.e., appraisal and attributions) shape emotional responses (Ellsworth & Scherer, 2003). In contrast, our work examines how affective, as well as cognitive, experiences emerge from the dynamical aspect of cognition, or, specifically, the fluency of perceiving, recognizing, categorizing, and recalling information. The structure of our chapter is roughly as follows. We start with an explanation of the concept of processing fluency and a general discussion of how fluency generates affective and cognitive experiences, such as feelings of familiarity. In this discussion, we argue that fluency typically comes with "hedonic marking"—intrinsic positivity. Next, we show how this idea explains several preference phenomena that have long intrigued psychologists, including the mere-exposure and "beauty-in-averages" effects, and generates interesting new predictions, such as the preference for conceptually primed stimuli. We also argue that the idea of hedonic fluency and its association with familiarity may explain people's tendency to "recognize" positive stimuli. Throughout this discussion we pay special attention to the relationship between affect and memory systems, and we present psychological and neuroscientific evidence for a tight connection between these systems. Given the focus of this book, we especially highlight the contribution of affective and cognitive neuroscience to understanding the fluency–feeling connection, with special emphasis on how social neuroscience methods contribute to resolution of theoretical controversies that are hard to address using traditional approaches.

THE CONCEPT OF PROCESSING FLUENCY

When a person processes a stimulus, one type of available information is *what*, or the content of the processed information. However, the person also has information about *how*, or the processing itself. It is now widely accepted that perceivers monitor the quality of their own processing and use this information in a variety of judgments (for an overview see Metcalfe & Shimamura, 1994). One such qualitative aspect of processing is "fluency"—a general term referring to the relative ease of mental operations (Jacoby, Kelley, & Dywan, 1989; Winkielman, Schwarz, Fazendeiro, & Reber, 2003). Although we use the general term "fluency" throughout the chapter, it is useful to make a couple of distinctions. First, it is worth distinguishing between subjective and objective fluency. Subjective fluency simply refers to the experienced feeling of ease (Schwarz, 1998). Objective fluency refers to efficiency as reflected by some performance measure, such as speed or accuracy (Jacoby, 1983; Mandler, 1980). In addition, it is useful to differentiate between perceptual and conceptual fluency. Perceptual fluency refers to the efficiency of low-level, data-driven operations concerned primarily with the processing of "surface" features, such as stimulus form. Accordingly, perceptual fluency is typically manipulated by variables such as repetition, contrast, clarity, and duration (Jacoby, 1983). Conceptual fluency reflects the ease of higher level mental operations concerned primarily with the processing of meaning-related features. Accordingly, conceptual fluency is typically manipulated by variables such as semantic priming, linguistic predictability, and semantic ambiguity (Whittlesea, 1993).

THE FLUENCY–EXPERIENCE CONNECTION

The past two decades of research brought substantial evidence that changes in fluency can influence affective and cognitive experiences. The models that explain this influence fall into two categories: two-step models and hedonic models.

Two-Step Models

According to several models, fluency translates into experience via a two-step process. The models share logic with the two-factor theory of emotion, which proposes that a specific emotional experience (e.g., a feeling of anger) arises from a context-dependent interpretation of "raw," nonspecific arousal (Schacter & Singer, 1962). Thus, in the first step, there is a change in "raw" fluency of a stimulus (e.g., due to some manipulation). This change triggers a search for an explanation (Why is processing of this stimulus particularly easy?). In the second step, the "raw" fluency is interpreted in the context of available situational cues, which results in a particular phenomenal experience, such as "familiarity," if the task involves memory context, or "liking," if the task involves evaluative context (Bornstein & D'Agostino, 1994; Jacoby, et al., 1989; Mandler, Nakamura, & Van Zandt, 1987; Seamon, Brody, & Kauff, 1983).

Supporting the two-step models, many studies found that fluency effects are context-dependent. For example, when asked to assess the brightness of a stimulus, participants rated high-fluency stimuli as brighter than low-fluency stimuli; yet when asked to rate their darkness, they rated the same stimuli as darker (Mandler et al., 1987). Other studies have shown that fluency influences a variety of perceptual and conceptual judgments, including judgments of loudness (e.g., Jacoby, Allan, Collins, & Larwill, 1988), clarity (e.g., Whittlesea, Jacoby, & Girard, 1990), or duration (e.g., Witherspoon & Allan, 1985). Interestingly, some of the most powerful fluency effects are found in the domain of recognition memory. For example, participants are more likely to "remember" targets whose perception was facilitated with matching, rather than mismatching, subliminal primes (Jacoby & Whitehouse, 1989), greater presentation clarity (Whittlesea et al., 1990), or a semantically predictive sentence stem (Whittlesea, 1993).

Hedonic Models

A few years ago, we suggested that two-step models cannot fully explain fluency effects on evaluations. Instead, our hedonic-fluency model proposes that fluency is often hedonically positive (see Winkielman et al., 2003, for a more comprehensive treatment). The basic idea behind this proposal is that fluency can function as a signal of a positive state of affairs, either within the cognitive system or in the world. More specifically, fluency can signal (1) good progress in processing and likelihood of achieving the current cognitive goal (e.g., Carver & Scheier, 1990), (2) availability of appropriate knowledge structures to interpret the stimulus (e.g., Schwarz, 1981), and (3) previous experience with the stimulus and thus lower likelihood that the stimulus is harmful (Zajonc, 1968). In addition to its signaling value, fluency processing might be intrinsically positive because it involves greater harmony or less perceptual and conceptual conflict (Fernandez-Duque, Baird, & Posner, 2000).

Our initial tests of the hedonic-fluency idea relied on the focus-of-judgment manipulations that had been used in testing the two-step models. In one study (Reber, Winkielman, et al., 1998, Study 2), we asked some participants to judge the "prettiness" of the targets, but asked other participants to judge the "ugliness" of the targets. In another study (Reber, Stark, et al., 1998, Study 3), we asked some participants to make "liking" judgments but asked others to make "disliking" judgments. In both studies, increased perceptual fluency resulted in higher judgments of "prettiness" and "liking" and lower judgments of "ugliness" and "disliking," as reflected in significant interactions of fluency and judgment focus. In combination, these findings indicate that increased fluency does not facilitate more extreme evaluations in general but selectively increases positive judgments.

One possible criticism of the above-mentioned studies is that judgments of disliking or ugliness may be less "natural" than judgments of liking and prettiness. In fact, Mandler et al. (1987) suggested that in their studies, repeated exposure did not lead to greater disliking, because "disliking is a complex judgment, often based on the absence of a liking response. Linguistically, liking is the unmarked and disliking the marked end of the imputed continuum" (p. 647). In other words, it is possible that participants may prefer to initially evaluate prettiness or likeability of stimuli and only later reverse their response to report it along an ugliness or disliking scale. In order to address these concerns, we have drawn on the methods of social neuroscience in order to measure the presence and valence of affective state independent of self-report. Specifically, Winkielman and Cacioppo (2001) had participants watch pictures of everyday objects presented on a computer screen. The fluency with which these pictures were processed was manipulated through visual priming (Study 1) and presentation duration (Study 2). Simultaneously, facial electromyography (EMG) monitored activity over both the zygomaticus major (smiling) muscle, which is indicative of positive affect, and the corrugator supercilli (frowning) muscle, which is indicative of negative affect (see Cacioppo, Petty, Losch, & Kim, 1986, for more on facial EMG). The study found that high-fluency stimuli were associated with an increase in activity over the zygomaticus facial muscle, indicative of positive affect, but was not associated with an increase in activity over the corrugator supercilli muscle, indicative of negative affect. This study clearly suggests that manipulating fluency can lead to genuine hedonic reactions. As we discuss shortly, other studies using different fluency manipulations show similar results.

FLUENCY AND CLASSIC PREFERENCE PHENOMENA

Our lab and related labs have also explored whether the connection between fluency and affect can explain some classic preference phenomena.

In what follows we discuss the contribution of fluency, as well as familiarity, to preference for (1) repeated stimuli (mere-exposure effect) and (2) prototypical stimuli (beauty-in-averages effect).

The "Mere-Exposure" Effect

Historically, the connection between fluency and affect has received the most attention in the debates about the nature of the mere-exposure effect, that is, the observation that nonreinforced repetition can enhance liking for an initially neutral stimulus (for reviews, see Bornstein, 1989; Zajonc, 2001). Several authors proposed that the mere-exposure effect might reflect increases in perceptual fluency (e.g., Bornstein & D'Agostino, 1994; Jacoby et al., 1989; Seamon et al., 1983; Whittlesea, 1993). This proposal is consistent with the observation that repeated exposure speeds up stimulus perception and enhances judgments of stimulus clarity and presentation duration (e.g., Haber & Hershenson, 1965; Jacoby & Dallas, 1981; Witherspoon & Allan, 1985; Whittlesea et al., 1990).

Interestingly, some early mere-exposure studies seemed to argue against a fluency explanation, with repetition influencing liking but not recognition (Bornstein, 1989; Wilson, 1979; Zajonc, 2001). For example, Kunst-Wilson and Zajonc (1980) found that participants preferred a subliminally repeated stimulus even when they could not reliably discriminate between old and new items on a memory test. This finding runs counter to the fluency explanation because changes in fluency should be able to support familiarity-based recognition (as they have in the recognition memory studies by Jacoby, Whittlesea, and colleagues). However, other findings have shown that the mere-exposure effect is associated with a feeling of familiarity and that participants can be led to rely on this feeling to make recognition judgments. Specifically, Bonnano and Stillings (1986) asked participants to discriminate between old and new items based either on explicit recognition (actually remembering that they had seen the items previously) or on familiarity (the sense that an item feels "old"). The results showed that participants who were asked for explicit recognition could not reliably discriminate between old and new items. However, when they based their recognition judgments on their sense of familiarity, previously seen items were recognized as much as they were preferred. Building on these findings, Whittlesea and Price (2001) showed that the dissociation between the preference and memory judgment is a function of the type of strategy with which participants approach the respective judgments. When participants were encouraged to use a "default" analytic strategy for recognition, they performed at chance levels. However when they were encouraged to use a nonanalytic strategy, they could reliably recognize old versus new items. Likewise, when paticipants were biased toward using a "default" nonanalytic strategy for their pleasantness judgments, they exhibited a preference for repeated items; but this preference disappeared when they were biased toward using an analytic strategy. In short, the work on the mere-exposure effect suggests that a simple repetition of a stimulus enhances fluency, which appears to be a source of feelings of liking, as well as feelings of familiarity.

Importantly, the idea that the mere-exposure effect is based on fluency is perfectly compatible both with Zajonc's (2001) claim that mere exposure elicits genuine positive affect and with the hedonic-fluency proposal (Winkielman et al., 2003). Thus, in Mandler et al.'s (1987) studies, as well as a follow-up by Seamon, McKenna, and Binder (1998), repeated exposure increased judgments of liking but not judgments of disliking. Further, in a psychophysiological study by Harmon-Jones and Allen (2001), mere-exposed stimuli elicited greater EMG activity over the zygomaticus region (with no differences over the corrugator region). Interestingly, in this study, the exposure effects were also modified by individual differences in approach–avoidance motivation, as measured by cortical asymmetry. Specifically, participants with less left-sided frontal activity (associated with lower approach motivation) showed a greater mere-exposure effect than participants with more left-sided frontal activity. Overall, these data suggest that the mere-exposure effect involves a genuine affective reaction and is sensitive to variables that should modify affective responding.

The "Beauty-in-Averages" Effect

Another classic psychological effect that can be understood with the idea of hedonic fluency is preference for prototypical stimuli, or the "beauty-in-averages" effect. The best-known example of this phenomenon is preference for prototypical or average faces—an effect that is robust within and across cultures (Langlois & Roggman, 1990; Rhodes & Tremewan, 1996; Rhodes, Yoshikawa, et al., 2002). The "beauty-in-averageness" effect is often theoretically explained as reflecting a biological predisposition to interpret prototypicality as a cue to reproductive mate value, perhaps due to an association of prototypicality with health (Symons, 1979; Thornhill & Gangestad, 1993; but see Rhodes, et al., 2000). However, if people prefer prototypicality because it signals reproductive fitness, this phenomenon should not necessarily extend to fitness-irrelevant stimuli. Yet several studies show comparable effects in a wide variety of natural and artificial categories, including dogs, birds, fish, automobiles, watches (Halberstadt & Rhodes, 2000, 2003), color patches (Martindale & Moore, 1988), furniture (Whitfield & Slatter, 1979), and even paintings (Hekkert & van Wieringen, 1990).

The very broad nature of prototypicality preferences suggests that they might reflect a general cognitive mechanism. Fluency is a promising candidate because it has long been known that prototypes are processed fluently. For example, people are faster to classify more prototypical patterns (Posner & Keele, 1968) and perceive them using fewer neural resources

(Reber et al., 1998). Reflecting these considerations, we have recently conducted three experiments testing whether prototypes are attractive because of their fluency (Winkielman, Halberstadt, Fazendeiro, & Catty, 2006). In two experiments, participants were presented with random dot patterns (Experiment 1) or common geometric patterns (Experiment 2) that varied in levels of prototypicality and were asked to classify these patterns into two categories and rate their attractiveness (with task order counterbalanced). In both experiments, prototypicality was a predictor of both fluency (as measured by classification speed) and attractiveness. Critically, fluency mediated the effect of prototypicality on attractiveness, although some effect of prototypicality remained when fluency was controlled. Further, as in earlier work, we also tested whether fluent prototypical stimuli elicit a genuine liking response, as reflected in physiological responses (Experiment 3). This is important because self-reports of attractiveness could possibly reflect a "cold" evaluation of a stimulus's closeness to the category prototype. Specifically, we first presented participants with multiple exemplars from a category of abstract dot patterns (without showing the prototype) and then showed them several test patterns. As predicted, the prototype of the presented category elicited significantly more EMG activity over the zygomaticus (smiling) muscle than the control prototype pattern from a nonpresented category, thus suggesting that participants' liking responses to random prototypes reflect genuine affective reactions.

As in the research on "mere exposure," one question concerns the relationship between the impact of prototypicality on affect and familiarity. Halberstadt and Rhodes (2000, 2003) have reported that manipulated, as well as rated, averageness (a proxy for prototypicality) correlates not only with rated attractiveness but also with familiarity. This raises the question of whether a third variable—fluency—feeds into both memorial and affective responses, with specific impact controlled by judgmental context. Our recent work (Chenier & Winkielman, 2006) recently addressed this question using a paradigm similar to the just-described Experiment 3. Specifically, we first presented participants with multiple exemplars of a category of abstract dot patterns. Next, we presented participants with several test patterns and measured their subjective and objective fluency, memory, and affect. Specifically, participants saw unseen but prepared prototypes of the studied category, previously seen exemplars, and unseen exemplars from the studied category, as well as matched control patterns from a category that was not exposed. The results were very interesting. First, on the fluency measures, the prepared but unseen prototypes were as fluent as seen exemplar patterns, with both patterns being more fluent than unseen exemplars and control patterns. This was true for both objective measures of fluency, as indicated by classification latencies, and subjective measures, as indicated by judgments of perceptual clarity. This result demonstrates that merely being exposed to exemplars from a category is sufficient to enhance the subjective and objective fluency of the unseen prototype, with this enhancement comparable to actually having been exposed to a member of the category. More important, the unseen prototype patterns were claimed to be old as frequently and liked as much as seen exemplar patterns, with both being claimed old more frequently and liked more than the unseen exemplar patterns and control patterns. This result suggests that the enhancement of fluency with prototypicality manipulations may, depending on judgment context, increase feelings of familiarity or lead to more positive evaluations of the target stimulus.

CONCEPTUAL FLUENCY AND THE CONSCIOUS EXPERIENCE OF FAMILIARITY AND LIKING

The studies we have described so far suggest that fluency can enhance recognition judgments, as well as preferences, as reflected in liking judgments and physiological reactions. However, two important issues remain. First, all of the manipulations described so far have targeted perceptual, rather than conceptual, aspects of stimulus processing. Thus it is possible that hedonic reactions emerge only after facilitation of low-level aspects of cognition.[1] Further, the studies described so far assessed only immediate hedonic reactions to the stimulus. Thus it is possible that fluency does not change the perceiver's conscious phenomenological experience (i.e., subjective feelings).

We addressed both of these issues in a paradigm that manipulates conceptual fluency using cross-format semantic priming. In this paradigm, participants are first exposed to a series of intermixed words and pictures. During the next "test" phase, participants are presented with another set of words and pictures. Some of the test items are identical to study list items, some are completely new, and some are also new but semantically related to study list items and appear in a different perceptual format. For example, a participant might be initially shown the word "table" and later asked about a picture of a "chair." In one series of experiments using this paradigm, we focused on the impact of conceptual fluency on recognition (Fazendeiro, Winkielman, Luo, & Lorah, 2005). As predicted, conceptual fluency enhanced false recognition, as reflected by a greater number of false alarms to semantic lures (e.g., picture of a chair after seeing the word "table"). Importantly, in addition to collecting recognition judgments, we also assessed the role of fluency-based subjective experiences using attributional manipulations borrowed from the psychology of emotion. Specifically, during the experiment, we played ambiguous-sounding music in the background, and participants were told different (false) stories about the possible impact of this music. Some participants were told that the music would cause certain items to feel familiar and to ignore that feeling when making memory judgments. Other participants were told that the music would cause certain items to come to mind more easily (i.e., subjective fluency). Yet another group was told that the music might somehow influence them (most participants interpreted this as a warning about a possible effect on affective feelings). The results showed that only the warning about feelings of familiarity influenced participants' judgments, eliminating the false memory for semantically related pictures. Interestingly, there were no effects of warnings about other feelings, including feelings of subjective fluency or affective feelings. This pattern of findings suggests that the conscious experience generated by manipulations of *objective* conceptual fluency is a *subjective* feeling of familiarity.

Using this paradigm, Winkielman and Fazendeiro (2006) explored the effects of conceptual fluency on liking. The results showed that participants liked stimuli more when their processing was facilitated with cross-format semantic primes (e.g., a picture of a table was liked more after participants saw the word "chair"). This finding clearly suggests that the fluency effects on liking are not restricted to low-level aspects of processing (see also Whittlesea, 1993). The results of these studies also suggest that fluency influences participants' conscious affective experience. Specifically, in one condition we told participants that music being played in the background might influence their affective feelings. In this condition, the impact of conceptual fluency on liking judgments disappeared. Interestingly, in other conditions, the same manipulation, designed to make feelings of familiarity and feelings of subjective fluency nondiagnostic, had no influence on liking judgments. This pattern of results suggests that the participants did not rely on feelings of familiarity (or raw subjective fluency) when making their liking judgments, but rather that their subjective experience carried a hedonic tone. More generally, these results show that the actual subjective experiences that underlie recognition and liking judgments arise in a context-specific manner. The same manipulation (e.g., semantic priming) can lead to two different subjective experiences depending on the judgment context—feelings of liking and feelings of familiarity—each with its own unique judgmental consequences. Further, as emphasized by our hedonic-marking model, when fluency triggers the affective experience, the feeling is not "undifferentiated" but rather is positive, as reflected by more favorable judgments of conceptually fluent stimuli.

POSITIVITY BREEDS FAMILIARITY

The research reviewed so far demonstrates that fluency enhances feelings of familiarity and positivity and that the judgmental impact of these feelings can be dissociated using a variety of manipulations. However, the fact that both feelings spring from the same source (fluency) and often occur together implies that participants should occasionally confuse positive affect with familiarity. If so, manipulations of positive affect should influence familiarity. Several lines of research support this assertion. Monin

(2003) found a correlation between rated attractiveness and familiarity of faces and found that this correlation held even when the discriminability variable (i.e., distinguishing features and prototypicality) was partialed out (Study 1). Monin also reported that attractive faces tend to be recognized as "old" more than less attractive faces regardless of their actual old or new status (Study 2). Similarly, Garcia-Marques, Mackie, Claypool, and Garcia-Marques (2004) found that novel smiling faces were more likely to be falsely recognized than neutral faces and that novel words subliminally primed with smiling faces were more likely to be falsely recognized than those primed with neutral faces. Additionally, they found that participants in positive moods, as opposed to those in negative moods, judged subliminally presented sentences as more valid, which, the researchers surmised, may reflect feelings of familiarity. Phaf and Rotteveel (2005) extended these findings and found that priming neutral words with positive words creates more false recognition than priming with negative words and that inducing positive affect with a physical manipulation (i.e., participants held a coffee stirrer horizontally between their front teeth, causing a smiling expression) creates more false recognition of word stimuli than inducing negative affect (i.e., participants furrowed their brows, causing a frowning expression). Taken together, these studies suggest that positive affect and familiarity tend to co-occur and that a "warm glow" may serve as the basis for determining whether or not a stimulus has been encountered previously. Importantly, as Phaf and Rotteveel (2005) emphasize, this research does not necessarily assign priority to what comes first—affect or familiarity. Instead, they argue for a correspondence hypothesis according to which both experiences emerge from the same source—an early processing system designed to quickly determine both the value and novelty of the stimulus. We agree and suggest that this early processing system draws on a nonanalytic source of information—fluency (we discuss more details shortly).

MODERATING CONDITION: EMERGENCE AND USE OF FLUENCY-BASED EXPERIENCES

In our discussion so far, we have not considered conditions that determine (1) whether fluency results in affective and cognitive experiences and (2) whether the experience will be used in judgment. This brings us to the role of expectations and attributions.

Expectations

The emotion literature has long emphasized that feelings are stronger when an event is surprising (e.g., expected vs. unexpected success). Similarly, fluency is more likely to engender a subjective experience (familiarity, pleasure) if it exceeds the person's normative processing expectations (Whittle-sea & Williams, 1998, 2000).[2] For example, when we see a regular cashier at our grocery store we experience no feeling of familiarity, although we process the cashier's features quite fluently (because of repetition and con-gruous contextual cues). However, if we encounter the same individual in a different context, say, while browsing through a bookstore, we experience a strong sense of familiarity. An empirical test of this idea is offered by a study in which participants pronounced and recognized letter strings that were orthographically irregular nonwords (e.g., stofwus), regular non-words (e.g., hension), or regular words (Whittlesea & Williams, 1998, Experiment 3). The actual fluency (measured by pronunciation speed) of regular nonwords was similar to that of regular words and greater than the fluency of irregular nonwords. However, participants' expected fluency (measured by participants' judgments of similarity to English words) was much closer for regular and irregular nonwords and much lower than the fluency expected for regular words. As a result, the regular nonwords were unexpectedly fluent (with irregular words being expectedly disfluent and regular words being expectedly fluent). Presumably, this discrepancy be-tween the expected and actual fluency was responsible for the higher rate of false recognition (familiarity) for the orthographically regular nonwords than for words and orthographically irregular nonwords (see also Lloyd, Westerman, & Miller, 2003).

Unfortunately, we are not aware of any published research that tested the role of fluency expectations in the domain of evaluative reactions, though, theoretically, some situations should exhibit a similar pattern. This is particularly true when positive affect arises, because fluency indicates unexpectedly good progress in processing. More specifically, when partici-pants expect that perception or understanding of a stimulus will be easy, they should not experience much positive affect for the fluent stimulus. Nevertheless, we argue that in several situations, fluency should continue to be positive even when it is expected. First, fluency can be positive because it reflects low conflict (e.g., absence of cognitive dissonance is good, even when expected) or low effort (e.g., smooth performance is fun, even when expected). Second, fluency can be positive if it signals stimulus quality (e.g., easily recognizable foods are safer, even when expected). In short, we sus-pect that fluency makes people enjoy prototypical faces and clearly written papers even when they have accurate processing expectations for these stimuli.

Attributions

Once an affective experience is elicited by a fluent stimulus, its impact on preference judgments should be moderated by attributional processes. That is, people should not rely on fluency-based experiences when their informa-tional value is called into question. This assumption is consistent with earlier described findings showing that the impact of processing fluency on judgment is eliminated when participants attribute their affective reactions to an irrelevant source, such as a salient repetition scheme (e.g., Bornstein & D'Agostino, 1994; Van den Bergh & Vrana, 1998) or background music (e.g., Winkielman & Fazendeiro, 2006).

THE NEURAL BASIS OF THE FLUENCY, FAMILIARITY, AND AFFECT CONNECTION

Though there is plenty of behavioral evidence for a tight connection between fluency, familiarity, and affect, relatively few neuroscience studies have directly examined this link. This is surprising, especially given what we know about the close overlap between subcortical structures connecting affect and memory (e.g., the hippocampus, the amygdala, and the "reward system" structures are anatomically adjacent and highly interconnected).[3] However, even with the paucity of direct studies, there are several lines of relevant research.

One line of relevant studies comes from research on the dual-process theory of memory (Atkinson & Juola, 1973; Jacoby, 1991; Jacoby & Dallas, 1981; Mandler, 1980). This theory distinguishes between familiarity (defined as a sense of oldness, without recollection of specific details) and recognition (defined by recall of an item in its specific context). Evidence suggests that these processes are supported by distinct neural mechanisms (Rugg & Yonelinas, 2003; see Yonelinas, 2002, for a review). Specifically, familiarity might be supported by the parahippocampal cortex—a polymodal area that serves as a gateway to the hippocampus. Because of its connectivity to early perceptual areas and relatively dense, overlapping way of coding information, the parahippocampal cortex can support fast assessment of the novelty–familiarity dimension of the stimulus, but not for retrieval of specific information about the context of a previous encounter with that particular stimulus. Importantly, the basis of this early assessment could be some fluency-related, nonspecific aspect of processing. For example, computational models have demonstrated that novelty can be roughly assessed using dynamical parameters such as settling time, signal-to-noise ratio, neuronal differentiation, and volatility (Lewenstein & Nowak, 1989; Norman & O'Reilly, 2003). On the other hand, recollection of the item in its specific context may be supported by the hippocampus and more frontal cortical areas. The hippocampus employs a sparse, nonoverlapping way of coding information, which is better suited for storing specific information regarding the context of a memorial event. The frontal areas are associated with explicit processing of event details and use of strategic memory processes.

The dissociation between familiarity and recollection is supported by studies on effects of neuropsychological insults to the temporal lobe and adjacent subcortical structures. Those insults can occasionally produce amnesia on traditional tests of recognition memory but preserve mechanisms supporting familiarity (Moscovitch, Vriezen, & Gottstein, 1993). Importantly, those insults also tend to preserve affective responses to familiar items. For example, patients with Korsakoff syndrome tested with the mere-exposure paradigm show preference for old versus new melodies, despite greatly impaired levels of explicit recognition for the melodies (Johnson, Kim, & Risse, 1985).

Interestingly, other types of neuropsychological insults can preserve overt recognition but impair feelings of familiarity and positivity. Thus patients with Capgras syndrome can explicitly recognize a face but say that the face does not "feel" like the person they know, and they do not show differential autonomic activity to familiar versus unknown faces (Ellis, Young, Quayle, & de Pauw, 1997; Hirstein & Ramachandran, 1997). As a result, these patients claim that close acquaintances (e.g., mothers, spouses) have been replaced by impostors, robots, or aliens that look identical to their loved ones. Studies have shown that the brain areas affected in Capgras syndrome include the temporal cortex (Signer, 1994), as well as the right frontoparietal cortices (Benson, 1994). More specifically, Ellis & Young (1990) also proposed that the syndrome is caused by a failure in communication between areas of ventral stream processing in the temporal lobe (area IT and other face-sensitive areas around the superior temporal sulcus involved in recognition of faces) and the subcortical structures (limbic complex) responsible for generating "warm and familiar" feelings to faces.

Providing further support for a tight link between positive affect and memory, a very recent study found that activation of the medial prefrontal cortex (PFC; manipulated by a gambling task) enhances later recognition of a stimulus (Adcock, Thangavel, Whitfield-Gabrieli, Knutson, & Gabrieli, 2006). The authors propose that this effect is mediated by projections from the mesolimbic dopamine system (involved in reward) to the hippocampus. If so, this connection could underlie a tight link between familiarity and positive affect found in behavioral studies.

Finally, neuroscientific data can help us understand how fluency manipulations can enhance both preferences and familiarity and yet result in subjectively distinct experiences of liking and familiarity. For example, Elliot and Dolan (1998) presented participants with novel or repeated stimuli (the mere-exposure paradigm) under different judgment conditions (recognition and preference). The results showed that repeated, as opposed to novel, stimuli activated the parahippocampal cortex, an area known as a "gateway to memory," as we just discussed. This was true regardless of whether participants judged recognition or preference. However, when participants made recognition judgments, repeated stimuli activated the frontopolar and parietal cortex (areas involved in explicit memory). In contrast, when participants made preference judgments, repeated stimuli activated the medial PFC, an area known for its role in reward processing. These data suggest that in early stages of processing, as the stimuli enter the memory system, fluency (manipulated by repetition) has a nonspecific effect that is similar across different task conditions. However, later processing, shaped by the task context, leads to selective influence of fluency on memory (if the goal is to assess whether this stimulus was encountered previously) or on affect (if the goal is to evaluate stimulus value). Critically, as in studies from our lab, the affective response was genuine and positive, as reflected in activation of the brain's reward system.

SUMMARY AND CONCLUSIONS

In this chapter, we explored how affective and cognitive experiences can derive from the dynamics of information processing. First, we showed that manipulations of perceptual and conceptual fluency increase feelings of familiarity and positivity and argued that this effect underlies some classic preference phenomena, including the mere-exposure and beauty-in-averageness effects, and new phenomena, such as the effect of semantic priming on evaluative judgments. Second, we discussed evidence that positive affect increases feelings of familiarity. Third, we discussed how expectation and attribution can shape and constrain fluency effects on experience and judgments. Fourth, we reviewed some possible neuroscientific bases of the connection between fluency, familiarity, and affect. Throughout the chapter, we presented evidence that fluency is hedonically marked, as reflected in psychological and physiological measures (Winkielman et al., 2003).

We believe that the research reviewed in this chapter makes three general points about the nature of emotion and cognition. First, cognition is not only about *what*—the content of the stimulus—but also about *how*—the perceiver's processing experiences. Second, cognition is inherently "warm"—infused with a hedonic tone that informs the perceiver about the quality of its processing and the value of things in the world. Third, the connection between cognition and emotion is built deep into the neural structures—with intertwined brain mechanisms supporting perception, memory, and affect. Of course, we still know little about what specific brain mechanisms are involved in the connection between fluency, familiarity, and affect, both on the level of immediate reactions and the level of conscious feelings. Thus this research could significantly benefit from studies involving psychological measures, as well as neuroimaging and modeling techniques examining the causal links between fluent processing and affective and memory response. However, even at this point, it seems clear that as we learn more about the psychology and neuroscience of cognition and emotion, we discover more evidence for their interactive nature.

ACKNOWLEDGMENT

This research was supported by National Science Foundation Grant No. BCS-0217294 (to Piotr Winkielman).

NOTES

1. There is good evidence for the influence of conceptual fluency on familiarity. For example, Whittlesea (1993) embedded previously presented target words in either predictive sentences (e.g., "the stormy seas tossed the BOAT") or nonpredictive sentences (e.g., "she saved her money and bought a BOAT"). Targets (e.g., BOAT) embedded in the semantically predictive sentence were pronounced faster, indicating greater fluency, and were more often falsely recognized, indicating greater familiarity.
2. Jacoby and Dallas (1981) were the first to observe that, in making recognition decisions, people are less influenced by an item's absolute fluency and more by the difference between the item's actual fluency and the fluency that could normatively be expected for that item. Specifically, they found that prior study facilitated naming low-frequency words more than it facilitated naming high-frequency words. However, even with this facilitation from prior study, high-frequency words were still named faster than low-frequency words at test. Yet, when making a recognition judgment for a word, participants were apparently more impressed by how much their fluency was facilitated (boosted above baseline) than by their absolute fluency of processing, as low-frequency words were more likely judged to be old than high-frequency words.
3. Of course, we know plenty about the role of the amygdala and related structures in enhancing memory for emotional events (McGaugh, 2000).

REFERENCES

Adcock, R. A., Thangavel, A., Whitfield-Gabrieli, S., Knutson, B., & Gabrieli, J. D. E. (2006). Reward-motivated learning: Mesolimbic activation precedes memory formation. *Neuron, 50,* 507–517.

Atkinson, R. C., & Juola, J. F. (1973). Factors influencing the speed and accuracy of word recognition. In S. Kornblum (Ed.), *Attention and performance: IV* (pp. 583–612). New York: Academic Press.

Benson, D.F. (1994). *The neurology of thinking.* New York: Oxford University Press.

Bonanno, G. A., & Stillings, N. A. (1986). Preference, familiarity, and recognition after repeated brief exposures to random geometric shapes. *American Journal of Psychology, 99,* 403–415.

Bornstein, R. F. (1989). Exposure and affect: Overview and meta-analysis of research 1968–1987. *Psychological Bulletin, 106,* 265–289.

Bornstein, R. F., & D'Agostino, P. R. (1994). The attribution and discounting of perceptual fluency: Preliminary tests of a perceptual fluency/attributional model of the mere exposure effect. *Social Cognition, 12,* 103–128.

Cacioppo, J. T., Petty, R. E., Losch, M. E., & Kim, H. S. (1986). Electro-myographic activity over facial muscle regions can differentiate the valence and intensity of affective reactions. *Journal of Personality and Social Psychology, 50,* 260–268.

Carver, C. S., & Scheier, M. F. (1981). *Attention and self-regulation: A control-theory approach to human behavior.* New York: Springer-Verlag.

Chenier, T., & Winkielman, P. (2006). *Fluency, memory, and liking: How fluency gives raise to judgment and experience.* Manuscript in preparation.

Eich, E., Kihlstrom, J., Bower, G., Forgas, J., & Niedenthal, P. (2000). *Cognition and emotion.* New York: Oxford University Press.

Elliott, R., & Dolan, R. (1998). Neural response during preference and memory judgements for subliminally presented stimuli: A functional neuroimaging study. *Journal of Neuroscience, 18,* 4697–4704.

Ellis, H. D. & Young, A. W. (1990). Accounting for delusional misidentification. *British Journal of Psychiatry, 157,* 239–248.

Ellis, H. D., Young, A. W., Quayle, A. H., & de Pauw, K. W. (1997). Reduced autonomic responses to faces in Capgras delusion. *Proceedings of the Royal Society of London: Series B: Biological Sciences, 264,* 1085–1092.

Ellsworth, P. C., & Scherer, K. R. (2003). Appraisal processes in emotion. In R. J. Davidson, H. Goldsmith, & K. R. Scherer (Eds.), *Handbook of affective sciences* (pp. 572–595). New York: Oxford University Press.

Fazendeiro, T., Winkielman, P., Luo, C., & Lorah, C. (2005). False recognition across meaning, language, and stimulus format: Conceptual relatedness and the feeling of familiarity. *Memory and Cognition, 33,* 249–260.

Fernandez-Duque, D., Baird, J. A., & Posner, M. I. (2000). Executive attention and metacognitive regulation. *Consciousness and Cognition, 9,* 288–307.

Garcia-Marques, T., Mackie, D. M., Claypool, H., & Garcia-Marques, L. (2004). Positivity can cue familiarity. *Personality and Social Psychology Bulletin, 30,* 585–593.

Haber, R. N., & Hershenson, M. (1965). The effects of repeated brief exposures on growth of a percept. *Journal of Experimental Psychology, 69,* 40–46.

Halberstadt, J., & Rhodes, G. (2000). The attractiveness of nonface averages: Implications for an evolutionary explanation of the attractiveness of average faces. *Psychological Science, 4,* 285–289.

Halberstadt, J., & Rhodes, G. (2003). It's not just average faces that are attractive: Computer-manipulated averageness makes birds, fish and automobiles attractive. *Psychonomic Bulletin and Review, 10,* 149–156.

Harmon-Jones, E., & Allen, J. J. B. (2001). The role of affect in the mere exposure effect: Evidence from psychophysiological and individual-differences approaches. *Personality and Social Psychology Bulletin, 27,* 889–898.

Hekkert, P., & van Wieringen, P. C. W. (1990). Complexity and prototypicality as determinants of the appraisal of cubist paintings. *British Journal of Psychology, 81,* 483–495.

Hirstein, W., & Ramachandran, V. S. (1997). Capgras syndrome: A novel probe for understanding the neural representation and familiarity of persons. *Proceedings of the Royal Society of London: Series B. Biological Sciences, 264,* 437–444.

Jacoby, L. L. (1983). Perceptual enhancement: Persistent effects of an experience.

Journal of Experimental Psychology: Learning, Memory, and Cognition, 9, 21–38.

Jacoby, L. L. (1991). A process dissociation framework: Separating automatic and intentional uses of memory. *Journal of Memory and Language, 30,* 513–541.

Jacoby, L. L., Allan, L. G., Collins, J. C., & Larwill, L. K. (1988). Memory influences subjective experience: Noise judgments. *Journal of Experimental Psychology: Learning, Memory, and Cognition, 14,* 240–247.

Jacoby, L. L., & Dallas, M. (1981). On the relationship between autobiographical memory and perceptual learning. *Journal of Experimental Psychology: General, 110,* 306–340.

Jacoby, L. L., Kelley, C. M., & Dywan, J. (1989). Memory attributions. In H. L. Roediger & F. I. M. Craik (Eds.), *Varieties of memory and consciousness: Essays in honour of Endel Tulving* (pp. 391–422). Hillsdale, NJ: Erlbaum.

Jacoby, L. L., & Whitehouse, K. (1989). An illusion of memory: False recognition influenced by unconscious perception. *Journal of Experimental Psychology, 118,* 126–135.

Johnson, M. K., Kim, J. K., & Risse, G. (1985). Do alcoholic Korsakoff's syndrome patients acquire affective reactions? *Journal of Experimental Psychology: Learning, Memory and Cognition, 11,* 22–36.

Kunst-Wilson, W. R., & Zajonc, R. B. (1980). Affective discrimination of stimuli that cannot be recognized. *Science, 207,* 557–558.

Langlois, J. H., & Roggman, L. A. (1990). Attractive faces are only average. *Psychological Science, 1,* 115–121.

Lewenstein, M., & Nowak, A. (1989). Recognition with self-control in neural networks. *Physical Review, 40,* 4652–4664.

Lloyd, M. E., Westerman, D. L., & Miller, J. M. (2003). The fluency heuristic in recognition memory: The effect of repetition. *Journal of Memory and Language, 48,* 603–614.

Mandler, G. (1980). Recognizing: The judgment of previous occurrence. *Psychological Review, 87,* 252–271.

Mandler, G., Nakamura, Y., & Van Zandt, B. J. S. (1987). Nonspecific effects of exposure on stimuli that cannot be recognized. *Journal of Experimental Psychology: Learning, Memory, and Cognition, 15,* 646–648.

Martindale, C., & Moore, K. (1988). Priming, prototypicality, and preference. *Journal of Experimental Psychology: Human Perception and Performance, 14,* 661–670.

McGaugh, J. L. (2000). Memory: A century of consolidation. *Science, 287,* 248–251.

Metcalfe, J., & Shimamura, A. P. (1994). *Metacognition: Knowing about knowing.* Cambridge, MA: MIT Press.

Monin, B. (2003). The warm glow heuristic: When liking leads to familiarity. *Journal of Personality and Social Psychology, 85,* 1035–1048.

Moscovitch, M., Vriezen, E. R., & Gottstein, J. (1993). Implicit tests of memory in patients with focal lesions or degenerative brain disorders. In H. Spinnler & F. Boller (Eds.), *Handbook of neuropsychology* (Vol. 8; pp. 133–173). Amsterdam: Elsevier.

Norman, K. A., & O'Reilly, R. C. (2003). Modeling hippocampal and neocortical contributions to recognition memory: A complementary learning systems approach. *Psychological Review, 110,* 611–646.

Phaf, R. H., & Rotteveel, M. (2005). Affective modulation of recognition bias. *Emotion, 5,* 309–318.

Posner, M. I., & Keele, S. W. (1968). On the genesis of abstract ideas. *Journal of Experimental Psychology, 77,* 353–363.

Reber, P. J., Stark, C. E. L., & Squire, L. R. (1998). Cortical areas supporting category learning identified using functional MRI. *Proceedings of the National Academy of Sciences of the USA, 95,* 747–750.

Reber, R., Winkielman, P., & Schwarz, N. (1998). Effects of perceptual fluency on affective judgments. *Psychological Science, 9,* 45–48.

Rhodes, G., & Tremewan, T. (1996). Averageness, exaggeration, and facial attractiveness. *Psychological Science, 7,* 105–110.

Rhodes, G., Yoshikawa, S., Clark, A., Lee, K., McKay, R., & Akamatsu, S. (2001). Attractiveness of facial averageness and symmetry in non-Western cultures: In search of biologically based standards of beauty. *Perception, 30,* 611–625.

Rhodes, G., Zebrowitz, L. A., Clark, A., Kalick, S. M., Hightower, A., & McKay, R. (2001). Do facial averageness and symmetry signal health? *Evolution and Human Behavior, 22,* 31–46.

Rugg, M. D., & Yonelinas, A. P. (2003). Human recognition memory: A cognitive neuroscience perspective. *Trends in Cognitive Sciences, 7,* 313–319.

Schachter, S., & Singer, J. E. (1962). Cognitive, social and physiological determinants of emotional state. *Psychological Review, 69,* 379–399.

Schwarz, N. (1990). Feelings as information: Informational and motivational functions of affective states. In E. T. Higgins & R. M. Sorrentino (Eds.), *Handbook of motivation and cognition: Vol. 2. Foundations of social behavior* (pp. 527–561). New York: Guilford Press.

Schwarz, N. (1998). Accessible content and accessibility experiences: The interplay of declarative and experiential information in judgment. *Personality and Social Psychology Review, 2,* 87–99.

Seamon, J. G., Brody, N., & Kauff, D. M. (1983). Affective discrimination of stimuli that are not recognized: Effects of shadowing, masking, and central laterality. *Journal of Experimental Psychology: Learning, Memory and Cognition, 9,* 544–555.

Seamon, J. G., McKenna, P. A., & Binder, N. (1998). The mere exposure effect is differentially sensitive to different judgment tasks. *Consciousness and Cognition, 7,* 85–102.

Signer, S.F. (1994). Localization and lateralization in the delusion of substitution. *Psychopathology, 27,* 168–176.

Symons, D. (1979). *The evolution of human sexuality.* Oxford, UK: Oxford University Press.

Thornhill, R., & Gangestad, S. W. (1993). Human facial beauty. *Human Nature, 4,* 237–269.

van den Bergh, O., & Vrana, S. R. (1998). Repetition and boredom in a perceptual fluency/attribution model of affective judgments. *Cognition and Emotion, 12,* 533–553.

Whitfield, T. W., & Slatter, P. E. (1979). The effects of categorization and prototypicality on aesthetic choice in a furniture selection task. *British Journal of Psychology, 70,* 65–75.

Whittlesea, B., & Price, J. (2001). Implicit/explicit memory versus analytic/nonanalytic processing: Rethinking the mere exposure effect. *Memory and Cognition, 29,* 234–246.

Whittlesea, B., & Williams, L. (2000). The source of feelings of familiarity: The discrepancy-attribution hypothesis. *Journal of Experimental Psychology: Learning, Memory, and Cognition, 26,* 547–565.

Whittlesea, B. W. A. (1993). Illusions of familiarity. *Journal of Experimental Psychology: Learning, Memory, and Cognition, 19,* 1235–1253.

Whittlesea, B. W. A., Jacoby, L. L., & Girard, K. (1990). Illusions of immediate memory: Evidence of an attributional basis for feelings of familiarity and perceptual quality. *Journal of Memory and Language, 29,* 716–732.

Whittlesea, B. W. A., & Williams, L.D. (1998). Why do strangers feel familiar, but friends don't? The unexpected basis of feelings of familiarity. *Acta Psychologica, 98,* 141–166.

Wilson, W. R. (1979). Feeling more than we can know: Exposure effects without learning. *Journal of Personality and Social Psychology, 37,* 811–821.

Winkielman, P., & Cacioppo, J. T. (2001). Mind at ease puts a smile on the face: Psychophysiological evidence that processing facilitation increases positive affect. *Journal of Personality and Social Psychology, 81,* 989–1000.

Winkielman, P., & Fazendeiro, T. A. (2006). *The role of conceptual fluency in preference and memory.* Manuscript in preparation.

Winkielman, P., Halberstadt, J., Fazendeiro, T., & Catty, S. (2006). Prototypes are attractive because they are easy on the mind. *Psychological Science, 17,* 799–806.

Winkielman, P., Schwarz, N., Fazendeiro, T., & Reber, R. (2003). The hedonic marking of processing fluency: Implications for evaluative judgment. In J. Musch & K. C. Klauer (Eds.), *The psychology of evaluation: Affective processes in cognition and emotion.* (pp. 189–217). Mahwah, NJ: Erlbaum.

Witherspoon, D., & Allan, L. G. (1985). The effects of a prior presentation on temporal judgments in a perceptual identification task. *Memory and Cognition, 13,* 103–111.

Yonelinas, A. P. (2002). The nature of recollection and familiarity: A review of 30 years of research. *Journal of Memory and Language, 46,* 441–517.

Zajonc, R. B. (1968). Attitudinal effects of mere exposure. *Journal of Personality and Social Psychology* [Monograph Suppl.], *9,* 1–27.

Zajonc, R. B. (2001). Mere exposure: A gateway to the subliminal. *Current Directions in Psychological Science, 10,* 224–228.

14

The X- and C-Systems

THE NEURAL BASIS OF AUTOMATIC
AND CONTROLLED SOCIAL COGNITION

Matthew D. Lieberman

The distinction between automatic and controlled processing is one of the most important theoretical distinctions made in social cognition. Our understanding of stereotyping (Banaji & Hardin, 1996; Devine, 1989; Macrae, Milne, & Bodenhausen, 1994), attitudes (Wilson, Lindsey, & Schooler, 2000), persuasion (Chaiken, Liberman, & Eagly, 1989; Petty & Cacioppo, 1986), person perception (Gilbert, 1989; Trope, 1986), self-regulation (Wegner, 1994), and mood effects (Bless & Schwarz, 1999; Forgas, 1995) has been transformed through the use of cognitive measures to assess automaticity and control. These measures have included reaction-time measures, manipulating interstimulus intervals, introducing cognitive load, subliminal priming versus drawing attention to the possible consequences of priming, sequential priming, memory clustering, and word-stem completion, among others (Bargh & Chartrand, 2000). But as with all measures, these have their limits. In this chapter, I hope to suggest that social cognitive neuroscience (Ochsner & Lieberman, 2001) offers additional theoretical and methodological tools that can be marshaled in the effort to better understand the automatic and controlled bases of social cognition.

One of the most fundamental limitations of the dual-process literature (Chaiken & Trope, 1999) is that automaticity and control are defined as opposing anchors on a number of dimensions. Controlled processes are those that score high on dimensions of awareness, effort, intention, and inefficiency (Bargh, 1996). Automatic processes are those that score low on at least one and preferably most of these dimensions. Unfortunately, this mostly paints a picture of what automaticity is not, rather than focusing on what automaticity is.

Whether automatic and controlled processes are endpoints on a continuum or qualitatively distinct processes is an empirical question. However, the traditional measures available to assess automaticity and control do not address the question, instead assuming a dimensional approach from the start. For instance, adding a secondary task (i.e., a cognitive-load manipulation) to be performed concurrently with the process of interest allows for the assessment of efficiency. Processes that are more affected by the secondary task are less efficient and therefore more controlled than processes that are less affected. This analysis provides only relative positioning on the dimension of efficiency but does not and cannot qualitatively identify or even posit boundaries between automaticity and control. However, one can imagine very different accounts of efficiency differences. On the one hand, some task that is performed with great efficiency may have become more automatic over time, moving from one end of the continuum toward the other, with the process's internal structure becoming solidified and more efficient. Alternatively, different processes may simultaneously support the task when the task is performed at different degrees of efficiency. Some processes may be specialized for performing new tasks, but never with great efficiency. Other processes may operate very efficiently but require a great deal of task experience until they develop to the point of being able to support task performance alone.

At root, this latter account allows for the possibility that qualitatively distinct processes could be at work without easily being identified as such with current measures (cf. Logan, 1988). Moreover, on many cognitive measures a person who is impulsive because of heightened automatic impulses would be indistinguishable from someone who is impulsive because of deficient control processes. In both cases, one would conclude that the individual's cognitive activity is more automatic than controlled, but the causes would be qualitatively different in the two cases, as would the treatments if the impairment was sufficiently severe.

If automatic and controlled components of social cognition can be studied separately from one another, it may help address numerous questions, such as: What is the representational structure of each type of process? Why do attempts at self-control often have paradoxical effects? Why do automatic processes appear to be both rigid (Kawakami et al., 2000) and flexible (Lowery, Hardin, & Sinclair, 2001; Mitchell, Nosek, & Banaji, 2003)? How can controlled processes interfere with automatic processes?

THE COGNITIVE NEUROSCIENCE REVOLUTION

The issue of whether the differences between automatic and controlled social cognition should be conceived quantitatively or qualitatively is no different from many of the interpretive problems that have faced cognitive scientists for decades. Cognitive psychologists noted long ago that data from cognitive measures will always be consistent with multiple, and potentially infinite, theories or models (Anderson, 1978). Gilbert (1999) made the same assessment of dual-process models of social cognition and concluded that we may be limited to ruling out particular models without ever being able to determine the truth of the matter. Cognitive science's response to this limitation of cognitive measures provides hope. Starting in the 1980s, cognitive scientists began turning to brain data on a regular basis to contrast models of cognition and created the field of cognitive neuroscience in the process. In a long-standing debate over whether memory should be characterized as one or several systems, Schacter (1992) demonstrated with neuropsychological data, and later with neuroimaging data, that multiple memory systems exist. In another debate over whether visual imagery relies on the same or different processes as visual perception, Kosslyn (1994) used neuroimaging techniques to show that the same brain regions are involved in both and therefore that visual imagery recruits perceptual processes.

It is my hope that the study of automatic and controlled social cognition will similarly benefit from incorporating cognitive neuroscience approaches. To begin this process, my collaborators and I have developed a model of the neural bases of automatic and controlled social cognition (Lieberman, in press; Satpute & Lieberman, 2006). Our model starts from an assumption that automatic and controlled processes are qualitatively distinct, separately evolved, and functionally intertwined mechanisms. Importantly, this assumption is falsifiable and thus is a starting point rather than an ending point.

THE X- AND C-CYSTEMS

In characterizing what we believe to be the two neural systems responsible for automatic and controlled social cognition, we named one system the *X-system*, named for the *x* in reflexive, and the other the *C-system*, named for the *c* in reflective (Lieberman, Gaunt, Gilbert & Trope, 2002). Because the derivation of these two systems came from cognitive, phenomenological, and neural sources, there are many ways in which these systems are not simply automaticity and control with new names (for a review, see Lieberman et al., 2002). Nevertheless, it is fair to say that the X-system is largely responsible for social processes that would be designated as automatic and the C-system is largely responsible for social processes that would be designated as controlled. For the purposes of this chapter, I highlight the similarities more than the differences.

It is worth noting that the word "system" is being used in a loose rather than a strict sense here. That is to say, the X- and C-systems do not differ as much, are not as discrete, and are not as independent as, for instance, the visual system and the digestive system. The X- and C-systems are not conceived as hermetically sealed Fodorian modules. Both the X- and C-systems function to process socioemotional information, and these two systems often work hand in hand to achieve socioemotional goals. However, each system has a collection of qualities that are relatively absent in the other system, and, for the most part, the subregions of each system often coactivate when one system's particular qualities are most adapted to current demands.

In this section, I review the brain regions nominated to each system and the original rationale for including them. On a personal note, I must admit that there was a certain degree of exploration in the conceptual development of these systems because cognitive neuroscience had not yet shown much of an interest in social cognition. I asked researchers where we might expect to find activations associated with schemas, implicit prejudice, self-focused attention, and intuitive processing and discovered that these were largely unexplored issues in brain research. As a result, I have assumed that the early proposals for the X- and C-systems would seem incomplete, inaccurate, and probably naive through the eyes of history. However, the distinction between automaticity and control is so crucial to social cognition that it seemed imperative to map out this distinction as well as possible and then update it as required by the data.

The X-System

The main criterion for a system to be nominated for inclusion in the X-system was that it be activated under conditions that promote automatic, implicit, or nonconscious processing of social information. These structures also tend to be phylogentically older than structures in the C-system and are more conserved across species. According to these criteria, the X-system (see Figure 14.1) is composed of the amygdala, basal ganglia, lateral temporal cortex (LTC), ventromedial prefrontal cortex (VMPFC), and dorsal anterior cingulate cortex (dACC). The dACC is a recent addition to the X-system (Eisenberger & Lieberman, 2004) and is discussed in some detail later in the chapter, as it was originally included in the C-system, although always with certain caveats.

The amygdalae are almond-shaped subcortical structures located within the poles of each of the temporal lobes. There is ongoing debate about the amygdala's function; however, it does appear to be sensitive to novel and emotionally evocative stimuli (LeDoux, 1996; Wright et al., 2001). A recent meta-analysis suggests that it responds more to stimuli that are negatively rather than positively valenced (Wager, Phan, Liberzon, & Taylor, 2003). It is critical to fear conditioning in animals (Fanselow & LeDoux, 1999). Additionally, for individuals who have amygdala lesions, there can be major disturbances of automatic social cognition (Heberlein & Adolphs,

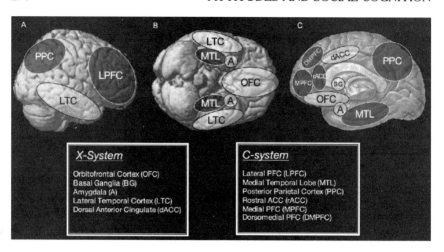

FIGURE 14.1. Neural correlates of the C-system and X-system displayed on a canonical brain rendering from (A) side, (B) bottom, and (C) medial views. Note: the hippocampus, nucleus accumbens, and amygdala are subcortical structures that are displayed here on the cortical surface for ease of presentation.

2004). This region projects to various other regions that allow it to serve as something of an alarm, triggering top-down controlled processes in prefrontal cortex and autonomic nervous system responses that shift energy resources in the body to prepare for fight or flight. Most relevant to the X-system, however, are the numerous studies that have demonstrated that the amygdala responds to subliminal and unseen presentations of threatening images (Cunningham et al., 2004; Liddell et al., 2005; Morris, Öhman, & Dolan, 1999; Pasley, Mayes, & Schultz, 2004; Whalen et al., 1998).

The basal ganglia are curved horn-like subcortical structures that appear to be involved in the automatic components of affect, cognition, and behavior. The basal ganglia are best known for their central role in movement disorders such as Parkinson's disease and Huntington's disease; however, these disorders also lead to various social and affective deficits, including deficits in nonverbal communication (Lieberman, 2000a). In the past decade, a number of neuropsychological and neuroimaging studies have established that the caudate, a substructure within the basal ganglia, is involved in implicit learning of abstract sequential patterns that may subserve human intuition (Knowlton, Mangels, & Squire, 1996; Lieberman, Chang, Chiao, Bookheimer, & Knowlton, 2004). Finally, the ventral striatum, another subregion of the basal ganglia, has been linked to positive affective responses to stimuli ranging from drugs to money to pictures of romantic partners (Bartels & Zeki, 2000; Breiter et al., 1997; Zalla et al., 2000).

VMPFC is the region of cortex at the intersection of the medial wall of prefrontal cortex and the orbital or bottom surface of prefrontal cortex. The damage to the famous patient Phineas Gage was primarily in VMPFC, and Gage's deficits in social cognition are well known (Damasio, 1994). It is only in the past decade, however, that data are beginning to demonstrate that the deficits associated with VMPFC damage are more automatic in nature. Damasio and colleagues (Bechara, Damasio, Tranel, & Damasio, 1997) have suggested that this region is involved in social intuition because it is critical to learning the long-term value of different alternatives in a gambling paradigm. For those who have VMPFC intact, accurate intuitions are formed about the different alternatives before explanations can be generated for the fact that some alternatives are better than others. Thus the learning appears to be implicit, as in the basal ganglia, at least for some period of time. Milne and Grafman (2001) have also observed that patients with VMPFC damage do not show evidence of implicit gender stereotyping on the Implicit Association Test (IAT; Greenwald, McGhee, & Schwartz, 1998). Most recently, Deppe et al. (2005) demonstrated that susceptibility to framing effects is positively related to activity in VMPFC. Framing effects have been considered a consequence of capitalizing on operational properties of intuitive over deductive reasoning (Kahneman, 2003), further supporting the role of VMPFC in conjunction with the basal ganglia in the formation of automatic intuitions. Finally, a recent ERP study (Carretie, Hinojosa, Mercado, & Tapia, 2005) localized early responses (~150 millieconds) to subliminally presented threat stimuli to VMPFC meeting two criteria of the X-system in sensitivity of subliminal presentations and speed of response.

Unlike the other regions of the X-system, LTC, consisting of the lateral and inferior portions of the temporal lobes as well as the temporal poles, is primarily associated with semantic rather than affective processes. A degenerative brain disorder called semantic dementia (or the temporal variant of frontotemporal dementia) selectively affects LTC and produces major deficits in semantic knowledge while largely sparing memory for particular episodes (Garrard & Hodges, 2000; Mummery et al., 2000). A number of studies have now observed LTC activations associated with implicit semantic processing (Crinion, Lambon-Ralph, Warburton, Howard, & Wise, 2003; Mummery, Shallice, & Price, 1999; Rissman, Eliassen, & Blumstein, 2003; Rossell, Bullmore, Williams, & David, 2001) and have found that explicit or intentional semantic processes recruit lateral prefrontal cortex in addition to LTC (Lee, Robbins, Graham, & Owen, 2002; Xu et al., 2002). Additionally, the multistaged pathway from visual cortex to the temporal poles is massively parallel (Suzuki, Saleem, & Tanaka, 2000; Vogels, 1999), an architecture that appears to promote efficient but nonsymbolic processes (Smolensky, 1988). Lastly, the posterior superior temporal sulcus, a subregion of LTC, is critical to nonverbal decoding of facial expressions, a process that is probably automatic given how little effort or intention is applied in determining the implication of most facial expressions (Ambady & Rosenthal, 1992).

The C-System

Nominating brain regions for the C-system required much less of an exploratory approach (guesswork) than the X-system because cognitive neuroscientists were already examining various networks relevant to controlled processing in their study of conflict detection, working memory, and episodic memory. From these lines of research, the C-system was posited to consist of anterior cingulate cortex (ACC), lateral prefrontal cortex (LPFC), posterior parietal cortex (PPC), and the hippocampus and surrounding medial temporal lobe region (MTL). In the current formulation, only the rostral anterior cingulate cortex (rACC) is included in the C-system, as is discussed in the next section. Medial prefrontal cortex (MPFC), particularly the medial portion of Brodmann's area 10, may be another good candidate region for the C-system, as it appears to be involved in self-focused attention (Gusnard, Akbudak, Shulman, & Raichle, 2001) and is a region that is disproportionately larger in humans than in other animals (Semendeferi, Schleicher, Zilles, Armstrong, & Van Hoesen, 2001).

LPFC is the heart of the C-system, as it is involved in numerous higher cognitive processes that are experienced as intentional and effortful, including working memory, implementation of top-down goals and plans, episodic retrieval, inhibition, and self-control (Cabeza & Nyberg, 2000). Though only rarely linked experimentally, working memory processes and controlled processes operate under similar constraints—functioning serially, rather than in parallel; operating on discrete symbolic representations and propositions; and limited by motivation, intention, and effort (Baddeley, 1986). Whereas X-system processes may be linked to our ongoing experience of the world, coloring in the semantic and affective aspects of the stream of consciousness, the C-system, and LPFC in particular, appears to be linked to our experience of responding to the world and our own impulses with our freely exerted "will" (Lau, Rogers, Ramnani, & Passingham, 2004).

Lateral posterior parietal cortex (LPPC) is thought to support many of the same functions attributed to LPFC, including working memory, controlled processing, and logic (Cabeza & Nyberg, 2000). A number of recent neuroimaging studies also suggest that medial PPC is involved in self-focused attention (Gusnard et al., 2001; Kelley, et al., 2002, Lieberman & Pfeifer, 2005), as well as in distinguishing one's own perspective from that of another (Ruby & Decety, 2001), both tasks that require effort and symbolic representations.

The hippocampus and surrounding MTL are included in the C-system because of their role in supporting episodic memory and the relation of episodic memory to controlled processing. One of the general functions of the frontal lobe and controlled processing is to exert control and override the X-system (and other habit-based processes such as motor functions) when the habits and impulses of the X-system are insufficient or contextually inappropriate (McClelland, McNaughton, & O'Reilly, 1995; Miller & Cohen, 2001; Sloman, 1996). Although the C-system is enormously flexible in its ability to create and implement new symbolic solutions in these situations, the C-system is also fragile because it processes information serially, which limits its speed and the number of problems that can be handled simultaneously. Additionally, there is growing evidence to suggest that controlled processes are analogous to muscles in that they can tire with continuous or intense use (Baumeister, Bratslavsky, Muraven, & Tice, 1998).

One way to greatly enhance the efficiency of the C-system would be to keep a repository of memories for the different times that the C-system was invoked to override the X-system. Such a repository would be called on when the same situation was encountered again, allowing the C-system to focus on implementing a plan rather than having to first deliberate to generate the plan anew. If a situation is encountered frequently enough, the X-system will change its habits to accommodate the situation; but the X-system is very slow to change, and thus these C-system memories would be very useful in the interim. Episodic memory can be characterized, in part, as a storehouse of memories for specific episodes when the C-system was engaged because things were running counter to expectations and one's habits were insufficient to guide behavior in a particular situation.

Since the 1970s, cognitive psychologists have known that "depth of processing" correlates with the strength of episodic memories; the more cognitive elaboration performed, the more likely the episodic memory will be successfully retrieved later (Craik & Tulving, 1975). The studies of patients like H.M., who are amnesic because of lesions to MTL, have suggested that MTL serves as the representational storehouse for episodic memories. Recent neuroimaging research has demonstrated that the success of episodic retrieval is predicted by the amount of activity in MTL, as well as LPFC (Brewer, Zhao, Desmond, Glover, & Gabrieli, 1998; Wagner et al., 1998). Moreover, the link between depth of processing and subsequent encoding has been tied to processing in the MTL and other regions of the C-system (Fujii et al., 2002). It appears, then, that the more work that is performed by the LPFC to override X-system habits, the better the long-term episodic memory is for that information.

Dorsal and Rostral ACC

In previous discussions of the X- and C-systems, the anterior cingulate cortex (ACC) was included as a C-system structure, but always with caveats. The ACC functions, in part, as a conflict monitor detecting when expectations are violated or contextually inappropriate responses might be made (Botvinick, Braver, Barch, Carter, & Cohen, 2001). As such, the ACC is something of an alarm system, triggering controlled processes, particularly in LPFC, to override contextually inappropriate responses. The prototypical example of ACC function is demonstrated in the Stroop task, when, for instance, one is required to say the ink color of a word (*blue*) although the word itself spells out another color ("R-E-D"). The ACC is thought to be critical in notifying LPFC that it needs to override the prepotent word-reading response. As the starting point in detecting the need for and triggering many controlled processes, it seemed appropriate to include the ACC in the C-system. However, part of the elegance of the connectionist models of ACC function is that the models explain how the ACC can detect conflict automatically, without having to posit an autonomous homunculus inside the ACC that guides the ACC through symbolic decision processes. One of the natural outputs of connectionist architectures is a tension parameter that reflects the total amount of tension in the system (Cohen, Dunbar, & McClelland, 1990; Hopfield, 1982).

More recently, Eisenberger and Lieberman (2004) have suggested that the dACC should be identified as an X-system structure, whereas the rACC should remain as part of the C-system. Eisenberger and Lieberman reviewed a number of cognition, affect, and pain studies and found that in each of these domains, dACC activations were associated with processes that could be characterized by nonsymbolic tension processes, whereas rACC activations were associated with processes for which a symbolic representation of what would or did constitute expectancy violations was explicitly held in mind. For instance, unexpected pain stimulation tends to activate dACC, whereas anticipation of pain activates rACC (Ploghaus, Becerra, Borras, & Borsook, 2003). Similarly, negative emotions, which are focused on a specific object or outcome, tend to activate rACC, whereas anxiety, which has been defined as similar to fear but without explicit focus on a specific object or outcome, tends to activate dACC. Additionally, Smith (1945) observed that in macaques, the entire ACC was morphologically analogous to human dACC. In other words, primates that lack the capacity for true symbolic processing (Thompson & Oden, 2000) have no rACC. More recent evidence points to "spindle cells" (Nimchinsky et al., 1999) that appear in rACC but not dACC and that are present in diminishing densities in the ACC of children and other primates paralleling the diminished symbolic capacities in these groups (Craig, 2004).

EVIDENCE FOR INDEPENDENCE OF THE SYSTEMS

The data used to nominate the brain regions to the X- and C-systems were largely obtained by considering the properties of each system separately. A number of more recent studies have specifically examined how neural activity in these systems changes as processing conditions are altered to favor automatic or controlled processing. By and large, these studies suggest that conditions favoring automatic processing tend to promote X-system activation with little C-system activation, whereas conditions favoring controlled processing tend to promote C-system activation with little X-system activation. It should be remembered that, whereas experimental tasks can be created that emphasize the processes of one system or the other, in everyday life, these two systems are often working together and simultaneously.

Category Learning

In one early study, Rauch et al. (1995) had participants perform a sequence learning task in which cues appeared in a nonrandom but nonobvious sequence of locations on the screen and participants produced location-specific responses as quickly as possible. Approximately half of the participants reported becoming aware of the pattern. Both aware and unaware participants showed evidence of sequence learning, as indicated by slowed reaction times when the learned sequence was interrupted and replaced by a random sequence; however, the brain activations were different for participants who were aware and those who were unaware. Participants who were unaware activated the basal ganglia in the X-system during task performance, whereas participants who were aware of the sequence did not activate the basal ganglia but instead activated the LPFC in the C-system.

In a similar study, Aizenstein et al. (2000) had participants perform a pattern learning task. In the first half of the study, participants were unaware that the dot arrays presented were all variations on a never-presented prototype (Posner & Keele, 1968). In this condition, implicit learning was associated with activation of the LTC in the X-system. Subsequently, participants were run through another block of trials, but this time they were informed that there was a pattern to be learned. Under these explicit learning conditions, the LTC activation disappeared and was replaced by C-system activations in LPFC, MTL, and PPC.

Attitudinal Prejudice

A number of fMRI studies have looked at the neural underpinnings of race-related processes. The general finding across these studies is greater amygdala activity to African American (AA) faces than to Caucasian American (CA) faces (Hart et al., 2000; Cunningham et al., 2004; Lieberman, Hariri, Jarcho, Eisenberger, & Bookheimer, 2005; Phelps et al., 2000) which is consistent with the negative stereotype of African Americans and the amygdala's responsiveness to negative or threatening stimuli. Several findings suggest that the amygdala's response to AA faces reflects an automatic rather than a controlled process. First, Phelps et al. (2000) observed that the magnitude of the amygdala response to AA faces varied as a function of implicit, but not explicit, attitudes toward African Americans. Additionally, Cunningham et al. (2004) found that subliminal presentation of

AA faces produced greater amygdala activity than supraliminal presentation of AA faces. Finally, Lieberman et al. (2005) found that African American participants also showed greater amygdala activity in response to AA faces than to CA faces. This is consistent with the behavioral research showing that African Americans have negative implicit attitudes but positive explicit attitudes toward African Americans (Nosek, Banaji, & Greenwald, 2002).

Alternatively, when negative stereotypes and attitude objects were processed verbally, enhanced activity occurred in right LPFC, but no significant activity occurred in the amygdala. Cunningham et al. (2003) found that judging the attitudinal valence of infamous names such as Adolf Hitler produced right LPFC activity; however, judging whether these were the names of living or dead individuals did not produce this activity. That this effect emerged only when judging valence is important because it indicates that the LPFC activity was dependent on explicit consideration of one's attitudes toward the targets rather than a simple result of reading the names, which would produce implicit effects as well. In the Lieberman et al. (2005) study of race-related processing, a second condition required participants to categorize faces according to race using verbal labels. In this condition, there was activity in right LPFC very close to the region found in the Cunningham et al. (2003) study during verbal categorization of AA faces compared with CA faces. Finally, in a neuroimaging study of automatic behavior (Lieberman, Eisenberger, & Crockett, 2006), the processing of words related to the negative stereotype of the elderly produced greater right LPFC activity in the same region seen in the previous studies when compared with the processing of words related to the relatively positive stereotype of intelligence.

Self-Knowledge

Another area in which a significant amount of social cognitive neuroscience research has been conducted is the domain of self-knowledge (for reviews, see Lieberman & Eisenberger, 2004; Lieberman & Pfeifer, 2005). The most reliable findings are that self-judgments tend to be associated with MPFC and medial PPC. Given that these are the same regions that tend to be observed in studies of self-focused attention (Eisenberger, Lieberman, & Satpute, 2005; Gusnard et al., 2001), it is unclear whether these activations are associated with self-knowledge per se or with the retrieval of self-knowledge through self-focused processing.

Lieberman, Jarcho, and Satpute (2004) recently conducted an fMRI study in which self-knowledge judgments in high-experience and low-experience domains were compared. Our assumption was that actors would tend to be schematic for actor-relevant traits and nonschematic for athlete-relevant traits, whereas athletes would tend to show the opposite relationship (Markus, 1977). In other words, we expected each group to process high-experience words more automatically than low-experience words, and indeed, reaction-time data bore out this assumption. Additionally, high-experience self-judgments activated VMPFC, basal ganglia, amygdala, and LTC in the X-system, along with PPC in the C-system. Alternatively, low-experience judgments produced only a C-system activation in LPFC.

Further inspection of the reaction-time data in this study indicated that approximately half of our participants did not show evidence of schematicity in their high-experience domain. Even though we selected people who clearly have much more experience in one domain than the other, some simply may not have had or used schemas in their high-experience domain. Consequently, all of the data were analyzed separately for schematics and nonschematics. When schematics made high-experience self-judgments, they produced increased activity in the VMPFC, basal ganglia, amygdala, LTC, and PPC and decreased activity in MTL and MPFC. Thus schematics tended to activate X-system structures and deactivate C-system structures when they made high-experience self-judgments. Nonschematics showed nearly the opposite pattern when they made high-experience self-judgments. Nonschematics produced increased activity in MTL, LPFC, MPFC, PPC, and LTC, along with no increases in X-system activity.

The results of this study provide strong evidence that automatic processes are not merely faster, quieter versions of controlled processes. If the representations used during automatic and controlled processes were the same, then one might expect controlled processing regions to show decreases for high-experience judgments without any concomitant increases elsewhere. In fact, some nonsocial forms of automaticity seem to follow this pattern (Jansma, Ramsey, Slagter, & Kahn, 2001). However, in our study, C-system decreases were matched by X-system increases, suggesting that two separate systems actively process social information under different conditions.

Personality

Extraversion has been frequently associated with positive affect and happiness, whereas neuroticism has been associated with negative affect and anxiety. There is also some evidence to suggest that extraverts and neurotics tend to differ with respect to automatic and controlled processing. Across several studies, extraverts were found to have greater working memory efficiency than introverts and thus were better able to handle multiple social-interaction goals simultaneously (Lieberman, 2000b; Lieberman & Rosenthal, 2001; Oya, Manalo, & Greenwood, 2004). Alternatively, trait anxiety, which is a construct similar to neuroticism, has been associated with greater automatic interference effects (Egloff & Hock, 2001) and diminished working-memory efficiency (Darke, 1988).

Eisenberger, Lieberman, and Satpute (2005) examined the neural reactivities associated with neuroticism and extraversion in an oddball task that combined conflict detection with exertion of control through response inhibition. As described earlier, we believe dACC and rACC to be involved in nonsymbolic and symbolic conflict detection, respectively, whereas LPFC is involved in response inhibition. In this study, neuroticism was positively correlated with the dACC response to conflict detection and negatively correlated with the rACC response to conflict detection. In contrast, extraversion was negatively correlated with the dACC response to conflict detection but positively correlated with the rACC, LPFC, and PPC responses to conflict detection. These results approximately replicate those of Gray and Braver (2002), who found similar personality correlations with the dACC and rACC. Together, these results suggest that extraverts tend to emphasize C-system processing, whereas neurotics tend to emphasize components of X-system processing, particularly those involved in automatic detection of threats and conflict.

EVIDENCE FOR C-SYSTEM REGULATION OF THE X-SYSTEM

The previous section reviewed research that suggests that during different kinds of social cognition, structures associated with the X- and C-systems tend to coactivate more with other structures from the same system than with structures from the other system. Additionally, these studies show that under processing conditions that favor automatic processing, X-system structures tend to be more active than C-system structures, whereas during conditions that favor controlled processing, C-system structures tend to be more active than X-system structures. These data suggest that qualitatively distinct systems support automatic and controlled social cognition. Although the conditions that are typically associated with eliciting automatic or controlled processing tend to vary in terms of awareness of stimuli and cognitive load, a central component of the X- and C-system's model is that the C-system has largely evolved to override the X-system when the habits and impulses of the X-system are contextually inappropriate. In this section, I review studies that demonstrate not only that the C-system is activated under different conditions than the X-system but also that the magnitude of C-system activity in these conditions is negatively correlated with X-system activity. In other words, these studies suggest that C-system activity can inhibit X-system activity.

Emotion Regulation

A number of recent studies have looked at intentional attempts at emotion regulation in neuroimaging paradigms (Beauregard, Levesque, & Bourgouin, 2001; Levesque et al., 2003; Ochsner et al., 2004; Schaefer et al., 2003; Small et al., 2001). In general, these studies show the same pattern of X- and C-system activity as reviewed earlier, with greater amygdala activity during passive viewing of emotionally evocative images and greater LPFC activity during attempts at emotion regulation by way of reappraisal or suppression (Gross, 1998). One of these studies has looked at the relationship between X- and C-system regions during reappraisal attempts at emotion regulation. Ochsner, Bunge, Gross, and Gabrieli (2002) asked participants to passively view negatively valenced images in one condition and observed activation in the amygdala and VMPFC. However, in a second condition, participants were asked to reappraise each image by reinterpreting the photo "so that it no longer elicited a negative response" (p. 1225). In this condition, LPFC was active, but neither of the amygdala or VMPFC activations observed in the passive viewing condition were present.

In subsequent functional connectivity analyses, Ochsner et al. (2002) examined the between-subject differences in the C- and X-system activity during reappraisal. Ochsner et al. (2002) found that the greater the magnitude of the LPFC response was during reappraisal, the smaller the magnitude of the amygdala and VMPFC responses were during reappraisal. In other words, during reappraisal, some participants activated the LPFC a lot and others just a little. The more any participant activated LPFC, the greater the reduction in X-system activity. This analysis suggests that the C-system is not merely "speaking more loudly" than the X-system. Rather, it appears that, under certain circumstances, while the C-system is speaking up, it is also taking away the X-system's "microphone," so that its volume is diminished.

Affect Labeling

Another set of studies have examined the effects of affective labeling on the amygdala's response to negatively valenced images (Hariri, Bookheimer, & Mazziotta, 2000; Lange et al., 2003; Lieberman et al., in press; Taylor, Phan, Decker, & Liberzon, 2003). Philosophers have long suggested that thinking explicitly about one's affect can dampen the affect that is being reflected on (James, 1890/1950; Spinoza, 1675/1949). Although thinking about or labeling one's affect is not an emotion-regulation strategy per se, it may be a mechanism by which other emotion-regulation strategies have their effect. In other words, part of reappraisal's effectiveness may be due to the fact that it involves linguistic processing of affective stimuli and thus recruits the brain regions involved in affective labeling.

Similar to the studies of overt emotion regulation, these studies of linguistic regulation of emotion tend to find amygdala activity present during passive viewing of negatively valenced images, but this activity is absent or attenuated during explicit or linguistic processing of the images' affective content ("affect labeling"). During affect labeling, amygdala activity is replaced by right LPFC activity. In two of these studies (Hariri et al., 2000, Lieberman et al., in press), functional connectivity between LPFC and the amygdala during affect labeling was assessed and found to be significantly negative; the greater the LPFC activity during labeling, the weaker the amygdala activity. These data suggest that merely activating this C-system region may be sufficient to down-regulate X-system activity, even in the absence of any explicit intention to self-regulate.

Attitudinal Prejudice

Some of the previously described studies of attitudes also examined functional connectivity. In each of the studies, during controlled processing of attitudinal objects, LPFC activity was negatively correlated with amygdala activity. Cunningham et al. (2004) found that in response to supraliminal but not subliminal presentations of AA faces, increases in right LPFC predicted reductions in the magnitude of amygdala response. Lieberman et al. (2005) observed that right ventral LPFC activity while linguistically labeling the race of AA faces was negatively correlated with amygdala activity. Finally, in a study of automatic behavior (Lieberman, Eisenberger, & Crockett, 2006), right ventral LPFC activity during linguistic processing of stereotypes about elderly people was negatively correlated with amygdala activity. This pattern was not observed when participants processed words related to the intelligence stereotype, again suggesting that this effect may be specific to negatively valenced language.

It should also be noted that this study used the sentence-unscrambling task (Bargh, Chen, & Burrows, 1996) that requires linguistic processing of stereotypes without bringing the relevance of the stereotype to mind for participants. Thus there is no reason to assume participants were engaged in any kind of intentional emotion regulation.

Implicit Learning

Although research on the neural correlates of implicit learning has been decidedly nonsocial in nature, the implications for social psychology are substantial (Lewicki, 1986; Lieberman, 2000a). It is then of interest that a number of studies—neuroimaging studies in humans and lesion studies in rodents—have suggested that the basal ganglia and MTL function competitively (Poldrack & Packard, 2003). Packard, Hirsh, and White (1989) lesioned either the basal ganglia or the MTL in rodents and then had the rodents perform tasks that depend on one or the other of these brain regions. Not surprisingly, rats with basal ganglia lesions performed poorly on the basal-ganglia-specific task, and rats with MTL lesions performed poorly on the MTL-specific task. What is surprising is that the rats with basal ganglia lesions performed *better than normal* on the MTL specific task, and the rats with MTL lesions performed better than normal on the basal-ganglia-specific task. In other words, the presence of a normally functioning MTL tends to interfere with performance on tasks that strongly rely on the basal ganglia, and thus performance on these tasks are enhanced when the MTL is removed.

Poldrack et al. (2001) found negative functional connectivity between the basal ganglia and MTL in humans during a category learning task that involves both explicit and implicit learning to some extent, such that the participants who activated MTL more during this task activated the basal ganglia less. Lieberman, Chang, Chiao, et al. (2004) extended this finding by using a paradigm in which trials promoting the use of implicit and explicitly learned cues were distinguishable and could be compared. On trials in which explicitly learned cues were likely to drive performance, greater MTL activity was associated with diminished basal ganglia activity. It should be noted that, on these trials, the implicitly learned cues were still relevant to accurate performance—more relevant in fact, than the explicitly learned cues—but with basal ganglia activity diminished under these conditions, behavioral performance suffered.

FUTURE DIRECTIONS: REFLECTIVE AND REFLEXIVE *MODES* OF SOCIAL SOGNITION

> It is a contrast between two modes of practice. One is the pushing, slam-bang, act-first and think-afterwards mode, to which events may yield as they give way to any strong force. The other mode is wary, observant . . . and inhibited . . . an ineffective Hamlet in performance.
> —DEWEY, *Experience and Nature* (1925, p. 256)

The research reviewed in this chapter suggests that the X- and C-systems are differentially recruited during automatic and controlled processes of social cognition. The pattern of results seen across these studies indicates that, within the domain of social cognition, automatic processes are qualitatively distinct from controlled processes, as the activation patterns associated with automatic social cognition do not merely look like controlled processes with increased efficiency. If that were the case, one would expect to see efficiency associated primarily with decreased C-system activity. The fact that conditions that promote automaticity lead to increased activity in regions not associated with controlled processing indicates that distinct processes are being recruited. Additionally, evidence was presented to suggest that C-system activations can disrupt X-system activity. Thus the systems are independent in the sense that they rely on different neural structures, but they are not independent in the sense that there is no interaction between them. In most everyday experiences, it is likely that both systems are operating and contributing to ongoing thought and behavior, albeit in different ways.

Given that C-system activity can interfere with X-system activity under certain processing conditions, one might conclude that C-system activity leads to a self-sustaining *reflective mode* of social cognition and behavior in which the C-system has greater control over thought and behavior. One might also reasonably conclude that in situations that do not recruit signifi-

cant C-system activity, there may exist a *reflexive mode* of social cognition
and behavior. What has not been examined in this chapter is the possibility that the reflexive mode is also self-sustaining, tending to inhibit C-system activity. There are indeed some tantalizing hints that this might be the
case.

Noradrenaline serves as one of the major agents of physiological and
neural arousal, helping to increase attention, vigilance, and autonomic
readiness in response to potential threats (Berridge & Foote, 1991; Bouret,
Duvel, Onat, & Sara, 2003). Over the past decade, numerous studies by
Arnsten (1998) have demonstrated the deleterious consequences of noradrenaline and other catecholamines on the processing efficiency of LPFC.
LPFC seems to follow an inverted-U processing efficiency curve with
respect to noradrenaline such that increases from low to moderate levels
enhance LPFC processing efficiency. This is thought to occur because the
α2-receptor responds to noradrenaline in low concentrations and tends to
facilitate neural efficiency. Once past a moderate level of noradrenaline,
further increases tend to diminish LPFC processing efficiency. This is
thought to occur because the α1-neuroadrenaline receptor is receptive only
to high concentrations of noradrenaline and tends to inhibit or mute the
function of LPFC.

Consistent with this account, Callicott et al. (1999) observed an
inverted-U response in LPFC and PPC to increasing levels of stress during a
working-memory task. Activity in these regions increased parametrically
with task difficulty up to a point, but then became less active with higher
levels of stress. Alternatively, the dACC in the X-system was one of the few
regions found to increase activity linearly across all levels of task difficulty.
Beversdorf, White, Chever, Hughes, and Bornstein (2002) also found
evidence that general cognitive flexibility, a hallmark of LPFC function, diminished with the administration of an adrenergic agonist and
was enhanced with the administration of an adrenergic antagonist. Thus
the C-system region seems to get "tired" or "frazzled" consistent with
Baumeister's claims about the draining effects of self-regulation on further
self-regulation attempts (Baumeister et al., 1998).

There is no evidence that X-system structures get frazzled from high
arousal in the same way that LPFC does. To the contrary, amygdala activity enhances the noradrenaline production in the medulla (Dayas & Day,
2001) and locus coeruleus (Bouret et al., 2003), two major centers of
noradrenaline production in the brain. Additionally, high levels of noradrenaline and stress are associated with enhanced amygdala function
(McIntyre, Hatfield, & McGaugh, 2002; Shors & Mathew, 1998). Though
the adrenergic effect of the amygdala on the prefrontal cortex is presumably mediated by the locus coeruleus, there is evidence that electric stimulation of the amygdala does result in noradrenaline increases in the neocortex
(Kapp, Supple, & Whalen, 1994).

The tradeoff between the X- and C-system responses to arousal
extends to the long-term consequences of chronic stress as well. There is

ample evidence that chronic stress damages MTL neurons (McEwen, 1999), producing dendritic shortening (Conrad, Galea, Kuroda, & McEwen, 1996). However, recently it has also been discovered that chronic stress facilitates neuronal growth in the amygdala, producing dendritic lengthening (Vyas, Mitra, Shankaranarayana Rao, & Chattarji, 2002). These findings linking stress, arousal, and noradrenaline suggest that C-system structures function best at low to moderate levels of arousal, whereas the X-system may function better at higher levels of arousal, especially when we consider that at higher levels of arousal, C-system structures may be less able to regulate X-system activity. These findings are quite reminiscent of Zajonc's finding that arousal facilitates dominant responses but impairs nondominant responses (Bond & Titus, 1983; Yerkes & Dodson, 1908; Zajonc, 1965) and may explain why dominant responses are facilitated by stress. If response dominance is considered equivalent to habit strength, then it would be reasonable to say that X-system responses are more dominant than C-system responses.

Why would humans and other mammals have evolved these two modes controlled by arousal or stress level? If arousal is assumed, among other things, to index the intensity and immediacy of potential threats, then having these two modes triggered by arousal would be highly adaptive. When threats are not imminent, people are best served by gathering new information and flexibly considering options. However, our ability to think and learn flexibly comes at a cost: time and effort. When threats are imminent, especially the kind of threats that were relevant in our evolutionary past, taking the time to think through options might put one's life at risk. Thus, when threats are imminent and arousal is high, our brain takes the decision out of the hands of the C-system and leaves it to the X-system. If the X-system has strong contextually appropriate habits and impulses, then the individual will likely escape unharmed. If the situation is novel such that the individual lacks contextually appropriate habits and the threat is truly imminent, C-system processes may have proved too inefficient to be of service. Thus future work may examine the interaction of situational demands and arousal on the generation and maintenance of these two modes of social cognitive processing.

REFERENCES

Aizenstein, H. J., MacDonald, A. W., Stenger, V. A., Nebes, R. D., Larson, J. K., Ursu, S., et al. (2000). Complementary category learning systems identified using event-related functional MRI. *Journal of Cognitive Neuroscience, 12,* 977–987.

Ambady, N., & Rosenthal, R. (1992). Thin slices of expressive behavior as predictors of interpersonal consequences: A meta-analysis. *Psychological Bulletin, 111,* 256–274.

Anderson, J. R. (1978). Arguments concerning representations for mental imagery. *Psychological Review, 85,* 249–277.

Arnsten, A. F. T. (1998). Catecholamine modulation of prefrontal cortical cognitive function. *Trends in Cognitive Sciences, 2,* 436–447.

Baddeley, A. (1986). *Working memory.* Oxford, UK: Clarendon Press.

Banaji, M. R., & Hardin, C. D. (1996). Automatic stereotyping. *Psychological Science, 7,* 136-141.

Bargh, J. A. (1996). Principles of automaticity. In E. T. Higgins & A. W. Kruglanski (Eds.), *Social psychology: Handbook of basic principles* (pp. 169–183). New York: Guilford Press.

Bargh, J. A., & Chartrand, T. L. (2000). The mind in the middle: A practical guide to priming and automaticity research. In H. T. Reis & C. M. Judd (Eds.), *Handbook of research methods in social and personality psychology* (pp. 253–285). New York: Cambridge University Press.

Bargh, J. A., Chen, M., & Burrows, L. (1996). Automaticity of social behavior: Direct effects of trait construct and stereotype activation on action. *Journal of Personality and Social Psychology, 71,* 230–244.

Bartels, A., & Zeki, S. (2000). The neural basis of romantic love. *NeuroReport, 11,* 3829–3834.

Baumeister, R. F., Bratslavsky, E., Muraven, M., & Tice, D. M. (1998). Ego depletion: Is the self a limited resource? *Journal of Personality and Social Psychology, 65,* 317–338.

Beauregard, M., Levesque, J., & Bourgouin, P. (2001). Neural correlates of conscious self-regulation of emotion. *Journal of Neuroscience, 21,* 6993–7000.

Bechara, A., Damasio, H., Tranel, D., & Damasio, A. R. (1997). Deciding advantageously before knowing the advantageous strategy. *Science, 275,* 1293–1294.

Berridge, C. W., & Foote, S. L. (1991). Effects of locus coeruleus activation on electrocephalographic activity in neocortex and hippocampus. *Journal of Neuroscience, 11,* 3135–3145.

Beversdorf, D. Q., White, D. M., Chever, D. C., Hughes, J. D., & Bornstein, R. A. (2002). Central β-adrenergic modulation of cognitive flexibility. *NeuroReport, 13,* 2505–2507.

Bless, H., & Schwarz, N. (1999). Sufficient and necessary conditions in dual-process models: The case of mood and information processing. In S. Chaiken & Y. Trope (Eds.), *Dual-process theories in social psychology* (pp. 423–440). New York: Guilford Press.

Bond, C. F., Jr., & Titus, L. T. (1983). Social facilitation: A meta-analysis of 241 studies. *Psychological Bulletin, 94,* 265–292.

Botvinick, M. M., Braver, T. D., Barch, D. M., Carter, C. S., & Cohen, J. D. (2001). Conflict monitoring and cognitive control. *Psychological Review, 108,* 624–652.

Bouret, S., Duvel, A., Onat, S., & Sara, S. J. (2003). Phasic activation of locus ceruleus neurons by the central nucleus of the amygdala. *Journal of Neuroscience, 23,* 3491–3497.

Breiter, H. C., Gollub, R. L., Weisskoff, R. M., Kennedy, D. N., Makris, N., Berke, J. D., et al. (1997). Acute effects of cocaine on human brain activity and emotion. *Neuron, 19,* 591–611.

Brewer, J. B., Zhao, Z., Desmond, J. E., Glover, G. H., & Gabrieli, J. D. E. (1998). Making memories: Brain activity that predicts how well visual experience will be remembered. *Science, 281,* 1185–1187.

Cabeza, R., & Nyberg, L. (2000). Imaging cognition: II. An empirical review of 275 PET and fMRI studies. *Journal of Cognitive Neuroscience, 12,* 1–47.

Callicott, J. H., Mattay, V. S., Bertolino, A., Finn, K., Coppola, R., Frank, J. A., et al. (1999). Physiological characteristics of capacity constraints in working memory as revealed by functional MRI. *Cerebral Cortex, 9,* 20–26.

Carretie, L., Hinojosa, J. A., Mercado, F., & Tapia, M. (2005). Cortical response to subjective unconscious danger. *NeuroImage, 24,* 615–623.

Chaiken, S., Liberman, A., & Eagly, A. H. (1989). Heuristic and systematic processing within and beyond the persuasion context. In J. S. Uleman & J. A. Bargh (Eds.), *Unintended thought* (pp. 212–252). New York: Guilford Press.

Chaiken, S., & Trope, Y. (Eds.). (1999). *Dual-process theories in social psychology.* New York: Guilford Press.

Cohen, J. D., Dunbar, K., & McClelland, J. L. (1990). On the control of automatic processes: A parallel distributed processing model of the Stroop effect. *Psychological Review, 97,* 332–361.

Conrad, C. D., Galea, L. A., Kuroda, Y., & McEwen, B. S. (1996). Chronic stress impairs rat spatial memory on the Y maze, and this effect is blocked by tianeptine pretreatment. *Behavioral Neuroscience, 110,* 1321–1334.

Craig, A. D. (2004). Human feelings: Why are some more aware than others. *Trends in Cognitive Sciences, 8,* 239–241.

Craik, F. I. M., & Tulving, E. (1975). Depth of processing and retention of words in episodic memory. *Journal of Experimental Psychology: General, 104,* 268–294.

Crinion, J. T., Lambon-Ralph, M. A., Warburton, E. A., Howard, D., & Wise, R. J. S. (2003). Temporal lobe regions engaged during normal speech comprehension. *Brain, 126,* 1193–1201.

Cunningham, W. A., Johnson, M. K., Raye, C. L., Gatenby, J., Gore, J. C., & Banaji, M. R. (2004). Separable neural components in the processing of black and white faces. *Psychological Science, 15,* 806–813.

Cunningham, W. A., Johnson, M. K., Gatenby, J. C., Gore, J. C., & Banaji, M. R. (2003). Neural components of social evaluation. *Journal of Personality and Social Psychology, 85,* 639–649.

Damasio, A. R. (1994). *Descartes' error: Emotion, reason, and the human brain.* New York: Putnam.

Darke, S. (1988). Effects of anxiety on inferential reasoning task performance. *Journal of Personality and Social Psychology, 55,* 499–505.

Dayas, C. V., & Day, T. A. (2001). Opposing roles for medial and central amygdala in the initiation of noradrenergic cell responses to a psychological stressor. *European Journal of Neuroscience, 15,* 1712–1718.

Deppe, M., Schwindt, W., Kramer, J., Kugel, H., Plassmann, H., Kenning, P., et al. (2005). Evidence for a neural correlate of a framing effect: Bias-specific activity in the ventromedial prefrontal cortex during credibility judgments. *Brain Research Bulletin, 67,* 413–421.

Devine, P. G. (1989). Stereotypes and prejudice: Their automatic and controlled components. *Journal of Personality and Social Psychology, 56,* 680–690.

Dewey, J. (1925). *Experience and nature.* LaSalle, IL: Open Court Press.

Egloff, B., & Hock, M. (2001). Interactive effects of state anxiety and trait anxiety on emotional Stroop interference. *Personality and Individual Differences, 31,* 875–882.

Eisenberger, N. I., & Lieberman, M. D. (2004). "Why it hurts to be left out": The neurocognitive overlap between physical and social pain. *Trends in Cognitive Sciences, 8,* 294–300.

Eisenberger, N. I., Lieberman, M. D., & Satpute, A. B. (2005). Personality from a controlled processing perspective: An fMRI study of neuroticism, extraversion, and self-consciousness. *Cognitive, Affective, and Behavioral Neuroscience, 5,* 169–181.

Fanselow, M. S., & LeDoux, J. E. (1999). Why we think plasiticity underlying Pavlovian fear conditioning occurs in the basolateral amygdala. *Neuron, 23,* 229–232.

Forgas, J. P. (1995). Mood and judgment: The affect infusion model (AIM). *Psychological Bulletin, 117,* 39–66.

Fujii, T., Okuda, J., Tsukiura, T., Ohtake, H., Suzuki, M., Kawashima, R., et al. (2002). Encoding-related brain activity during deep processing of verbal materials: A PET study. *Neuroscience Research, 44,* 429–438.

Garrard, P., & Hodges, J. R. (2000). Semantic dementia: Clinical, radiological and pathological perspectives. *Journal of Neurology, 247,* 409–422.

Gilbert, D. T. (1989). Thinking lightly about others: Automatic components of the social inference process. In J. S. Uleman & J. A. Bargh (Eds.), *Unintended thought* (pp. 189–211). New York: Guilford Press.

Gilbert, D. T. (1999). What the mind's not. In S. Chaiken & Y. Trope (Eds.), *Dual-process theories in social psychology* (pp. 3–11). New York: Guilford Press.

Gray, J. R., & Braver, T. S. (2002). Personality predicts working-memory-related activation in the caudal anterior cingulate cortex. *Cognitive, Affective, and Behavioral Neuroscience, 2,* 64–75.

Greenwald, A. G., McGhee, D. E., & Schwartz, J. L. K. (1998). Measuring individual differences in implicit cognition: The Implicit Association Test. *Journal of Personality and Social Psychology, 74,* 1464–1480.

Gross, J. J. (1998). Antecedent- and response-focused emotion regulation: Divergent consequences for experience, expression, and physiology. *Journal of Personality and Social Psychology, 74,* 227–237.

Gusnard, D. A., Akbudak, E., Shulman, G. L., & Raichle, M. E. (2001). Medial prefrontal cortex and self-referential mental activity: Relation of a default mode of brain function. *Proceedings of the National Academy of Sciences of the USA, 98,* 4259–4264.

Hariri, A. R., Bookheimer, S. Y., & Mazziotta, J. C. (2000). Modulating emotional response: Effects of a neocortical network on the limbic system. *Neuroreport, 11,* 43–48.

Hart, A. J., Whalen, P. J., Shin, L. M., McInerney, S. C., Fischer, H., & Rauch, S. L. (2000). Differential response in the human amygdala to racial outgroup vs ingroup face stimuli. *Brain Imaging, 11,* 2351–2355.

Heberlein, A. S., & Adolphs, R. (2004). Impaired spontaneous anthropomorphizing despite intact perception and social knowledge. *Proceedings of the National Academy of Sciences of the USA, 19,* 7487–7491.

Hopfield, J. J. (1982). Neural networks and physical systems with emergent collective computational abilities. *Proceedings of the National Academy of Sciences of the USA, 79,* 2554–2558.

James, W. (1950). *Principles of psychology.* New York: Dover. (Original work published 1890)

Jansma, J. M., Ramsey, N. F., Slagter, H. A., & Kahn, R. S. (2001). Functional anatomical correlates of controlled and automatic processing. *Journal of Cognitive Neuroscience, 13*, 730–743.

Kahneman, D. (2003). A perspective on judgment and choice: Mapping bounded rationality. *American Psychologist, 58*, 697–720.

Kapp, B. S., Supple, W. F., & Whalen, P. J. (1994). Effects of electrical stimulation of the amygdaloid central nucleus on neocortical arousal in the rabbit. *Behavioral Neuroscience, 108*, 81–93.

Kawakami, K., Dovidio, J. F., Moll, J., Hermsen, S., & Russin, A. (2000). Just say no (to stereotyping): Effects of training in the negation of stereotypic associations on stereotype activation. *Journal of Personality and Social Psychology, 78*, 871–888.

Kelley, W. M., Macrae, C. N., Wyland, C. L., Caglar, S., Inati, S., & Heatherton, T. F. (2002). Finding the self? An event-related fMRI study. *Journal of Cognitive Neuroscience, 14*(5), 785–794.

Knowlton, B. J., Mangels, J. A., & Squire, L. R. (1996). A neostriatal habit learning system in humans. *Science, 273*.

Kosslyn, S. M. (1994). *Image and brain: The resolution of the imagery debate.* Cambridge, MA: MIT Press.

Lange, K., Williams, L. M., Young, A. W., Bullmore, E. T., Brammer, M. J., Williams, S. C. R., et al. (2003). Task instructions modulate neural response to fearful facial expressions. *Biological Psychiatry, 53*, 226–232.

Lau, H. C., Rogers, R. D., Ramnani, N., & Passingham, R. E. (2004). Willed action and attention to the selection of action. *NeuroImage, 21*, 1407–1415.

LeDoux, J. E. (1996). *The emotional brain: The mysterious underpinnings of emotional life.* New York: Simon & Schuster.

Lee, A. C. H., Robbins, T. W., Graham, K. S., & Owen, A. M. (2002). "Pray or prey?" Dissociation of semantic memory retrieval from episodic memory processing using positron emission tomography and a novel homophone task. *NeuroImage, 16*, 724–735.

Levesque, J., Eugene, F., Joanette, Y., Paquette, V., Mensour, B., Deaudoin., G., et al. (2003). Neural circuitry underlying voluntary suppression of sadness. *Biological Psychiatry, 53*, 502–510.

Lewicki, P. (1986). *Nonconscious social information processing.* San Diego, CA: Academic Press.

Liddell, B. J., Brown, K. J., Kemp, A. H., Barton, M. J., Das, P., Peduto, A., et al. (2005). A direct brainstem–amygdala–cortical "alarm" system for subliminal signals of fear. *NeuroImage, 24*, 235–243.

Lieberman, M. D. (in press). Social cognitive neuroscience: A review of core processes. *Annual Review of Psychology.*

Lieberman, M. D. (2000a). Intuition: A social cognitive neuroscience approach. *Psychological Bulletin, 126*, 109–137.

Lieberman, M. D. (2000b). Introversion and working memory: Central executive differences. *Personality and Individual Differences, 28*, 479–486.

Lieberman, M. D. (2003). Reflective and reflexive judgment processes: A social cognitive neuroscience approach. In J. P. Forgas, K. R. Williams, & W. von Hippel (Eds.), *Social judgments: Implicit and explicit processes* (pp. 44–67). New York: Cambridge University Press.

Lieberman, M. D., Chang, G. Y., Chiao, J. Y., Bookheimer, S. Y., & Knowlton,

B. J. (2004). An event-related fMRI study of artificial grammar learning in a balanced chunk strength design. *Journal of Cognitive Neuroscience, 16,* 427–438.

Lieberman, M. D., & Eisenberger, N. I. (2004). Conflict and habit: A social cognitive neuroscience approach to the self. In A. Tesser, J. V. Wood, & D. A. Stapel (Eds.), *On building, defending and regulating the self: A psychological perspective* (pp. 77–102). New York: Psychology Press.

Lieberman, M. D., Eisenberger, N. I., Crockett, M. J., Tom, S., Pfeifer, J. H., & Way, B. M. (in press). Putting feelings into words: Affect labeling disrupts amygdala activity to affective stimuli. *Psychological Science.*

Lieberman, M. D., Eisenberger, N. I., & Crockett, M. (2006). *An fMRI study of automatic behavior: Comparing ideomotor and disruption accounts.* Manuscript submitted for publication.

Lieberman, M. D., Gaunt, R., Gilbert, D. T., & Trope, Y. (2002). Reflection and reflexion: A social cognitive neuroscience approach to attributional inference. *Advances in Experimental Social Psychology, 34,* 199–249.

Lieberman, M. D., Hariri, A., Jarcho, J. J., Eisenberger, N. I., & Bookheimer, S. Y. (2005). An fMRI investigation of race-related amygdala activity in African-American and Caucasian-American individuals. *Nature Neuroscience, 8,* 720–722.

Lieberman, M. D., Jarcho, J. M., Berman, S., Naliboff, B., Suyenobu, B. Y., Mandelkern, M., & Mayer, E. (2004). The neural correlates of placebo effects: A disruption account. *NeuroImage, 22,* 447–455.

Lieberman, M. D., Jarcho, J. M., & Satpute, A. B. (2004). Evidence-based and intuition-based self-knowledge: An fMRI study. *Journal of Personality and Social Psychology, 87,* 421–435.

Lieberman, M. D., & Pfeifer, J. H. (2005). The self and social perception: Three kinds of questions in social cognitive neuroscience. In A. Easton & N. Emery (Eds.), *Cognitive neuroscience of emotional and social behavior* (pp. 195–235). Philadelphia: Psychology Press.

Lieberman, M. D., & Rosenthal, R. (2001). Why introverts can't always tell who likes them: Multi-tasking and nonverbal decoding. *Journal of Personality and Social Psychology, 80,* 294–310.

Logan, G. D. (1988). Toward an instance theory of automatization. *Psychological Review, 95,* 492–527.

Lowery, B. S., Hardin, C. D., & Sinclair, S. (2001). Social influence on automatic racial prejudice. *Journal of Personality and Social Psychology, 81,* 842–855.

Macrae, C. N., Milne, A. B., & Bodenhausen, G. V. (1994). Stereotypes as energy-saving devices: A peek inside the cognitive toolbox. *Journal of Personality and Social Psychology, 66,* 34–47.

Markus, H. R. (1977). Self-schemata and processing information about the self. *Journal of Personality and Social Psychology, 35,* 63–78.

McClelland, J. L., McNaughton, B. L., & O'Reilly, R. C. (1995). Why there are complementary learning systems in the hippocampus and neocortex: Insights from the successes and failures of connectionist models of learning and memory. *Psychological Review, 102,* 419–457.

McEwen, B. S. (1999). Stress and hippocampal plasticity. *Annual Review of Neuroscience, 22,* 105–122.

McIntyre, C. K., Hatfield, T., & McGaugh, J. L. (2002). Amygdala norepinephrine levels after training predict inhibitory avoidance retention performance in rats. *European Journal of Neuroscience, 16,* 1223–1226.

Miller, E. K., & Cohen, J. D. (2001). An integrative theory of prefrontal cortex function. *Annual Review of Neuroscience, 24,* 167–202.

Milne, E., & Grafman, J. (2001). Ventromedial prefrontal cortex lesions in humans eliminate implicit gender stereotyping. *Journal of Neuroscience, 21,* RC150 151–156.

Mitchell, J. P., Nosek, B. A., & Banaji, M. R. (2003). Contextual variations in implicit evaluation. *Journal of Experimental Psychology: General, 132,* 455–469.

Morris, J. S., Öhman, A., & Dolan, R. J. (1999). A subcortical pathway to the right amygdala mediating "unseen" fear. *Proceedings of the National Academy of Sciences of the USA, 96,* 1680–1685.

Mummery, C. J., Patterson, K., Price, C. J., Ashburner, J., Frackowiak, R. S. J., & Hodges, J. R. (2000). A voxel-based morphometry study of semantic dementia: Relationship between temporal lobe atrophy and semantic memory. *Annals of Neurology, 47,* 36–45.

Mummery, C. J., Shallice, T., & Price, C. J. (1999). Dual-process model in semantic priming: A functional imaging perspective. *NeuroImage, 9,* 516–525.

Nimchinsky, E. A., Gilissen, E., Allman, J. M., Perl, D. P., Erwin, J. M., & Hof, P. R. (1999). A neuronal morphological type unique to humans and great apes. *Proceedings of the National Academy of Sciences of the USA, 96,* 5268–5273.

Nosek, B.A., Banaji, M. R., & Greenwald, A. G. (2002). Harvesting implicit group attitudes and beliefs from a demonstration web site. *Group Dynamics: Theory, Research, and Practice, 6,* 101–115.

Ochsner, K. N., Bunge, S. A., Gross, J. J., & Gabrieli, J. D. (2002). Rethinking feelings: An FMRI study of the cognitive regulation of emotion. *Journal of Cognitive Neurosciences, 14,* 1215–1229.

Ochsner, K. N., & Lieberman, M. D. (2001). The emergence of social cognitive neuroscience. *American Psychologist, 56*(9), 717–734.

Ochsner, K. N., Ray, R. D., Cooper, J. C., Robertson, E. R., Chopra, S., Gabrieli, J. D. E., et al. (2004). For better or for worse: Neural systems supporting the cognitive down- and up-regulation of negative emotion. *NeuroImage, 23,* 483–499.

Oya, T., Manalo, E., & Greenwood, J. (2004). The influence of personality and anxiety on the oral performance of Japanese speakers of English. *Applied Cognitive Psychology, 18,* 841–855.

Packard, M. G., Hirsh, R., & White, N. M. (1989). Differential effects of fornix and caudate nucleus lesions on two radial maze tasks: Evidence for multiple memory systems. *Journal of Neuroscience, 9,* 1465–1472.

Pasley, B. N., Mayes, L. C., & Schultz, R. T. (2004). Subcortical discrimination of unperceived objects during binocular rivalry. *Neuron, 42,* 163–172.

Petty, R. E., & Cacioppo, J. T. (1986). The elaboration likelihood model of persuasion. *Advances in Experimental Social Psychology, 19,* 123–205.

Phelps, E. A., O'Connor, K. J., Cunningham, W. A., Funayama, E. S., Gatenby, J. C., Gore, J. C., et al. (2000). Performance on indirect measures of race evaluation predicts amygdala activation. *Journal of Cognitive Neuroscience, 12,* 729–738.

Ploghaus, A., Becerra, L., Borras, C., & Borsook, D. (2003). Neural circuitry underlying pain modulation: Expectation, hypnosis, placebo. *Trends in Cognitive Sciences, 7*, 197–200.

Poldrack, R. A., Clark, J., Par -Blagoev, E. J., Shohamy, D., Creso Moyano, J., Myers, C., et al. (2001). Interactive memory systems in the human brain. *Nature, 414*, 546–550.

Poldrack, R. A., & Packard, M. G. (2003). Competition among multiple memory systems: Converging evidence from animal and human studies. *Neuropsychologia, 41*, 245–251.

Posner, M. I., & Keele, S. W. (1968). On the genesis of abstract ideas. *Journal of Experimental Psychology, 77*, 353–363.

Rauch, S. L., Savage, C. R., Brown, H. D., Curran, T., Alpert, N. M., Kendrick, A., et al. (1995). A PET investigation of implicit and explicit sequence learning. *Human Brain Mapping, 3*, 271–286.

Rissman, J., Eliassen, J. C., & Blumstein, S. E. (2003). An event-related fMRI investigation of implicit semantic priming. *Journal of Cognitive Neuroscience, 15*, 1160–1175.

Rossell, S. L., Bullmore, E. T., Williams, S. C. R., & David, A. S. (2001). Brain activation during automatic and controlled processing of semantic relations: A priming experiment using lexical decision. *Neuropsychologia, 39*, 1167–1176.

Ruby, P., & Decety, J. (2001). Effect of subjective perspective taking during simulation of action: A PET investigation of agency. *Nature Neuroscience, 4*, 546–550.

Satpute, A. B., & Lieberman, M. D. (2006). Integrating automatic and controlled processing into neurocognitive models of social cognition. *Brain Research, 1079*, 86–97.

Schacter, D. L. (1992). Understanding implicit memory: A cognitive neuroscience approach. *American Psychologist, 47*, 559–569.

Schaefer, A., Collette, F., Philippot, P., Van der Linden, M., Laureys, S., Delfiore, G., et al. (2003). Neural correlates of "hot" and "cold" emotional processing: A multilevel approach to the functional anatomy of emotion. *NeuroImage, 18*, 938–949.

Semendeferi, K., Schleicher, A., Zilles, K., Armstrong, E., & Van Hoesen, G. W. (2001). Evolution of the hominoid prefrontal cortex: Imaging and quantitative analysis of area 10. *American Journal of Physical Anthropology, 114*, 224–241.

Shors, T. J., & Mathew, P. R. (1998). NMDA receptor antagonism in the lateral/basolateral but not central nucleus of the amygdala prevents the induction of facilitated learning in response to stress. *Learning and Memory, 5*, 220–230.

Sloman, S. A. (1996). The empirical case for two systems of reasoning. *Psychological Bulletin, 119*, 3–22.

Small, D. M., Zatorre, R. J., Dagher, A., Evans, A. C., & Jones-Gotman, M. (2001). Changes in brain activity related to eating chocolate. From pleasure to aversion. *Brain, 124*, 1720–1733.

Smith, W. (1945). The functional significance of the rostral cingular cortex as revealed by its responses to electrical excitation. *Journal of Neurophysiology, 8*, 241–255.

Smolensky, P. (1988). On the proper treatment of connectionism. *Behavioral and Brain Sciences, 11*, 1–74.

Spinoza, B. (1949). *Ethics.* New York: Hafner. (Original work published 1675)

Suzuki, W., Saleem, K. S., & Tanaka, K. (2000). Divergent backward projections from the anterior part of the inferotemporal cortex (area TE) in the macaque. *Journal of Comparative Neurology, 422*, 206–228.

Taylor, S. F., Phan, K. L., Decker, L. R., & Liberzon, I. (2003). Subjective rating of emotionally salient stimuli modulates neural activity. *NeuroImage, 18*, 650–659.

Thompson, R. K. R., & Oden, D. L. (2000). Categorical perception and conceptual judgments by nonhuman primates: The paleological monkey and the analogical ape. *Cognitive Science, 24*, 363–396.

Trope, Y. (1986). Identification and inferential processes in dispositional attribution. *Psychological Review, 93*, 239–257.

Vogels, R. (1999). Categorization of complex visual images by rhesus monkeys: Part 2. Single-cell study. *European Journal of Neuroscience, 11*, 1239–1255.

Vyas, A., Mitra, R., Shankaranarayana Rao, B. S., & Chattarji, S. (2002). Chronic stress induces contrasting patterns of dendritic remodeling in hippocampal and amygdaloid neurons. *Journal of Neuroscience, 22*, 6810–6818.

Wager, T. D., Phan, K. L., Liberzon, I., & Taylor, S. F. (2003). Valence, gender, and lateralization of functional brain anatomy in emotion: A meta-analysis of findings from neuroimaging. *NeuroImage, 19*, 513–531.

Wagner, A. D., Schacter, D. L., Rotte, M., Koutstaal, W., Maril, A., Dale, A. M., et al. (1998). Building memories: Remembering and forgetting of verbal experiences as predicted by brian activity. *Science, 281*, 1188–1191.

Wegner, D. M. (1994). Ironic processes of mental control. *Psychological Review, 101*, 34–52.

Whalen, P. J., Rauch, S. L., Etcoff, N. L., McInerney, S. C., Lee, M. B., & Jenike, M. A. (1998). Masked presentations of emotional facial expressions modulate amygdala activity without explicit knowledge. *Journal of Neuroscience, 18*, 411–418.

Wilson, T. D., Lindsey, S., & Schooler, T. Y. (2000). A model of dual attitudes. *Psychological Review, 107*, 101–126.

Wright, C. I., Fischer, H., Whalen, P. J., McInerney, S. C., Shin, L. M., & Rauch, S. L. (2001). Differential prefrontal and amygdala habituation to repeatedly presented emotional stimuli. *Neuroreport, 12*, 379–383.

Xu, B., Grafman, J., Gaillard, W. D., Spanaki, M., Ishii, K., Balsamo, L., et al. (2002). Neuroimaging reveals automatic speech code during perception of written word meaning. *NeuroImage, 17*, 859–870.

Yerkes, R. M., & Dodson, J. D. (1908). The relation of strength of stimulus to rapidity of habit-formation. *Journal of Comparative Neurology and Psychology, 18*, 459–482.

Zajonc, R. B. (1965). Social facilitation. *Science, 149*, 269–274.

Zalla, T., Koechlin, E., Pietrini, P., Basso, G., Aquino, P., Sirigu, A., et al. (2000). Differential amygdala responses to winning and losing: A functional magnetic resonance imaging study in humans. *European Journal of Neuroscience, 12*, 1764–1770.

15

An Evolutionary Perspective on Domain Specificity in Social Intelligence

Valerie E. Stone

Western culture has a long history of placing "man" above "beast" and emphasizing the huge gap between our species and all others, particularly when it comes to our mental capacities. Many people believe we are civilized and refined in our social behavior, certainly not like our screeching, teeth-baring cousins, the other primates. After years of observing politics, I have come to the conclusion that we may not be as different in our social behavior from other primates as we would like to think. Humans are animals. In particular, we are social animals, adapted to living in groups, descended from a long line of species that were also adapted to groups. Many of our social behaviors are shared with our primate cousins, thus so must be many of our social cognitive abilities. However, there are clearly some aspects of our social cognition that are unique to our species. In this chapter, I place both our shared and our unique cognition and behavior in an evolutionary perspective.

Social behavior is any interaction with members of one's own species. Social cognition, then, is the information-processing architecture that enables us to engage in social behavior. Social neuroscience is the study of how the brain implements the information-processing architecture for sociality. A key question, then, is to what extent brain systems that subserve social behavior are *domain specific*, consisting of neural processes that operate preferentially on social information, and to what extent they are *domain general*, relying on the same neural processes that subserve multiple areas of cognition. A domain-specific ability operates on particular types of input, uses certain types of representations, and performs certain types of computations on those representations (Tooby & Cosmides, 1992). Domain-general mechanisms can be characterized as content independent, able to operate on a wide variety of types of representations and to perform a variety of computations on them. Social behavior includes a number of different domains: parenting, mating, dominance hierarchy negotiations, kin relationships, intergroup interactions, cooperation and competition, and so forth. Specialized information-processing systems might subserve each of these domains, with different processing for each domain. Research with neurological patients can give us insight into domain specificity. Dissociations in patients can reveal either that social cognition can be impaired independently of more general cognitive processes or that deficits in social cognition are always accompanied by more general cognitive impairments. Neuroimaging can show us whether the brain areas active for different social tasks are in different locations in the brain and how much those systems overlap with areas involved in more general cognitive functions. Thus social neuroscience is in a unique position to answer questions about domain specificity in social cognition.

Whereas neuroscience provides us with methods to investigate domain specificity, an evolutionary perspective gives us some theoretical grounds for understanding domain specificity. Domain-specific cognitive systems are *adaptations*, mechanisms specialized for particular functions and designed by natural selection over millions of generations to have information-processing features specific to the cognitive problem being solved (Cosmides & Tooby, 1987). Cognitive systems specific to the social domain will have design features that make them most efficient at processing social information, rather than nonsocial information. Such design features might include specialized representations, such as visual representations of faces or eyes, or specialized processing, such as inferential rules that make certain social inferences rapidly and automatically. Because adaptations are so complex, each design feature must evolve layered onto previous features; special design in an adaptation thus takes a long evolutionary time to emerge (Williams, 1966; Dawkins, 1987). Much of our emotional life, our social motivations, and social intelligence are doubtless shared in common with other primates and mammals who faced the same adaptive problems. There have been tens or hundreds of millions of years to refine neural adaptations for those domains of behavior. See Figure 15.1 for information about times at which human evolution diverged from lineages leading to other primate species.

Abilities that are recent and unique to the hominid line, however, are not likely to depend solely on domain-specific systems. Tooby and Cosmides (1992) point out that "purely human-specific adaptive problems, such as extensive tool use or extensive reciprocation, would have . . . adaptations less exquisite than vision, hearing, maternal care, threat-perception, mate selection, foraging, emotional communication, and many other problems that have been with us for tens of millions of years" (1992, p. 60). The appropriate conclusion is not that our human-specific adaptations are inefficient kludges. Rather, our human-specific abilities represent merely the latest layer of innovation on abilities that were present in some form in ancestral species. They are unlikely to have evolved as much domain specificity as more ancient abilities. To understand social intelligence, we must look at how domain-specific systems that we share with other primates interact with more general cognitive abilities that are uniquely human.

Much of our social behavior is similar to that of other primates and other mammals. Parenting, attachment, and negotiating dominance hierarchies, for example, are all behaviors that we share with other social mammals and that appear to depend on specific neural systems. Evolution does not throw away adaptations unless they are costly to maintain and no longer needed, so it is parsimonious to assume that many of the brain systems that subserve social behavior in humans and in other social mammals with whom we share common descent are inherited from a common social mammal ancestor and will share common features.

With each domain of social cognition—attachment, hierarchy negotiation, cooperation, in-group–out-group categorization—one needs to define its components carefully, consider whether each is an aspect of cognition that we share with other social primates, and then do careful work to define whether each component is domain specific to social information processing or whether it depends on more general cognitive processes.

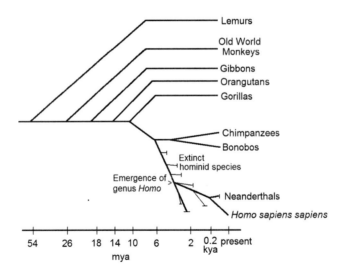

FIGURE 15.1. Our primate family tree, showing branching points leading to monkeys, great apes, hominids, and humans. Time is measured in mya = millions of years ago, except where marked kya = thousands of years ago. Information on when certain branchings occurred is based on genetic analyses and has been compiled from Yoder et al. (1996), Foley (1997), Gibbons (2000), and Wildman et al. (2003).

"Theory of mind" (ToM), the ability to infer others' mental states, has received much attention in the social neuroscience literature lately as a key social cognitive ability in humans. I argue that ToM depends on domain-specific social abilities that we share with other primates, but that its uniquely human component is not specifically social at all. Humans make complex, embedded ToM inferences regularly, for example, in political maneuvering: "If the Republican Senator thinks that the Democratic Senator believes that he wants to lower taxes, then if the Republican agrees to a small tax raise in a negotiation, the Democrat will believe this is a concession and think she owes the Republican something." This sort of complex inference happens every day on Capitol Hill, and indeed, we could not follow many spy stories or soap operas if we could not track such complex inferences. I believe this level of complexity in social cognition depends on uniquely human and therefore recent cognitive abilities. The crucial abilities for adult human ToM may not be domain-specific social processes but rather some very general and powerful cognitive abilities that are used in many other contexts besides social cognition. Our capacity for executive function, for embedding and recursion, and for metarepresentation enable not only our complex social cognition but also many of our other uniquely human abilities: symbolic language, syntax, future planning, episodic memory, and tool use, just to name a few (Suddendorf, 1999; Corballis, 2003). Yet these domain-general abilities would have no usefulness in the social world if they could not operate using the output of several more ancient domain-specific social abilities.

SOCIAL COGNITION IN MONKEYS, APES, AND HUMANS: COMPONENTS OF ToM

As an example of how to approach a topic in social neuroscience by looking at components and domain specificity, I review research on our ability to understand other people's mental states, the cognitive capacity known as theory of mind (ToM). Humans make inferences about others' mental states and interpret others' behavior in terms of their mental states, where mental states can mean emotions, desires, goals, intentions, attention, knowledge, and belief. ToM thus encompasses a variety of cognitive processes and takes several years to unfold in human development (Baron-Cohen, 1995; Wellman & Liu, 2004). By breaking ToM down into components, we can ask which of those components are shared with our primate relatives and which are uniquely human.

It will be helpful to clarify some issues of terminology, as different scholars and fields sometimes use the term "theory of mind" differently. Some argue that ToM refers specifically to the ability to represent the *contents* of others' mental states. Thus ToM is often seen as equivalent to *metarepresentation*, the ability to represent representations as representations, as in "He thinks that [his car is in the garage]" or "She saw that [the lion had escaped from its cage]" (Leslie, 1987; Perner, 1991; Baron-Cohen, 1995; Suddendorf, 1999; Leslie & Frith, 1990). Inferring another person's emotional state does not require metarepresentation, as one does not have to represent someone else's representations but only his or her external appearance: "She looks angry." For this reason, Leslie and Frith (1990) have argued that inferring emotional states should *not* be considered ToM. Inferring others' intentions, goals, and desires is another gray area for ToM terminology, as such inferences also do not necessarily require metarepresentation. Children can make these inferences much earlier than they can do metarepresentation (Suddendorf & Whiten, 2001). In social neuroscience, however, ToM is used broadly to mean inferring a variety of mental states, not necessarily limited to metarepresentation. Without having strong views on the proper use of the term, we can still attempt to be clear about which type of mental state is meant when using the term "theory of mind."

Developmental psychology can reveal the building blocks and components of ToM, and comparative ethology can tell us whether or not our mammal and primate relatives have each component (Saxe, Carey & Kanwisher, 2004; Suddendorf, 1999). The groundwork is then laid for neuroscience to investigate the brain systems involved in each component. This is not to say that ontogeny recapitulates phylogeny, but rather that both developmental and primatological studies can be helpful in mapping the components of such a complex cognitive ability. Many building blocks of theory of mind are present in old-world monkeys and in our ape relatives (Suddendorf, 1999; Suddendorf & Whiten, 2001; Hare, Call, Agnetta, & Tomasello, 2000; Leavens, Hopkins, & Thomas, 2004). Thus those building blocks at least are more ancient than the hominid line of the past 6 million years.

I outline how humans develop ToM, point to primate studies indicating which aspects of ToM we share with our monkey and ape cousins, and review the neuroscience data on the brain systems involved (see Table 15.1 for a summary). In reviewing the developmental literature, I remain agnostic on whether ToM develops through simulation, theory building, or modular maturation. That is not the focus of the review; rather, it focuses on what abilities emerge when, which abilities seem to be domain specific, and how domain-general abilities might depend on domain-specific ones to produce complex social cognition.

Building Blocks of ToM

Animacy Detection

ToM inferences are made only about animate entities; therefore, one of the fundamental components of any kind of social perception is the detection of animacy, that is, perceiving entities in the world as having self-propelled, goal-directed motion. Many animals readily detect the dif-

TABLE 15.1. Stages in ToM Development and Components of ToM

Cognitive ability	Age at which it emerges	Possible evolutionary age	Possibly relevant brain regions
Animacy detection	16–20 weeks	Mammals and primates, 54–85 million years	Superior temporal sulcus (STS), superior parietal, right middle frontal gyrus
Eye-direction detection	0–4 months	Mammals and primates, 54–85 million years	STS, amygdala
Gaze following	3–4 months	Primates, 26–54 million years	Unknown
Intention/goal detection	5–15 months	Primates, 26–54 million years	STS, orbitofrontal cortex
Gaze monitoring	9–18 months	Great apes, macaques, 14–26 million years	Unknown
Joint attention	18–24 months	Great apes, macaques, 14–26 million years	Unknown
Pretend play	18–24 months	Anecdotal evidence, chimps only, 5–7 million years	Unknown
Desire (mentalism)	18–24 months	Great apes, 7–14 million years	STS, temporal pole, temporo-parietal junction, orbitofrontal cortex, dorsomedial frontal cortex, amygdala
Implicit belief understanding (mentalism)	36–40 months	Great apes, 7–14 million years	STS, temporal pole, temporo-parietal junction, orbitofrontal cortex, dorsomedial frontal cortex, amygdala
Explicit belief understanding, metarepresentation	3.5–4 years	Uniquely human, 0.2–5 million years	STS, temporal pole, temporo-parietal junction, orbitofrontal cortex, dorsomedial frontal cortex, amygdala

ference between inanimate motion, in which something moves only by the laws of physics, such as a nut falling down from a tree or branches swaying in the wind, and animate motion, in which something moves in a way that can only be self-propelled: changing direction without an apparent force to change that direction, or moving against a force, say, by moving uphill. Detection of animacy is not limited to vision but can also be triggered by touch and hearing (Baron-Cohen, 1995). Vision, touch, and hearing can thus all provide cues that an animate agent is present. Infants as young as 16–20 weeks distinguish between visual displays of animate and inanimate motion (Crichton & Lange-Küttner, 1999), pointing to this ability being a very early building block in the emerging system of social perception.

In primates, Perrett et al. (1990) found cells in the superior temporal sulcus (STS) of rhesus macaque monkeys that were activated by unexpected touch. As there was no short-term habituation, these cells did not respond to novelty but instead to expectation. Even when the tactile stimulus was identical, these cells responded only when the touch was unexpected. Other cells in the STS were active only in response to the sight of others' hand movements, not to the sight of the monkey's own movements (Perrett et al., 1990). Thus the primate STS may contain networks of neurons for detecting visual or tactile contact with an animate agent. These networks require specific input to compute animacy—responding to unexpected but not expected touch, responding to others' hands but not to objects or the self. Thus this system seems to show design features indicating domain specificity for detecting animacy. Because rhesus macaques, with whom we diverged in evolution some 26 million years ago, also have such a system, our common ancestor must have had similar systems in place. Animacy detection, therefore, is an ancient part of our social-perception heritage.

Neuroimaging in humans points to the STS, as well as other areas, for animacy detection. In an fMRI study, inanimate motion (billiard-ball-type movement of one shape after another shape ran into it) specifically activated left and right posterior middle temporal gyrus and right intraparietal sulcus (Blakemore et al., 2003). In contrast, when participants saw animate motion (one shape started rotating only when another shape some distance away passed by a "window"), right and left superior parietal areas, right middle frontal gyrus, and left superior temporal sulcus were also activated. Inanimate motion primarily activated different areas than animate motion, indicating domain specificity. The brain processes animate objects differently from inanimate ones.

Inferring Goals and Intentions

Infants from very early on begin to distinguish actions that are intentional and to discern an actor's goal. Infants between 5 and 9 months can differentiate accidental from intentional behavior (Woodward, 1999), and by 15 months, infants classify actions according to the goal of an action (Csibra, Biro, Koos, & Gergely, 2003). These results show an implicit understanding of intentions and goals. Call and Tomasello (1998) showed that chimpanzees (Pan troglodytes) and orangutans (Pongo pygmaeus) could also distinguish visually between accidental and intentional actions. Monkeys do not seem to make this distinction. Assuming homology, this would put the date for this ability in a common ancestor at about 14 million years ago (Wildman, Uddin, Liu, Grossman, & Goodman, 2003).

Jellema, Baker, Wicker, and Perrett (2000) have begun to investigate the neural networks involved in detection of motor goals. They recorded cells in the anterior STS of macaque monkeys that responded to the sight of an agent reaching for something, but only when the agent was looking at the point reached for, with "looking at" indicated by eye gaze, head orientation, and upper body orientation. They propose that these cells integrate input from cells that respond to gaze direction with cells that respond to limb movement direction (Jellema et al., 2000). Such an integration is a necessary part of the cognitive architecture of detecting goals, which is the first step in understanding intentional action. Only social information—that is, information about others' eye-gaze direction, head and body orientation, and body movements—was found to activate this set of computations in macaques. A neural response only to a specific type of stimulus is one indicator of domain-specific cognitive processing; thus these results point to domain-specific computations for goal detection.

Eye Gaze Detection and Gaze Following

Once the brain's sensory systems have detected another agent, how does the brain then go about building up inferences about that agent's mental states? Implicit inferences about others' attention and gaze direction may be one of the first levels of mental-state inference. Certainly, prey animals need to be able to detect whether or not a predator is paying attention to them, and predators need to be able to detect whether their prey has seen them or not. Chickens, plovers, and hog-nosed snakes can all differentiate between direct and averted eye gaze (Burghardt, 1990; Gallup, Cummings, & Nash, 1972; Ristau, 1990, 1991), and dogs and mountain goats appear to track conspecifics' gaze (Tomasello, Hare, & Fogleman, 2001). Thus detecting and responding to gaze direction is likely to be quite an ancient ability. In humans, eye-gaze direction and head orientation are key cues used to determine what another person is paying attention to, what he or she might want, or what his or her intentions might be. Thus one of the earliest building blocks of ToM is the ability simply to detect direction of gaze, or "eye direction detection" (Baron-Cohen, 1995), and to refocus one's attention where another person is looking, known as "gaze following." Newborn infants are sensitive to direct eye contact versus averted gaze at 2–5 days after birth. Infants also follow gaze by age 3–4 months (Farroni, Mansfield, Lai, & Johnson, 2003). Electrophysiological methods show that the brains of 4-month-olds show distinct activity patterns to direct versus averted gaze (Farroni, Csibra, Simion, & Johnson, 2002).

Primates are clearly sensitive to eye gaze and eye contact. Several species of macaques (pig-tailed, stumptailed, and rhesus) can follow gaze from cues of a human experimenter's or conspecific's eye direction alone, as well as eye and head orientation together (Anderson & Mitchell, 1999; Ferrari, Kohler, Fogassi, & Gallese, 2000; Tomasello et al., 2001; but see Itakura, 1996, for conflicting results on rhesus macaques). Baboons have been observed to track others' gaze spontaneously, without training in using eye gaze as a cue (Vick & Anderson, 2003). Chimpanzees, orangutans, and sootey mangabeys have also been found to follow human gaze, though only adult chimps have been found to use eye direction alone (Tomasello et al., 2001; Okamoto et al., 2002).

These results on diverse species enable us to specify a phylogenetic age for gaze following, as opposed to simple detection of gaze direction. Apes clearly show the behavior (Tomasello et al., 2001), and we can be relatively certain that if apes and humans share the ability, that we share it because of common descent. Gaze following seems to be present in old-world monkeys as diverse as sootey mangabeys, baboons, and macaques, with whom we share a common ancestor 26 million years ago, but does not seem to be present in lemurs (Tomasello, Call, & Hare, 1998; Anderson & Mitchell, 1999; Tomasello et al., 2001; Ferrari et al., 2000). This pattern would specify the date of common descent for this ability as 26 million years ago, more recently than their common ancestor with lemurs 54 million years ago (Yoder, Cartmill, Ruvolo, Smith, & Vilgalys, 1996; Foley, 1997; Wildman et al., 2003).

The temporal lobes seem to be the key area for gaze-direction detection. In rhesus macaques, cells in the STS respond differentially to certain directions of eye gaze and head angle, and lesions in STS impair the ability to differentiate gaze direction (Perrett et al., 1990; Campbell, Heywood, Cowey, Regard, & Landis, 1990). Cells in the macaque amygdala respond selectively to direct eye contact as well, if the animal displaying the eye-gaze cues is a dominant animal (David Amaral, personal communication, May 1997). In human adults, there is evidence from neuroimaging studies that the STS and amygdala are activated specifically in tasks involving detecting direction of gaze (Kawashima et al., 1999; Hoffman & Haxby, 2000). Young et al. (1995) also found that a patient with bilateral amygdala lesions was not able to correctly detect whether someone in a photograph was looking right at her. The brain systems involved in eye-direction detection in humans appear to be similar to those in monkeys and thus may be shared through common descent. As with goal detection, these systems require a particular kind of visual input, the image of eyes or a head looking in a certain direction. In fact, Campbell et al. (1990) used a control stimulus of white circles with black dots in the middle of them and, even with such a perceptually similar stimulus, they did not find the same effects they found with eye gaze. Thus these gaze-detection systems seem to be domain specific for processing a very particular subset of social stimuli.

I know of no research to date on the neural systems involved in gaze *following*, as opposed to gaze-direction detection. Gaze following represents a distinct and important behavior, showing that infants and primates are doing something with information about gaze direction, that is, using it to seek information in the world. Jellema et al.'s (2000) study on goal detection points to some possibly relevant systems. They reported cells in the anterior STS that integrated input from cells responding to gaze direction with cells responding to limb-movement direction. A similar type of integration might be required for gaze following. A system in the brain that integrates the output of cells that respond to gaze direction with cells that control the viewer's own gaze direction would be necessary. Thus the STS might be involved, as well as areas to which STS "gaze-direction cells" project. Activation in the frontal eye fields and any other areas involved in control of one's own gaze direction would have to be integrated with STS activity. This remains an open area for study.

Eye Gaze as Implicit Information about Mental States

Gaze monitoring. Young children, however, do more with gaze direction than just follow it. They also gradually begin to interpret it to mean something about others' mental states. Between 9 and 24 months of age, children begin not just to follow gaze reflexively but also to actively monitor others' gaze direction as a source of information. Children 9–18 months old will look at an adult's eyes when presented with an ambiguous situation, indicating that they have an implicit understanding that direction of eye gaze can give them information about the world (Phillips, Baron-Cohen, & Rutter, 1992). Butterworth and Jarrett (1991) demonstrated that infants will look where an adult is looking if it is within the infant's own visual field by age 12 months and will monitor an adult's gaze outside of their own visual field later, between 12 and 18 months. Baldwin (1993) found that children ages 14–19 months were successful at learning novel words for novel objects if they could rely on the speaker's direction of gaze to find the correct referent for the word. Thus, during this time, from roughly 9 to 19 months, infants are becoming more sophisticated in using adult eye gaze as a source of information. This new stage could be called "gaze monitoring" and involves actively seeking out information about others' gaze direction instead of merely following it when presented with the visual stimulus of another's gaze.

In order for this stage to happen, the child must understand implicitly that others' focus of attention can be different from their own. Infants, toddlers, or primates who engage in gaze monitoring demonstrate their implicit assumptions about the *cause* of ambiguous behavior. They do not look for the cause of such events by looking at all the moving parts of the other person, as they would with artifacts. Rather, they look for the cause in the actors' *minds*, in their perception and attention as revealed through eye gaze. We see the emergence of an implicit understanding that mental states cause behavior. Causes of ambiguous behavior are sought in the social rather than the physical world; thus gaze monitoring is another indicator of domain specificity.

Some level of decoupling from immediate perception is also implied by gaze monitoring, as the child must have an implicit understanding that his or her own mental state could be different if he or she looked where an adult is looking. The child must hold a representation that is decoupled from the child's current perceptual reality, or there would be no reason to seek further information through eye gaze. Such decoupled representations are referred to as "secondary representations" to indicate their difference from primary perceptual representations (representations of immediate perceptual reality; Perner, 1991; Suddendorf, 1999; Suddendorf & Whiten, 2001).

Joint attention. Gradually, children start to treat another's gaze direction not just as a source of information but as being indicative of that person's focus of attention. "Joint attention" emerges between 18 and 24 months and involves the child taking another active step beyond gaze monitoring to calling adults' attention to particular objects by pointing or holding up something for them to see. It is worth noting that they do not always *successfully* bring things to adults' attention, as children at this age still fail perspective-taking tasks. They may hold something up or point to something without realizing that an adult cannot see what they are looking at. Thus there is still no evidence that children at this stage can correctly understand the *contents* of others' mental states. Nevertheless, children at this stage become active in trying to affect others' attention. Establishing empirically that a child is using joint attention usually depends on clear evidence that the child has either moved an object deliberately into another person's line of view or that the child is using "protodeclarative pointing," that is, pointing to something and alternating gaze between another person and the object (Baron-Cohen, 1995; Franco & Butterworth, 1996). Pointing can be used in several ways, not all of which indicate joint attention—such as pointing simply to request an object or pointing to count and keep track of objects one is sorting. Thus pointing that clearly indicates reference is the "acid test" of joint attention. At this stage, children must understand implicitly not only that others' attentional focus can be different from their own but also that others' attentional focus can be engaged and controlled to some degree by the child's own actions.

Joint attention also requires a secondary representation that is decoupled from the child's primary representation of reality. Baron-Cohen (1995) suggests that such a representation must simultaneously include both the relationship between an agent and an object and that between the self and an object. The child must be able to compute that he or she and another person are paying attention *to the same thing*. Baron-Cohen (1995) argues that this stage also requires what he terms "triadic representations," because they include three types of information: about agent and object, about self and object, and about agent and self:

grown-up –sees→ [I –see→ the dog].

However, such a representational format implies that the child is representing the contents of the adult's mental state of seeing and also implies such young children can do embedding and recursion, neither of which seems to be the case. Children who have joint attention nevertheless make systematic errors about what others can and cannot see (Mossler, Marvin, & Greenberg, 1976; Liben, 1978; Flavell et al., 1981), and call adults' attention to things the adult cannot see (such as holding up a watch and saying to a parent on the phone, "Mommy, look at my new watch!"). It seems that children do *not* have any kind of representation at this stage that is embedded, that allows them to represent the contents of others' mental states (Suddendorf, 1999). Thus I believe it is more parsimonious to assume the child has only a secondary representation for integrating information about whether or not an adult is paying attention (binary yes/no) and about the rough location of objects in space and a repertoire of actions that generally succeed in engaging adult's attention (holding things up, pointing). Thus what may have emerged at the joint attention stage is not only a new domain-specific ability but also a new domain-general ability, the capacity to form secondary representations. This domain-general ability can take the output of domain-specific systems for gaze direction and goal detection and integrate them with the child's own actions.

What evidence is there for gaze monitoring and joint attention in primates? Kumashiro, Ishibashi, Itakura, and Iriki (2002) have presented suggestive evidence that a Japanese macaque monkey (*Macaca fuscata*) in their lab engaged in gaze monitoring and learned to use protodeclarative pointing. The monkey, named Pin, looked at the human experimenter's gaze direction to determine which item to choose in an ambiguous two-item choice task, evidence of gaze monitoring. She seemed to use joint attention spontaneously, pointing "with an index finger, to food while alternating her gaze between the food and the human. Pin also pointed at a TV screen while both she and the human were watching a movie" (p. 3). Another monkey in the same lab was unable to use human eye gaze as information. In a later study, the same lab found that monkeys that had been trained to learn this kind of joint attention could imitate complex motions by human experimenters, whereas monkeys that did not engage in joint attention did not imitate a human experimenter (Kumashiro et al., 2003). There are no reported examples of monkeys using protodeclarative gestures in the wild, in their natural social development. Nevertheless, it is still informative that a monkey has the capacity to be trained to use referential pointing and that this capacity seems to be linked to the capacity for imitation. Imitation, like joint attention, requires secondary representations (Suddendorf, 1999; Suddendorf & Whiten, 2001). Thus it may be that monkeys, as well as great apes, have this level of cognitive ability.

Chimpanzees and orangutans have clearly been observed to engage in gaze monitoring, as they respond differently to situations in which another animal or human experimenter can see an object clearly and to situations in which the other's gaze is occluded (Hare et al., 2000; Suddendorf & Whiten, 2001, 2003). There are also many anecdotes of strategic deception in apes, such as a female chimpanzee sneaking off into the bushes to mate with a nondominant male, monitoring to make sure that the dominant male cannot see (Byrne, 2001). There is behavioral evidence that apes, like young children, can understand that another animal is paying attention or not paying attention or that another animal has seen or not seen something; as with children, there is no evidence that they understand the contents of someone else's mental states based on what that individual can see. Evidence is somewhat mixed, but the majority of studies find that chimpanzees and orangutans treat situations in which another's gaze is occluded differently from situations in which another can see (Suddendorf & Whiten, 2001, 2003; Povinelli, Theall, Reaux, & Dunphy-Lelii, 2003). Chimpanzees also seem to use gestures differently when a human experimenter is or is not looking at a food item they desire (Povinelli et al., 2003). Though apes have been found to use gaze monitoring, apes, like monkeys, do not seem to use referential pointing spontaneously in their natural environment. Even apes in captivity usually use pointing only to request an object (Povinelli & O'Neill, 2000). It seems likely that macaque monkeys and apes might, in their natural social environment, rely more on gaze direction and gaze monitoring for something like joint attention, and not on gestures such as pointing (Stone, 2005). These abilities are at least 14 million years old if only shared with apes and possibly 26 million years old if also shared with monkeys.

I know of no study to date that focuses specifically on systems that might mediate joint attention in the brain. Because joint attention represents a significant stage in ToM development, this is a striking omission in social neuroscience. The empirical assay used to assess joint attention in children, monkeys, and apes involves shifts in eye-gaze direction and pointing; thus it might be difficult to come up with an empirical paradigm that would work well in a scanner or in neuropsychological testing of patients. However, in this search, I believe a less domain-specific approach might be helpful. Good research always depends on having the right control conditions. Understanding some of our social cognitive abilities as an interaction between domain-specific and domain-general abilities can suggest necessary control conditions.

In looking for brain systems that underlie joint attention, I suggest a different approach than the sort that has been used in the studies cited earlier for animacy, goal, and gaze detection, an approach not focused specifically on joint attention. If one *key* cognitive ability underlying joint attention, the ability to form secondary representations, is not specific to joint attention, then looking for a "joint attention network" in the brain requires taking this into account. Any study looking at joint attention in neuroimaging paradigms or in patient research should include control tasks that require the same key cognitive ability. Perhaps the search should be not for brain systems that mediate joint attention but for brain systems that mediate secondary representations. Although secondary representations may enable some crucial aspects of social cognition and behavior to emerge, their usefulness is not restricted to the social domain. The ability to form secondary representations applies across a number of cognitive abilities that emerge in children at the same time, such as means–end problem solving or searching for hidden objects (Suddendorf & Whiten, 2001). In each of these abilities, an alternative mental model of the world can be held online and kept distinct from the primary representation of reality. Apes can do many of these tasks; thus the ability to form secondary representations seems to be one we share with great apes (Suddendorf, 1999; Suddendorf & Whiten, 2001).

Perhaps the most significant other example of the non-ToM uses of secondary representations is found in the fact that the child is beginning to learn language at the same time. Learning to associate arbitrary symbolic sounds to objects and actions in the world and to understand that one "refers" to the other implies some form of decoupled secondary representation. This is particularly true because the child has to simultaneously understand that sounds he or she hears and sounds he or she makes both refer to the same object. (In this sense, language learning is similar to reciprocal imitation.) This level of secondary representation seems to be a cognitive ability we share with apes, as they can be taught to make symbolic associations between objects or actions and symbols on a picture board or hand signs (for a review, see Snowdon, 2001).[1]

Such nonsocial tasks that require secondary representations could be used as control tasks in neuroimaging or patient studies. If a patient has difficulty with joint attention, but not with these other tasks requiring secondary representations, then we would have strong evidence for areas involved specifically in joint attention. If an area is active for joint attention and these other tasks, then that may be an area subserving domain-general functions; but if another area is active only for joint attention and not for, say, searching for hidden objects, then that would be a candidate area to be specific to joint attention.

Pretend Play

In this same age range (18–24 months), children begin to engage in pretend play. Pretending involves decoupling the pretend reality ("this is my baby") from perceptual reality ("this is an inanimate doll"). There is considerable debate in developmental psychology over what children understand about pretense as a mental state. Leslie (1987) argues strongly that pretense involves representing one's own and others' mental states, that is, that children have a representation such as "Mommy is pretending that → [the doll is a baby]," that is, that they have some form of metarepresentation. However, children at this age still fail perspective-taking tasks and make systematic errors about what others can and cannot see (Mossler et al., 1976; Liben, 1978; Flavell et al., 1981). Thus it is difficult to make a convincing case that they can represent the *contents* of a playmate's mental states. Furthermore, younger children do not always understand the role of mental states in pretense (Lillard et al., 2000). In debates over whether children at this age truly understand the representational nature of pretend play, the more parsimonious alternative hypothesis is that they treat pretense as a special kind of action (e.g., Wellman & Lagattuta, 2000). Neuroscience research into the brain substrates for pretense might help resolve this debate. If an understanding of pretense is just a special kind of action, then areas involved in pretense might overlap with areas involved in representing actions not currently being done, for example, the supplementary motor area. If pretense does involve representing the contents of others' mental states, then the same areas active for full metarepresentational ToM should be active for pretense. In this case, studies of the neural substrate of pretend play and ToM tasks could inform theories about cognitive representations in pretense. German et al. (2004) have found that in adults, the same regions active for higher order ToM are active during pretense, but no neuroscience studies of pretense in children have yet been reported.

Seeing Leads to Knowing

Up to the third year of life, it seems that children can understand attention and lack of attention, or looking at and not looking at, but they are not able to understand the *contents* of someone else's mental states based on what that person can see. Understanding the contents of another's mental states may depend on metarepresentation, discussed later. I include a discussion of the mentalistic significance of eye gaze here, as it represents the last stage in how domain-specific representations of eye gaze contribute to ToM. At this latest stage of representing eye gaze, gaze direction is not simply inferred or used to guide a child's actions; the mentalistic significance of eye gaze seems to be explicitly represented—that is, seeing leads to knowing, looking equates to attending.

By ages 3–4, sighted children begin to interpret eye gaze explicitly to imply other mental states besides attention and seem to have explicit knowledge of the mental states implied by eye gaze, rather than just the implicit understanding evidenced earlier. From age 3 years 4 months, children in one study could say that someone who is looking into a box knows what is in the box, whereas someone who is merely touching the box but not looking in it does not know (Pratt & Bryant, 1990). Four-year-olds can say that someone who is looking at something intends to act on that thing (Baron-Cohen, Campbell, Karmiloff-Smith, Grant, & Walker, 1995).

It has been easier to come up with tasks to use in neuroscience paradigms that tap into the ability to interpret eye-gaze direction mentalistically than to come up with gaze-monitoring or joint-attention tasks. Baron-Cohen et al. (1999) used a task called Reading the Mind in the Eyes, which requires participants to choose one of four adjectives describing mental states to describe pictures of the eye region of several faces. Using fMRI, the researchers scanned participants while they performed the task and found greater activation in the amygdala and superior temporal gyrus (STG) during this task compared with a control task in normal participants but did not find this differential activation in individuals with Asperger's syndrome (Baron-Cohen et al., 1999). However, whereas an earlier version of the task (Baron-Cohen, Joliffe, Mortimore, & Robertson, 1997) had included both items about emotion (nervous vs. calm) and items about attention and mental states (looking at you vs. looking at someone else, or daydreaming vs. paying attention), the version of the task used in the scanner included only items about emotion. Thus these results can show only that amygdala and STG are involved in inferring emotional states from the eyes.

Evidence indicates that the amygdala may not be involved in inferring more complex mental states from the eyes. Stone, Baron-Cohen, Calder, Keane, and Young (2003) tested the older version of the Eyes task, including both mental-state items and emotional items, in two patients with bilateral amygdala damage. We found that patients were impaired on both types of items, though the low number of mental-state items (eight) means that this is not firm evidence that the amygdala is involved in the mentalistic interpretation of eye gaze. More convincing evidence is presented by Adolphs, Baron-Cohen, and Tranel (2002), who used a similar task measuring the ability to identify social emotions (e.g., arrogant, guilty), basic emotions (e.g., sad, angry), and complex mental states (e.g., interested, quizzical, bored) from pictures of the eyes. They found that patients with bilateral amygdala damage were impaired in identifying social emotions relative to controls and patients with unilateral amygdala damage but were not impaired in identifying basic emotions or complex mental states. Thus it is possible that although the amygdala may be involved in detecting gaze direction and in identifying expressions of social emotions, it is not involved in inferring the mentalistic significance of eye gaze. Further tests using tasks that directly test amygdala patients' ability to infer that "seeing leads to knowing" and using seeing-leads-to-knowing tasks in neuroimaging paradigms will provide more information about this question.

There is the possibility that orbitofrontal cortex (OFC) might be involved in the mentalistic significance of gaze. Gregory et al. (2002) tested patients with OFC damage from frontotemporal dementia (FTD) on a series of ToM tasks, including the version of the Reading the Mind in the Eyes test that included both emotion and mental-state items. These patients were impaired on this task relative to controls matched on the Mini-Mental State Exam and education and to patients with Alzheimer's disease and were impaired on both mental-state and emotional items. Snowden et al. (2003) tested patients with OFC damage from FTD and patients with Huntington's disease on the Charlie and the Chocolates task (Baron-Cohen et al., 1995), measuring whether a participant can say whether someone who is looking at an object likes or intends to act on that object, and found that the group with FTD were specifically impaired in understanding preference and intention from gaze but had no difficulty determining eye-gaze direction. Thus OFC, but not the amygdala, may be involved in inferring mental states, particularly *intentions*, from direction of eye gaze. Both of these tasks used with FTD patients are explicit ToM tasks, but they are quite different from traditional ToM tasks, discussed later. Neuroimaging studies of the ability to infer knowledge or attention from eye gaze, using the ability to detect direction of gaze as a control task, should be used to further explore brain areas that might be involved in this ability.

Implicit Mentalistic Understanding: Acting Based on Others' Mental States

Desire

Beginning at around age 2, children readily use language about desire: "I want," "she likes" (Wellman & Lagattuta, 2000; Wellman, Cross, & Watson, 2001). They seem to understand that people's attitudes and emotions toward various objects can be used to predict what they will do (Wellman & Lagattuta, 2000). Thus understanding desire may develop out of an understanding of intentions and goals in development. At this age, children can also understand that different people's desires are distinct—that, for example, they don't want to eat their vegetables but that grown-ups seem to like this yucky-tasting stuff. When given information about what another person likes or wants and asked, for example, "Which snack would this other person want?", young children simply answer with their own desire; but from 18 to 24 months, children can say that someone else would choose the snack he or she likes best (Wellman & Woolley, 1990; Repacholi & Gopnik, 1997; Wellman & Liu, 2004). Understanding such *diverse desires* is something that may also depend on decoupled secondary representations. The child has to understand two relations:

$$\text{agent } -\text{likes} \rightarrow \text{object,}$$
$$\text{self } -\text{likes} \rightarrow \text{other object}$$

and understand that the two agent–object relations are different. Thus understanding diverse desire may not develop until after the ability to form secondary representations has emerged.

However, an understanding of desire also implies something beyond secondary representations. Likes, wants, and desires are private mental states that are changeable. A person's likes and wants can change independent of external reality changing. Unlike eye-gaze direction, desires inherently cannot be observed directly but must be inferred from behavior. A state of liking or wanting must be inferred from the coupling of intention plus affect. This mentalistic understanding of desire is a particular aspect of ToM development that I believe cannot be explained in domain-general terms alone. Secondary representations about agent–object relations are not sufficient; a representation of desire needs to specify some additional information about the nature of that agent–object relation. The relation *desire* in "agent –desire→ object" is a special kind of relation, different from "agent –looks at→ object." "Looking at" can represent a state of perceptual reality, eyes open, eyes directed toward object, no occlusion between eyes and object. Gaze monitoring and joint attention depend on an observable mental quality, perception and attention as revealed through eye gaze. "Looking at" does not change unless perceptual reality changes. "Desire," however, can change without external reality changing. Thus this developmental step represents the first stage at which children display understanding of something that is uniquely *mental*, private, unobservable, and changeable. This implicit understanding of the private and changeable nature of mental things, which could be called "mentalism," is a genuinely new development in ToM and is specific to ToM, not explainable by reference to general cognitive abilities such as forming secondary representations. I believe this aspect of ToM cognition, mentalism, is domain specific. Understanding desire thus may set the stage for the next step in ToM development at age 3 (Wellman, 1990; Wellman & Liu, 2004).

Belief and Knowledge

Adult human ToM involves understanding knowledge and beliefs. Like desire, knowledge is also changeable, though knowledge is cumulative compared with desire. When someone "knows" something that can be untrue or uncertain, we call that "belief." If people see something new or are told something new, they know about that thing; their knowledge state has changed. If something in the world changes, but a person does not see the change, then his or her knowledge state does not change and does not reflect the current state of reality. Knowledge and belief are thus decoupled from reality. The ability to form decoupled secondary representations is a necessary precursor to representing knowledge states, but mentalism is crucial as well, an understanding of the private and changeable nature of these mental states. Children show an *implicit* understanding of knowledge and belief before they can talk about it or understand it explicitly.

To test whether children or primates know about someone else's knowledge state, one has to distinguish their representation of someone else's mental state from their representation of the state of reality. If one probes what a participant thinks someone else knows and what the participant knows is true, it is always possible that the participant is just responding with what he or she knows him- or herself. Thus testing whether a participant can understand that someone else holds a false belief has long been held to be the key test of ToM. But what does it mean to understand false belief? Does someone understand it if he or she can act based on someone else's false belief but can't talk about it, or does someone have to be able to talk or answer verbal questions about it explicitly? Understanding false belief, it appears, can be either implicit or explicit. Two basic kinds of false belief tasks have been used with children: *location-change* tasks and *unexpected-contents* tasks.[2] In a location-change task, the person is told a short story (and shown pictures to go with the story; or the story is acted out with toy figures) in which character A puts an object in location 1 and then turns away or goes out of the room. Character B moves the object to location 2 while A cannot see (or, if the object is animate, such as a pet, it moves itself), and then the person is asked where A will look for the object, in location 1 or location 2. Children usually pass this test some time between late in the third year of life and age 4, but it is rare that 3-year-olds can pass it (Wellman & Liu, 2004; Wellman et al., 2001).

Perner and Garnham (2001) used an ingenious test to assess whether younger children who could not yet pass a standard false-belief task could nevertheless understand another person's false belief implicitly. In their study, the child was told that another person was going to slide down one of two slides and that the child was supposed to place a mat so the person could land safely at the bottom of the slide he or she was going to come down. The researchers manipulated the situation so that sometimes the person who was supposed to slide down had a true belief about which slide he or she was supposed to come down and sometimes had a false belief and would therefore come down the wrong slide. The task was set up so that the children had to act quickly, without time for deliberation. The 36-month-olds in this study were likely to place the mat under the correct slide, showing that they had an implicit ability to track the other person's belief state, true or false. These same children failed a standard false-belief task that asked for an explicit choice of which slide the person would come down. It is also worth noting, for comparison, that Pratt and Bryant (1990; discussed earlier) found that 40-month-olds could pass a "seeing-leads-to-knowing" test, which may be an implicit belief task, at an age when children generally cannot pass explicit false-belief tasks (Wellman & Liu, 2004). Thus an implicit understanding of the fact that knowledge can change and that such changes are linked to perception and decoupled from reality seems to emerge around age 3. Three-year-olds seem to be able to use mentalism to solve such tasks implicitly.

Chimpanzees (*Pan troglodytes*) can also solve an implicit task testing understanding of knowledge and ignorance. If two chimpanzees both see the same food source, the more dominant animal almost always gets it, or else a conflict ensues. In this study, chimpanzees were given a choice to head toward one of two food items, one that a dominant animal could see and one that it couldn't see, or one location in which the dominant animal had seen food being hidden but had not seen it being moved (Hare, Call, & Tomasello, 2001). The "subject," the nondominant chimp, could see what the dominant animal had or had not seen. In each case, the chimp preferentially chose to head toward food about which the dominant animal was ignorant or had a false belief as to location (Hare et al., 2001). Thus chimpanzees seem to be able to act on an implicit understanding of other animals' knowledge and ignorance when testing conditions are ecologically valid (competition for food), and their behavior must be guided by tracking other animals' knowledge (Suddendorf & Whiten, 2003).

Like understanding desire, this stage of implicit belief understanding cannot be explained simply by the operation of secondary representations. It requires an understanding that others' mental states can change or not change over time and that this is distinct from how reality changes. This is what is meant by "mentalism," an implicit understanding of the relationship between mental states and reality, that mental states are private, internal, and can change or not change independent of reality. In this sense, the mentalism that emerges with the understanding of desire is further extended into an implicit understanding of belief (cf. Wellman, 1990). However, there is still no watertight evidence that either 3-year-old children or apes can represent the *contents* of others' mental states explicitly. Indeed, the fact that children this age still fail perspective-taking tasks (even with controls for nonmentalizing task demands) is evidence that they cannot track the actual content of others' mental states (Mossler et al., 1976; Liben, 1978; Flavell et al., 1981). To represent others' mental contents, another cognitive ability must emerge first.

ToM Proper:
Metarepresentation, Recursion, and Executive Function

Although 3-year-olds and chimpanzees can demonstrate implicit tracking of others' belief states, this does not mean that they understand the representational nature of beliefs. Knowledge and belief are about knowledge representations and referents: agent −represents→ [proposition]. Understanding this representational nature of knowledge and belief means understanding the way that epistemic mental states refer to propositions about the world. Mentalism does not suffice for understanding representation. Rather, a new step in ToM development must occur, "metarepresentation," the ability to explicitly represent representations *as representations* (Perner, 1991; Leslie, 1994; Baron-Cohen, 1995). It is metarepresentation that enables children to pass explicit false-belief tasks, and it is metarepresentation that apes lack (Suddendorf, 1999). The child at this stage can understand that beliefs refer to propositions about the world, can explicitly represent the contents of those beliefs, and thus can represent explicitly that beliefs can be mistaken. Passing an explicit false-belief task has been seen as certain evidence of ToM capacities (Dennett, 1978).

However, the converse is not true. Many other cognitive abilities also contribute to being able to pass an explicit false-belief task. Thus if a person fails a false-belief task, it does not necessarily mean that he or she lacks metarepresentation. It might be that he or she lacks one of the other cognitive abilities on which successful false-belief task performance depends. In particular, solving false-belief tasks depends on executive control, on being able to inhibit the inappropriate response, that is, what the participant knows to be the true state of reality, in order to answer with the perhaps less salient correct response, that is, what the other person's mental state is (Carlson & Moses, 2001; Flynn, O'Malley, & Wood, 2004; Carlson, Moses, & Claxton, 2004). In fact, children can pass false-belief tasks slightly earlier if the task demands are changed so that less inhibitory control is required, for example, by making the current state of reality less salient (Wellman & Lagattuta, 2000). False-belief tasks also depend on working memory and sequencing, as the participant has to keep in mind all the elements of the story as it unfolds in order, and how those elements are changing with respect to each other (Keenan, 1998; Stone, Baron-Cohen, & Knight, 1998). Thus someone who has deficits in inhibiting a prepotent response or in working memory could easily fail a false-belief task even while having intact metarepresentational abilities.

Furthermore, metarepresentation also depends on a more general cognitive ability, embedding/recursion. To explicitly represent "X represents → [proposition]" requires the ability to embed one proposition in another. If metarepresentation depends on recursion, then difficulties with recursion could cause failures on the false-belief task (Corballis, 2003). There are many other cognitive tasks besides ToM that use metarepresentation and recursion: complex syntax, self-representation, creativity, episodic memory and future planning (a.k.a. "mental time travel"), metamemory, and counterfactual reasoning (Shimamura, Janowsky & Squire, 1990; Knight & Grabowecky, 1995; Suddendorf, 1999; Suddendorf & Fletcher-Flinn, 1999; De Villiers, 2000; Shimamura, 2000; Corballis, 2003). Thus recursion and metarepresentation appear to be domain-general cognitive abilities, not limited to social cognition, that interact with mentalism to produce what we call explicit ToM.

As an example of metarepresentation and recursion in another domain, De Villiers (2000) argues that the ability to form embedded sentence complements, that is, utterances of the form "agent −says→ subordinate clause," for example, "He said that he finished his peas," or "She says that she saw the movie," provides the representational structure needed for explicitly representing belief and knowledge. Sentences such as "Agent says that X," however, are about observable things, utterances, rather than about private and changeable things, such as mental states. Thus the metarepresentational ability that is needed for sentence complements is distinct from mentalism, from understanding the relationship between mental states and reality. In development, the ability to use and understand sentence complements and embedded relative clauses precedes the ability to pass false-belief tests (De Villiers & Pyers, 2002; Smith, Apperly & White, 2003).

The idea that explicit ToM is dependent on the metarepresentational competence needed for such complex grammatical structures is consistent with results on the cognitive abilities of chimps. Currently, chimps have been found to fail an explicit false-belief task (Call & Tomasello, 1999). Chimpanzees who have been taught to use signs and symbols to refer to things have never been observed to use complex syntax at all, much less sentence complements (Snowdon, 2001). Apes also do not show any evidence of either episodic memory or future planning (Suddendorf, 1999; Suddendorf & Busby, 2003). Thus metarepresentation and recursion may be uniquely human capacities (Suddendorf, 1999; Corballis, 2003).

Until the development of metarepresentation, ToM's building blocks consist mostly of specific social abilities: animacy detection, gaze-direction detection and gaze following, gaze monitoring and joint attention, and mentalism. Each of these abilities is domain specific. They depend on particular input formats and lead to certain kinds of implicit causal inferences. However, without the development of two domain-general abilities, the ability to form secondary representations and the ability to form metarepresentations, ToM as we define it in adult humans could not emerge. It is ironic that metarepresentation, the very aspect of adult ToM that some researchers have treated as the "defining characteristic" of ToM proper (e.g., Leslie, 1994), may turn out not to be specific to the domain of mental state inferences at all. It is crucial for having a fully functioning adult ToM, yet it is also crucial for complex syntax, future-oriented thinking, and many other abilities (Suddendorf, 1999; Corballis, 2003). The most advanced *domain-specific* aspect of ToM is the implicit mentalism that we share with toddlers and great apes. Thus human ToM is an integration of our domain-specific abilities and our powerful domain-general abilities. Any search for ToM in the brain must take both types of abilities into account.

UNIQUELY HUMAN AND DOMAIN-GENERAL COGNITION: ToM IN THE BRAIN

The union of two kinds of abilities—domain-specific mentalism, that is, an implicit understanding of the changeable nature of mental states, and the domain-general abilities of recursion, metarepresentation, and executive cognitive control—may result in an explicit ToM in humans. However, metarepresentation, recursion, and executive control are not at all limited to ToM. The generality of these cognitive abilities makes the search for ToM in the brain a difficult one: Do we search for ToM, or do we search for metarepresentation, recursion, and executive function?

Social neuroscience has been studying ToM for less than a decade, and thus neuroscience research on ToM is still very much in its infancy. Much ToM research in neuroscience has not been done with proper controls for working memory, inhibitory demands of tasks, or other executive functions, nor has it been done with a clear definition of which types of mental states (e.g., intention, belief, desire) are being tapped by various tasks (Stone, 2005; Apperly, Samson, & Humphreys, 2005). I include my own research in this criticism. The body of research in this area claims variously that ToM might be processed in superior temporal areas, the temporal pole, the amygdala, the temporoparietal junction (TPJ), the medial frontal cortex, the orbitofrontal cortex (OFC), and/or the frontal pole (Goel, Grafman, Sadato, & Hallett, 1995; Fletcher et al., 1995; Stone et al., 1998; Gallagher et al., 2000; Fine, Lumsden, & Blair, 2001; Happé, Mahli, & Checkley, 2001; Stuss, Gallup, & Alexander, 2001; Gallagher, Jack, Roepstorff, & Frith, 2002; Gregory et al., 2002; Frith & Frith, 2003; Snowden et al., 2003; Stone et al., 2003; Grèzes, Frith, & Passingham, 2004; Liu, Saabagh, Gehring, & Wellman, 2004; Samson, Apperly, Chiavarino, & Hymphreys, 2004; Saxe, Carey, & Kanwisher, 2004). At least we know ToM is not superior parietal or occipital! Perhaps so many candidate brain areas have emerged as important for ToM because different areas subserve different aspects of ToM, some subserving domain-general functions, some domain-specific.

Elsewhere, I have argued that understanding the brain basis of ToM requires that social neuroscientists answer the three questions that follow (Stone, 2005) to establish whether some aspect of ToM (e.g., mentalism) is separate from domain-general abilities and to establish whether the brain areas involved in inferring belief, desire, and other mental states are the same or different. Each of these questions can be addressed by using patient research to look for dissociations and neuroimaging to investigate commonalities and differences in areas activated by different kinds of tasks.

1. *Do patients fail ToM tasks because of non-ToM task demands?* Do any patients show deficits on a ToM task but not a control task that has the same executive function (EF) demands or verbal-comprehension demands? Does changing the task to lessen the executive or comprehension demands improve patients' performance? For example, Stone et al. (1998) suggested that dorsolateral frontal cortex (DFC) was not crucial for false-belief performance after showing that patients with left DFC lesions did poorly on false-belief tasks only when the tasks included working-memory and sequencing demands. Many studies of ToM in patients with frontal lesions have not controlled for executive demands of ToM tasks (e.g., Stuss et al., 2001). Ironically, in patients with lesions elsewhere, when it may not be as crucial to control for EF, better EF controls have been done. Samson et al. (2004) reported specific ToM deficits in patients with lesions in temporoparietal junction (TPJ) and no deficits in control tasks with matched memory and inhibitory demands but no belief attribution required. Thus the TPJ patients' poor false-belief task performance is more clearly attributable to deficits in ToM rather than to non-ToM demands.

2. *Is ToM independent of EF, metarepresentation, and recursion?* Do patients' deficits in ToM correlate with deficits on EF measures that tap into relevant areas of EF: inhibitory control and working memory? Are

there patients who perform highly on relevant EF measures while being impaired in ToM? Are there patients with EF deficits who can perform well on ToM tasks that minimize executive demands? Some studies have reported that patients with medial frontal or OFC damage who have poor ToM scores also have EF deficits, but these studies have not reported the direct relationship between scores on ToM tasks and on EF tasks (e.g., Stone et al., 1998; Happé et al., 2001; Snowden et al., 2003), thus leaving open the question of independence in these patients. Furthermore, one patient with massive medial frontal damage showed no ToM impairments whatsoever, calling into question whether medial frontal cortex plays a crucial role in ToM at all (Bird, Castelli, Malik, Frith, & Husain, 2004).

There are, however, examples of patients with orbitofrontal damage, possibly extending into medial frontal damage, who demonstrate impaired ToM without impaired EF (Fine et al., 2001; Gregory et al., 2002; Lough, Gregory, & Hodges, 2002; Stone, Cosmides, Tooby, Kroll, & Knight, 2002; Apperly, Samson, Chiavarino, & Humphreys, 2004). Apperly and colleagues have devised a nonverbal version of the false-belief task with reduced demands in EF that allows for a more precise answer to this question in patient groups with executive or language deficits and found that some patients with TPJ lesions were impaired on this task without corresponding executive deficits (Apperly et al., 2004; Apperly et al., 2005). Some TPJ patients also have difficulty with false-belief tasks but not with tasks requiring counterfactual reasoning, which depends on recursion (Samson et al., 2004). Thus, using false-belief tasks, it does seem possible to separate ToM from EF and possibly recursion.

However, can ToM be separated from a general ability for meta-representation? Here, neuroimaging and patient studies lead to opposite conclusions. Saxe and Kanwisher (2003) looked at separability of ToM and metarepresentation in fMRI by using a nonmentalistic task requiring metarepresentation: the false-photograph task. Activation in the TPJ, superior temporal pole, and medial portions of frontal pole was significantly greater during false-belief tasks than false-photograph tasks. However, there was some difference in the difficulty of the two types of task (Saxe & Kanwisher, 2003). Patients with TPJ damage who show a specific deficit on false-belief tasks compared with EF and counterfactual reasoning are a good test group for establishing separability of ToM and metarepresentation. However, Apperly et al. (2005) report that when given false-photograph tests, every such patient with TPJ damage has deficits equivalent to their deficits on false-belief tasks. Neuroimaging of the exact versions of the tasks used by Apperly and colleagues will do much to clarify this issue. For the moment, however, it appears that there is no strong evidence for ToM being a separate ability from general metarepresentation (Stone & Gerrans, 2006).

3. *Does inferring belief require different brain systems as inferring other mental states (e.g., desire or intention), or are the same brain areas involved?* Are there patients who perform poorly on measures that tap

explicit metarepresentation of belief while still being able to perform well on tasks that measure an understanding of desire or intention, and vice versa? Patients with damage in OFC perform poorly on a ToM task requiring an understanding of whether others' actions are unintentional, but they perform well on a variety of false-belief tasks, including first-, second-, and third-order belief inferences, thus indicating that any ToM problems they have are not with metarepresentation (Stone et al., 1998; Stone, 2000; Gregory et al., 2002; Stone, 2005). One patient with OFC, temporal pole, and amygdala damage was selectively impaired in the ability to tell whether someone might cheat another person, that is, in inferring others' intentions, but the patient performed normally on false-belief tasks and on a nonsocial control task matched exactly for executive and nonexecutive task demands (Stone et al., 2002). Separating belief and desire has been more difficult, as many ToM tasks used with patients tap into both belief and desire inferences (e.g., Happé et al., 2001). Fine, Lumsden, and Blair (2001) reported that a patient with amygdala damage had difficulty both on tasks that tap only belief and on tasks that tap belief, desire, and other mental states. The amygdala may be involved when people make inferences about a variety of mental states, and OFC may be involved in inferences about intentions but not beliefs.

The Maturation of ToM Research in Neuroscience

Social neuroscience research on ToM is beginning to learn methodological lessons from developmental research demonstrating that children can have difficulty with false-belief tasks because of limitations in non-ToM cognitive abilities. We are also beginning to make distinctions between ToM and other related abilities, such as recursion and metarepresentation. Finally, we are beginning to look at different *kinds* of ToM inferences, belief, desire, intentions, and emotions.

Mentalism, the understanding of the nature of mental things, should be carefully distinguished from recursion and metarepresentation of belief, because these abilities emerge at different points in development and evolution. I suggest that if there is a brain network that mediates what is specifically *social* about high-level ToM inferences, then it would mediate the mentalism required to understand private and changeable belief states and desires. As such, the computations carried out by these areas would be maturing between 24 and 40 months of age in human children and could be those shared with great apes. To the extent that brain regions are involved in *specifically social* computations, they may not be involved in *uniquely human* computations.

Uniquely human cognition is not likely to be socially specific. Evolutionary psychology clarifies that domain-specific cognitive adaptations by definition are complex and thus must have evolved over vast spans of time. Special design for a particular cognitive function requires the gradual evolution of design features useful for that function layered on top of preexisting design features over tens of millions of years of natural selection (Tooby & Cosmides, 1992). Since our last common ancestor with the great apes, there have been only 5–7 million years, or roughly 330,000–460,000 generations, enough time for significant evolutionary change but not enough time for the gradual, layered, complex design necessary for domain specificity to have occurred through natural selection (Stone, 2003, 2004). The highest level social inferences that we can make are unique to our species, having emerged in this recent evolutionary time span: explicit ToM inferences using recursion and metarepresentation and requiring executive function, working memory, and inhibition. Recent human evolution seems to have involved expansion in these domain-general cognitive capacities (Stone, 2003, 2006). However, these general cognitive abilities do not operate in a vacuum and would not be useful for social cognition unless they were layered on top of domain-specific social abilities that emerged earlier (Stone & Gerrans, 2006).

ToM and social intelligence require the coordination of ancient domain-specific abilities with more evolutionarily recent domain-general abilities. We share gaze-direction detection in the STS with other mammals, at least, so this domain-specific ability is more than 54 million years old. Gaze following and detection of intentions and goals is shared with other social primates and thus may be 26–54 million years old. Such abilities are ancient enough to be domain specific. The interaction of these abilities with the domain-general ability to form secondary representations—which we share with great apes (7–14 million years old)—gave apes and hominids even more complex social cognition. This level of domain-general thought allowed for further elaboration into other domain-general abilities in the hominid line of the past 5–7 million years—recursion, metarepresentation, complex syntax and symbolic representation, and expanded EF (Suddendorf, 1999; Corballis, 2003; Stone, 2006). Over this same time period, the frontal and temporal lobes were increasing in size and developmental complexity (Semendeferi, Armstrong, Schleicher, Zilles, & Van Hoesen, 2001; Lieberman, McBratney, & Krovitz, 2002; Stone, in press). Uniquely human aspects of language, for example, depend on recursion (Corballis, 2003), and such complex syntactic abilities seem to involve areas in left temporoparietal cortex and inferior frontal regions (Cooke et al., 2001; Caplan et al., 2002). EF involves the prefrontal cortex. Thus these brain regions may be the seat of the domain-general abilities that are the hallmark of *Homo sapiens sapiens*.

Evolution is a tinkerer, not an optimizing engineer. Every change that takes place in an organism has to be advantageous within the context of the traits that organism already had. Thus our domain-general abilities were useful because they could flexibly combine the output of many different domain-specific mechanisms. They were useful for social cognition because they could use such domain-specific mechanisms as gaze-direction detection or goal detection to build up more complex, embedded inferences about mental states. They may have been useful for syntax, tool use, and mental time travel because they could combine representations from nonsocial domain-specific mechanisms. Thus increased complexity in social cognition was probably only one of many reasons why these domain-general abilities were selected for. The remarkable changes that have taken place in hominid brain evolution enabled expansion of our general cognitive capacities, but these capacities worked with the domain-specific social-cognitive abilities that were the legacy of our primate ancestors to produce our species' unique brand of social cognition.

NOTES

1. Obviously, there is a great deal more to language than this ability—this is only one building block. Children between 1 and 2 have very limited language, and apes who have been taught sign language have not been found to learn vocabularies of more than 300 or so symbols. Apes also seem able to combine symbols in sentences of only about three elements, as in subject–verb–object, and never spontaneously ask to learn new symbols for objects they do not already know how to refer to (Pinker, 1994; Snowdon, 2001). However limited its scope, for this stage of social and symbolic development, the key cognitive ability may be the ability to form secondary representations. This domain-general ability may be what underlies the early stages of both ToM and symbolic thought, working together with domain-specific representations of eye gaze in the case of early ToM. Truly complex syntax and more advanced ToM do not emerge for another year in development.

2. In an unexpected-contents task, the participant is shown a container that is clearly labeled as if it contains one kind of thing; for example, a candy box clearly indicates that it contains candy. The participant is shown that it really contains a quite different thing (e.g. there are pencils inside the candy box). Then the participant is asked what another person, who hasn't seen what's inside the box, will think is in there. Control questions usually ask about what was true originally, what the subject thought originally, and what is true right now.

REFERENCES

Adolphs, R., Baron-Cohen, S., & Tranel, D. (2002). Impaired recognition of social emotions following amygdala damage. *Journal of Cognitive Neuroscience, 14*(8), 1264–1274.

Anderson, J., & Mitchell, R. (1999). Macaques but not lemurs co-orient visually with humans. *Folia Primatologica, 70*(1), 17–22.

Apperly, I. A., Samson, D., Chiavarino, C. & Humphreys, G. W. (2004). Frontal and temporo-parietal lobe contributions to theory of mind: Neuropsychological evidence from a false-belief task with reduced language and executive demands. *Journal of Cognitive Neuroscience, 16*(10), 1773–1784.

Apperly, I. A., Samson, D., & Humphreys, G. W. (2005). Domain-specificity and theory of mind: Evaluating evidence from neuropsychology. *Trends in Cognitive Science, 9,* 572–577.

Baldwin, D. (1993). Infants' ability to consult the speaker for clues to word reference. *Journal of Child Language, 20(2),* 395–418.

Baron-Cohen, S. (1995). *Mindblindness: An essay on autism and theory of mind.* Cambridge, MA: MIT Press.

Baron-Cohen, S., Campbell, R., Karmiloff-Smith, A., Grant, J., & Walker, J. (1995). Are children with autism blind to the mentalistic significance of the eyes? *British Journal of Developmental Psychology, 13(4),* 379–398.

Baron-Cohen, S., Joliffe, T., Mortimore, C., & Robertson, M. (1997). Another advanced test of theory of mind: Evidence from very high-functioning adults with autism or Asperger's syndrome. *Journal of Child Psychology and Psychiatry, 38,* 813–822.

Baron-Cohen, S., Ring, H. A., Wheelwright, S., Bullmore, E. T., Brammer, M. J., & Simmons, A. (1999). Social intelligence in the normal and autistic brain: An fMRI study. *European Journal of Neuroscience, 11,* 1891–1898.

Bird, C. M., Castelli, F., Malik, O., Frith, U., & Husain, M. (2004) The impact of extensive medial frontal lobe damage on "theory of mind" and cognition. *Brain, 127(4),* 914–928.

Blakemore, S. J., Boyer, P., Pachot-Clouchard, M., Meltzoff, A., Segebarth, C., & Decety, J. (2003). The detection of contingency and animacy from simple animations in the human brain. *Cerebral Cortex, 13(8),* 837–844.

Burghardt, G. (1990). Cognitive ethology and critical anthropomorphism: A snake with two heads and hog-nosed snakes that play dead. In C. Ristau (Ed.), *Cognitive ethology: The minds of other animals* (pp. 53–90). New York: Erlbaum.

Butterworth, G., & Jarrett, N. (1991). What minds have in common is space: Spatial mechanisms serving joint visual attention in infancy. *British Journal of Developmental Psychology, 9(1),* 55–72.

Byrne, R. W. (2001). Social and technical forms of primate intelligence. In F. deWaal (Ed.), *Tree of origin: What primate behavior can tell us about human social evolution* (pp. 147–172). Cambridge, MA: Harvard University Press.

Call, J., & Tomasello, M. (1998). Distinguishing intentional from accidental actions in orangutans (*Pongo pygmaeus*), chimpanzees (*Pan troglodytes*) and human children (*Homo sapiens*). *Journal of Comparative Psychology, 112(2),* 192–206.

Call, J., & Tomasello, M. (1999). A nonverbal false belief task: The performance of children and great apes. *Child Development, 70(2),* 381–395.

Campbell, R., Heywood, C., Cowey, A., Regard, M., & Landis, T. (1990). Sensitivity to eye gaze in prosopagnosic patients and monkeys with superior temporal sulcus ablation. *Neuropsychologia, 28(11),* 1123–1142.

Caplan, D., Vijayan, S., Kuperberg, G., West, C., Waters, G., Greve, D. D. et al. (2002). Vascular responses to syntactic processing: Event-related fMRI study of relative clauses. *Human Brain Mapping, 15(1),* 26–38.

Carlson, S., & Moses, L. (2001). Individual differences in inhibitory control and children's theory of mind. *Child Development, 72(4),* 1032–1053.

Carlson, S., Moses, L., & Claxton, L. (2004). Individual differences in executive functioning and theory of mind: An investigation of inhibitory control and planning ability. *Journal of Experimental Child Psychology, 87(4),* 299–319.

Cooke, A., Zurif, E. B., DeVita, C., Alsop, D., Koenig, P., Detre, J., et al. (2001). Neural basis for sentence comprehension: Grammatical and short-term memory components. *Human Brain Mapping, 15*, 80–94.

Corballis, M. (2003). Recursion as the key to the human mind. In K. Sterelny & J. Fitness (Eds.), *From mating to mentality: Evaluating evolutionary psychology* (pp. 155–171). New York: Psychology Press.

Cosmides, L., & Tooby, J. (1987). From evolution to behavior: Evolutionary psychology as the missing link. In J. Dupre (Ed.), *The latest on the best: Essays on evolution and optimality* (pp. 277–306). Cambridge, MA: MIT Press.

Crichton, M., & Lange-Küttner, C. (1999). Animacy and propulsion in infancy: Tracking, waving, and reaching to self-propelled and induced moving objects. *Developmental Science, 2*(3), 318–324.

Csibra, G., Biro, S., Koos, O., & Gergely, G. (2003). One-year-old infants use teleological representations of actions productively. *Cognitive Science, 27*(1), 111–133.

Dawkins, R. (1987). *The blind watchmaker*. New York: Norton.

De Villiers, J. (2000). Language and theory of mind: What are the developmental relationships? In S. Baron-Cohen, H. Tager-Flusberg, & D. Cohen (Eds.), *Understanding other minds: Perspectives from developmental cognitive neuroscience* (2nd ed., pp. 83–123). Oxford, UK: Oxford University Press.

De Villiers, J., & Pyers, J. (2002). Complements to cognition: A longitudinal study of the relationship between complex syntax and false-belief understanding. *Cognitive Development, 17*(1), 1037–1060.

Dennett, D. (1978). Beliefs about beliefs. *Behavioral and Brain Sciences, 1*, 568–570.

Farroni, T., Csibra, G., Simion, F., & Johnson, M. (2002). *Proceedings of the National Academy of Sciences of the USA, 99*(14), 9602–9605.

Farroni, T., Mansfield, E., Lai, C., & Johnson, M. (2003). Infants perceiving and acting on the eyes: Tests of an evolutionary hypothesis. *Journal of Experimental Child Psychology, 85*, 199–212.

Ferrari, P. F., Kohler, E., Fogassi, L., & Gallese, V. (2000). The ability to follow eye gaze and its emergence during development in macaque monkeys. *Proceedings of the National Academy of Sciences of the USA, 97*(25), 13997–14002.

Fine, C., Lumsden, J., & Blair, J. (2001). Dissociation between "theory of mind" and executive functions in a patient with early left amygdala damage. *Brain, 124*, 287–298.

Flavell, J., Everett, B., Croft, K., & Flavell, E. (1981). Young children's knowledge about visual perception: Further evidence for the Level 1–Level 2 distinction. *Developmental Psychology, 17*, 99–103.

Fletcher, P., Happé, F., Frith, U., Baker, S., Dolan, R. J., Frackowiak, R. et al. (1995). Other minds in the brain: A functional imaging study of "theory of mind" in story comprehension. *Cognition, 57*(2), 109–128.

Flynn, E., O'Malley, C., & Wood, D. (2004). A longitudinal, microgenetic study of the emergence of false belief understanding and inhibition skills. *Developmental Science, 7*(1), 103–115.

Foley, R. (1997). *Humans before humanity*. London: Blackwell.

Franco, F., & Butterworth, G. (1996). Pointing and social awareness: Declaring and requesting in the second year. *Journal of Child Language, 23*(2), 307–336.

Frith, U., & Frith, C. D. (2003). Development and neurophysiology of mentalizing. *Philosophical Transactions of the Royal Society of London: Series B. Biological Sciences, 358*, 459–473.

Gallagher, H.L., Happé, F., Brunswick, N., Fletcher, P., Frith, U., et al. (2000). Reading the mind in cartoons and stories: An fMRI study of "theory of the mind" in verbal and nonverbal tasks. *Neuropsychologia, 38*(1), 11–21.

Gallagher, H. L., Jack, A. I., Roepstorff, A., & Frith C. D. (2002). Imaging the intentional stance in a competitive game. *NeuroImage, 16*, 814–821.

Gallup, G., Cummings, W., & Nash, R. (1972). The experimenter as an independent variable in studies of animal hypnosis in chickens (*Gallus gallus*). *Animal Behaviour, 20*, 166–169.

German, T., Niehaus, J., Roarty, M., Giesbrecht, B., & Miller, M. (2004). Neural correlates of detecting pretense: Automatic engagement of the intentional stance under covert conditions. *Journal of Cognitive Neuroscience, 16*(10), 1805–1817.

Gibbons, A. (2002). In search of the first hominids. *Science, 295*(5558), 1214–1219.

Goel, V., Grafman, J., Sadato, N., & Hallett, M. (1995). Modeling other minds. *Neuroreport, 6*(13), 1741–1746.

Gregory, C. , Lough, S., Stone, V. E., Erzinclioglu, S., Martin, L., Baron-Cohen, S. et al. (2002). Theory of mind in frontotemporal dementia and Alzheimer's disease: Theoretical and practical implications. *Brain, 125*, 752–764.

Grèzes, J., Frith, C. D., & Passingham, R. E. (2004). Inferring false beliefs from the actions of oneself and others: An fMRI study. *NeuroImage, 21*, 744–750.

Happé, F., Mahli, G. S., & Checkley, S. (2001). Acquired mind-blindness following frontal lobe surgery: A single case study of impaired "theory of mind" in a patient treated with stereotactic anterior capsulotomy. *Neuropsychologia, 39*, 83–90.

Hare, B., Call, J., Agnetta, B., & Tomasello, M. (2000). Chimpanzees know what conspecifics do and do not see. *Animal Behaviour, 59*, 771–785.

Hare, B., Call, J., & Tomasello, M. (2001). Do chimpanzees know what conspecifics know? *Animal Behaviour, 61*, 139–151.

Hoffman, E. A., & Haxby, J. V. (2000). Distinct representations of eye gaze and identity in the distributed human neural system for face perception. *Nature Neuroscience, 3*(1), 80–84.

Itakura, S. (1996). An exploratory study of gaze-monitoring in non-human primates. *Japanese Psychological Research, 38*, 174–180.

Jellema, T., Baker, C. I., Wicker, B., & Perrett, D. I. (2000). Neural representation for the perception of the intentionality of actions. *Brain and Cognition, 44*(2), 280–302.

Kawashima, R., Sugiura, M., Kato, T., Nakamura, A., Hatano, K., Ito, K., et al. (1999). The human amygdala plays an important role in gaze monitoring: A PET study. *Brain, 122*(4), 779–783.

Keenan, T. (1998). Memory span as a predictor of false belief understanding. *New Zealand Journal of Psychology, 27*(2), 36–43.

Knight, R. T., & Grabowecky, M. (1995). Escape from linear time: Prefrontal cortex and conscious experience. In M.S. Gazzaniga (Ed.), *The cognitive neurosciences* (pp. 570–581). Cambridge, MA: MIT Press.

Kumashiro, M., Ishibashi, H., Itakura, S., & Iriki, A. (2002). Bidirectional communication between a Japanese monkey and a human through eye gaze and pointing. *Current Psychology of Cognition, 21*(1), 3–32.

Kumashiro, M., Ishibashi, H., Uchiyama, Y., Itakura, S., Murata, A., & Iriki, A. (2003). Natural imitation induced by joint attention in Japanese monkeys. *International Journal of Psychophysiology, 50*, 81–99.

Leavens, D.A., Hopkins, W. D., & Thomas, R. K. (2004). Referential communication by chimpanzees (*Pan troglodytes*). *Journal of Comparative Psychology, 118*(1), 48–57.

Leslie, A. M. (1987). Pretence and representation: The origins of "theory of mind." *Psychological Review, 94*, 412–426.

Leslie, A. M. (1994). Pretending and believing: Issues in the theory of ToMM. *Cognition, 50*, 211–238.

Leslie, A. M., & Frith, U. (1990). Prospects for a cognitive neuropsychology of autism: Hobson's choice. *Psychological Review, 97*(1), 122–131.

Liben, L. S. (1978). Perspective-taking skills in young children: Seeing the world through rose-colored glasses. *Developmental Psychology, 14*(1), 87–92.

Lieberman, D. E., McBratney, B. M., & Krovitz, G. (2002). The evolution and development of cranial form in *Homo sapiens. Proceedings of the National Academy of Sciences of the USA, 99*(3), 1134–1139.

Lillard, A., Zeljo, A., Curenton, S., & Kangars, A. (2000). Children's understanding of the animacy constraint on pretense. *Merrill-Palmer Quarterly, 46*(1), 21–44.

Liu, D., Sabbagh, M. A., Gehring, W. J., & Wellman, H. (2004). Decoupling beliefs from reality in the brain: An ERP study of theory of mind. *Neuroreport, 15*(6), 991–995.

Lough, S., Gregory, C., & Hodges, J. (2002). Dissociation of social cognition and executive function in frontal variant frontotemporal dementia. *Neurocase, 7*(2), 123–130.

Mossler, D. G., Marvin, R. S., & Greenberg, M. T. (1976). Conceptual perspective taking in 2- to 6-year-old children. *Developmental Psychology, 12*(1), 85–86.

Okamoto, S., Tomonaga, M., Ishii, K., Kawai, N., Tanaka, M., & Matsuzawa, T. (2002). An infant chimpanzee (*Pan troglodytes*) follows human gaze. *Animal Cognition, 5*(2), 107–114.

Perner, J. (1991). *The representational theory of mind.* Cambridge, MA: MIT Press.

Perner, J., & Garnham, W. A. (2001). Actions really do speak louder than words— but only implicitly: Young children's understanding of false belief in action. *British Journal of Developmental Psychology, 19*(3), 413–432.

Perrett, D., Harries, M., Mistlin, A., Hietanen, J., Benson, P., Bevan, R., et al. (1990). Social signals analyzed at the single cell level: Someone is looking at me, something touched me, something moved! *International Journal of Comparative Psychology, 4*(1), 25–55.

Phillips, W., Baron-Cohen, S., & Rutter, M. (1992). The role of eye contact in the detection of goals: Evidence from normal toddlers and children with autism or mental handicap. *Development and Psychopathology, 4*, 375–383.

Pinker, S. (1994). *The language instinct.* New York: Morrow.

Povinelli, D. J., & O'Neill, D. K. (2000). Do chimpanzees use their gestures to instruct each other? In S. Baron-Cohen, H. Tager-Flusberg, & D. Cohen (Eds.),

Understanding other minds: Perspectives from developmental cognitive neuroscience (2nd ed., pp. 459–487). Oxford, UK: Oxford University Press.

Povinelli, D. J., Theall, L. A., Reaux, J. E., & Dunphy-Lelii, S. (2003). Chimpanzees spontaneously alter the location of their gestures to match the attentional orientation of others. *Animal Behaviour, 66*(1), 71–79.

Pratt, C., & Bryant, P. (1990). Young children understand that looking leads to knowing (so long as they are looking into a single barrel). *Child Development, 61*(4), 973–982.

Repacholi, B. M., & Gopnik, A. (1997). Early reasoning about desires: Evidence from 14- and 18-month-olds. *Developmental Psychology, 33*(1), 12–21.

Ristau, C. A. (1990). Aspects of the cognitive ethology of an injury-feigning plover. In C. A. Ristau (Ed.), *Cognitive ethology: The minds of other animals* (pp. 91–126). New York: Erlbaum.

Ristau, C. A. (1991). Before mindreading: Attention, purposes and deception in birds. In A. Whiten (Ed.), *Natural theories of mind* (pp. 209–222). London: Blackwell.

Samson, D., Apperly, I.A., Chiavarino, C., & Humphreys, G.W. (2004). The left temporoparietal junction is necessary for representing someone else's belief. *Nature Neuroscience, 7*(5), 499–500.

Saxe, R., Carey, S., & Kanwisher, N. (2004). Understanding other minds: Linking developmental psychology and functional neuroimaging. *Annual Review of Psychology, 55,* 87–124.

Saxe, R., & Kanwisher, N. (2003). People thinking about people: The role of the temporo-parietal junction in "theory of mind." *NeuroImage, 19,* 1835–1842.

Semendeferi, K., Armstrong, E., Schleicher, A., Zilles, K., & Van Hoesen, G.W. (2001). Prefrontal cortex in humans and apes: A comparative study of area 10. *American Journal of Physical Anthropology, 114*(3), 224–241.

Shimamura, A. P. (2000). Toward a cognitive neuroscience of metacognition. *Consciousness and Cognition, 9,* 313–323.

Shimamura, A. P., Janowsky, J. S., & Squire, L. R. (1990). Memory for the temporal order of events in patients with frontal lobe lesions and amnesic patients. *Neuropsychologia, 28*(8), 803–813.

Smith, M., Apperly, I., & White, V. (2003). False belief reasoning and the acquisition os relative clause sentences. *Child Development, 74*(6), 1709–1719.

Snowden, J. S., Gibbons, Z., Blackshaw, A., Doubleday, E., Thompson, J., Craufurd, D., et al. (2003). Social cognition in frontotemporal dementia and Huntington's disease. *Neuropsychologia, 41,* 688–701.

Snowdon, C. T. (2001). From primate communication to human language. In F. deWaal (Ed.), *Tree of origin: What primate behavior can tell us about human social evolution* (pp. 195–227). Cambridge, MA: Harvard University Press.

Stone, V.E. (2000). The role of the frontal lobes and the amygdala in theory of mind. In S. Baron-Cohen, H. Tager-Flusberg, & D. Cohen (Eds.), *Understanding other minds: Perspectives from developmental cognitive neuroscience* (2nd ed., pp. 253–273). Oxford, UK: Oxford University Press.

Stone, V. E. (2003). Footloose and fossil-free no more: Evolutionary psychology needs archaeology. *Behavioral and Brain Sciences, 25*(3), 420–421.

Stone, V. E. (2004, August). *The evolution of brain ontogeny in primates and homi-*

nids. Paper presented at the annual Australasian Winter Conference on Brain Research, Otago, New Zealand.

Stone, V. E. (2005). Theory of mind and the evolution of social intelligence. In J. Cacciopo (Ed.), *Social neuroscience: People thinking about people* (pp. 103–130). Cambridge, MA: MIT Press.

Stone, V. E. (2006). The evolution of ontogeny and human cognitive uniqueness: Selection for extended brain development in the hominid line. In J. P. Keenan, S. Platek, & T. Shackelford (Eds.), *Evolutionary cognitive neuroscience* (pp. 65–94). Cambridge, MA: MIT Press.

Stone, V. E., Baron-Cohen, S., Calder, A. C., Keane, J., & Young, A. W. (2003). Acquired theory of mind impairments in individuals with bilateral amygdala lesions. *Neuropsychologia, 41,* 209–220.

Stone, V. E., Baron-Cohen, S., & Knight, R. T. (1998). Frontal lobe contributions to theory of mind. *Journal of Cognitive Neuroscience, 10,* 640–656.

Stone, V. E., Cosmides, L., Tooby, J., Kroll, N., & Knight, R. T. (2002). Selective impairment of reasoning about social exchange in a patient with bilateral limbic system damage. *Proceedings of the National Academy of Sciences of the USA, 99*(17), 11531–11536.

Stone, V. E., & Gerrans, P. (2006). Does the normal brain have a theory of mind? *Trends in Cognitive Sciences, 10*(1), 3–4.

Stuss, D. T., Gallup, G., & Alexander, M. (2001). The frontal lobes are necessary for "theory of mind." *Brain, 124*(2), 279–286.

Suddendorf, T. (1999). The rise of the metamind. In M. C. Corballis & S. Lea (Eds.), *The descent of mind: Psychological perspectives on hominid evolution* (pp. 218–260). London: Oxford University Press.

Suddendorf, T., & Busby, J .(2003). Mental time travel in animals? *Trends in Cognitive Sciences, 7*(9), 391–396.

Suddendorf, T., & Fletcher-Flinn, C. M. (1999). Children's divergent thinking improves when they understand false beliefs. *Creativity Research Journal, 12,* 115–128.

Suddendorf, T., & Whiten, A. (2001). Mental evolution and development: Evidence for secondary representation in children, great apes and other animals. *Psychological Bulletin, 127*(5), 629–650.

Suddendorf, T., & Whiten, A. (2003). Reinterpreting the mentality of apes. In J. Fitness & K. Sterelny (Eds.), *From mating to mentality: Evaluating evolutionary psychology* (pp. 173–196). New York: Psychology Press.

Tomasello, M., Call, J., & Hare, B. (1998). Five primate species follow the visual gaze of conspecifics. *Animal Behaviour, 55*(4), 1063–1069.

Tomasello, M., Hare, B., & Fogleman, T. (2001). The ontogeny of gaze following in chimpanzees, *Pan troglodytes,* and rhesus macaques, *macaca mulatto. Animal Behaviour, 61*(2), 335–343.

Tooby, J., & Cosmides, L. (1992). The psychological foundations of culture. In J. Barkow, L. Cosmides, & J. Tooby (Eds.), *The adapted mind: Evolutionary psychology and the generation of culture* (pp. 19–136). New York: Oxford University Press.

Vick, S., & Anderson, J. (2003). Use of human visual attention cues by Olive baboons (*Papio anubis*) in a competitive task. *Journal of Comparative Psychology, 117*(2), 209–216.

Wellman, H. (1990). *The child's theory of mind.* Cambridge, MA: MIT Press.

Wellman, H., Cross, D., & Watson, J. (2001). Meta-analysis of theory-of-mind development: The truth about false belief. *Child Development, 72*(3), 655–684.

Wellman, H., & Lagattuta, K. H. (2000). Developing understandings of mind. In S. Baron-Cohen, H. Tager-Flusberg, & D. Cohen (Eds.), *Understanding other minds: Perspectives from developmental cognitive neuroscience* (2nd ed., pp. 21–49). Oxford, UK: Oxford University Press.

Wellman, H., & Liu, D. (2004). Scaling theory of mind tasks. *Child Development, 75*(2), 523–541.

Wellman, H., & Wooley, J. (1990). From simple desires to ordinary beliefs: The early development of everyday psychology. *Cognition, 35*(3), 245–275.

Wildman, D. E., Uddin, M., Liu, G., Grossman, L. I., & Goodman, M. (2003). Implications of natural selection in shaping 99.4% nonsynonymous DNA identity between humans and chimpanzees: Enlarging genus *Homo. Proceedings of the National Academy of Sciences of the USA, 100*(12), 7181–7188.

Williams, G. C. (1966). *Adaptation and natural selection: A critique of some current evolutionary thought.* Princeton, NJ: Princeton University Press.

Woodward, A. (1999). Infants' ability to distinguish between purposeful and non-purposeful behaviors. *Infant Behavior and Development, 22*(2), 145–160.

Yoder, A. D., Cartmill, M., Ruvolo, M., Smith, K., & Vilgalys, R. (1996). Ancient single origin for Malagasy primates. *Proceedings of the National Academy of Sciences of the USA, 93*(10), 5122–5126.

Young, A. W., Aggleton, J. P., Hellawell, D., Johnson, M., Broks, P. & Hanley, J. R. (1995). Face processing impairments after amygdalotomy. *Brain, 118*, 15–24.

V

PERSON PERCEPTION, STEREOTYPING, AND PREJUDICE

16

Mechanisms for the Regulation of Intergroup Responses

INSIGHTS FROM A SOCIAL NEUROSCIENCE APPROACH

David M. Amodio, Patricia G. Devine,
and Eddie Harmon-Jones

Issues of prejudice and stereotyping have been at the forefront of social-psychological inquiry for much of the field's history. The psychological phenomenon of racial bias embodies the confluence of social psychology's major themes: how elements of the situation interact with attitudes, emotions, motivations, and beliefs to influence behavior, and, more recently, how these influences may operate in automatic or more controlled fashions. For this reason, the area of prejudice and stereotyping has provided a rich context for studying the interplay of social-psychological variables, in addition to addressing important sociopolitical issues. The basic psychological variables underlying prejudice and stereotyping were first formally articulated by Allport in his classic treatise *The Nature of Prejudice* in 1954, and since that time, volumes of research on the topic have been published (Dovidio, Glick, & Rudman, 2005). However, although much has been accomplished in the understanding of intergroup bias, some major questions remain, such as, How is the process of prejudice control initiated in the first place? For such questions that probe the interface of basic cognitive mechanisms and social attitudes, traditional social-psychological theory and methods have limited explanatory power. These limitations have led many social psychologists to expand their approach to include theory and methods from the related areas of cognitive neuroscience and psychophysiology. In this chapter, we review how research from the social neuroscience perspective has contributed to the literature on prejudice and stereotyping. We begin with a brief history of social neuroscience research in the area of prejudice and stereotyping and then describe in more detail how we have used the social neuroscience approach to address important theoretical questions in our own research. Finally, we discuss what we think are some important guidelines for ensuring the successful development of the field of social neuroscience.

A BRIEF HISTORY OF SOCIAL NEUROSCIENCE INVESTIGATIONS OF PREJUDICE AND STEREOTYPING

American history is rife with racial conflict, most notably between the white majority and the black minority. When psychologists first began to study the nature of prejudice and stereotyping in the 1920s and 1930s, discrimination against black people was the norm. In their seminal surveys of racial beliefs, Katz and Braly (1933) found widespread, candid endorsement of African American stereotypes at the time, suggesting that in the 1930s, there were few, if any, normative pressures to appear nonprejudiced (see also LaPiere, 1934). However, as social norms began to shift toward favoring civil rights in the post–World War II era (Schuman, Steeh, Bobo, & Krysan, 1997), respondents grew increasingly reluctant to express prejudice overtly (Crosby, Bromley, & Saxe, 1980). The earliest use of physiological measures in research on racial attitudes was to circumvent deliberate efforts to conceal racial biases. Rankin and Campbell (1955; see also Vidulich & Krevanick, 1966) measured white participants' galvanic skin response, an index of sympathetic nervous system arousal, as they interacted with either a white or a black experimenter. They found larger galvanic skin responses toward black experimenters than white experimenters, suggesting an underlying bias against black people. More recently, facial electromyography (EMG) has been used to measure facial muscle activity associated with affective reactions, such as frowns (corrugator supercillii) and smiles (zygomaticus), during interracial interactions (Vanman, Paul, Ito, & Miller, 1997; Vrana & Rollock, 1998). EMG provides a continuous and unobtrusive measure of emotional responses that is sensitive enough to detect facial expressions unobservable by the naked eye. Participants in these studies showed facial muscle responses toward black individuals that indicated negative affect despite reporting high levels of liking (Vanman et al., 1997; Vrana & Rollock, 1998). Thus, up through the 1990s, physiological measures were used primarily as unobtrusive markers for racial bias (Guglielmi, 1999). In addition, some social psychologists began to incorporate theories from cognitive and behavioral neuroscience without necessarily using physiological measures. For example, Monteith (1993) integrated Gray's (1982; see also Fowles, 1980) neurophysiological model of the behavioral activation and behavioral inhibition systems with social-psychological theories of self-regulation (e.g., Carver & Scheier, 1990; Rokeach, 1973; Pyszczynski & Greenberg, 1987) to break new ground in understanding the mechanisms of prejudice control.

Since the publication of Guglielmi's (1999) review, social neuroscience research on prejudice and stereotyping has increasingly focused on applying neuroscientific models to probe the sociocognitive mechanisms that underlie different aspects of race bias. For example, research using startle-eyeblink methodology and functional magnetic resonance imaging (fMRI) studies have indicated that the amygdala, a neural structure associated with the detection of threat and fear learning, was more strongly activated when participants viewed out-group (vs. in-group) faces (Amodio, Harmon-Jones, & Devine, 2003; Hart et al., 2000; Phelps et al., 2000). By considering the function of amygdala-based learning and memory, theorists can infer that basic emotional forms of race bias (e.g., implicit prejudice) follow the dynamics of classical conditioning in that they are learned quickly with little cognitive mediation and may be difficult to extinguish. In other research, event-related potential (ERP) studies of expectancy violation and multiple categorization have revealed forms of implicit stereotyping (Bartholow, Fabiana, Gratton, & Bettencourt, 2001) and evaluation (Ito, Thompson, & Cacioppo, 2004) in rapidly activated patterns of neural activity. By using ERPs to track changes in brain activity on the order of milliseconds, these researchers have gained new insights into the time course of implicit and explicit forms of race bias activation and have already shown that stereotype-based processing is evident within 100 milliseconds of encountering a stigmatized group member (e.g., Ito et al., 2004). More recently, researchers using ERP and fMRI measures have linked frontal cortical mechanisms to the regulation of a prejudiced response (Amodio et al., 2004; Cunningham et al., 2004; Richeson et al., 2003). This research has begun to unpack the subprocesses involved in response control, suggesting increasingly refined models of how different personal and situational factors may affect different aspects of control. Taken as a whole, the social neuroscience approach has begun to make important strides in shedding new light on the sociocognitive mechanisms of prejudice and stereotyping. In the following section, we describe our own research on the neurocognitive substrates of prejudice control and discuss its theoretical implications in some detail.

A SOCIAL NEUROSCIENCE APPROACH TO MECHANISMS OF RACE-BIAS CONTROL

For many white Americans, an interracial interaction constitutes a significant self-regulatory challenge. Research has shown that the vast majority of Americans are familiar with the societal stereotypes of African Americans, regardless of whether they believe them to be true (Devine & Elliot, 1995).

Because familiarity with stereotypes leads to their automatic activation, all Americans are susceptible to the influence of stereotypes on their behavior (Devine, 1989). For this reason, people with egalitarian beliefs must effortfully override the influence of automatic stereotypes in order to respond consistently with their beliefs. Furthermore, the initiation of regulatory processes must occur rapidly and with little deliberation in order to facilitate a smooth social interaction.

Several social-psychological models have been proposed to account for the regulation of automatically activated race-biased tendencies (e.g., Bodenhausen & Macrae, 1998; Devine, 1989; Devine & Monteith, 1993; Monteith, 1993). These models posit detailed accounts of stereotype inhibition and response control, yet they have been limited in that they assume that regulatory processes are initiated only after conscious reflection on one's biased course of action. Thus they have limited applicability to the rapid flow of a real-life interaction. Monteith's (1993) model is notable for acknowledging that regulation may be deployed rapidly in the course of an unfolding response to preempt a race-biased behavior, although its focus is on the process of self-regulation that arises from a prejudiced response to prevent future transgressions. Hence previous social-psychological models have not yet addressed the critical step in the regulatory process by which race bias is detected and overridden in a single, rapidly unfolding response. One reason that this step has received little attention may be that the traditional tools of the social psychologist—self-reports, behavioral observation, computerized reaction-time tasks—are poorly equipped for measuring rapid changes in underlying cognitive processes that may be observable only through measures of neural activity. These factors led us to incorporate recent theoretical and methodological advances from the cognitive neuroscience and psychophysiological literatures that were capable of addressing this gap in the prejudice control literature.

Neurocognitive Model of Control

Botvinick, Braver, Barch, Carter, and Cohen's (2001) influential model of cognitive control proposed that two distinct neurocognitive systems work in concert to successfully regulate responses. The first is *conflict-monitoring system* (sometimes referred to as conflict detection), which monitors ongoing responses for conflicts between alternative response tendencies. Research suggests that this system is constantly active, requires few cognitive resources, and operates below conscious awareness (Berns, Cohen, & Mintun, 1997; Nieuwenhuis, Ridderinkhof, Blom, Band, & Kok, 2001). When conflict is detected, a second, resource-dependent *regulatory system* is signaled. The regulatory system draws on more deliberative processing to ensure that one's intended response prevails over the conflicting alternative tendency.

The conflict-monitoring and regulatory systems have been linked to distinct neural substrates. Conflict monitoring has been associated with activity in the anterior cingulate cortex (ACC) in fMRI and ERP investigations, and fMRI data link the regulatory system with activity in the prefrontal cortex (Botvinick, Nystrom, Fissel, Carter, & Cohen, 1999, Carter et al., 1998, Dehaene, Posner, & Tucker, 1994; Kerns et al., 2004; van Veen & Carter, 2002a). This research has shown that ACC activity is heightened when prepotent responses are at odds with one's consciously intended response, such as in the color-naming Stroop task and the Eriksen flankers task (in which a participant must identify a target stimulus [e.g., S] amid inconsistent flankers [HHSHH] versus consistent flankers [SSSSS]).

When applied to the context of race bias, the neurocognitive model of control suggests two ways that automatic stereotypes can make their way into the behavior of a person with low prejudice. The first possibility is that a discrepancy between one's automatic stereotyping tendency and one's egalitarian intentions does not activate the conflict-monitoring system, and therefore the regulatory system is never signaled. The second possibility is that the regulatory system is signaled but is unable to orchestrate the intended egalitarian response needed to override the unwanted stereotyping tendency. Although the theorized role of the *regulatory system* in prejudice control has been addressed in social-psychological research examining the effects of cognitive load (e.g., Gilbert & Hixon, 1991; Spencer, Fein, Wolfe, Fong, & Dunn, 1998), the role of *conflict monitoring* in prejudice control has not been investigated. Thus we were particularly interested in whether conflict monitoring might provide a theoretical account of how regulatory processes aimed at responding without prejudice are initiated in rapidly unfolding behaviors that involve little conscious deliberation. Having identified a useful theoretical framework, our next step was to identify a measure capable of assessing rapid changes in conflict-related ACC activity that could be used in conjunction with a task that reliably elicited response conflicts between automatic stereotypes and the desire to respond in an unbiased manner.

Measuring Conflict Monitoring with ERPs

ERP methods provide the highest resolution of localizable neural activity available among noninvasive neuroimaging techniques. Whereas fMRI and PET typically measure changes in neural activity on the order of seconds, ERPs, derived from either EEG or magnetoencephalography, measure changes on the order of milliseconds. ERPs refer to patterns of neuronal activity that are detectable using electrodes placed on the scalp (see Luck, 2005, for an excellent and highly accessible ERP sourcebook; Fabiani, Gratton, & Coles, 2000, for a review chapter). To observe ERPs, very subtle electrical changes on the scalp are recorded using EEG while a participant responds to events in an experimental task. By recording changes in scalp voltage using EEG at a high sampling rate (e.g., 2000 Hz), ERPs can provide an extremely high-resolution measure of brain activity. Because EEG picks up neural signals from a wide range of neural processes, only a subset of which are related to task events, EEG must be collected from many trials and averaged, such that extraneous EEG signals are "canceled out" and only the signals associated with the experimental event are preserved. When averaging, it is critical that epochs of EEG are aligned with respect to the event of interest (e.g., at the onset of a stimulus or behavioral response) to ensure optimal signal-to-noise ratio of the desired ERP component. This process of averaging is illustrated in Figure 16.1.

Several different ERP components have been identified in the experimental literature, each corresponding to a specific pattern of voltage change detected on the scalp, which in turn reflects a particular underlying pattern of neural activity that is evoked by a specific psychological, perceptual, or behavioral event (for a review, see Coles, Gratton, & Fabiani, 1990). An ERP component that has been shown previously to reflect conflict-related activity in the ACC is the *error-related negativity* (ERN; Gehring & Fencsik, 2001; Falkenstein, Hohnsbein, Hoorman, & Blanke, 1991). The ERN is a response-locked wave, meaning that epochs of EEG for each trial are aligned to the moment a response is made for the averag-

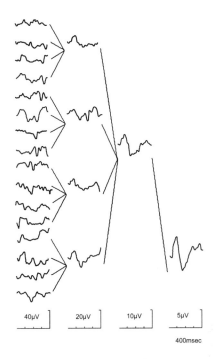

40μV   20μV   10μV   5μV

400msec

FIGURE 16.1. An illustration of the averaging process used to extract ERPs from epochs of scalp-recorded voltage measured using EEG, adapted from Picton (1980). Several epochs of raw EEG signals are illustrated on the left side of the diagram. As more epochs of raw signal are included in the average, the overall amplitude of the signal diminishes, while a clear event-related "signal" begins to emerge from the background "noise."

ing process. The ERN is characterized by its negative-polarity voltage deflection that peaks approximately at the time a response is made (Gehring, Goss, Coles, Meyer, & Donchin, 1993). It is most strongly pronounced at frontocentral midline scalp sites and originates from the ACC (Dehaene et al., 1994; van Veen & Carter, 2002a). ERNs are specifically sensitive to conflicts that lead to response errors (i.e., failed control; Yeung, Holroyd, & Cohen, 2004), making them particularly useful for examining failures in response regulation. However, conflict monitoring associated with response errors has been shown to arise from the same ACC neural generator as conflict monitoring that leads to successful regulation (Yeung et al., 2004), and therefore an individual's average ERN response provides an index of the general sensitivity of the conflict-monitoring system, which may then be used to predict patterns of successful control (e.g., Gehring et al., 1993; Pailing, Segalowitz, Dywan, & Davies, 2002).

Behavioral Task

A good behavioral task serves two purposes in a neuroscience experiment: (1) it elicits the neural response of interest and (2) it provides behavioral data that can corroborate one's interpretation of the elicited neural response. Furthermore, because a particular neural structure is often involved in multiple psychological processes (Cacioppo, Tassinary, & Berntson, 2000), it is advisable to choose behavioral tasks that offer several measures of related processes to permit an assessment of convergent and discriminant validity. With these considerations in mind, we needed a task that could (1) provide separate, theoretically independent indices of automatic stereotyping and controlled response patterns, (2) elicit a sufficient number of errors across trial conditions to permit reliable analyses of accuracy and ERP averages, (3) elicit ERN waves concurrently with behavioral responses, and (4) be completed with minimal head movement, thereby enabling artifact-free EEG recording. After considering several different tasks, we chose to use Payne's (2001) weapons identification task because it best suited these requirements.

The weapons identification task is a sequential priming task designed to elicit high- versus low-conflict stereotype-related responses in a way that is conceptually similar to the Stroop or flankers tasks. On each trial of the weapons identification task, a black or a white face is presented for 200 milliseconds, followed by a picture of either a handgun or a hand tool, presented for 200 milliseconds and then masked (Figure 16.2). Participants must quickly categorize each target as a gun or a tool via button press. Because white Americans tend to associate black faces with danger and hostility (Devine & Elliot, 1995), black face primes tend to facilitate correct categorization of guns. By the same token, because a black face primes a gun response, it interferes with the correct categorization of tools, thereby eliciting high levels of response conflict. By this logic, black–gun trials may be thought of as low-conflict trials, whereas black–tool trials may be

A

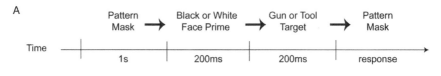

B

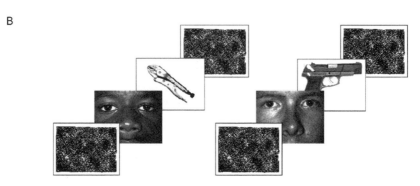

FIGURE 16.2. Schematic of weapons identification task, adapted from Payne (2001), illustrating the time course of events (A) and stimuli (B).

thought of as high-conflict trials. Because white faces are not typically associated with either guns or tools, they should not differentially affect responses to targets.

Conventional response facilitation indices of automaticity (e.g., degree of response facilitation) may be derived from responses on the weapons identification task (Fazio, 1990), and levels of response control may be inferred from measures of post-error slowing and accuracy (Rabbit, 1966). However, response facilitation scores are limited in their ability to index purely automatic or controlled processes because any deliberative response (such as a key press) involves some degree of control, and therefore response-latency measures provide somewhat ambiguous indicators of automatic versus controlled processing (Jacoby, 1991). With this limitation in mind, the weapons identification task was designed to provide theoretically independent measures of automatic processing (e.g., stereotype-based responding) versus controlled processing (e.g., accuracy-based responding), as inferred from patterns of error rates according to the processes dissociation (PD) procedure (Payne, 2001). According to the PD framework, the independent effects of automatic and controlled processes can be dissociated using tasks that place these processes in opposition to one another. For example, when a correct response is congruent with automatic tendencies (e.g., choosing "gun" following a black face), automatic and controlled processes act in concert. When a correct response is incongruent with automatic tendencies (e.g., choosing "tool" following a black face), automatic and controlled processes act in opposition. By assessing accuracy performance across congruent (black–gun) and incongruent (black–tool) trial types, independent estimates of automatic and controlled processes may be obtained (see Payne, 2001, for PD formulas), which permits us to assess the convergent and discriminant validity of the ERN as a measure of conflict monitoring.

A Neural Mechanism for Recruiting Prejudice Control

The preceding paradigm was initially used by Amodio et al. (2004) to demonstrate the role of conflict monitoring in the process of prejudice control. Although participants reported low-prejudice attitudes on average, they exhibited a pattern of automatic race bias on the weapons identification task such that black faces facilitated responses to guns and interfered with responses to tools relative to white faces. These results suggested that enhanced control was needed to override the prepotent tendency to erroneously choose "gun" on black–tool trials. Next, we examined participants' ERN amplitudes to test whether levels of behavioral control could be explained by individual differences in conflict monitoring. As illustrated in Figure 16.3, error responses to all trial types elicited the typical ERN wave relative to correct responses, consistent with the idea that a response error generally conflicts with one's intention to respond accurately. However, the ERN was significantly larger on black–tool trials, on which automatic stereotypes created high response conflict, compared with the other trial types, supporting the hypothesis that the need to control stereotypes elicits activity of the neural system for conflict monitoring. To further validate the meaning of the ERN effect, we examined correlations between ERN ampli-

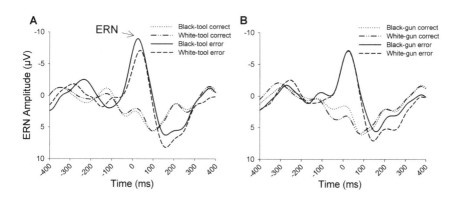

FIGURE 16.3. Response-locked event-related potential waveforms for correct and incorrect tool (A) and gun (B) trials as a function of race of face. The larger error-related negativity (ERN) elicited on black–tool trials reflects the heightened activity of the conflict-monitoring system when an automatic stereotyping tendency conflicts with participants' intention to correctly categorize the target as "tool." (Zero indicates the time of the key press.)

tudes and PD estimates of automatic and controlled responding. Consistent with predictions, larger ERN amplitudes were associated with higher levels of PD control, as well as longer posterror response latency and accuracy. On the other hand, ERNs were uncorrelated with the PD estimate of automatic processing, consistent with the idea that all participants would show similar levels of automatic bias, independent of whether they engaged controlled processing.

Taken together, these findings demonstrated that conflict-monitoring processes are activated in response to automatic race-biased tendencies at very early stages of response execution. In a broader sense, the findings identified an important component of prejudice control that had not been addressed in previous social-psychological models. Hence, this work suggested a new theoretical framework and methodology for addressing some enduring questions regarding the regulation of behavior in response to race bias.

APPLYING A NEW MECHANISM TO OLD QUESTIONS

The next step in our program of research was to apply the findings of Amodio et al. (2004) to a question that has captured the attention of prejudice researchers for years: Why do racial biases sometimes appear in the behavior of well-intentioned egalitarians? And why do some low-prejudice people have more trouble responding without prejudice than others with similarly low-prejudice beliefs? Amodio et al.'s (2004) findings raised the possibility that individual differences in the ability to control bias may be rooted in the conflict-monitoring process. In the next section, we describe how we applied the conflict-monitoring model of prejudice control to address this question.

Individual Differences in the Ability to Respond without Prejudice

All people who are truly low in prejudice desire to respond without prejudice, yet some tend to be more effective than others (e.g., Devine, Monteith, Zuwerink, & Elliot, 1991; Dovidio, Kawakami, & Gaertner, 2002; Gaertner & Dovidio, 1986; Moskowitz, Gollwitzer, Wasel, & Schaal, 1999). Research has shown that this variability is related to the motivations behind people's efforts to respond without prejudice (Amodio et al., 2003; Devine, Plant, Amodio, Harmon-Jones, & Vance, 2002). For example, some people are internally motivated to respond without prejudice—they inhibit race biases primarily for personal reasons. Others are externally motivated—they inhibit bias primarily to avoid social disapproval (Plant & Devine, 1998). Some people may be motivated for both reasons, whereas still others are simply not motivated for either reason. Research examining the effects of these motivations on people's ability to control bias has characterized good regulators as people low in prejudice who respond without prejudice primarily because it is personally important to them (i.e., high internal, low external motivation). Poor regulators are people low in prejudice who respond without prejudice for personal reasons but also because they are worried about social disapproval (i.e., high internal, high external motivation). Finally, one may think of nonregulators as people high in prejudice who are simply uninterested in responding without prejudice for internal reasons (although some nonregulators might feel the need to conceal their prejudice in social situations to avoid disapproval; see Devine, Brodish, & Vance, 2005; Plant, Vance, & Devine, 2006).

Amodio, Devine, and Harmon-Jones (2006) proposed that individual differences in the conflict-monitoring process might account for differences between good and poor regulators. They hypothesized that the neural systems of poor regulators may be less sensitive to conflict between an automatic race-biased tendency and an egalitarian response intention compared with good regulators. To test this hypothesis, they recruited participants who fit the profiles of good, poor, and nonregulators based on their scores on the Internal and External Motivation to Respond Without Prejudice scales, as in past research (Plant & Devine, 1998), and then tested for differences in these groups' average ERN responses as they completed the weapons identification task. As in past work, the researchers found that all participants showed evidence of automatic stereotyping (i.e., elevated PD-automatic scores for black vs. white faces), yet good and poor regulators reported equally positive attitudes toward black people. Thus good and poor regulators needed to regulate their responses, whereas nonregulators did not. However, an examination of response control (PD-control estimate) showed that good regulators were significantly better at responding without bias than poor regulators. As hypothesized, the difference between good and poor regulators in behavioral control corresponded to their differences in conflict monitoring on trials in which control was needed to overcome bias. That is, good regulators exhibited an enhancement in ERN amplitudes when responses required the control of automatic stereotypes (i.e., on black–tool trials; see Figure 16.4), but poor regulators did not. Indeed, the difference in behavioral control between good and poor regulators was found to be fully mediated by their ERN amplitudes, suggesting that poor regulators are less effective in regulating their intergroup responses because their conflict-monitoring systems were relatively insensitive to discrepancies between a tendency to use stereotypes and their intention to respond without bias. By considering the neurocognitive mechanisms involved in the control of race bias, these results were able to address what has been an enduring and often puzzling question in the prejudice literature.

Our findings (Amodio et al., 2005) indicated that poor regulators may respond with prejudice for different reasons than nonregulators and that,

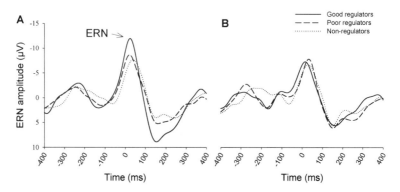

FIGURE 16.4. Error-related negativity (ERN) amplitudes associated with black–tool (A) and black–gun trials (B) as a function of regulation group. Good regulators showed larger ERNs only on trials requiring the inhibition of a stereotype-based response. ERNs did not vary by group when responses did not require stereotype inhibition. (Zero represents the time of key press.)

therefore, different prejudice-reduction strategies could be targeted for these two groups. Whereas past efforts at prejudice reduction have focused on influencing people's consciously held attitudes and beliefs, our findings suggest that for people who fit the "poor regulator" profile, efforts should focus on enhancing the strength of the conflict-monitoring signal in situations in which control is needed. One must ask, Why were conflict processes lower among the poor regulators? One possibility is that poor regulators' brains are simply less sensitive to response conflicts; however, this explanation is not supported by the data. For example, the ERNs of poor regulators did not differ from those of other groups when response conflict was unrelated to race-bias control (e.g., on black–gun trials). A more plausible possibility is that situations requiring control do not strongly activate belief-based response tendencies at automatic levels of processing among poor regulators compared with good regulators and therefore prejudice-reduction strategies should focus on automatizing responses to cues that control is needed. At the theoretical level, Monteith (1993) emphasized the importance of learning to recognize such "regulatory cues" (see also Devine & Monteith, 1993), although this work focused on more deliberative forms of cue processing. Our findings highlight the important role of the more automatic processing of regulatory cues (e.g., Kawakami, Dovidio, Moll, Hermsen, & Russin, 2000; Monteith, Ashburn-Nardo, Voils, & Czopp, 2002; Moskowitz et al., 1999). One way to accomplish automatic cue sensitivity is through repetition training, in which a person practices identifying stimuli that might normally elicit unwanted stereotypic associations. Kawakami et al. (2000) showed that this type of training is effective in enhancing behavioral control. A next step in this line of research would be to test whether this type of training affects the conflict-monitoring system.

Using Social Neuroscience to Uncover
New Neural Mechanisms of Control

Our previous work has focused on how people regulate their race-biased behavior in private, when concerns about social disapproval are not an issue. Yet much research has shown that normative pressures can have a profound influence on people's behavior as well (Cialdini & Trost, 1998). For example, some people high in prejudice have been shown to change their behavior in order to appear nonprejudiced when giving responses in public (Plant & Devine, 1998; Plant, Devine, & Brazy, 2003). However, the mechanism by which highly externally motivated individuals control prejudice in public situations is unknown. Does enhanced control occur via a preconscious mechanism, such as conflict monitoring? Or does it reflect a conscious, deliberative effort to modify one's behavior?

To investigate how mechanisms of prejudice control might operate differently when motivated by internal versus external concerns, we conducted a study in which participants completed the weapons identification task either privately or while being observed by an ostensibly non-prejudiced experimenter (i.e., in public; Amodio, Kubota, Harmon-Jones, & Devine, 2006). Because people vary in their sensitivity to external pressures (e.g., Plant & Devine, 1998), we recruited participants who reported either very high or very low levels of external motivation to respond without prejudice. By considering this combination of situational and dispositional factors, we could make the focused prediction that neural mechanisms of control that operate specifically in response to normative pressures should emerge most strongly in the public condition and only among participants high in sensitivity to external social pressures.

As described earlier, cognitive neuroscience research has identified the conflict-monitoring process, measured via the ERN, as a preconscious mechanism for eliciting control. In contrast, social-psychological theory has emphasized a postconscious mechanism of control that is recruited when an individual becomes consciously aware of an initial response error and that leads to a more careful style of responding (Devine, 1989; Monteith, 1993; Monteith et al., 2002; Bodenhausen & Macrae, 1998). Recent work has shown that the postconscious awareness of a response error on a cognitive conflict task, referred to as *error perception*, is associated with the error-positivity (P_e) ERP wave (see Figure 16.5a; Nieuwenhuis et al., 2001). Thus, the ERP literature has identified two separate neural processes linked to different aspects of control. The P_e is a positive-polarity wave that immediately follows the ERN. Whereas the ERN is generated by the dorsal ACC, the P_e has been linked to activity of the rostral ACC (Kiehl, Liddle, & Hopfinger, 2001; van Veen & Carter, 2002), an area associated with affect and awareness in response to error commission (Bush, Luu, & Posner, 2000). However, few studies have found an association between P_e amplitude and changes in behavioral measures of control, and therefore the functional significance of the error-perception process is not well understood.

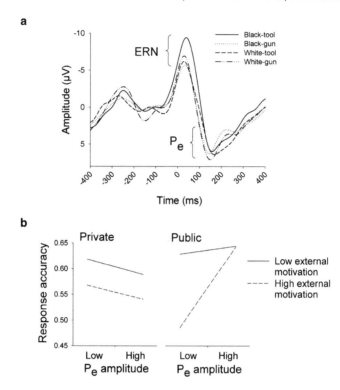

FIGURE 16.5. Error-related negativity (ERN) and error-positivity (P_e) waveforms (see labels) elicited during weapons identification task (Panel A; zero indicates the time of the key press). Panel B illustrates predicted values for behavioral control as predicted by error-positivity (P_e) amplitudes as a function of private versus public response condition for participants reporting high vs. low external motivation to respond without prejudice. Behavioral control represents a probability estimate of control derived using the process-dissociation (PD) procedure. Predicted values of PD control show that P_e amplitudes predicted control only among externally sensitive participants who responded in the public condition.

We proposed that prejudice control motivated by external concerns would involve the error-perception process because the error-perception process could theoretically support more conscious forms of conflict appraisal associated with complex social contingencies (Amodio & Frith, 2006). We therefore predicted that whereas the ERN reflects a basic mechanism for recruiting control across situations, the P_e reflects an additional process that emerges only when external cues, such as the presence of normative social pressures to respond without prejudice, are used to evaluative one's performance and regulate behavior.

Our primary interest in this research was in the association between alternative neural processes and behavioral control. Specifically, we examined the effect of the ERN and P_e waves on behavioral control on the weapons identification task. As in past work, we found that ERN amplitudes predicted behavioral control across conditions, corroborating the important role of conflict monitoring in eliciting control regardless of the social situation. However, the association between P_e amplitude and behavioral control followed a different pattern: The P_e wave predicted control only among highly externally motivated participants who responded in the public condition (Fig. 16.5b). This pattern of effects was replicated when the dependent measure was response accuracy (see Amodio et al., 2006). These findings suggest that the error-perception process elicits control specifically when behavior must be modulated according to external social cues, beyond the effects of conflict monitoring found in previous work.

The results of this research suggest that two processes, pre- and postconscious, are at work when behavior is controlled in response to normative pressures. Based on these findings, prejudice researchers may develop new hypotheses regarding how situational factors affect people's ability to control prejudice. For example, past work suggests that the conflict-monitoring process does not rely on cognitive resources. On the other hand, error-perception processes may rely heavily on cognitive resources. Therefore, cognitive load may have a deleterious effect on the ability to control prejudice in public for people high in external motivation but not for those low in external motivation, as reported by Lambert et al. (2003). At a broader level, this research is noteworthy because it suggests a function for a pattern of neural activity that emerges only in certain social situations. That is, although past work had identified the P_e wave as a potential elicitor of control, a consideration of situational factors and individual differences helped to elucidate the parameters of its function.

As a whole, our program of research on prejudice control has combined many important elements of the social neuroscience approach. Our initial questions arose from theoretical issues in the prejudice and stereotyping literature. To address these questions, we incorporated neurocognitive theory on the conflict-monitoring component of control and adopted psychophysiological methods of measurement that were most appropriate for assessing our theoretical construct. After establishing a paradigm for examining the role of conflict monitoring in prejudice control (Amodio et al., 2004), we used the paradigm to address questions about individual differences in the ability to control prejudice. Here, we demonstrated that error-detection processes accounted for individual differences in the ability of people with low prejudice to override the influence of automatic stereotypes on their behavior. These findings then raised new questions of how mechanisms of control are affected by external social pressures to respond in a nonprejudiced way. Our research on the effects of external pressures identified a new mechanism of behavioral control, the error-perception process, as having a targeted effect on control that emerges only among people who are sensitive to normative pressures when those pressures are salient. Finally, these findings have generated new hypotheses regarding methods of prejudice reduction tailored to individuals with a particular motivational profile (e.g., poor regulators). We believe that the findings from this program of research could only have resulted from a social neuroscience approach.

IMPORTANT ISSUES FOR THE DEVELOPMENT OF SOCIAL NEUROSCIENCE

In this section, we describe what we think are some of the important issues that social neuroscientists will need to address in order for the field to develop successfully. We begin with a few suggested guidelines for conducting social neuroscience research.

1. *Social neuroscience research should be theory driven.* Science is a theory-based endeavor. Hypotheses are formed based on previous observations and theory, submitted to empirical tests, and then revised as needed. Much of the cachet that social neuroscience research has enjoyed in recent years appears to arise from its innovative methodology. However, the longevity of social neuroscience as an approach will no doubt depend on its ability to contribute to theory. As in other areas of research, it will be important for social neuroscientists to let their theoretical questions drive their use of methodology and not vice versa.

2. *Neural correlates of social-psychological processes should be validated with behavioral and/or individual-difference measures.* The brain is an extremely complex organ, and measurable neural activations are almost always likely to be multiply determined. That is, many different factors can contribute to activity of a particular neural region at any given time. Although many scientists have relied on subtraction procedures in fMRI and ERP research to isolate task-specific activations, the subtraction procedure may not be sufficient to establish validity of the neural response. For most investigations involving social psychology, the best way to validate the meaning of a pattern of neural activity is to show that neural activations obtained using subtraction are correlated with theoretically related behavior. Alternatively, experimental precision may be gained through the use of individual-difference factors in interaction designs, whereby a hypothesized neural response occurs only among certain individuals under specific conditions.

3. *Social neuroscience research should focus on mechanisms of social processes.* The ability to address questions of mechanism is one of social neuroscience's greatest assets. Social neuroscience researchers are not typically interested in brain mapping but rather in the implications of known neural functions for understanding social processes. By applying knowledge of functional and anatomical interconnectivity in the brain, researchers

may develop new theories of how basic mechanisms interact to produce social-psychological phenomena. Moreover, neuroimaging methods such as fMRI and ERP provide powerful tools for measuring the activity of neural mechanisms directly and unobtrusively. We believe that the unique potential of social neuroscience for addressing questions about psychological mechanisms is what will ultimately make it indispensable to the field.

4. *Social neuroscience research should integrate the theory and methods of neuroscience and social psychology.* A truly integrative approach combines theoretical perspectives to form novel hypotheses, tests them using a multidisciplinary set of methods, and offers interpretations of findings that make use of the theoretical traditions of each constituent field. That is, integrative research goes beyond using new methods to measure existing constructs; it incorporates ideas from other literatures to better understand a construct from one's own literature. For example, many researchers have discovered physiological markers of prejudice, such as amygdala activity indexed by fMRI or startle-eyeblink modulation. However, simply using a new method does not in itself reveal something new about the underlying process. By associating prejudice with amygdala activity, one can access the large literature on the role of the amygdala in emotional learning and its neural interconnectivity to broaden understanding of the phenomenon of prejudice and to generate interesting new hypotheses. Much of the potential of social neuroscience to have a lasting impact rests on researchers' success in drawing inferences from diverse perspectives in this way.

Contributions of Social Neuroscience to Cognitive Neuroscience

Social neuroscience research has already advanced our understanding of several important social-psychological phenomena, such as prejudice activation and control, emotions, and attitudes. Indeed, it can be argued that most research taking the social neuroscience approach is geared toward understanding social and affective processes. But what has social neuroscience done for cognitive neuroscience lately? Our research on the function of the error-perception process in externally motivated prejudice control provides one example of how a consideration of social factors may elucidate a basic neurocognitive mechanism. As another example, Eisenberger and Lieberman (2004; Eisenberger, Lieberman, & Williams, 2003) showed that the ACC is involved in social exclusion, a form of "social" pain, suggesting a more elaborate function of the previously delineated pain circuit. Recent work by Taylor and colleagues has expanded on the known functions of the hormone oxytocin through a consideration of social factors (Taylor et al., 2004; Taylor & Gonzaga, Chapter 21, this volume). By comparing levels of oxytocin with profiles of participants' personal relationships and psychological stress levels, they found evidence that oxytocin is involved in social distress and may serve to motivate social behavior rather than being a consequence of affectionate social interaction, as previously believed. Finally, research by Harmon-Jones and his colleagues (e.g., Harmon-Jones & Allen, 1998) has addressed a debate over the interpretation of frontal cortical asymmetry effects by examining the role of a uniquely social emotion: anger. Previously, some theorists have described frontal asymmetry as reflecting the valence of one's emotional state, with left-sided activity relating to positive emotions and right-sided activity relating to negative emotions (e.g., Silberman & Weingartner, 1986). Other theorists have described the asymmetry as reflecting one's motivational orientation, such that left-sided activity is associated with approach and right-sided activity with withdrawal (Davidson, 1992). Unfortunately, research had examined only the effects of stimuli that were either positive *and* approach-related or negative *and* withdrawal-related, thereby confounding any attempts to disentangle the alternative interpretations. Harmon-Jones and his colleagues proposed that anger—a negative emotion that is approach-oriented—would provide the critical test of these competing views (see Harmon-Jones, 2003, for a review). Across several studies, they found that anger was linked to greater left-sided activity, supporting the motivation account. These recent lines of research provide examples of how the social neuroscience approach may lead to theoretical advances in cognitive neuroscience, psychoneuroimmunology, and psychophysiology.

Importance of Social Neuroscience Findings for the Nonneuroscientist

An important role for social neuroscientists to take is that of the interpreter. It is incumbent on social neuroscientists to communicate the implications of their findings for other theoretical perspectives, such as traditional social psychology, cognitive psychology, neuroscience, and psychoneuroimmunology, so that researchers in these fields can (1) integrate new findings obtained through a social neuroscience approach into their existing theories and (2) appreciate the value of social neuroscience. Effective communication of social neuroscience's contributions will be essential for its survival as an emerging field.

Conclusion

Social neuroscience holds great promise for advancing the understanding of the mind and brain. As an emerging field, the social neuroscience approach is still developing, finding its identity, and occasionally experiencing growing pains. Nevertheless, the social neuroscience approach has already led to many important contributions to prejudice research and to psychological science more broadly, as detailed throughout the present volume, and there continues to be much enthusiasm among students for interdisciplinary training in social psychology and neuroscience. Ultimately, like previous hybrid fields such as "social cognition," "cognitive neuroscience," and "psychoneuroimmunology," the greatest potential contribution of social neuroscience lies in its ability to bring together researchers with diverse backgrounds who are working toward the common goal of understanding mind, body, and behavior in order to make discoveries that could only be achieved through their joint effort.

REFERENCES

Allport, G. W. (1954). *The nature of prejudice*. Reading, MA: Addison-Wesley.

Amodio, D. M., & Frith, C. D. (2006). Meeting of minds: The role of medial frontal cortex in social cognition. *Nature Reviews Neuroscience, 7*, 268–277.

Amodio, D. M., Harmon-Jones, E., & Devine, P. G. (2003). Individual differences in the activation and control of affective race bias as assessed by startle eyeblink responses and self-report. *Journal of Personality and Social Psychology, 84*, 738–753.

Amodio, D. M., Harmon-Jones, E., Devine, P. G., Curtin, J. J., Hartley, S. L., & Covert, A. E. (2004). Neural signals for the detection of unintentional race bias. *Psychological Science, 15*, 88–93.

Amodio, D. M., Kubota, J. T., Harmon-Jones, E., & Devine, P. G. (2006). Alternative mechanisms for regulating racial responses according to internal vs. external cues. *Social Cognitive and Affective Neuroscience, 1*, 26–36.

Bartholow, B. D., Fabiani, M., Gratton, G., & Bettencourt, B. A. (2001). A psychophysiological analysis of cognitive processing of and affective responses to social expectancy violations. *Psychological Science, 12*, 197–204.

Berns, G. S., Cohen, J. D., & Mintun, M. A. (1997). Brain regions responsive to novelty in the absence of awareness. *Science, 276*, 1272–1275.

Bodenhausen, G. V., & Macrae, C. N. (1998). Stereotype activation and inhibition. In R. S. Wyer, Jr. (Ed.), *Advances in social cognition* (Vol. 11, pp. 1–52). Mahwah, NJ: Erlbaum.

Botvinick, M. M., Braver, T. S., Barch, D. M., Carter, C. S., & Cohen, J. D. (2001). Conflict monitoring and cognitive control. *Psychological Review, 108*, 624–652.

Botvinick, M. M., Nystrom, L. E., Fissel, K., Carter, C. S., & Cohen, J. D. (1999). Conflict monitoring versus selection-for-action in anterior cingulate cortex. *Nature, 402*, 179–181.

Bush, G., Luu, P., & Posner, M. I. (2000). Cognitive and emotional influences in anterior cingulate cortex. *Trends in Cognitive Science, 4*, 215–222.

Cacioppo, J. T., Tassinary, L. G., & Berntson, G. G. (2000). Psychophysiological Science. In J. T. Cacioppo, L. G. Tassinary, & G. G. Berntson (Eds.), *Handbook of psychophysiology* (pp. 53–84). New York: Cambridge University Press.

Carter, C. S., Braver, T. S., Barch, D. M., Botvinick, M. M., Noll, D., & Cohen, J. D. (1998). Anterior cingulate cortex, error detection, and the online monitoring of performance. *Science, 280*, 747–749.

Carver, C. S., & Scheier, M. F. (1990). Origins and functions of positive and negative affect: A control process view. *Psychological Review, 97*, 19–35.

Cialdini, R. B., & Trost, M. R. (1998). Social influence: Social norms, conformity and compliance. In D. T. Gilbert, S. T. Fiske, & G. Lindzey (Eds.), *The handbook of social psychology* (4th ed., pp. 151–192). New York: McGraw-Hill.

Coles, M. G. H., Gratton, G., & Fabiani, M. (1990). Event-related brain potentials. In J. T. Cacioppo & L. G. Tassinary (Eds.), *Principles of psychophysiology* (pp. 413–455). New York: Cambridge University Press.

Crosby, F., Bromley, S., & Saxe, L. (1980). Recent unobtrusive studies of Black and White discrimination and prejudice: A literature review. *Psychological Bulletin, 87,* 546–563.

Cunningham, W. A., Johnson, M. K., Raye, C. L., Gatenby, J. C., Gore, J. C., & Banaji, M. R. (2004). Dissociated conscious and unconscious evaluations of social groups: An fMRI Investigation. *Psychological Science, 15,* 806–813.

Davidson, R. J. (1992). Emotion and affective style: Hemispheric substrates. *Psychological Science, 3,* 39–43.

Dehaene, S., Posner, M. I., & Tucker, D. M. (1994). Localization of a neural system for error detection and compensation. *Psychological Science, 5,* 303–305.

Devine, P. G. (1989). Prejudice and stereotypes: Their automatic and controlled components. *Journal of Personality and Social Psychology, 56,* 5–18.

Devine, P. G. & Elliot, A. J. (1995). Are racial stereotypes really fading? The Princeton Trilogy revisited. *Personality and Social Psychology Bulletin, 21,* 1139–1150.

Devine, P. G., & Monteith, M. J. (1993). The role of discrepancy associated affect in prejudice reduction. In D. M. Mackie & D. L. Hamilton (Eds.), *Affect, cognition, and stereotyping: Interactive processes in intergroup perception* (pp. 317–344). San Diego, CA: Academic Press.

Devine, P. G., Monteith, M., Zuwerink, J. R., & Elliot, A. J. (1991). Prejudice with and without compunction. *Journal of Personality and Social Psychology, 60,* 817–830.

Devine, P. G., Plant, E. A., Amodio, D. M., Harmon-Jones, E., & Vance, S. L. (2002). The regulation of explicit and implicit race bias: The role of motivations to respond without prejudice. *Journal of Personality and Social Psychology, 82,* 835–848.

Dovidio, J. F., Glick, P. G., & Rudman, L. (Eds.). (2005). *On the nature of prejudice: Fifty years after Allport.* Malden, MA: Blackwell.

Dovidio, J. F., Kawakami, K., & Gaertner, S. L. (2002). Implicit and explicit prejudice and interracial interaction. *Journal of Personality and Social Psychology, 82,* 62–68.

Eisenberger, N. I., & Lieberman, M. D. (2004). Why rejection hurts: A common neural alarm system for physical and social pain. *Trends in Cognitive Sciences, 8,* 294–300.

Eisenberger, N. I., Lieberman, M. D., & Williams, K. D. (2003). Does rejection hurt? An fMRI study of social exclusion. *Science, 302,* 290–292.

Fabiani, M., Gratton, G., & Coles, M. G. H. (2000). Event-related brain potentials: Methods, theory, and applications. In J. T. Cacioppo, L. G. Tassinary, & G. G. Berntson (Eds.), *Handbook of psychophysiology* (pp. 53–84). New York: Cambridge University Press.

Falkenstein, M., Hohnsbein, J., Hoorman, J., & Blanke, L. (1991). Effects of crossmodal divided attention on late ERP components: II. Error processing in choice reaction tasks. *Encephalography and Clinical Neurophysiology, 78,* 447–455.

Fazio, R. H. (1990). A practical guide to the use of response latency in social psychological research. In C. Hendrick & M. S. Clark (Eds.), *Research methods in personality and social psychology* (pp. 74–97). Thousand Oaks, CA: Sage.

Fowles, D. C. (1980). The three-arousal model: Implications of Gray's two-factor learning theory for heart rate, electrodermal activity, and psychopathy. *Psychophysiology, 17,* 87–104.

Gaertner, S. L., & Dovidio, J. F. (1986). The aversive form of racism. In J. F. Dovidio & S. L. Gaertner (Eds.), *Prejudice, discrimination, and racism* (pp. 61–89). San Diego, CA: Academic Press.

Gehring, W. J., & Fencsik, D. E. (2001). Functions of the medial frontal cortex in the processing of conflict and errors. *Journal of Neuroscience, 21,* 9430–9437.

Gerhing, W. J., Goss, B., Coles, M. G. H., Meyer, D. E., & Donchin, E. (1993). A neural system for error detection and compensation. *Psychological Science, 4,* 385–390.

Gilbert, D. T., & Hixon, J. G. (1991). The trouble of thinking: Activation and application of stereotypic beliefs. *Journal of Personality and Social Psychology, 60,* 509–517.

Gray, J. A. (1982). *The neuropsychology of anxiety: An enquiry into the functions of the septohippocampal system.* New York: Oxford University Press.

Guglielmi, R. S. (1999). Psychophysiological assessment of prejudice: Past research, current status, and future directions. *Personality and Social Psychology Review, 3,* 123–157.

Hart, A. J., Whalen, P. J., Shin, L. M., McInerney, S. C., Fischer, H., & Rauch, S. L. (2000). Differential response in the human amygdala to racial outgroup vs. ingroup face stimuli. *Neuroreport, 11,* 2351–2355.

Harmon-Jones, E. (2003). Clarifying the emotive functions of asymmetrical frontal cortical activity. *Psychophysiology, 40,* 838–848.

Harmon-Jones, E., & Allen, J. J. B. (1998). Anger and frontal brain activity: EEG asymmetry consistent with approach motivation despite negative affective valence. *Journal of Personality and Social Psychology, 74,* 1310–1316.

Ito, T. A., Thompson, E., & Cacioppo, J. T. (2004). Tracking the time course of social perception: The effects of racial cues on event-related brain potentials. *Personality and Social Psychology Bulletin, 30,* 1267–1280.

Jacoby, L. L. (1991). A process dissociation framework: Separating automatic from intentional uses of memory. *Journal of Memory and Language, 30,* 513–541.

Kawakami, K., Dovidio, J. F., Moll, J., Hermsen, S., & Russin, A. (2000). Just say no (to stereotyping): Effects of training on the negation of stereotypic associations on stereotype activation. *Journal of Personality and Social Psychology, 78,* 871–888.

Katz, D., & Braly, K. (1933). Racial stereotypes of one hundred college students. *Journal of Abnormal Psychology, 30,* 175–193.

Kerns, J. G., Cohen, J. D., MacDonald, A. W., Cho, R. Y., Stenger, V. A., & Carter, C. S. (2004). Anterior cingulate conflict monitoring and adjustments in control. *Science, 303,* 1023–1026.

Kiehl, K. A., Liddle, P. F., & Hopfinger, J. B. (2001). Error processing and the rostral anterior cingulate: An event-related fMRI study. *Psychophysiology, 37,* 216–223.

Lambert, A. J., Payne, B. K., Jacoby, L. L., Shaffer, L. M., Chasteen, A. L., & Khan, S. R. (2003). Stereotypes as dominant responses: On the "social facilitation" of prejudice in anticipated public contexts. *Journal of Personality and Social Psychology, 84,* 277–295.

LaPiere, R. T. (1934). Attitudes vs. actions. *Social Forces, 13,* 230–237.

Luck, S. J. (2005). *An introduction to the event-related potential technique.* Cambridge, MA: MIT Press.

Monteith, M. J. (1993). Self-regulation of stereotypical responses: Implications for progress in prejudice reduction. *Journal of Personality and Social Psychology, 65,* 469–485.

Monteith, M. J., Ashburn-Nardo, L., Voils, C. I., & Czopp, A. M. (2002). Putting the brakes on prejudice: On the development and operation of cues for control. *Journal of Personality and Social Psychology, 83,* 1029–1050.

Moskowitz, G. B., Gollwitzer, P. M., Wasel, W., & Schaal, B. (1999). Preconscious control of stereotype activation through chronic egalitarian goals. *Journal of Personality and Social Psychology, 77,* 167–184.

Nieuwenhuis, S., Ridderinkhof, K. R., Blom, J., Band, G. P. H., & Kok, A. (2001). Error-related brain potentials are differently related to awareness of response errors: Evidence from an antisaccade task. *Psychophysiology, 38,* 752–760.

Pailing, P. E., Segalowitz, S. J., Dywan, J., & Davies, P. L. (2002). Error negativity and response control. *Psychophysiology, 39,* 198–206.

Payne, B. K. (2001). Prejudice and perception: The role of automatic and controlled processes in misperceiving a weapon. *Journal of Personality and Social Psychology, 81,* 181–192.

Phelps, E. A., O'Connor, K. J., Cunningham, W. A., Funayama, S., Gatenby, J. C., Gore, J. C., et al. (2000). Performance on indirect measures of race evaluation predicts amygdala activation. *Journal of Cognitive Neuroscience, 12,* 729–738.

Picton, T. W. (1980). The use of human event-related potentials in psychology. In I. Martin & P. H. Venables (Eds.), *Techniques in psychophysiology* (pp. 357–395). Chicester, UK: Wiley.

Plant, E. A., & Devine, P. G. (1998). Internal and external motivation to respond without prejudice. *Journal of Personality and Social Psychology, 75,* 811–832.

Plant, E. A., Devine, P. G., & Brazy, P. C. (2003). The bogus pipeline and motivations to respond without prejudice: Revisiting the fading and faking of racial prejudice. *Group Processes and Intergroup Relations, 6,* 187–200.

Pyszczynski, T., & Greenberg, J. (1987). Self-regulatory preservation and the depressive self-focusing style: A self-awareness theory of reactive depression. *Psychological Bulletin, 102,* 122–138.

Rabbit, P. M. A. (1966). Errors and error correction in choice-response tasks. *Journal of Experimental Psychology, 71,* 264–272.

Rankin, R. E., & Campbell, D. T. (1955). Galvanic skin response to Negro and white experimenters. *Journal of Abnormal and Social Psychology, 51,* 30–33.

Richeson, J. A., Baird, A. A., Gordon, H. L., Heatherton, T. F, Wyland, C. L., Trawalter, S., et al. (2003). An fMRI examination of the impact of interracial contact on executive function. *Nature Neuroscience, 6,* 1323–1328.

Rokeach, M. (1973). *The nature of human values.* New York: Free Press.

Schuman, H., Steeh, C., Bobo, L., & Krysan, M. (1997). *Racial attitudes in America: Trends and interpretations.* Cambridge, MA: Harvard University Press.

Silberman, E. K., & Weingartner, H. (1986). Hemispheric lateralization of functions related to emotion. *Brain and Cognition, 5*, 322–353.

Spencer, S. J., Fein, S., Wolfe, C. T., Fong, C., & Dunn, M. A. (1998). Automatic activation of stereotypes: The role of self-image threat. *Personality and Social Psychology Bulletin, 24*, 1139–1152.

Taylor, S. E., Gonzaga, G. C., Cousino Klein, L., Hu, P., Greendale, G. A., & Seeman, T. E. (2006). Relation of oxytocin to psychological and biological stress responses in older women. *Psychosomatic Medicine, 68*, 238–245.

van Veen, V., & Carter, C. S. (2002). The timing of action-monitoring processes in the anterior cingulate cortex. *Journal of Cognitive Neuroscience, 14*, 593–602.

Vanman, E. J., Paul, B. Y., Ito, T. A., & Miller, N. (1997). The modern face of prejudice and structural features that moderate the effect of cooperation on affect. *Journal of Personality and Social Psychology, 73*, 941–959.

Vidulich, R. N., & Krevanick, F. W. (1966). Racial attitudes and emotional response to visual representations of the Negro. *Journal of Social Psychology, 68*, 85–93.

Vrana, S. R., & Rollock, D. (1998). Physiological response to a minimal social encounter: Effects of gender, ethnicity, and social context. *Psychophysiology, 35*, 462–469.

Yeung, N., Botvinick, M. M., & Cohen, J. D. (2004). The neural basis of error detection: Conflict monitoring and the error-related negativity. *Psychological Review, 111*, 931–959.

17

Social Cognitive Neuroscience of Person Perception

A SELECTIVE REVIEW FOCUSED ON
THE EVENT-RELATED BRAIN POTENTIAL

Bruce D. Bartholow and Cheryl L. Dickter

Although social psychologists have long been interested in understanding the cognitive processes underlying social phenomena (e.g., Markus & Zajonc, 1985), their methods for studying them traditionally have been rather limited. Early research in person perception, like most other areas of social-psychological inquiry, relied primarily on verbal reports. Researchers using this approach have devised clever experimental designs to ensure the validity of their conclusions concerning social behavior (see Reis & Judd, 2000). The cognitive revolution of the 1970s and 1980s provided a new conceptual model derived in part from a computer metaphor of human thought, involving input (perception), information processing (cognition), and output (behavior), as well as new methods for examining the mental operations underlying social behavior that did not depend on participants' self-reports (e.g., response latency; see Fazio, 1990).

Recently, another conceptual shift has occurred, based on the notion that complex human behaviors cannot be fully explicated by either a strictly biological or a strictly social-psychological approach (e.g., Cacioppo, Berntson, Sheridan, & McClintock, 2000). That is, although human beings (and therefore human behaviors) are inherently social, a purely social level of analysis may ignore or misrepresent important biological events that mediate human action. At the same time, reducing behavior to its biological underpinnings generally does not satisfactorily account for situational differences in behavioral expression. In contrast, a social neuroscience (or social cognitive neuroscience) approach is based on the premise that the most comprehensive understanding of a host of psychological processes is achieved only by examining them at social, cognitive, and neural levels of analysis (Ochsner, 2004; Ochsner & Lieberman, 2001). The aim of this chapter is to review recent developments in social cognitive neuroscience associated with one admittedly narrow topic in the field of social psychology, that of person perception, and specifically to review work that examines this topic through one primary technique—the event-related brain potential (ERP). We begin with a brief overview of ERP theory and measurement (for more comprehensive reviews of the theory and methods of ERP research, see Fabiani, Gratton, & Coles, 2000) and conclude by reviewing recent research in which ERPs have been used as a tool for addressing theoretical questions in person perception.

ERPs AND HUMAN INFORMATION PROCESSING

Background and Theory

Hans Berger (1929) first demonstrated that it is possible to record the electrical activity of the human brain (the electroencephalogram; EEG) by placing a pair of electrodes on the surface of the scalp connected to a differential amplifier. When stimuli are presented during EEG recording, epochs of the EEG that are time-locked to stimulus onset can be defined. With repeated samplings of data from epochs time-locked to the same stimulus (or stimulus class), EEG activity that is not time-locked to stimulus onset will vary randomly across epochs and thus tend to average to zero; the remaining average waveform reflects activity associated directly with processing of the stimulus in question (i.e., the ERP). Physiologically, ERPs are assumed to reflect the postsynaptic activity of groups of neurons that are active synchronously and that share an electrical field orientation that permits their effects at the scalp to cumulate. Psychologically, ERP components—positive and negative voltage deflections in the waveform—reflect various sensory, cognitive, and motor processes based on their responsiveness to experimental manipulations (see Fabiani et al., 2000; Friedman & Johnson, 2000; Rugg & Coles, 1995; Stern, Ray, & Quigley, 2001).

Deriving the ERP

ERPs are recorded with an array of electrodes placed on the scalp (usually fixed in a nylon-lycra cap) according to standard location conventions (e.g., the 10–20 international electrode placement system; Jasper, 1958). The electrodes are connected to amplifiers, and the outputs of the amplifiers are converted to numbers using an analog-to-digital converter. Electrical potentials are generally sampled at a frequency ranging from 100 to 10,000 Hz (samples per second); sampling rates of 250–1,000 Hz are common. Potentials may be recorded continuously during an experimental session (in which case epochs are defined later) or during predefined epochs around stimulus or response events. Deriving the ERP from the raw EEG begins with attenuating (filtering) portions of the EEG that are not of interest. A typical filter setting for recording ERPs will attenuate frequencies above 30–40 Hz (low-pass filter) and those below approximately 0.5 Hz (high-pass filter). Large artifacts in the data, typically defined as voltage deflections larger than some criterion (e.g., 100 μV), also must be removed or attenuated; this is typically accomplished with automated, regression-based procedures (e.g., Semlitsch, Anderer, Schuster, & Presslich, 1986).

ERP Components and their Interpretation

Components are typically described according to their polarity (positive or negative) and the latency (in milliseconds) at which they typically peak. Component amplitude reflects the extent of neural activation associated with a particular cognitive operation, whereas component latency reflects the time required to carry out that operation (e.g., Gehring, Gratton, Coles, & Donchin, 1992; Rugg & Coles, 1995). Although a group of very short-latency *exogenous* components is elicited in the ERP, most social neuroscientists focus on the longer latency *endogenous* components (see Figure 17.1), which are associated with higher cognitive processes such as those typically of interest to social psychologists (e.g., attention, memory, evaluation, categorization).

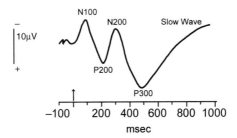

FIGURE 17.1. A schematic representation of endogenous ERP components elicited by a novel visual stimulus. Very early components (approximately 0–100 ms after stimulus onset; i.e., *exogenous* components) tend to be described with a different nomenclature and are not typically examined in social neuroscience research. The vertical arrow on the timeline represents stimulus onset (i.e., time zero); the 100 milliseconds preceding time zero represents a hypothetical prestimulus baseline period. Negative voltage is plotted up as a matter of convention, though ERPs are not always presented this way.

Notable endogenous components include the N100, P200, N200, and P300. Both the N100 and P200 (also sometimes called the P1 because it is the first notable positive peak) have been linked to attentional processes (see Fabiani et al., 2000; Rugg & Coles, 1995), with increasing amplitude of the components reflecting increased direction of implicit attention to a stimulus (e.g., Hopfinger & Mangun, 2001; Mangun, Hillyard, & Luck, 1993). In social neuroscience work, the N100 and P200 have been associated with automatic direction of attention to negative relative to positive information (Bartholow, Pearson, Gratton, & Fabiani, 2003; Smith, Cacioppo, Larsen, & Chartrand, 2003) and increased attention to outgroup relative to in-group members (Ito, Thompson, & Cacioppo, 2004; Ito & Urland, 2003). The N200 has been associated both with stimulus infrequency (e.g. (Nieuwenhuis, Yeung, Van Den Wildenberg, & Ridderinkhof, 2003; Squires, Squires, & Hillyard, 1975) and with conflict between the response demands associated with concurrent tasks (i.e., *response conflict*; see Botvinick, Braver, Barch, Carter, & Cohen, 2001).

One of the most widely studied endogenous components of the ERP is the P300, a large positive component that usually peaks between 300 and 800 milliseconds. The P300 has been associated with the brain's response to novelty (Friedman, Cycowicz, & Gaeta, 2001) in that P300 amplitude increases as the subjective probability of an eliciting event decreases (e.g., Donchin & Coles, 1988; Duncan-Johnson & Donchin, 1977; Squires et al., 1975; see also Nieuwendhuis, Aston-Jones, & Cohen, 2005). The P300 has been described as a manifestation of context updating in working memory, based on numerous studies indicating better subsequent memory for stimuli that elicit larger P300 amplitude (e.g., Donchin, 1981; Donchin & Coles, 1988; Friedman & Johnson, 2000). The latency at which the P300 peaks serves as a neural indicator of stimulus evaluation or categorization time, with longer latencies indicating more effortful categorization (see Coles, 1989). It is not uncommon for the P300 to peak substantially later than 300 milliseconds; in tasks involving complex social or emotional stimuli, peaks often occur between 550 and 800 milliseconds. Thus, some researchers refer to this component more generically as the "late positive potential," or LLP, to refer to its general time course and polarity without reference to a specific temporal anchor (e.g., see Cacioppo, Crites, Gardner, & Berntson, 1994, 1995; Ito, Larsen, Smith, & Cacioppo, 1998).

Why Use ERPs to Study Person Perception?

Person perception research has a deep and important history in social psychology, involving such seminal topics as stereotyping, causal attribution, impression formation, and expectancy effects, to name just a few (see Jones, 1990, for a review). It goes without saying that the behavioral methods typically used in person perception research, including recall (i.e., person memory), response latency, and self-reported evaluations (among others; see Olson, Roese, & Zanna, 1996), have provided a strong foundation for advancing our understanding of how people come to know what others are "really like" (Jones, 1990). However, the nature of the cognitive and affective processes thought to be important in driving person perception makes certain theoretical questions difficult to address when using such methods alone. For example, when participants are better able to recall information about people in one condition versus another, we infer that the information in the former condition received more extensive processing than the information in the latter condition. In this sense, recall represents one *outcome* of some cognitive activity associated with memory, but a number of processes likely intervene between stimulus encoding and recall that are not well represented in a memory measure. ERPs can provide a direct index of such intervening processes.

A related issue concerns the temporal specificity of cognitive measures. A number of theoretical models (e.g., Brewer, 1988; Fiske & Neuberg, 1990) posit multiple steps or stages of person perception, each of which may represent a distinct cognitive process or set of processes. Given that most social cognitive processes are assumed to unfold very quickly (e.g., Bargh, 1997; Higgins, 1996), behavioral and self-report measures are not especially well suited to represent them as they happen. In contrast, the temporal specificity of the ERP makes it an ideal measure for examining hypothesized sequential components of information processing involved in person perception (e.g., see Ito et al., 2004), allowing identification of various stages of processing that mediate the link between perception and overt behavior (e.g., see Rugg & Coles, 1995). Even the act of responding to stimuli (as with a response latency measure) can introduce noise into the data associated with response preparation and execution, effectively confounding relevant cognitive processes with irrelevant motor-related processes. In this regard, P300 latency provides an advantage over more traditional measures of processing time (e.g., response latency) in that it is independent of behavioral responses (though it often correlates with response latency; see McCarthy & Donchin, 1981). Thus this measure serves as an indicator of stimulus categorization time that is not confounded with the duration of response-related motor processes or task-relevant response selection requirements (Ito & Cacioppo, 2000; Kutas, McCarthy, & Donchin, 1975; McCarthy & Donchin, 1981; Smid, Mulder, Mulder, & Brands, 1992). This issue is particularly relevant for researchers interested in separating relatively automatic from more controlled processes. Another advantage is that the brain activity represented by ERPs generally is less controllable than self-reported data, thereby reducing concerns with self-presentational biases and permitting examination of the effects of a stimulus that individuals are either unable or unwilling to report.

P300 amplitude is particularly relevant for research in person perception for several reasons. First, the P300 can index the effects of probabilistic beliefs such as stereotypes and expectancies on perceivers' implicit reactions to others (see Ito & Cacioppo, 2007). Second, given the link between the P300 and working memory processes (see Friedman & Johnson, 2000), P300 amplitude can serve as an online, neural marker for person memory effects (see Bartholow, Fabiani, Gratton, & Bettencourt, 2001). Third, the P300 is known to index evaluative categorization (e.g., Ito & Cacioppo, 1999), a fundamental aspect of differentiating friend from foe. Finally, research suggests that the P300 can reveal task-irrelevant categorization processes (Ito & Cacioppo, 2000) and therefore may indicate implicit cognitive processes of which the participant is unaware.

In addition to these cognitive processes, affective processes also play a central role in many models of person perception. As one example, some models of expectancy processes (e.g., Burgoon, 1993; Mandler, 1990) predict that perceivers experience affective arousal when others behave in unexpected ways. However, the precise nature of these affective reactions has been debated. Some models (e.g., Mandler, 1990; Olson et al., 1996) predict that expectancy violations will always result in negative affect for the perceiver (at least initially) because unpredictability and uncertainty are generally unpleasant. Other models (e.g., Bettencourt, Dill, Greathouse, Charlton, & Mulholland, 1997; Kernahan, Bartholow, & Bettencourt, 2000), however, predict that the affective reaction to an expectancy violation depends on the valence of the violating information. As we review later, the temporal specificity of electrophysiological measures can allow direct tests of these theoretical assertions that have been difficult to obtain with self-report measures.

ERP STUDIES OF PERSON PERCEPTION

Cacioppo and his colleagues (Cacioppo, Crites, Berntson, & Coles, 1993) were among the first to study social perception using ERPs. These researchers reasoned that because the P300 serves as an index of subjective probability in categorization processes (e.g., Donchin & Coles, 1988; Friedman et al., 2001), it also should mark the implicit categorization of evaluatively consistent and inconsistent attitude objects. Early research by this group (e.g., Cacioppo, Crites, Berntson, & Coles, 1993) supported this hypothesis, showing that P300 amplitude was enhanced when participants implicitly categorized attitude words that differed in valence from a preceding context established by other attitude words. Similar research showed that the P300 to evaluative categorization (e.g., good, bad) differs from that to nonevaluative categorization (e.g., vegetable, nonvegetable; Crites & Cacioppo, 1996). Extending this paradigm to person perception, Cacioppo, Crites, Gardner, and Berntson (1994) showed that the P300 also indexes evaluative categorization of positive and negative personality traits and that this effect is associated with categorization per se rather than with response processes (Crites, Cacioppo, Gardner, & Berntson, 1995), suggesting that the P300 might assess implicit interpersonal attitudes.

Expectancies and Expectancy Violation

Based in part on the findings of Cacioppo and colleagues, Bartholow et al. (2001) reasoned that cognitive activity associated with interpersonal expectancy violations also should be manifest in P300 amplitude. A large literature in social and developmental psychology indicates that expectancy-violating information about people tends to be recalled better than expectancy-confirming information (e.g., Stangor & McMillan, 1992). Theoretical models (e.g., Srull & Wyer, 1989) posit that this recall advantage reflects updating of working memory that occurs as people attempt to reconcile the discrepancy between new information and existing "person concepts," a process generally known as *inconsistency resolution*. The long-standing notion that the P300 is an electrocortical index of working memory updating (e.g., Donchin, 1981; Donchin & Coles, 1988; Friedman & Johnson, 2000) suggests that the amplitude of this component should reflect the neural processes associated with inconsistency resolution.

To test these assertions, Bartholow and colleagues (2001) asked participants to read paragraph descriptions of several fictitious individuals in order to form impressions of them and then to read sentences (presented one word at a time on a computer monitor) depicting behaviors that were either consistent or inconsistent with those impressions. The valence of trait information was varied so that physiological responses to both positive and negative expectancy violations could be compared (Bettencourt et al., 1997; Olson et al., 1996). To examine affective reactions to expectancy violations, Bartholow et al. (2001) recorded the electrical activity of the *corrugator supercilii* muscle (under the brow) using electromyography (EMG). Previous research had established activity of the *corrugator* as an index of negative affective reactions that may be too small or too fleeting to be noticed with the "naked eye" (e.g., Cacioppo, Petty, Losch, & Kim, 1986; see also, e.g., Dimberg & Petterson, 2000; Hess, Blairy, & Kleck, 2000; Vanman, Paul, Ito, & Miller, 1997).

As predicted, Bartholow et al. (2001) found that expectancy-violating behaviors elicited larger P300 amplitude than did expectancy-consistent behaviors (see Figure 17.2). Similarly, expectancy-violating behaviors subsequently were recalled better than expectancy-consistent behaviors, supporting the idea that the P300 reflects working memory updating during person perception. Moreover, although earlier research suggested that the P300 to evaluatively inconsistent words was similar in amplitude regardless of word valence (Cacioppo et al., 1993), Bartholow et al. (2001) found that P300 effects were larger to inconsistent negative behaviors than to inconsistent positive behaviors (see Figure 17.2, bottom panel), consistent with the literature on positive–negative asymmetry in person perception (e.g.,

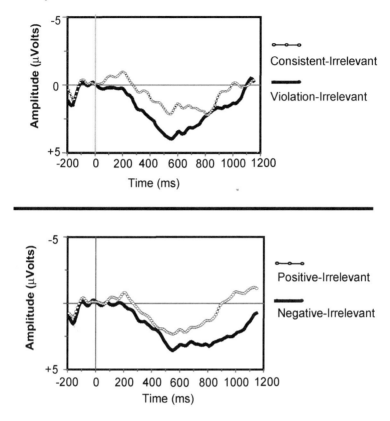

FIGURE 17.2. Difference waveforms representing effects of expectancy violation (top panel) and behavior valence (bottom panel) in the ERP recorded at the Pz (midline parietal) electrode site. Difference waveforms were created by subtracting amplitudes elicited by irrelevant behaviors from those elicited by expectancy-violating and expectancy-consistent behaviors (top panel), and from negative and positive behaviors (bottom panel). From Bartholow, Fabiani, Gratton, and Bettencourt (2001). Copyright 2001 by the Association for Psychological Science. Reprinted by permission.

Peeters & Czapinski, 1990; Reeder & Coovert, 1986; Ybarra, Schaberg, & Keiper, 1999) and with other ERP evidence that supports an implicit negativity bias (Ito, Larsen, Smith, & Cacioppo, 1998). Finally, facial EMG data indicated that the *corrugator* was activated by negative but not by positive expectancy-violating behaviors, supporting the notion that valence is an important determinant of affective reactions to expectancy violation (e.g., Bettencourt et al., 1997).

Bartholow et al.'s (2001) findings indicated that the recall advantage long known to accompany expectancy violations (e.g., Stangor & McMillan, 1992) results from evaluative categorization processes occurring very rapidly following perception and strongly implicates a role for working memory—one of a host of so-called executive cognitive functions thought to be mediated by activity in the prefrontal cortex—in the process of inconsistency resolution (see also Macrae, Bodenhausen, Schloersheidt, & Milne, 1999). To further explore the role of executive working memory in the inconsistency resolution processes reflected in the P300, Bartholow et al. (2003) conducted an experiment in which participants consumed either a moderate (0.40 g/kg ethanol) or high (0.80 g/kg ethanol) dose of alcohol or a placebo beverage just prior to engaging in the person-perception task used by Bartholow et al. (2001). Theory (e.g., Steele & Josephs, 1990) and research (e.g., Herzog, 1999) on the effects of alcohol has suggested that controlled processes are impaired following consumption but that automatic processes are relatively unaffected. Inconsistency resolution arguably involves both automatic (e.g., early direction of attention to novel or salient information) and controlled (e.g., comparison of new information with preexisting person concepts) components. Moreover, alcohol's effects on interpersonal behaviors are commonly attributed to impairment of executive cognitive functions thought to be mediated by the prefrontal cortex (e.g., Hoaken, Giancola, & Pihl, 1998; Peterson, Rothfleisch, Zelazo, & Pihl, 1990; Steele & Josephs, 1990). Given these factors and the evidence suggesting an important role for executive function in person perception (e.g., Macrae et al., 1999), Bartholow et al. (2003) reasoned that inconsistency resolution might be impaired during intoxication and used ERPs to specify which processes would be affected.

The main findings from this experiment are presented in Figure 17.3. For participants in the placebo condition, the ERP results largely replicated those of the earlier report (Bartholow et al., 2001), in that (negative) expectancy-violating behaviors presented in a positive context elicited enhanced P300 amplitude compared with expectancy-consistent behaviors, whereas (positive) expectancy-violating behaviors presented in a negative context did not. This finding is consistent with other data indicating that negative expectancy violations elicit more processing than do positive expectancy violations (e.g., Sherman & Frost, 2000; Trafimow & Finlay, 2001; Ybarra, Schaberg, & Keiper, 1999; see also Ybarra, 2002). For participants in the alcohol conditions, however, the opposite pattern emerged, with generally larger expectancy-violation effects associated with positive behaviors presented in a negative context. This reversal likely reflects the effects of alcohol-induced activation of the cerebral reward system on working memory operations associated with processing reward-congruent stimuli (see London, Ernst, Grant, Bonson, & Weinstein, 2000). These differential patterns of processing as a function of valence were corroborated by recall data. Whereas participants in the placebo condition recalled more negative expectancy-violating behaviors, those in the alcohol conditions recalled more positive expectancy-violating behaviors. Importantly, though, alcohol did not appear to disrupt the direction of attention to nega-

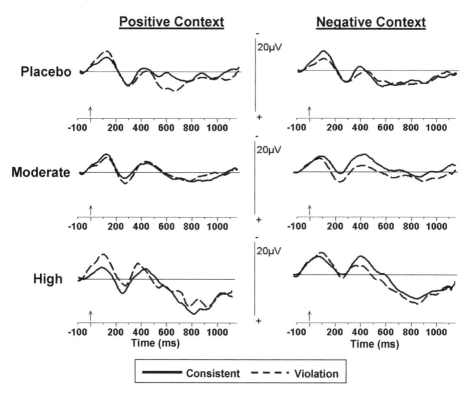

FIGURE 17.3. Event-related brain potential waveforms measured at the Pz (midline parietal) electrode as a function of alcohol dose, valenced expectancy context, and consistency of behaviors with expectancies. The vertical arrow on the timeline represents stimulus onset. From Bartholow, Pearson, Gratton, and Fabiani (2003). Copyright 2003 by American Psychological Association. Reprinted by permission.

tive information in early processing stages. The N100 component was larger to negative than to positive behaviors among all participants, regardless of alcohol dose. This finding is consistent with prior research suggesting that alcohol does not disrupt relatively automatic aspects of person perception (Herzog, 1999) and that, instead, its effects are limited to somewhat later, more effortful processing stages associated with working memory updating. Distinguishing alcohol's effects on these two stages of processing would not have been possible in this paradigm using a recall measure alone. This study also illustrates the use of alcohol as a tool in social neuroscience research. Given that many social cognitive phenomena are presumed to be mediated by prefrontal cortical activity, examining social cognitive processes in healthy individuals temporarily impaired by alcohol provides a method for bridging gaps between research in neuropsychology, social cognition, and cognitive neuroscience, literatures that traditionally have been largely segregated (see also Macrae et al., 1999).

Social Categorization: Processes and Consequences

A major focus of person perception research over the past 50 years has been on understanding the influence of perceiving others as members of social categories. However, this research is made difficult by participants' unwillingness or inability to divulge their true reactions to others, particularly on issues pertaining to out-group prejudice. In this regard, ERPs can provide relevant information concerning how differential categorization covertly influences information processing and ultimately behavioral responses.

A study by Osterhout, Bersick, and McLaughlin (1997) provided an early example of the use of ERPs to study the covert effects of social categorization. Participants were presented with sentences that violated definitional (e.g., "The fireman took a shower after *she* got home") or stereotypical (e.g., "Our aerobics instructor gave *himself* a break") noun–pronoun agreement (or violated neither) while ERPs were recorded. The results showed that both definitionally and stereotypically incongruent sentences elicited enhanced P300 amplitude. Moreover, these ERP effects were independent of participants' judgments of grammatical and syntactical acceptability, highlighting the effectiveness of ERPs in revealing implicit judgment processes.

In a more recent series of experiments, Ito and her colleagues (Ito & Cacioppo, 2000; Ito et al., 2004; Ito & Urland, 2003) have used ERPs to examine implicit and explicit aspects of categorization (for a more comprehensive review of physiological measures of implicit cognition, see Ito & Cacioppo, 2007). In one such study, Ito and Cacioppo (2000) found enhanced P300 amplitude to negative images and to images of people (compared with objects), regardless of whether participants were explicitly categorizing the images. Also, consistent with many of the studies reviewed here (see also Bartholow et al., 2001; Bartholow et al., 2003; Ito et al., 1998), Ito and Cacioppo (2000) found larger effects of evaluative inconsistency with negative as compared with positive targets. In two follow-up experiments, Ito and Urland (2003) showed that several ERP components are sensitive to implicit racial and gender categorization processes. Early components, such as the N100 and P200, appeared sensitive to processing of race and gender information, with larger amplitudes indicating more cognitive resources devoted to processing images of blacks and men, respectively. Later working memory-related processes, as indexed by the P300, were activated by individuals whose racial or gender categories differed from that of the social context established by the preceding images. Another recent study by this group (Ito et al., 2004) showed that the evaluative categorization effects reflected in the P300 correlated with perceivers' level of explicit prejudice toward out-group members, establishing P300 amplitude as an implicit measure of out-group bias that, unlike other implicit measures (e.g., Implicit Association Test; see Greenwald, McGhee, & Schwartz, 1998), requires no behavioral response.

When combined with behavioral measures, ERPs can also reveal the cognitive processes associated with the behavioral expression of racial bias. Because racial stereotypes are so pervasive in American culture, the behavior of white Americans—even those who believe themselves to be egalitarian—is often unintentionally biased against blacks. In other words, whites who are low in prejudice often face situations in which their egalitarian goals are in conflict with behavioral tendencies engendered by the automatic activation of stereotypes (e.g., Plant & Devine, 1998). Such situations exemplify *response conflict*—that is, prepotent, well-learned responses are in conflict with less automatic, goal-driven behaviors (see Botvinick et al., 2001). Two neural systems are posited to produce intended behaviors when conflict arises: a *conflict-detection* system that monitors ongoing responses for occasions of conflict and a *regulatory control* system designed to implement intended responses once conflict has been detected.

Amodio and his colleagues (2004) used ERPs to examine whether race-biased responses occur because the conflict-detection system fails to recognize that a given behavior is at odds with an individual's non-prejudiced beliefs. These researchers presented participants with trials in which a black or white face prime was followed by an image of either a gun or a tool. The participants' task was to categorize the second image (gun or tool) by pressing one of two buttons. Previous research using this paradigm (e.g., Payne, 2001) had established that participants are more likely to miscategorize tools as guns following black primes than following white primes, revealing racial bias associated with the stereotype that blacks are violent. As a neural index of conflict detection associated with this bias, Amodio et al. (2004) measured the amplitude of the error-related negativity (ERN) on miscategorization trials. The ERN is a response-locked ERP component that peaks within 100 milliseconds after a response and is thought to reflect activation of the conflict-detection system (see Botvinick et al., 2001; but also see Bartholow et al., 2005). As predicted, the conflict-detection system was more strongly engaged on trials in which a tool was mistaken for a gun following black primes (black–tool error) than following White primes (White-tool error). Nevertheless, participants were much more likely to mistake a tool for a gun on Black prime trials (see Amodio et al., 2004, Figure 2), indicating that racially biased responses occur despite the brain's detection of the conflict inherent in those responses and suggesting that bias might result from failure of the regulatory control system to overcome well-learned (though unintentional) response tendencies.

In a recent test of this latter possibility, Bartholow, Dickter, and Sestir (2006) examined the influence of stereotype activation on biased responding using a task designed to assess the role of the regulatory control system in withholding prejudiced responses. An important aspect of self-regulation of behavior is the ability to inhibit well-learned but potentially maladaptive responses in favor of other responses that are more appropriate in a given context (e.g., MacDonald, Cohen, Stenger, & Carter, 2000). Experimental tests of inhibitory control often involve the use of "go–stop" paradigms that engage participants in responding to "go" signals while "stop" signals occasionally inform them to withhold their responses (see Logan & Cowan, 1984). In such paradigms, responding in the presence of a stop signal represents a failure of the regulatory control system to implement top-down inhibitory control.

Bartholow et al. (2006) used a go–stop racial priming paradigm in which participants responded to trait adjectives associated with stereotypes of blacks (e.g., *violent, athletic*) and whites (e.g., *educated, uptight*) or to control words (descriptors of houses) following pictures of black or white faces or pictures of houses. Their task was to indicate (via a key press) whether or not each word could ever be true of the person (or house) that preceded it (see Dovidio, Evans, & Tyler, 1986). On one-fourth of the trials, a stop signal appeared shortly after the trait adjective, indicating that no response should be made. To the extent that face primes activate racial stereotypes, stereotype-consistent responses should be facilitated and more inhibitory control should be required to withhold responses on stereotype-consistent stop trials (e.g., a black face followed by *violent*) than on stereotype-violation stop trials (e.g., a black face followed by *educated*). Bartholow et al. (2006) measured the frequency of inhibition errors (i.e., failures to inhibit) in participants' responses, as well as the amplitude of the negative slow wave (NSW), a stimulus-locked ERP component that develops late in trial epochs (see Figure 17.1) and indexes activity in the regulatory control system (see West & Alain, 1999).

As an additional manipulation of cognitive control of inhibition, Bartholow et al. (2006) assigned participants to one of three alcohol dose conditions, as in previous research (Bartholow et al., 2003). A substantial number of studies have indicated that moderate doses of alcohol significantly impair behavioral inhibition but have no effect on the activation and implementation of responses (e.g., Easdon & Vogel-Sprott, 2000; Fillmore & Vogel-Sprott, 2000; Mulvihill, Skilling, & Vogel-Sprott, 1997) and that these effects stem specifically from alcohol's impairment of the regulatory cognitive control system (Abroms, Fillmore, & Marczinski, 2003; Easdon & Vogel-Sprott, 2000). Recent ERP evidence (Curtin & Fairchild, 2003) has shown that these effects are evident in an alcohol-induced reduction of NSW amplitude that correlates with behavioral undercontrol. Therefore, alcohol provides an excellent tool for testing hypotheses associated with the role of regulatory control in expression of racial bias. Bartholow et al. (2006) reasoned that alcohol's effects on regulatory control should result in a dose-dependent increase in the frequency of inhibition errors, but only (or primarily) on stereotype-consistent trials, which should be most difficult to inhibit. This pattern of impairment also was predicted for NSW amplitude, with smaller amplitude of the component reflecting less effective implementation of regulatory cognitive control.

The primary findings from Bartholow et al.'s (2006, Experiment 2) study are presented in Figure 17.4. As predicted, the inhibition error data (Figure 17.4a) indicated a linear increase in failures to inhibit on stereotype-consistent trials as a function of alcohol dose, but no significant effect of alcohol on stereotype-violation trials. The ERP waveforms (Figure 17.4b) nicely mirrored the behavioral data. First, the amplitude of the NSW was significantly reduced by alcohol, consistent with the idea that alcohol impairs cognitive control (Curtin & Fairchild, 2003). More important, stereotype-consistent trials elicited larger NSW amplitude than did stereotype-violation trials, but only among those in the placebo group. This finding supports the idea that withholding dominant, prejudiced responses engages more regulative cognitive control resources and that this process is impaired following alcohol consumption. Although the data presented in Figure 17.4a are restricted to the middle fronto-central electrode location, this effect was fairly broadly distributed over frontal, central, and anterior parietal scalp regions. These data indicate that intact regulatory control is a critical component of inhibiting unintentional race-biased behaviors. These data also suggest that motivation to control prejudice (e.g., Plant & Devine, 1998; Monteith, Ashburn-Nardo, Voils, & Czopp, 2002) is only part of what determines whether or not bias will be expressed; a high level of motivation to exert control might not be enough to ensure unbiased responding when regulatory control is impaired. These findings, along with those of Amodio et al. (2004), provide important evidence of the neural underpinnings of racial bias and its control.

Racial Priming Effects: ERP Evidence of Response Conflict

In a number of the studies just described, various priming techniques were used to demonstrate the effects of automatic stereotype activation on behavior. It has long been argued that racial primes facilitate stereotype-consistent responses because of *spreading activation*, the process through which activation of particular constructs (e.g., racial category labels) increases the accessibility of related constructs (e.g., stereotypically associated traits) in semantic memory and decreases the accessibility of unrelated constructs (e.g., counterstereotypic traits; see Higgins, 1996; Schank & Abelson, 1977). This hypothesized memory structure provides a concise explanation for the faster response latencies typically associated with stereotype-consistent prime-word pairs, which are assumed to reside near one another in semantic space and thus require less time to "spread" activation from the category to the trait, compared with stereotype-violating prime-word pairs, which are assumed to occupy more distant semantic

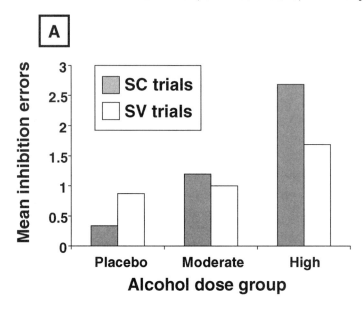

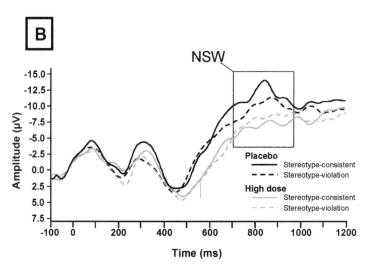

FIGURE 17.4. Inhibition errors (panel A) and ERP waveforms elicited over the midline frontocentral cortex (panel B) on stop trials as a function of alcohol dose and trial type. Increased inhibition errors (panel A) on stereotype-consistent (SC) trials relative to stereotype-violating (SV) trials indicate difficulty inhibiting race-biased behaviors. The larger negative slow wave (NSW) amplitude associated with stereotype-consistent trials in the placebo group (panel B) indicates greater implementation of cognitive control resources to inhibiting responses on those trials. Time zero indicates onset of the stop signal. The decrease in NSW amplitude associated with the high alcohol dose indicates alcohol-induced impairment of cognitive control. Adapted from Bartholow, Dickter, and Sestir (2006).

spaces (e.g., Dovidio et al., 1986; Fazio, Jackson, Dunton, & Williams, 1995; Gaertner & McLaughlin, 1983).

Recent evidence from cognitive neuroscience studies of response conflict suggests an alternative explanation for response facilitation in priming paradigms. As discussed previously, response conflict occurs when a well-learned or prepotent response must be overridden by an alternative response in order to respond correctly in a given context. A classic paradigm used to induce response conflict is the Eriksen flanker task (Eriksen & Eriksen, 1974), in which a target stimulus (e.g., a letter) is flanked by so-called noise stimuli. The participant's task is to categorize the target by pressing one of two keys. A very robust response facilitation is produced in this task on low-conflict, compatible trials (when the target and flankers are identical; e.g., *HHHHH*) compared with high-conflict, incompatible trials (when the target and flankers represent opposing categories; e.g., *SSHSS*). Research shows that the lateralized readiness potential (LRP)—a response-locked component of the ERP that reflects motor cortex activity associated with instigating behavioral responses—reveals initial activation of incorrect response channels preceding activation of the correct response on high-conflict trials in this task (for a review, see Coles, Smid, Scheffers, & Otten, 1995). This initial activation of the incorrect response requires some degree of effort (and time) to reverse, leading to longer response latencies on high-conflict trials (see Gratton, Coles, Sirevaag, Eriksen, & Donchin, 1988). To the extent that responding to stereotype-incongruent prime-word pairs induces response conflict, incorrect response activation that occurs on such trials could provide an alternative account for the longer response latencies in racial priming experiments. This response activation should be evident in the LRP.

To test this assertion, Bartholow and Dickter (2006) recently conducted a series of experiments using a modified Eriksen flanker task in which the targets were facial photos of blacks and whites and the flankers were words associated with cultural stereotypes for blacks and whites. In this case, compatible trials were defined as those in which the race of the target was congruent with the stereotypicality of the flanker words (e.g., a black face flanked by *violent*) and incompatible trials were those in which the target's race was incongruent with the stereotypicality of the flanker words (e.g., a white face flanked by *violent*). The participants' task was simply to categorize the target person as white or black by pressing one of two keys, while attempting to ignore the flanker words.

In their first experiment, Bartholow and Dickter (2006) simply measured response latencies on compatible and incompatible trials. The data showed that participants were faster to categorize targets by race when they were flanked by stereotype-congruent than by stereotype-incongruent words, suggesting that response conflict occurs in this version of the paradigm even though the flankers were not associated with either response and shared only an implicit semantic relationship with the targets. However, these data do not directly address whether the slowed categorization of incongruent flankers results from initial activation of the incorrect response channel. (See Amodio, Chapter 16, this volume, for a fuller account of this and related studies.)

To address this question, Bartholow and Dickter (2006) added LRP measures in Experiment 2. These waveforms are presented in Figure 17.5. According to the logic of the LRP (see Coles et al., 1995), cortical activity associated with incorrect response activation results in a positive-going waveform, whereas correct response activation is associated with negative voltage (see also DeJong, Liang, & Lauber, 1994; Gratton et al., 1988). As shown in Figure 17.5, correctly categorized incompatible trials tended to elicit a small (but significant) degree of incorrect response activation (seen as the initial positive-going "dip" in the waveform around 50 ms) prior to the activation of the correct response. In contrast, compatible trials were associated only with correct response activation. LRP activity also can be used to infer when behavioral responses will be emitted (see Gratton et al., 1988). The horizontal dotted lines in Figure 17.5 represent hypothetical response thresholds for commission of correct (upper line) and incorrect (lower line) responses. Examining the point at which the LRP waveform crosses this threshold in each condition provides a visual representation of

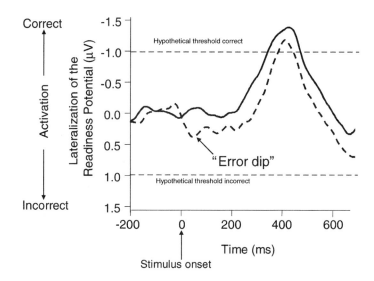

FIGURE 17.5. Lateralized readiness potential (LRP) waveforms elicited on stereotype-congruent trials (i.e., compatible trials; solid line) and stereotype-incongruent trials (incompatible trials; dashed line), measured over left and right motor cortex areas. The "error dip" evident in the incompatible-trials waveform indicates initial activation of the incorrect response at the neural level prior to the correct response being activated and emitted.

the delay in response latency caused by initial incorrect response activation in the incompatible condition. Thus these data suggest that stereotype-incongruent trials result in slower behavioral responses because they initially engender activation of the incorrect response, delaying activation of the correct response. This interpretation is at odds with notions from spreading activation theory that stereotype-incongruent constructs are activated slowly because of their distance from racial categories in semantic memory. Instead, these data support a response-conflict account, whereby responses are activated quickly at the neural level but the initial activation is incorrect. It is this "confused" activation of both response channels that slows response latency. This finding has a number of implications. For our purposes here, one important implication is that ERPs provide a more complete understanding of the apparent interference caused by stereotype-related contextual information during racial categorization than could be gained with reaction time measures alone. In this way, this study stands as a clear example of the promise of the social-cognitive neuroscience approach, which holds that processes of interest can be best understood when examined at the social, cognitive, and neural levels of analysis (see Ochsner & Lieberman, 2001).

CONCLUSIONS

The aim of this chapter was to outline ways in which electrocortical measures can be used to answer important theoretical questions in person perception. As the research reviewed here demonstrates, ERPs provide an additional tool for the experimental social psychologist's arsenal of methods. We contend, however, that ERPs are most fruitfully employed in conjunction with more traditional behavioral methods. Most important, ERPs are only as effective in solving theoretical dilemmas as the experimental designs in which they are applied (e.g., Cacioppo et al., 2003; Willingham & Dunn, 2003). It is our hope that this chapter, along with the other chapters in this volume, will inform researchers as to the potential value of including the ERP and other physiological measures in their research programs.

In closing, it is important to briefly address when researchers should choose ERPs as opposed to other measures of brain function. A host of other psychophysiological measures not discussed in this review, including (but not limited to) brain imaging techniques designed to specify which brain structures and systems underlie social cognitive processes (e.g., functional magnetic resonance imaging; fMRI), also are now important tools for social neuroscientists interested in person perception (e.g., see Phelps et al., 2000; Richeson et al., 2003). Deciding which kind of neural measure(s) to use is driven by theoretical, as well as practical, considerations. On the practical side, electrophysiological measures (such as ERPs) can be employed at far less cost than fMRI and can be incorporated into a social cognition lab with relatively modest physical renovations and technical expertise. Acquiring fMRI technology requires a substantial, often institution-wide, commitment of financial and personnel resources to purchase and operate a magnet and construct a space in which to house it. More important, ERPs and fMRI are simply suited to addressing different theoretical questions. In general, ERPs are among the best tools available for specifying the temporal sequence of cognitive processes associated with social perception, but their usefulness for determining the neural sources of these processes is limited (but see Koles, 1998). In contrast, fMRI provides exceptional spatial resolution but, at least at present, poor temporal resolution (on the order of 4–6 seconds poststimulus). An ideal scenario for many researchers would involve the combined use of ERPs and fMRI in order to specify both spatial and temporal parameters of the neural events underlying person perception. Some relatively new technologies combining these properties already have been applied in cognitive neuroscience (e.g., see Gratton & Fabiani, 1998). Use of such techniques has promise for fostering further links between social and biological approaches and for advancing our understanding of the neural machinery driving social-psychological phenomena.

REFERENCES

Abroms, B. D., Fillmore, M. T., & Marczinski, C. A.. (2003). Alcohol-induced impairment of behavioral control: Effects on the alteration and suppression of prepotent responses. *Journal of Studies on Alcohol, 64,* 687–695.

Amodio, D. M., Harmon-Jones, E., Devine, P. G., Curtin, J. J., Hartley, S. L., & Covert, A. E. (2004). Neural signals for the detection of unintentional race bias. *Psychological Science, 15,* 88–93.

Bargh, J. A. (1997). The automaticity of everyday life. In R.S. Wyer, Jr. (Ed.), *Advances in social cognition: Vol. 10. The automaticity of everyday life* (pp. 1–61). Mahwah, NJ: Erlbaum.

Bartholow, B. D., & Dickter, C. L. (2006). *A response conflict account of response facilitation in stereotype priming paradigms.* Manuscript in preparation.

Bartholow, B. D., Dickter, C. L., & Sestir, M. (2006). Stereotype activation and control of prejudiced responses: Cognitive control of inhibition and its impairment by alcohol. *Journal of Personality and Social Psychology, 90,* 272–287.

Bartholow, B. D., Fabiani, M., Gratton, G., & Bettencourt, B. A. (2001). A psychophysiological analysis of cognitive processing of and affective responses to social expectancy violations. *Psychological Science, 12,* 197–204.

Bartholow, B. D., Pearson, M. A., Dickter, C., Sher, K. J., Fabiani, M., & Gratton, G. (2005). Strategic control and medial frontal negativity: Beyond errors and response conflict. *Psychophysiology, 42,* 33–42.

Bartholow, B. D., Pearson, M. A., Gratton, G., & Fabiani, M. (2003). Effects of alcohol on person perception: A social cognitive neuroscience approach. *Journal of Personality and Social Psychology, 85,* 627–638.

Berger, H. (1929). Über das Elektrenkephalogramm das Menchen. *Archiv für Psychiatrie, 87,* 527–570.

Bettencourt, B. A., Dill, K. E., Greathouse, S. A., Charlton, K., & Mulholland, A. (1997). Evaluations of in-group and out-group members: The role of category-based expectancy violation. *Journal of Experimental Social Psychology, 33,* 244–275.

Botvinick, M. M., Braver, T. S., Barch, D. M., Carter, C. S., & Cohen, J. D. (2001). Conflict monitoring and cognitive control. *Psychological Review, 108,* 624–652.

Brewer, M. (1988). A dual process model of impression formation. In T. Srull & R. Wyer, Jr. (Eds.), *Advances in social cognition* (Vol. 1, pp. 1–36). Hillsdale, NJ: Erlbaum.

Burgoon, J. K. (1993). Interpersonal expectations, expectancy violations, and emotional communication. *Journal of Language and Social Psychology, 12,* 30–48.

Cacioppo, J. T., Berntson, G. G., Lorig, T. S, Norris, C. J., Rickett, E., & Nusbaum, H. (2003). Just because you're imaging the brain doesn't mean you can stop using your head: A primer and set of first principles. *Journal of Personality and Social Psychology, 85,* 650–651.

Cacioppo, J. T., Berntson, G. G., Sheridan, J. F., & McClintock, M. K. (2000). Multilevel integrative analyses of human behavior: Social neuroscience and the complementing nature of social and biological approaches. *Psychological Bulletin, 126,* 829–843.

Cacioppo, J. T., Crites, S. L., Jr., Berntson, G. G., & Coles, M. G. H. (1993). If attitudes affect how stimuli are processed, should they not affect the event-related brain potential? *Psychological Science, 4*(2), 108–112.

Cacioppo, J. T., Crites, S. L., Gardner, W. L., & Berntson, G. G. (1994). Bioelectrical echoes from evaluative categorizations: I. A late positive brain potential that varies as a function of trait negativity and extremity. *Journal of Personality and Social Psychology, 67,* 115–125.

Cacioppo, J. T., Petty, R. E., Losch, M. E., & Kim, H. S. (1986). Electromyographic activity over facial muscle regions can differentiate the valence and intensity of affective reactions. *Journal of Personality and Social Psychology, 50,* 260–268.

Coles, M. G. H. (1989). Modern mind–brain reading: Psychophysiology, physiology, and cognition. *Psychophysiology, 26,* 251–269.

Coles, M. G. H., Smid, H. G. O. M., Scheffers, M. K., & Otten, L. J. (1995). Mental chronometry and the study of human information processing. In M. D. Rugg & M. G. H. Coles (Eds.), *Electrophysiology of mind: Event-related brain potentials and cognition* (pp. 86–131). New York: Oxford University Press.

Crites, S. L., & Cacioppo, J. T. (1996). Electrocortical differentiation of evaluative and nonevaluative categorizations. *Psychological Science, 7,* 318–321.

Crites, S. L., Cacioppo, J. T., Gardner, W. L., & Berntson, G. G. (1995). Bioelectrical echoes from evaluative categorization: II. A late positive brain potential that varies as a function of attitude registration rather than attitude report. *Journal of Personality and Social Psychology, 68,* 997–1013.

Curtin, J. J., & Fairchild, B. A. (2003). Alcohol and cognitive control: Implications for regulation of behavior during response conflict. *Journal of Abnormal Psychology, 112,* 424–436.

De Jong, R., Liang, C. C., & Lauber, E. (1994). Conditional and unconditional automaticity: A dual process model of effects of spatial stimulus–response correspondence. *Journal of Experimental Psychology: Human Perception and Performance, 20,* 731–750.

Dimberg, U., & Petterson, M. (2000). Facial reactions to happy and angry facial expressions: Evidence for right hemisphere dominance. *Psychophysiology, 37,* 693–696.

Donchin, E. (1981). Surprise!...Surprise? *Psychophysiology, 18,* 493-513.

Donchin, E., & Coles, M. G. (1988). Is the P300 component a manifestation of context updating? *Behavioral and Brain Sciences, 11,* 357–427.

Dovidio, J. F., Evans, N., & Tyler, R. B. (1986). Racial stereotypes: The contents of their cognitive representations. *Journal of Experimental Social Psychology, 22,* 22–37.

Duncan-Johnson, C. C., & Donchin, E. (1977). On quantifying surprise: The variation of event-related potentials with subjective probability. *Psychophysiology, 14,* 456–467.

Easdon, C. M., & Vogel-Sprott, M. (2000). Alcohol and behavioral control: Impaired response inhibition and flexibility in social drinkers. *Experimental and Clinical Psychopharmacology, 8,* 387–394.

Eriksen, B. A., & Eriksen, C. W. (1974). Effects of noise letters upon the identification of a target in a nonsearch task. *Perception and Psychophysics, 16,* 143–149.

Fabiani, M., Gratton, G., & Coles, M. G. H. (2000). Event-related brain potentials. In L. G. Tassinary & J. T. Cacioppo (Eds.), *Handbook of psychophysiology* (2nd ed., pp. 53–84). New York: Cambridge University Press.

Fazio, R. H. (1990). A practical guide to the use of response latency in social psychological research. In M. S. Clark & C. Hendrick (Eds.), *Review of personality and social psychology* (Vol. 11, pp. 74–97). Thousand Oaks, CA: Sage.

Fazio, R. H., Jackson, J. R., Dunton, B. C., & Williams, C. J. (1995). Variability in automatic activation as an unobtrusive measure of racial attitudes: A bona fide pipeline? *Journal of Personality and Social Psychology, 69,* 1013–1027.

Fillmore, M. T., & Vogel-Sprott, M. (2000). Response inhibition under alcohol: Effects of cognitive and motivational conflict. *Journal of Studies on Alcohol, 61,* 239–246.

Fiske, S. T., & Neuberg, S. L. (1990). A continuum of impression formation, from category-based to individuated processes: Influences of information and motivation on attention and interpretation. In M. P. Zanna (Ed.), *Advances in experimental social psychology* (Vol. 23, pp. 1–74). New York: Academic Press.

Friedman, D., Cycowicz, Y. M., & Gaeta, H. (2001). The novelty P3: An event-related brain potential (ERP) sign of the brain's evaluation of novelty. *Neuroscience and Biobehavioral Reviews, 25,* 355–373.

Friedman, D., & Johnson, R., Jr. (2000). Event-related potential (ERP) studies of memory encoding and retrieval: A selective review. *Microscopy Research and Technique, 51,* 6–28.

Gaertner, S. L., & McLaughlin, J. P. (1983). Racial stereotypes: Associations and ascriptions of positive and negative characteristics. *Social Psychology Quarterly, 46,* 23–30.

Gehring, W. J., Gratton, G., Coles, M. G., & Donchin, E. (1992). Probability effects on stimulus evaluation and response processes. *Journal of Experimental Psychology: Human Perception and Performance, 18,* 198–216.

Gratton, G., Coles, M. G., Sirevaag, E. J., Eriksen, C. W., & Donchin, E. (1988). Pre- and poststimulus activation of response channels: A psychophysiological analysis. *Journal of Experimental Psychology: Human Perception and Performance, 14,* 331–334.

Gratton, G., & Fabiani, M. (1998). Dynamic brain imaging: Event-related optical signal (EROS) measures of the time course and localization of cognitive-related activity. *Psychonomic Bulletin and Review, 5,* 535–563.

Greenwald, A. G., McGhee, D. E., & Schwartz, J. L. K. (1998). Measuring individual differences in implicit cognition: The Implicit Association Test. *Journal of Personality and Social Psychology, 74,* 1464–1480.

Herzog, T. A. (1999). Effects of alcohol intoxication on social inferences. *Experimental and Clinical Psychopharmacology, 7,* 448–453.

Hess, U., Blairy, S., & Kleck, R. E. (2000). The influence of facial emotion displays, gender, and ethnicity on judgments of dominance and affiliation. *Journal of Nonverbal Behavior, 24,* 265–283.

Higgins, E. T. (1996). Knowledge activation: Accessibility, applicability, and salience. In E. T. Higgins & J. A. Bargh (Eds.), *Social psychology: Handbook of basic principles* (pp. 133–168). New York: Guilford Press.

Hoaken, P. N. S., Giancola, P. R., & Pihl, R. O. (1998). Executive cognitive functions as mediators of alcohol-related aggression. *Alcohol and Alcoholism, 33,* 47–54.

Hopfinger, J. B., & Mangun, G. R. (2001). Electrophysiological studies of reflexive attention. In C. L. Folk & B. S. Gibson (Eds.), *Attraction, distraction, and action: Multiple perspectives on attentional capture* (pp. 3–26). Amsterdam: Elsevier Science.

Ito, T. A., & Cacioppo, J. T. (1999). The psychophysiology of utility appraisals. In D. Kahneman, E. Diener, & N. Schwartz (Eds.), *The foundations of hedonic psychology* (pp. 470–488). New York: Russell Sage Foundation.

Ito, T. A., & Cacioppo, J. T. (2000). Electrophysiological evidence of implicit and explicit categorization processes. *Journal of Experimental Social Psychology, 36,* 660–676.

Ito, T. A., & Cacioppo, J. T. (2007). Attitudes as mental and neural states of readiness: Using psychological measures to study implicit attitudes. In B. Wittenbrink & N. Schwartz (Eds.), *Implicit measures of attitudes* (pp. 125–158). New York: Guilford Press.

Ito, T. A., Larsen, J. T., Smith, N. K., & Cacioppo, J. T. (1998). Negative information weighs more heavily on the brain: The negativity bias in evaluative categorizations. *Journal of Personality and Social Psychology, 75,* 887–900.

Ito, T. A., Thompson, E., & Cacioppo, J. T. (2004). Tracking the time course of social perception: The effects of racial cues on event-related brain potentials. *Personality and Social Psychology Bulletin, 30,* 1267–1280.

Ito, T. A., & Urland, G. R. (2003). Race and gender on the brain: Electrocortical measures of attention to the race and gender of multiply categorizable individuals. *Journal of Personality and Social Psychology, 85,* 616–626.

Jasper, H. H. (1958). The ten–twenty electrode system of the International Federation. *Electroencephalography and Clinical Neurophysiology, 10,* 371–375.

Jones, E. E. (1990). *Interpersonal perception.* New York: Freeman.

Kernahan, C. A., Bartholow, B. D., & Bettencourt, B. A. (2000). Effects of category-based expectancy violation on affect-related evaluations: Toward a comprehensive model. *Basic and Applied Social Psychology, 22,* 85–100.

Koles, Z. J. (1998). Trends in EEG source localization. *Electroencephalography and Clinical Neurophysiology, 106,* 127–137.

Kutas, M., McCarthy, G., & Donchin, E. (1975). Differences between sinistrals' and dextrals' ability to infer a whole from its parts: A failure to replicate. *Neuropsychologia, 13*(4), 455–464.

Logan, D. G., & Cowan, W. B. (1984). On the ability to inhibit thought and action: A theory of an act of control. *Psychological Review, 91,* 295–327.

London, E. D., Ernst, M., Grant, S., Bonson, K., & Weinstein, A. (2000). Orbitofrontal cortex and human drug abuse: Functional imaging. *Cerebral Cortex, 10,* 334–342.

MacDonald, A. W., Cohen, J. D., Stenger, V. A., & Carter, C. S. (2000). Dissociating the role of the dorsolateral prefrontal and anterior cingulate cortex in cognitive control. *Science, 288,* 1835–1838.

Macrae, C. N., Bodenhausen, G. V., Schloersheidt, A. M., & Milne, A. B. (1999). Tales of the unexpected: Executive function and person perception. *Journal of Personality and Social Psychology, 76,* 200–213.

Mandler, G. (1990). A constructivist theory of emotion. In N. L. Stein & B. Leventhal (Eds.), *Psychological and biological approaches to emotion* (pp. 21–43). Hillsdale, NJ: Erlbaum.

Mangun, G. R., Hillyard, S. A., & Luck, S. J. (1993). Electrocortical substrates of visual selective attention. In S. Kornblum & D. E. Meyer (Eds.), *Attention and performance: Vol. 14. Synergies in experimental psychology, artificial intelligence, and cognitive neuroscience* (pp. 219–243). Cambridge, MA: MIT Press.

Markus, H., & Zajonc, R. B. (1985). The cognitive perspective in social psychology. In G. Lindzey & E. Aronson (Eds.), *Handbook of social psychology* (3rd ed., pp. 137–230). New York: Random House.

McCarthy, G., & Donchin, E. (1981). A metric for thought: A comparison of P300 latency and reaction time. *Science, 211,* 77–80.

Monteith, M. J., Ashburn-Nardo, L., Voils, C. I., & Czopp, A. M. (2002). Putting the brakes on prejudice: On the development and operation of cues for control. *Journal of Personality and Social Psychology, 83,* 1029–1050.

Mulvihill, L. E., Skilling, T. A., & Vogel-Sprott, M. (1997). Alcohol and the ability to inhibit behavior in men and women. *Journal of Studies on Alcohol, 58,* 600–605.

Nieuwenhuis, S., Aston-Jones, G., & Cohen, J. D. (2005). Decision making, the P3, and the locus coeruleus-norepinephrine system. *Psychological Bulletin, 131,* 510–532.

Nieuwenhuis, S., Yeung, N., Van Den Wildenberg, W., & Ridderinkhof, K. R. (2003). Electrophysiological correlates of anterior cingulate function in a go/no-go task: Effects of response conflict and trial type frequency. *Cognitive, Affective and Behavioral Neuroscience, 3,* 17–26.

Ochsner, K. N. (2004). Current directions in social cognitive neuroscience. *Current Opinion in Neurobiology, 14,* 254–258.

Ochsner, K. N., & Lieberman, M. D. (2001). The emergence of social cognitive neuroscience. *American Psychologist, 56,* 717–734.

Olson, J. M., Roese, N. J., & Zanna, M. P. (1996). Expectanices. In E. T. Higgins

& A. W. Kruglanski (Eds.), *Social psychology: Handbook of basic principles* (pp. 211–238). New York: Guilford Press.

Osterhout, L., Bersick, M., & McLaughlin, J. (1997). Brain potentials reflect violations of gender stereotypes. *Memory and Cognition, 25*, 273–285.

Payne, B. K. (2001). Prejudice and perception: The role of automatic and controlled processes in misperceiving a weapon. *Journal of Personality and Social Psychology, 81*, 181–192.

Peeters, G., & Czapinksi, J. (1990). Positive-negative asymmetry in evaluations: The distinction between affective and informational negativity effects. *European Review of Social Psychology, 1*, 33–60.

Peterson, J. B., Rothfleisch, J., Zelazo, P. D., & Pihl, R. O. (1990). Acute alcohol intoxication and cognitive functioning. *Journal of Studies on Alcohol, 51*, 114–122.

Phelps, E. A., O'Connor, K. J., Cunningham, W. A., Funayama, E. S., Gatenby, J. C., Gore, J. C., et al. (2000). Performance on indirect measures of race evaluation predicts amygdala activation. *Journal of Cognitive Neuroscience, 12*, 729–738.

Plant, E. A., & Devine, P. G. (1998). Internal and external motivation to respond without prejudice. *Journal of Personality and Social Personality, 75*, 811–832.

Reeder, G. D., & Coovert, M. D. (1986). Revising an impression of morality. *Social Cognition, 4*, 1–7.

Reis, H. T., & Judd, C.M. (Eds.). (2000). *Handbook of research methods in social and personality psychology*. New York: Cambridge University Press.

Richeson, J. A., Baird, A. A., Gordon, H. L., Heatherton, T. F., Wyland, C. L., Trawalter, S., et al. (2003). An fMRI investigation of the impact of interracial contact on executive function. *Nature Neuroscience, 6*, 1323–1328.

Rugg, M. D., & Coles, M. G. H. (Eds.). (1995). *Electrophysiology of mind: Event-related brain potentials and cognition*. New York: Oxford University Press.

Schank, R. C., & Abelson, R. P. (1979). *Scripts, plans, goals, and understanding: An inquiry into human knowledge structures*. Oxford, UK: Erlbaum.

Semlitsch, H.V., Anderer, P., Schuster, P., & Presslich, O. (1986). A solution for reliable and valid reduction of ocular artifacts, applied to the P300 ERP. *Psychophysiology, 23*, 695–703.

Sherman, J. W., & Frost, L. A. (2000). On the encoding of stereotype-relevant information under cognitive load. *Personality and Social Psychology Bulletin, 26*, 26–34.

Smid, H. G., Mulder, G., Mulder, L. J., & Brands, G. J. (1993). A psychophysiological study of the use of partial information in stimulus–response translation. *Journal of Experimental Psychology: Human Perception and Performance, 18*, 1101–1119.

Smith, N. K., Cacioppo, J. T., Larsen, J. T., & Chartrand, T. L. (2003). May I have your attention, please: Electrocortical responses to positive and negative stimuli. *Neuropsychologia, 41*, 171–183.

Squires, N. K., Squires, K. C., & Hillyard, S. A. (1975). Two varieties of long-latency positive waves evoked by unpredictable auditory stimuli in man. *Electroencephalography and Clinical Neurophysiology, 38*, 387–401.

Srull, T. K., & Wyer, R. S., Jr. (1989). Person memory and judgment. *Psychological Review, 96*, 58–83.

Stangor, C., & McMillan, D. (1992). Memory for expectancy-congruent and expectancy-incongruent information: A review of the social and social developmental literatures. *Psychological Bulletin, 111,* 42–61.

Steele, C. M., & Josephs, R. A. (1990). Alcohol myopia: Its prized and dangerous effects. *American Psychologist, 45,* 921–933.

Stern, R. M., Ray, W. J., & Quigley, K. S. (2001). *Psychophysiological recording* (2nd ed.). New York: Oxford University Press.

Trafimow, D., & Finlay, K. A. (2001). An investigation of three models of multitrait representations. *Personality and Social Psychology Bulletin, 27,* 226–241.

Vanman, E. J., Paul, B. Y., Ito, T. A., & Miller, N. (1997). The modern face of prejudice and structural features that moderate the effect of cooperation on affect. *Journal of Personality and Social Psychology, 73,* 941–959.

West, R., & Alain, C. (1999). Event-related neural activity associated with the Stroop task. *Cognitive Brain Research, 8,* 157–164.

Willingham, D. T., & Dunn, E. W. (2003). What neuroimaging and brain localization can do, cannot do, and should not do for social psychology. *Journal of Personality and Social Psychology, 85,* 662–671.

Ybarra, O. (2002). Naïve causal understanding of valenced behaviors and its implications for social information processing. *Psychological Bulletin, 128,* 421–441.

Ybarra, O., Schaberg, L., & Keiper, S. (1999). Favorable and unfavorable target expectancies and social information processing. *Journal of Personality and Social Psychology, 77,* 698–709.

18

Social Neuroscience and Social Perception

NEW PERSPECTIVES ON CATEGORIZATION, PREJUDICE, AND STEREOTYPING

Tiffany A. Ito, Eve Willadsen-Jensen, and Joshua Correll

From a resource-conservation perspective, our ability to categorize individuals into meaningful social groups, then to use whatever information we associate with the group to guide impressions about and behavior toward those individuals greatly facilitates our ability to make sense of the people around us (Brewer, 1988; Fiske & Neuberg, 1990). Although a single outcome such as a behavioral response can represent this process, fully understanding the mechanisms that produce this outcome requires access to the multiple underlying processes that constitute social perception. Due to rapid increases in technology, neuroscience measures are increasingly being used to do this. In this chapter, we focus in particular on the application of event-related brain potentials (ERPs) to understanding social perception. We first provide a short background on the recording and interpretation of ERPs. We then review specific ERP studies that examine how individuals are categorized into social groups and how prejudices and stereotypes are activated and influence behavior. We hope both to highlight the way these findings integrate with existing theories of social perception and to suggest new directions for future research.

RECORDING ERPS: A BRIEF REVIEW

ERPs are changes in brain electrical activity that occur in response to discrete events such as a stimulus or onset of a response. They can be recorded noninvasively from the surface of the scalp and are thought to reflect summated postsynaptic potentials from large sets of synchronously firing neurons in the cerebral cortex (Fabiani, Gratton, & Coles, 2000). The recorded electrical waveform is a time-by-voltage function composed of a series of positive and negative deflections.[1] Time-locked deflections in the waveform are referred to as *components*. The importance of ERPs to the study of psychological processes derives from the association of individual ERP components with distinct information-processing operations (Gehring, Gratton, Coles, & Donchin, 1992). Component amplitude is thought to reflect the extent to which the associated psychological operation has been engaged, and latency of the component's peak is thought to reflect the point in time by which the operation has been completed.

Cognitive psychologists have been at the forefront of ERP research, so components associated with processes of relevance in cognitive psychology (e.g., attention, memory) have received the most attention. Fortunately, many of these same psychological processes are of relevance in understanding social behavior. For instance, components sensitive to covert orienting processes (e.g., N100, P200, and N200) may be used to assess attention to social cues. Similarly, a number of components have been associated with executive control process (e.g., N200, N400, the negative slow wave), which should prove useful in understanding how social behavior is regulated, and components associated with attitudes and affective processes (e.g., the P300) can be used to understand attitudes and affective responses toward other people. In other cases, components uniquely associated with social processes have been identified (e.g., structural encoding of conspecifics has been associated with the N170).[2]

In addition to the identification of components that are sensitive to relevant psychological processes, ERPs provide several additional advantages. One is their excellent temporal resolution (on the order of milliseconds), which allows them to assess operations occurring very early in processing. ERPs are also useful in assessing both explicit and implicit processes. The latter is made possible because ERPs can be recorded without informing participants of what is being assessed or requiring them to accurately or honestly report their reactions (cf., Greenwald & Banaji, 1995). Moreover, some components are known to be insensitive to manipulations in overt response; even when participants purposely misreport their explicit answer, ERPs reflect the underlying true response (Crites, Cacioppo, Gardner, & Berntson, 1995; Farwell & Donchin, 1991; Rosenfeld, Angell, Johnson, & Qian, 1991). This has not been demonstrated for all components, but it can often be reasonably assumed for components occurring early enough in processing, where the influence of response manipulation strategies is less likely. Finally, although the spatial resolution of ERPs is lower than that with techniques such as fMRI and PET, the scalp distribution of observed activity can be used to obtain estimates of the neuroanatomical location of the source of activity.

With this brief background on ERPs in mind, we next review what ERPs have revealed about the process of social perception. Our focus is on understanding how perceivers are influenced by the social category membership of the individuals they perceive. We accordingly divide the remainder of the chapter into three main sections: perception of social category information (social categorization), the activation of biased evaluative responses (prejudice), and the activation of category-based beliefs (stereotyping) and their influence on behavior.

SOCIAL CATEGORIZATION

Many models of person perception assume that social category information is encoded automatically, especially for frequently used and socially emphasized dimensions such as race, gender, and age (Brewer, 1988; Fiske & Neuberg, 1990; Macrae & Bodenhausen, 2000). But because stereotypes and prejudice can be so easily activated by social category information, it can be difficult to examine encoding of social cues independent of the beliefs and feelings they activate. Consequently, the fact that a stereotype has been applied or a biased evaluation has been made is often used to infer that categorization has occurred, but the processes supporting the assignment of an individual into one or more social groups are not examined directly. This neglect has made it difficult to assess theoretically relevant issues such as the degree of malleability in the encoding of social category information. Fortunately, for the reasons reviewed in the previous section, ERPs are well suited to addressing these issues.

An initial assessment of the automaticity of social categorization was provided by Mouchetant-Rostaing and colleagues, who showed participants blocks of pictures containing either faces or body parts (hands and torsos; Mouchetant-Rostaing, Giard, Bentin, & Aguera, 2000). Within each block, the pictures were either from a single gender group (hands or body parts of women only) or from both males and females. Finally, task also varied across the blocks, with some blocks requiring an explicit gender categorization task (whether the hand or body part belongs to a man or woman) and other blocks requiring a nongender classification (presence of eyeglasses in the face blocks, presence of torsos in the body-parts blocks). This design allowed a comparison of the processing of faces and of other body parts. It also compared explicit gender categorization to a situation in which gender category was homogeneous (i.e., when all faces or body parts were from the same gender) and to a situation in which any gender categorization was implicit (when making the glasses or torsos categorization in the mixed-gender blocks).

Mouchetant-Rostaing et al. (2000) found that brain activity was sensitive to gender categorization from faces but not hands starting at around 145 milliseconds at central–frontal areas. This was shown as differences in a positive-going component in blocks including both male and female faces as compared with blocks containing only one gender. That is, ERPs differed when gender differentiation was possible as compared with when it was not. Moreover, this occurred during both explicit and implicit gender categorization; the effects occurred in the mixed-gender blocks both when participants made explicit gender judgments and when they were explicitly attending to eyeglasses. By contrast, viewing same-gender or mixed-gender pictures had no effect when viewing body parts. These effects have also been replicated for age categorization from faces (Mouchetant-Rostaing & Giard, 2003).

Ito and Urland (2003) found similarly early social category effects at central brain areas for gender categorization and also extended the effects to racial categorization. In addition, whereas Mouchetant-Rostaing and colleagues (Mouchetant-Rostaing et al., 2000; Mouchetant-Rostaing & Giard, 2003) examined responses as a function of whether gender or age differentiation was possible (i.e., whether there was variability in the faces along those dimensions), Ito and Urland (2003) examined responses as a function of the specific target group being viewed. This was done by showing participants pictures of black and white males and females, then examining whether components known to reflect visual attention differed as a function of target race and gender. Specifically, Ito and Urland (2003) quantified the amplitude of the N100, P200, and N200 components, which have been shown to vary as a function of covert orienting to task-relevant and/or salient features (Czigler & Geczy, 1996; Eimer, 1997; Kenemans, Kok, & Smulders, 1993; Naatanen & Gaillard, 1983; Wijers, Mulder, Okita, Mulder, & Scheffers, 1989).

Several processing differences to black versus white and male versus female faces were observed. Race first modulated responses in the N100 component. Peaking with a mean latency of around 120 milliseconds after face onset, N100s were larger to blacks than to whites. This continued into the next component, the P200 (mean peak latency around 180 ms), with larger P200s to blacks than to whites. Target gender did not begin to affect processing until the P200, when responses were larger to males than to females. The third temporally occurring component, the N200, peaked around 260 milliseconds. The direction of both race and gender effects was reversed in the N200, with larger N200s to whites and females than to blacks and males, respectively. Given the association of these early components with attentional selection, these results suggest initially greater attention to blacks and males but subsequently greater attention to whites and females. Moreover, all effects occurred regardless of whether participants were explicitly categorizing faces in terms of race or gender, indicating that these early attentional effects do not require an explicit focus on that social dimension.

In addition to components that are sensitive to attention, Ito and Urland (2003) also examined the P300 component. P300 amplitude typically increases as a function of the discrepancy between a given stimulus and preceding stimuli along salient dimensions. This has led to the conclusion that P300 amplitude reflects working memory updates that serve to maintain an accurate mental model of the external environment (Donchin, 1981). To allow an examination of how social category information affects working memory, stimuli were systematically varied so that responses could be analyzed, not only in terms of the race and gender of the target picture but also in terms of the race and gender of the face that preceded it.

Consistent with past P300 research (e.g., Donchin, 1981), P300s were larger when a target individual's social category membership differed from that of preceding individuals on the *task-relevant* dimension (as compared with matching the preceding faces). For instance, for participants categorizing faces in terms of *gender*, P300s were larger to a male face that was preceded by several female faces as compared with several male faces. Not surprisingly, then, working memory processes were sensitive to the social category dimension along which categorization was occurring explicitly. In addition, as expected based on the implicit attentional effects seen in the earlier components, implicit working memory effects were also seen. P300 amplitude increased when a target picture differed from the individuals pictured in preceding pictures along the *task-irrelevant* dimension. For instance, for participants categorizing faces in terms of *gender*, P300s were larger to a black face preceded by several white faces as compared with several black faces.

Several conclusions are suggested by these initial studies examining social categorization. First, they confirm assumptions that social category information is encoded automatically. Race, gender, and age all moderated ERP responses by 145 milliseconds at the latest, and this occurred even when participants were attending to another social category dimension or a category-irrelevant physical cue (presence of eyeglasses). There is also evidence that these effects reflect processes specialized for extracting physiognomic features from faces and not from body parts more generally. This is seen in the specificity of gender categorization effects in Mouchetant-Rostaing et al. (2000) to faces and not body parts. Race effects were also found to emerge faster than gender and age effects. Whereas gender and age moderated ERP responses between 145 and 180 milliseconds, race effects occurred as early as 120 milliseconds.[3] Of interest, this race effect was observed with both color and grayscale stimuli that were equated for luminance and contrast (Ito & Urland, 2003). This decreases the likelihood that the greater observed potency of race is due to a confound with low-level visual features (e.g., that black and white faces differ in some nonsocial feature such as luminance more so than do male and female faces). Finally, results from Ito and Urland (2003) suggest that what is considered a single social categorization outcome at the behavioral level—the determination of the groups to which individuals belong—actually consists of multiple, possibly dissociable processing stages. This is shown by the changing direction of attention throughout processing. Greater attention is initially directed to blacks and males (as seen in larger N100s to blacks and larger P200s to blacks and males), but greater attention is subsequently directed to whites and females (as seen in larger N200s).

Effects of Levels of Processing

Studies of social perception have often followed a trajectory of identifying a process that can occur automatically, then examining conditions under which automatic processing can be moderated (see Blair, 2002, for a review of this trajectory in the domain of stereotyping and prejudice). The same issues can be addressed here. The studies reviewed in the previous section demonstrate that race, gender, and age can be encoded even when attention is not explicitly directed at those dimensions, but this was examined under relatively limited conditions. In the Ito and Urland (2003) studies, participants were always explicitly attending to either race or gender, raising the possibility that attending to one social dimension sensitized participants to attend to all social category information. The studies of Mouchetant-Rostaing and colleagues did include conditions in which participants were attending to the presence and absence of eyeglasses, so these studies provide a stronger test of the automaticity of social category encoding. However, eyeglass detection still focuses perceivers on the physical characteristics of a face. Consequently, these initial studies do not provide the strongest tests of the degree to which automatic encoding of social category information can be moderated.

As a starting point to more systematically examining the issue of moderation, Ito and Urland (2005) had participants view faces of black and white males and females as they performed tasks previously shown to attenuate stereotype activation, which is presumed to depend on social categorization. ERPs were examined to determine whether these tasks can also affect the ways in which the individual's category membership is initially encoded. In one study, the effects of focusing attention at a level either more shallow or more deep than the social category were examined. The more shallow level of processing was encouraged by having some participants perform a visual-feature detection task, requiring detection of the presence or absence of a white dot on each face. Macrae, Bodenhausen, Milne, Thorn, and Castelli (1997) showed that this task, which focuses attention away from the social nature of the stimulus person altogether, is successful in attenuating stereotype activation. The deeper level of processing was encouraged by having the remaining participants perform an individuating task, judging whether each individual they saw would like various kinds of vegetables. This task was chosen because it, too, has been shown to decrease stereotype activation. It also attenuates differences in amygdala activation to racial out-group than in-group faces, which are thought to reflect greater negativity toward the out-group (Wheeler &

Fiske, 2005). As a partial replication, a second study examined the effects of another individuating task. Participants in this study made introversion–extraversion judgments about each individual. This task was chosen because it was assumed to be engaging and easy for participants to perform, thereby easily directing attention away from social category cues and encouraging more person-based than category-based encoding.

Even with these very different processing goals, ERP effects were very similar to those obtained by Ito and Urland (2003) when participants were explicitly attending to race and gender. P200s were larger to blacks and males, N200s were larger to whites and females, and the P300 was sensitive to the match between a target's race and gender and the race and gender of preceding faces. At the same time, although processing goals did not affect ERP responses that occurred after 180 milliseconds (i.e., after the P200), N100 differences were attenuated. Whereas N100s were larger to blacks when participants explicitly attended to race or gender (Ito & Urland, 2003), race did not affect the N100 when participants attended to dots or performed the vegetable preference task. It is not yet clear, though, whether this reflects a processing or a stimulus effect. This is because stimulus presentation was more complex in both tasks. The dot task required placing dots on some of the faces, and the vegetable task required presenting the name of the vegetable about which the preference judgment was to be made before each face. It is notable that stimulus presentation for participants performing the introversion–extraversion task was identical to the studies in Ito and Urland (2003) and that N100s here were larger to blacks than to whites. This suggests that increased visual complexity, more so than level of processing, may have been responsible for the delay of race effects from the N100 to the P200.

Categorization of Biracial Individuals

Much of the research on stereotyping and prejudice has examined the effects of racial categories, and most of that research has studied reactions to individuals who can be clearly identified as belonging to a single racial category. Although this increases experimental control, it does not fully address real-world social processing, which often occurs with people whose social category membership is less clear (e.g., people who are biracial). Even among targets who are consensually viewed as belonging to a single racial group, trait inferences are influenced by variations in facial features such as skin tone (Blair, Judd, Sadler, & Jenkins, 2002; Livingston & Brewer, 2002; Maddox & Gray, 2002). This suggests that studies of racial perception should address how the process operates across a range of facial cues.

ERPs have been used to examine this question in two studies that digitally morphed together photos of black and white males and Asian and white males. This process created realistic photos of faces possessing features intermediate to the two "parent" racial groups (Willadsen-Jensen & Ito, in press). In order to examine responses to faces that were maximally racially ambiguous, morphs that were a 50–50 blend of a black face and a white face or an Asian face and a white face were created. These were then pilot-tested to determine that they were subjectively perceived as falling in between the two racial extremes used to create them and not simply perceived as some other racial group. ERPs were then recorded as white participants viewed the racially ambiguous black–white morphs, as well as unambiguously black and white faces, in one study and the racially ambiguous Asian–white morphs, as well as unambiguously Asian and White faces, in another study. In both studies, participants made dichotomous race judgments about the faces, choosing between *black* and *white* in the first study and *Asian* and *white* in the second study.

P200s were larger to blacks and Asians than to whites, and N200s were larger to whites than to blacks and Asians. This both replicates past findings with black and white targets and extends the effects to another racial target group (e.g., Asians). Interestingly, P200 and N200 responses to the racially ambiguous faces were indistinguishable from responses to whites in both studies. It was not until the P300, peaking at around 500 milliseconds, that responses to whites and the racially ambiguous faces diverged. Participants' explicit categorization decisions also differentiated the racially ambiguous faces from both the faces of whites and blacks or Asians (e.g., black–white morphs were categorized as white 50% of the time), indicating subjective ambiguity in explicit categorization.

All participants in these studies were white, so the similarity of P200 and N200 responses to white and racially ambiguous faces appears to represent assimilation of racially ambiguous faces to the in-group. This is interesting in light of the P300 and explicit categorization data. At these later points in processing, the racially ambiguous faces were being perceived in a manner consistent with their objective status as 50–50 blends between two racial groups. P200 and N200 results are also interesting in light of research showing that if the perception of racially ambiguous individuals is shifted away from the objective midpoint of a racial continuum, the shift occurs in the direction of assimilation to the out-group (Blascovich, Wyer, Swart, & Kilber, 1997; Castano, Yzerbyt, & Bourguignon, 2002). Labeled the "in-group overexclusion effect," this is thought to derive from the motivation to protect one's own racial identity by showing caution over who is accepted as an in-group member (Leyens & Yzerbyt, 1992). The absence of assimilation to the out-group in the ERP data may indicate a lack of strong racial in-group identification among the participants or lack of strong consequences for erroneously categorizing someone as an in-group member. In addition, lack of assimilation to the out-group at earlier processing stages may again point to the apparent multifaceted nature of social categorization. Even though a racially ambiguous face may ultimately be identified as racially ambiguous (as in Willadsen-Jensen & Ito, in press) or assimilated to the out-group (when in-group identity is strong, as in Blascovich et al., 1997, and Castano et al., 2000), the overlap in physical features between the in-group and some biracial individuals may lead to initial processing of biracial individuals in a manner similar to the way in-group faces are processed. This also suggests that processing of social category information is initially more gross than fine-grained. The interval in which processing of racially ambiguous faces switches from being similar to that of in-group members (the N200) to being different from the processing of both in-group and out-group members (the P300) may signal a change to more finely tuned processing.

What ERPs Tell Us about Social Categorization

These initial studies examining how social category information is processed help us to better understand the larger process of person perception. Results consistently demonstrate the ease and speed with which race, gender, and age are processed. It is particularly striking that sensitivity to social cues occurs across a range of tasks: when perceivers are attending to (1) another social dimension (e.g., race effects occur even when perceivers explicitly attend to gender), (2) a nonsocial cue (searching for dots on faces), or (3) individual characteristics that foster person-based as opposed to category-based impressions. This invites the conclusion that early perceptual aspects of social categorization are relatively obligatory, driven more by the properties of the individual being perceived than by the goals and intentions of the perceiver.

What do these results imply about the mechanism by which processing manipulations are able to attenuate stereotyping and prejudice? And does this mean that social category information must always be encoded? These are essentially questions regarding the locus of attentional selection and may therefore profit from considering research on attentional selection. Consider the dot task. This task could be successfully accomplished if attentional selection is employed early in processing to differentiate between relevant and irrelevant cues, with full processing applied to only relevant information. This account, which corresponds to an early-selection view of attention, treats perceptual processing capabilities as limited and therefore requiring selection between to-be-attended-to and to-be-ignored items early in processing (e.g., Broadbent, 1958; Triesman, 1969). Alternatively, successful performance of a dot-detection task could be accomplished by automatically processing both dot and face cues, then employing attentional selection later in processing only when a behavioral response must be produced. This account, which corresponds to a late-selection view of attention, treats perceptual capacity as unlimited and therefore supporting full, parallel processing of all stimuli in the perceptual field (Deutch & Deutch, 1963; Norman, 1968).

The effects of processing manipulations at one point (stereotype activation or application) but not at an earlier point (encoding of social category information) suggests that these manipulations have later-attentional-selection effects. That is, the behavioral effects appear to be driven by attentional effects that occur after completion of rudimentary physical analyses that provide information about social category membership. An integration of early- and late-selection views also suggests manipulations that may be successful in diminishing attention to social category information. According to Lavie (1995), perceptual capacity is limited (consistent with early selection) but operates automatically and in parallel (consistent with late selection) until capacity is exceeded. The important feature of this model for our purposes is the finding that perceptual load is necessary to exhaust capacity and trigger early selection; in the absence of perceptual load, automatic attentional allocation cannot be inhibited. From this perspective, then, automatic encoding of social category information should be attenuated only when perceptual demands are high. This is consistent with the failure of the processing manipulations in Ito and Urland (2005) to eliminate social category effects; these tasks were primarily directed at changing the level of processing and probably did not exhaust processing capacity. However, in implementing the visual-feature detection task and the individuating task that involved judgments about vegetable preferences, the visual complexity of the stimuli was increased, increasing perceptual demands. Consistent with Lavie's perceptual load perspective, N100 race effects were attenuated in these conditions.

PREJUDICE

The studies reviewed to this point capitalize primarily on ERP components that are sensitive to attentional processes or on the P300's sensitivity to salient category distinctions. Additional processes are also obviously of interest in understanding social perception, including the way in which identification of an individual's social category membership influences the activation of category-based evaluative responses. Although the measurement of this process with ERPs has received less empirical attention, Ito, Thompson, and Cacioppo (2004) recently showed that category-based evaluative reactions can be assessed with the P300.

In the studies discussed to this point, P300 amplitude was used to measure the difference between the social category of a target individual and individuals that preceded him or her. More generally, P300 amplitude will vary as a function of the distance between a target and preceding stimuli along salient (e.g., task-relevant) dimensions. If participants are making evaluative decisions, P300 amplitude will reflect evaluative distance (Cacioppo, Crites, Berntson, & Coles, 1993; Cacioppo, Crites, Gardner, & Berntson, 1994). Capitalizing on this, Ito et al. (2004) showed participants pictures of black and white males that were embedded in a context of either positive items (e.g., cute puppies, appetizing foods) or negative items (e.g., dead animals, rotting food). After viewing each picture, participants were asked to register their explicit evaluative response, indicating how much they liked what was shown. Participants also completed a self-report measure of prejudice toward blacks (the Modern Racism Scale [MRS]; McConahay, Hardee, & Batts, 1981). All participants in these studies were white.

When faces were seen in a context of positive pictures, a bias score was computed to reflect the degree to which P300s were larger to black than to white faces. This represents the degree to which blacks were seen as more evaluatively discrepant with positive things than were whites. When faces were seen in a context of negative pictures, a bias score was computed to reflect the degree to which P300s were larger to white than to black faces. This represents the degree to which whites were seen as more evaluatively discrepant with negative things than were blacks. These bias scores were significantly related to MRS scores such that greater explicit reports of bias were associated with greater in-group bias in ERP responses. By contrast, P300 bias scores were unrelated to the liking judgments participants provided of each individual.

This correlation of the P300 to one type of evaluative response (the MRS) and not another (self-reported liking of the individual) may reflect a social judgability effect. With only physical information on which to base their judgments, participants may not have felt entitled to use category-based expectancies in their explicit liking judgments (Yzerbyt, Schadron, Leyens, & Rocher, 1994). By contrast, category-level evaluations are the very thing assessed by the MRS. The category level of measurement also makes the expression of any bias less personally directed toward an individual, which may diminish participants' concerns about expressing some dislike. The temporal information provided by ERPs helps us understand the timing of these processes. The P300 peaked at approximately 500 milliseconds after stimulus onset, and explicit liking judgments were made after picture offset, which occurred at 1000 milliseconds. This indicates that not long after the differential evaluative responses shown in the P300, processes that shape explicit responses such as social judgability were in operation.

STEREOTYPING AND BEHAVIOR

Consistent perhaps with the role cognitive psychologists have played in ERP research, processes related to stereotyping have received greater attention than those related to prejudice. Initial work in this area by Osterhout, Bersick, and McLaughlin (1997) showed that ERPs are sensitive to stereotype incongruency in much the same way that they are sensitive to definitional incongruency. They found that a sentence containing a stereotype violation ("The nurse prepared *himself* for the operation") elicited a large positive wave starting at about 500 milliseconds, similar to the response elicited by sentences containing definitional violations between a pronoun and its antecedent ("The wealthy queen built *himself* a castle"). Moreover, this effect occurred even when participants judged the stereotype-incongruent sentences to be semantically coherent and grammatically correct. This implies that even when perceivers view a gender-stereotypical behavior as possible (e.g., that men can be nurses), they still perceive it to be erroneous on some level. In a conceptually similar demonstration, Bartholow and colleagues created behavioral expectations by having participants read paragraphs that strongly conveyed a particular trait (Bartholow, Fabiani, Gratton, & Bettencourt, 2001). ERPs recorded during the reading of subsequent sentences that violated the trait expectation showed a larger positivity between 450 and 650 milliseconds than sentences that confirmed the trait expectation (see also Bartholow & Dickter, Chapter 17, this volume).

More recent studies have used ERPs to examine how stereotypes influence behavior by examining the process of behavior regulation, which is thought to involve a two-part system (Botvinick, Braver, Barch, Carter, & Cohen, 2001; Carter et al., 1998). The first component consists of the monitoring of conflict in activated representations during ongoing information processing. This is thought to occur continuously, often at a preconscious level, and to provide information for the second part of the system, which consists of a regulatory system that responds to detected conflict with the implementation of higher-order control. This model has been particularly applied to understanding how race affects decisions to shoot an individual.

Work in this area was originally stimulated by several high-profile shootings between 1999 and 2001 in which police officers shot and killed unarmed black men. In response to concerns that racial stereotypes influenced the officers' behavior, Correll, Park, Judd, and Wittenbrink (2002) created a simulation in which participants view pictures of black and white men who are holding either guns or innocuous objects such as wallets and cell phones. Participants make speeded decisions to "shoot" armed targets by pressing one button and "don't shoot" unarmed targets by pressing another. Behavioral results show a consistent bias against blacks relative to whites. Participants in Correll et al. (2002) were faster and more accurate in "shooting" armed blacks as compared with armed whites. By contrast, they were faster and more accurate in "not shooting" unarmed whites than unarmed blacks. This bias was also associated with perceptions of the cultural stereotype of blacks and whites. A stronger association of violence and aggression with blacks as compared with whites was associated with greater behavior bias. Similar findings have been obtained using slightly different procedures (Greenwald, Oakes, & Hoffman, 2003).

One of the main determinants of behavior in this task is obviously the identity of the object held by the targets. However, given the ease with which stereotypes can be activated following the mere perception of a group exemplar, representations related to racial stereotypes are also likely to be active when performing this task. According to the two-part model of behavior regulation, the degree of conflict in these activated representations is important to understanding racial bias. Given strong cultural and personal stereotypes about race, seeing a white individual may more strongly activate representations about safety, whereas seeing a black person may activate representations more evocative of threat and danger. If so, greater conflict would be generated when a white than when a black target is seen holding a gun. Thus, although conflict monitoring may be occurring when making decisions regarding whom to shoot, it might not be occurring equally for black and white targets.

Investigation of these issues is aided by the association of several anteriorly distributed, negative-going ERP components with the two systems thought to be involved in behavior regulation. Detection of conflict during successful behavior regulation (e.g., when correct behavior is implemented) has been associated with an N200 (Nieuwenhuis, Yeung, Van Den Wildenberg, & Ridderinkhof, 2003). Neuroimaging research implicates the anterior cingulate cortex (ACC) and areas of prefrontal cortex in conflict monitoring and cognitive control, respectively (e.g., Botvinick et al., 2001; Carter et al.,1998; MacDonald, Cohen, Stenger, & Carter, 2000). Consistent with this, source modeling of the N200 implicates the ACC and other areas of the prefontal cortex (Liotti, Woldorff, Perez, & Mayberg, 2000; Nieuwenhuis et al., 2003).

To examine whether behavior regulation processes differentiate between black and white targets in the decision to shoot, Correll, Urland, and Ito (2006) recorded ERPs as participants played the shooter video game developed by Correll et al. (2002). Consistent with past behavioral studies, participants displayed a biased pattern of response latencies; they were faster to "shoot" armed blacks than whites, but faster to "not shoot" unarmed whites than blacks.

Of greater interest, ERP responses showed differences in conflict monitoring as a function of target race. Specifically, the N200, associated with conflict monitoring during successful behavior regulation, was larger to white than to black targets. Because of converging factors such as the general bias toward detecting the presence rather than the absence of a stimulus (e.g., Treisman & Gelade, 1980), task instructions, and the explicit reward structure of the game,[4] shooting tends to be the dominant response in the Correll et al. (2002) video game. Participants are, in fact, typically faster and more accurate in making shoot than not-shoot decisions. Coupled with prevailing stereotypes more strongly linking blacks than whites with violence, greater conflict monitoring for white than black targets suggests the detection of greater conflict between White targets and the tendency to make a shoot response. When the targets are armed, this should result in facilitation of the "shoot" response for blacks relative to whites. By contrast, when the targets are unarmed, this should facilitate the "don't shoot" response for whites relative to blacks.

In models of behavior regulation, conflict monitoring is integral to successful behavior. Thus, if the N200 effects observed by Correll et al. (2006) reflect differential detection of conflict for white and black targets, this should predict subsequent behavior. Indeed, the degree to which N200s to whites exceeded those to blacks predicted racial bias in response latencies. Moreover, although racial stereotypes were also correlated with racial bias in response latencies, the N200 conflict monitoring difference mediated this relation. That is, participants who more strongly associated blacks than whites with violence were more biased in their behavior, and this was accounted for by stronger neural signals associated with conflict monitoring to whites than to blacks.

Further evidence of differential behavior regulation to whites and blacks was obtained by Ito, Correll, and Urland (2005). Whereas Correll et al. (2006) examined behavior regulation processes when participants made correct decisions to shoot armed targets and not shoot unarmed ones, Ito et al. (2005) examined conflict monitoring when behavior regulation fails—that is, when behavior is inaccurate. This was done by quantifying the error-related negativity (ERN), a component sensitive to conflict monitoring following erroneous behavioral choices, when participants shot unarmed targets or failed to shoot armed ones. The ERN is a response-locked component observed 50–100 milliseconds after a response characterized by high conflict, such as when a prepotent response is inconsistent with an accurate response (Falkenstein, Hohnsbein, & Hoormann, 1995; Falkenstein, Hoormann, & Hohnsbein, 1999; Gehring, Coles, Meyer, & Donchin, 1995; Gehring, Goss, Coles, Meyer, & Donchin, 1993; Scheffers & Coles, 2000). Consistent with an ACC localization for conflict monitoring processing, dipole modeling has located the source of the ERN to the medial temporal area (Dehaene, Posner, & Tucker, 1994).

Behavioral responses replicated Correll et al. (2002). For unarmed targets, more errors were made to black than to white targets. That is, unarmed black men were more likely to be erroneously "shot" than were unarmed white men. At the neural level, erroneous "shoot" and "don't shoot" responses were associated with increased conflict, as reflected in larger ERNs on erroneous than correct trials. However, race also moderated the effect. Specifically, when participants made an erroneous "don't shoot" response to *armed* targets, ERNs were larger to armed blacks than to whites. By contrast, ERNs were equally large following erroneous shooting of *unarmed* blacks and whites.

The specific pattern of results differs in these last two studies, but they show conceptually similar sensitivity to stereotype content. When considering correct responses, the bias to shoot conflicts most with the absence of violence and aggression in the stereotype about whites. Conflict monitoring that is integral to subsequent accurate behavior is therefore greatest in this condition. When considering reactions following incorrect responses, making a "don't shoot" response is most incongruent with the presence of violence and aggression in the stereotype about blacks. Conflict monitoring sensitive to the congruency between stimulus-activated representations and subsequent behavior is therefore greater in this condition than when a comparable error is made about an armed white.

Differences in conflict monitoring as a function of race have also been observed by Amodio et al. (2004). These researchers also used a task designed to assess whether race biases weapon detection, this time with a sequential priming paradigm (Payne, 2001). In this task, brief presentations of black or white faces precede pictures of objects that participants had to classify as either guns or tools. Participants were faster and more accurate in identifying guns when primed with a black face but faster and more accurate in identifying tools when primed with a white face. ERN responses suggested greater sensitivity in conflict monitoring to race-biased response tendencies. Specifically, when tools were incorrectly classified as guns, ERNs were larger on trials primed with black than with white faces (see also Amodio, Devine, & Harmon-Jones, Chapter 16, this volume).

These last two studies focusing on conflict detection following incorrect responses show similar elevations in conflict detection in a racially biased condition (i.e., when shooting unarmed blacks or when misclassifying a tool as a gun following a black prime). However, results differ in the conditions that can be viewed as the omission of a racially biased response: failing to shoot armed blacks and misclassifying guns as tools following a black prime. Conflict detection was elevated in the former but not the latter case. This difference likely reflects the nature of the tasks. The effects of racial stereotypes may be broader in the shoot–don't shoot task developed by Correll et al. (2002), influencing responses to all black targets, whereas their effects may be more focused in the sequential priming task developed by Payne (2001). In addition, sensitivity to black–tool errors in Amodio et al. (2004) was heightened by telling participants that responding "gun" to a tool primed by a black face would reflect racial bias. It is interesting to note that, despite possible differences in the psychological concerns they activate, the two tasks produce conceptually similar behavioral outcomes. Both tasks show that black men facilitate the detection of weapons, but these similar outcomes may be achieved through different mechanisms.

CONCLUSION

Although the area of social neuroscience is relatively new, the chapters in this volume attest to the many domains in which it has been applied. One of the greatest promises of social neuroscience is the advancement of social-psychological theorizing through the integration of tools and ideas from other levels of analysis. To be maximally beneficial, then, social neuroscience should go beyond the mere adoption of neuroscience methods by social psychologists to tangible theoretical advancement in social-psychological knowledge. Toward this end, we have tried in this chapter to focus on insights that ERP research provides in understanding social perception.

When applied to the issue of social categorization, social neuroscience research confirms long-standing assumptions that information about an individual's race, gender, and age are processed automatically. This research also extends previous theoretical models in two important ways. First, although all possible moderating conditions have not been investigated, all findings so far point to relatively obligatory encoding of social category information. Attending to another social category, other features of the face (e.g., eyeglasses), personality characteristics, or nonsocial physical features (e.g., a dot on the photo) can sometimes delay effects, but in no case was attention to social category information eliminated (Ito & Urland, 2003, 2005; Mouchetant-Rostaing et al., 2000; Mouchetant-Rostaing & Giard, 2003). This helps us to better understand the locus of moderating effects in person perception. For the types of tasks investigated so far (tasks that manipulate processing goals), any beneficial effects on stereotype and prejudice activation seem to occur after encoding of the social category information on at least some basic level.

Second, the studies on social categorization suggest that the encoding of social category information is a multistage process. Initial stages appear more gross than fine-grained, as shown, for instance, in the apparent assimilation of racially ambiguous faces to the in-group during early processing, even though the faces are differentiated from the in-group later in processing (e.g., as seen in the P300 and in explicit category judgments; Willadsen-Jensen & Ito, 2005). The greater initial attention to racial out-group members (Ito & Urland, 2003, 2005) may also reflect a more coarse level of analysis that scans the environment for more threatening and/or more novel stimuli.

ERP studies examining prejudice have been less numerous, but those studies that have been done can be related to the issue of how implicit and explicit processes are related. Although lack of congruency on factors such as level of measurement (e.g., processing at the level of exemplar vs. category; Olson & Fazio, 2003) and whether more affective or cognitive processes are assessed (Wittenbrink, Judd, & Park, 2001) can attenuate relations between implicit and explicit measures, Ito et al. (2004) found a correlation between measures that differed in both factors. That is, ERP responses that reflected evaluative responses to individuals were correlated with more cognitive responses to the entire group. It is reasonable that measurement factors should moderate relations among different types of measures, but at the same time, there should be overlap among the different representations. The relatively unconstrained processing goal employed by Ito et al. (2004) may have made this overlap easier to detect. This suggests that previously identified measurement dimensions used to explain relations among implicit prejudice measures and between implicit and explicit measures may be expanded to include a consideration of the breadth of processing of the category-related information that is allowed.

ERP research that examines how stereotypes affect behavior highlights the benefit of applying behavior regulation models to understanding social perception. Consideration of behavior regulation processes in social perception is not new (e.g., Dunton & Fazio, 1997; Monteith, 1993; Plant & Devine, 1998), but models informed by neuroscience research detail another level of analysis and provide methods for measuring key mechanisms. Moreover, prior research has tended to emphasize the regulation of behavior toward stigmatized groups. The finding that greater conflict monitoring to whites than to blacks precedes correct responses in a shoot–don't shoot video simulation (Correll et al., 2006) demonstrates the importance of also examining behavior regulation to members of nonstigmatized groups. Overall, we think the research reviewed here and in this volume illustrates the exciting promise of social neuroscience and the nature of advancement possible when neuroscientific and social-psychological perspectives are integrated.

NOTES

1. Polarity of the signal is determined by the polarity of the electrical potential at that location at that point in time relative to the reference electrode(s).
2. Although it is relevant to understanding the broader process of social perception, N170 research is not reviewed in this chapter because it is not clear whether social category information influences initial face encoding (for a review, see Ito & Urland, 2005).
3. The difference in latency for gender effects in Mouchetant-Rostaing et al. (2000) and Mouchetant-Rostaing and Giard (2003), 145 milliseconds, as compared with Ito and Urland (2003), 120 milliseconds, could be due to the slightly different psychological processes being assessed. Mouchetant-Rostaing and colleagues assessed sensitivity to the heterogeneity in face gender, whereas Ito and Urland assessed differential attention to males versus females.
4. To motivate performance, a cumulative score based on performance is displayed after every trial. Correct detection of an unarmed target earns 5 points, correct detection of an armed target earns 10 points, incorrect detection of an unarmed target costs 20 points, and incorrect detection of an armed target costs 40 points.

REFERENCES

Amodio, D. M., Harmon-Jones, E., Devine, P. G., Curtin, J. J., Hartley, S. L., & Covert, A. E., (2004). Neural signals for the detection of unintentional race bias. *Psychological Science, 15,* 88–93.

Bartholow, B. D., Fabiana, M., Gratton, G., & Bettencourt, B. A. (2001). A psychophysiological examination of cognitive processing of and affective responses to social expectancy violations. *Psychological Science, 12,* 197–204.

Blair, I. V. (2002). The malleability of automatic stereotypes and prejudice. *Personality and Social Psychology Review, 6,* 242–261.

Blair, I. V., Judd, C. M., Sadler, M. S., & Jenkins, C. (2002). The role of Afrocentric features in person perception: Judging by features and categories. *Journal of Personality and Social Psychology, 83,* 5–25.

Blascovich, J., Wyer, N. A., Swart, L. A., & Kibler, J. L. (1997). Racism and racial categorization. *Journal of Personality and Social Psychology, 72,* 1364–1372.

Botvinick, M. M., Braver, T. S., Barch, D. M., Carter, C. S., & Cohen, J. D. (2001). Conflict monitoring and cognitive control. *Psychological Review, 108,* 624–652.

Brewer, M. C. (1988). A dual process model of impression formation. In R. Wyer & T. Scrull (Eds.), *Advances in social cognition* (Vol. 1, pp. 1–36). Hillsdale, NJ: Erlbaum.

Broadbent, D. E. (1958). *Perception and communication.* London: Oxford University Press.

Cacioppo, J. T., Crites, S. L., Jr., Berntson, G. G., & Coles, M. G. H. (1993). If attitudes affect how stimuli are processed, should they not affect the event-related brain potential? *Psychological Science, 4,* 108–112.

Cacioppo, J. T., Crites, S. L., Jr., Gardner, W. L., & Berntson, G. G. (1994). Bioelectrical echoes from evaluative categorizations: I. A late positive brain potential that varies as a function of trait negativity and extremity. *Journal of Personality and Social Psychology, 67,* 115–125.

Carter, C. S., Braver, T. S., Barch, D. M., Botvinick, M. M., Noll, D., & Cohen, J. D. (1998). Anterior cingulate cortex, error detection, and the online monitoring of performance. *Science, 280,* 747–749.

Castano, E., Yzerbyt, V., & Bourguignon, D. (2002). Who may enter? The impact of in-group identification on in-group/out-group categorization. *Journal of Experimental Social Psychology, 38,* 315–322.

Correll, J., Park, B., Judd, C. M., & Wittenbrink, B. (2002). The police officer's dilemma: Using ethnicity to disambiguate potentially threatening individuals. *Journal of Personality and Social Psychology, 83,* 1314–1329.

Correll, J., Urland, G. R., & Ito, T. A. (2006). Event-related potentials and the decision to shoot: The role of threat perception and cognitive control. *Journal of Experimental Social Psychology, 42,* 120–128.

Crites, S. L., Jr., Cacioppo, J. T., Gardner, W. L., & Berntson, G. G. (1995). Bioelectrical echoes from evaluative categorizations: II. A late positive brain potential that varies as a function of attitude registration rather than attitude report. *Journal of Personality and Social Psychology, 68,* 997–1013.

Czigler, I., & Geczy, I. (1996). Event-related potential correlates of color selection and lexical decision: Hierarchical processing or late selection? *International Journal of Psychophysiology, 22,* 67–84.

Dehaene, S., Posner, M. I., & Tucker, D. M. (1994). Localization of a neural system for error detection and compensation. *Psychological Science, 5,* 303–305.

Deutch, J. A., & Deutch, D. (1963). Attention: Some theoretical considerations. *Psychological Review, 70,* 80–90.

Donchin, E. (1981). Surprise! . . . Surprise? *Psychophysiology, 18,* 493–513.

Dunton, B. C., & Fazio, R. H. (1997). An individual difference measure of motivation to control prejudiced reactions. *Personality and Social Psychology Bulletin, 23,* 316–326.

Eimer, M. (1997). An event-related potential (ERP) study of transient and sustained visual attention to color and form. *Biological Psychology, 44,* 143–160.

Fabiani, M., Gratton, G., & Coles, M. G. H. (2000). Event-related brain potentials. In J. T. Cacioppo, L. G. Tassinary, & G. G Berntson (Eds.), *Handbook of psychophysiology* (2nd ed., pp. 53–84). Cambridge, UK: Cambridge University Press.

Falkenstein, M., Hohnsbein, J., & Hoormann, J. (1995). Event-related potential correlates of errors in reaction tasks. *Perspectives of Event-Related Potentials Research* (EEG Suppl. 44), 287–296.

Falkenstein, M., Hoormann, J., & Hohnsbein, J. (1999). ERP components in Go/Nogo tasks and their relation to inhibition. *Acta Psychologica, 101,* 267–291.

Farwell, L. A., & Donchin, E. (1991). The truth will out: Interrogative polygraphy ("lie detection") with event-related brain potentials. *Psychophysiology, 28,* 531–547.

Fiske, S. T., & Neuberg, S. L. (1990). A continuum of impression formation, from category-based to individuating processes: Influences of information and motivation on attention and interpretation. *Advances in Experimental Social Psychology, 23,* 1–73.

Gehring, W. J., Coles, M. G. H., Meyer, D. E., & Donchin, E. (1995). A brain potential manifestation of error-related processing. *Perspectives of Event-Related Potentials Research* (EEG Suppl. 44), 261–272.

Gehring, W. J., Goss, B., Coles, M. G. H., Meyer, D. E., & Donchin, E. (1993). A neural system for error detection and compensation. *Psychological Science, 4,* 385–390.

Gehring, W. J., Gratton, G., Coles, M. G. H., & Donchin, E. (1992). Probability effects on stimulus evaluation and response processes. *Journal of Experimental Psychology: Human Perception and Performance, 18,* 198–216.

Greenwald, A. G., & Banaji, M. R. (1995). Implicit social cognition: Attitudes, self-esteem, and stereotypes. *Psychological Review, 102,* 4–27.

Greenwald, A. G., Oakes, M. A., & Hoffman, H. G. (2003). Targets of discrimination: Effects of race on responses to weapons holders. *Journal of Experimental Psychology, 39,* 399–405.

Ito, T. A., Correll, J., & Urland, G. R. (2005). [Detection of conflict between stereotypes and behavior: The role of behavior regulation in racial bias]. Unpublished raw data.

Ito, T. A., Thompson, E., & Cacioppo, J. T. (2004). Tracking the time course of social perception: The effects of racial cues on event-related brain potentials. *Personality and Social Psychology Bulletin, 30,* 1267–1280.

Ito, T. A., & Urland, G. R. (2003). Race and gender on the brain: Electrocortical measures of attention to race and gender of multiply categorizable individuals. *Journal of Personality and Social Psychology, 85,* 616–626.

Ito, T. A., & Urland, G. R. (2005). The influence of processing objectives on the perception of faces: An ERP study of race and gender perception. *Cognitive, Affective, and Behavioral Neuroscience, 5,* 21–36.

Kenemans, J. L., Kok, A., & Smulders, F. T. Y. (1993). Event-related potentials to conjunctions of spatial frequency and orientation as a function of stimulus parameters and response requirements. *Electroencephalography and Clinical Neurophysiology, 88,* 51–63.

Lavie, N. (1995). Perceptual load as a necessary condition for selection attention. *Journal of Experimental Psychology, Human Perception and Performance, 21,* 451–468.

Leyens, J.-P., & Yzerbyt, V.Y. (1992). The ingroup overexclusion effect: Impact of valence and confirmation on stereotypical information search. *European Journal of Social Psychology, 22,* 549–569.

Liotti, M., Woldorff, M. G., Perez, R., & Mayberg, H. S. (2000). An ERP study of the temporal course of Stroop color–word interference effect. *Neuropsychologia, 38,* 701–711.

Livingston, R. W., & Brewer, M. B. (2002). What are we really priming? Cue-based versus category-based processing of facial stimuli. *Journal of Personality and Social Psychology, 82,* 5–18.

MacDonald, A. W., III, Cohen, J. D., Stenger, V. A., & Carter, C. S. (2000). Dissociating the role of the dorsolateral prefrontal and anterior cingulate cortex in cognitive control. *Science, 288,* 1835–1838.

Macrae, C. N., & Bodenhausen, G. V. (2000). Social cognition: Thinking categorically about others. *Annual Review of Psychology, 51,* 93–120.

Macrae, C. N., Bodenhausen, G. V., Milne, A. B., Thorn, T. M. J., & Castelli, L. (1997). On the activation of social stereotypes: The moderating role of processing objectives. *Journal of Experimental Social Psychology, 33,* 471–489.

Maddox, K. B., & Gray, S. A. (2002). Cognitive representations of Black Americans: Reexploring the role of skin tone. *Personality and Social Psychology Bulletin, 28,* 250–259.

McConahay, J. B., Hardee, B. B., & Batts, V. (1981). Has racism declined in America? It depends on who is asking and what is asked. *Journal of Conflict Resolution, 25,* 563–579.

Monteith, M. J. (1993). Self-regulation of prejudiced responses: Implications for progress in prejudice-reduction efforts. *Journal of Personality and Social Psychology, 65,* 469–485.

Mouchetant-Rostaing, Y., & Giard, M. H. (2003). Electrophysiological correlates of age and gender perception on human faces. *Journal of Cognitive Neuroscience, 15,* 900–910.

Mouchetant-Rostaing, Y., Giard, M. H., Bentin, S., & Aguera, P. E. (2000). Neurophysiological correlates of face gender processing in humans. *European Journal of Neuroscience, 12,* 303–310.

Naatanen, R., & Gaillard, A. W. K. (1983). The orientating reflex and the N2 deflection of the event-related potential (ERP). In A. W. K. Gaillard & W. Ritter (Eds.), *Tutorials in ERP research: Endogenous components* (pp. 119–141). New York: North-Holland.

Nieuwenhuis, S., Yeung, N., Van Den Wildenberg, W., & Ridderinkhof, K.R. (2003). Electrophysiological correlates of anterior cingulate function in a go/no-go task: Effects of response conflict and trial type frequency. *Cognitive, Affective and Behavioral Neuroscience, 3,* 17–26.

Norman, D. A. (1968). Toward a theory of memory and attention. *Psychological Review, 75,* 522–536.

Olson, M. A., & Fazio, R. H. (2003). Relations between implicit measures of prejudice: What are we measuring? *Psychological Science, 14,* 636–639.

Osterhout, L., Bersick, M., & McLaughlin, J. (1997). Brain potentials reflect violations of gender stereotypes. *Memory and Cognition, 25,* 273–285.

Payne, B. K. (2001). Prejudice and perception: The role of automatic and controlled processes in misperceiving a weapon. *Journal of Personality and Social Psychology, 81,* 181–192.

Plant, E. A., & Devine, P. G. (1998). Internal and external motivation to respond without prejudice. *Journal of Personality and Social Psychology, 75*, 811–832.

Rosenfeld, J. P., Angell, A., Johnson, M., & Qian, J. (1991). An ERP-based, control-question lie detector analog: Algorithms for discrimination effects within individuals' average waveforms. *Psychophysiology, 28,* 319–335.

Scheffers, M. K., & Coles, M. G. H. (2000). Performance monitoring in a confusing world: Error-related brain activity, judgments of response accuracy, and types of errors. *Journal of Experimental Psychology: Human Perception and Performance, 26,* 141–151.

Treisman, A. M. (1969). Strategies and models of selective attention. *Psychological Review, 76,* 282–299.

Treisman, A. M., & Gelade, G. (1980). A feature-integration theory of attention. *Cognitive Psychology, 12,* 97–136.

Wheeler, M. E., & Fiske, S. T. (2005). Controlling racial prejudice: Social cognitive goals affect amygdala and stereotype activation. *Psychological Science, 16,* 56–63.

Wijers, A., Mulder, G., Okita, T., Mulder, L. J. M., & Scheffers, M. (1989). Attention to color: An analysis of selection, controlled search, and motor activation, using event-related potentials. *Psychophysiology, 26,* 89–109.

Willadsen-Jensen, E. C., & Ito, T. A. (in press). Ambiguity and the time course of racial perception. *Cognition and Emotion.*

Wittenbrink, B., Judd, C. M., & Park, B. (2001). Spontaneous prejudice in context: Variability in automatically activated attitudes. *Journal of Personality and Social Psychology, 81,* 815–827.

Yzerbyt, V. Y., Schadron, G., Leyens, J. P., & Rocher, S. (1994). Social judgeability: The impact of meta-informational cues on the use of stereotypes. *Journal of Personality and Social Psychology, 66,* 48–55.

VI

INTERPERSONAL RELATIONSHIPS

19

Neuropeptides and the Protective Effects of Social Bonds

C. Sue Carter

During the 20th century, biomedical research focused on mechanisms underlying illness. However, the major challenge for science in the 21st century is developing an understanding of the processes and mechanisms responsible for health. It is increasingly clear that health is not simply the absence of illness but that it includes active processes, maintained in part by social interactions and social bonds. The goal of this chapter is to review our current understanding of the biological basis of social bonds. This knowledge may, in turn, suggest mechanisms through which social experiences can be both protective and restorative in the face of the challenges of life.

IDENTIFYING THE QUESTION

The benefits of social support and social bonds have been described in epidemiological studies. Perceived social support is often negatively correlated with various illnesses, ranging from mental illness to heart disease and cancer (Uchino, Cacioppo, & Kiecolt-Glaser, 1996; Knox & Uvnas-Moberg, 1998; Singer & Ryff, 2001). However, correlative studies do not address the mechanisms through which social behaviors and social experience help to maintain good health.

Social support is difficult to define operationally, especially in a manner that is meaningful for studies of the nervous system. In addition, neurobiology is most often studied in animals that do not form selective social bonds. For these reasons, the analysis of neural and endocrine factors that underlie social bonding has focused on two types of animal models: mother–infant interactions (most notably in sheep) and adult–adult social bonds (found in socially monogamous or cooperatively breeding mammals such as prairie voles; Carter, DeVries, & Getz, 1995). Studies of these models have implicated shared neuroendocrine processes in social behavior and in the buffering of reactivity to challenges. The physiological bases of social support and social bonds are most readily understood in the context of their adaptive role in human natural history and evolution. This chapter uses examples, primarily drawn from voles, to illustrate the role of social experience and the neurobiological factors that influence social bonding in the regulation of good health.

NATURAL HISTORY AND THE ADAPTIVE FUNCTIONS OF SOCIAL BONDS

Why Are Social Bonds Important and When Do They Form?

Most mammals—and especially primates—cannot live alone. Among primates, humans are particularly dependent on selective social interactions and have been described as *cooperative breeders* (Hrdy, 1999). For example, in human societies, individuals other than or in addition to the biological parents may share in the care of young. Humans elicit social interactions as early as the first day of postnatal life and normally continue to seek social engagement throughout their lives (Porges, 2003a, 2003b). Humans form many different social relationships, with both costs and benefits to social interactions, and although some relationships may be negative and potentially detrimental to health, others are positive and generally beneficial (Kiecolt-Glaser, Preacher, MacCallum, Malarkey, & Glaser, 2003). Evidence for the importance of social bonds is so strong that, in humans, the inability to form social bonds is usually considered indicative of psychopathology.

Social bonds are capable of promoting both survival and reproduction. Clues to the causes and consequences of social bonds are interwoven with an understanding of reproduction and reproductive hormones. Most mammalian species experience internal fertilization, pregnancy, and live birth. This is important to consider because the physiological substrates for human social bonds are shared with those for sexual behavior, birth, and lactation. Social bonds also may be of particular relevance to young mammals because there is an inherent nutritional and social interdependence between the mammalian mother and infant. Human infants were historically reliant on human milk and thus on physical contact with their biological mothers or a lactating caretaker. Mechanisms for maintaining proximity between a mother and an infant could promote genetic fitness of the parent and the immediate survival of the offspring. In addition, there are survival and fitness benefits to social bonds, and endocrine adaptations to an ever-changing and stressful environment also play a role in social bonding.

What Are Social Bonds?

Social bonds are hypothetical constructs: No one has ever seen a social bond, although evidence for their existence is strong. Social bonds are commonly defined by behavioral processes, measured by selective social behaviors, or indexed by self-report or autonomic responses. The tendency to prefer a partner, to seek contact with the partner, and in some cases to show emotional distress in the absence of the preferred partner are all considered indicative of a social bond. The most common measures of social bonding rely on approach and contact behaviors. Humans and other animals are discriminating in their willingness to show social contact. For example, in socially monogamous species such as prairie voles, there is a strong tendency for adult animals to select one partner (typically one made familiar by prior association or mating) and to ignore or reject other partners. In young mammals that are mobile and thus capable of expressing a preference, the preferred partner may be the mother or a familiar caretaker.

The presence of social bonds is most dramatically documented by the intense emotional reactions that follow separation from or the loss of an attachment figure. However, most animals, including many primate species, do not show selective reactions to the presence or absence of a partner. Therefore, animal models for infant separation responses generally have been limited to species such as guinea pigs or sheep that are capable of expressing distress or seeking behaviors in the absence of the mother (Panksepp, Nelson, & Bekkedal, 1997; Carter & Keverne, 2002).

What Conditions Lead to the Formation of Social Bonds?

The capacity to form a social bond is species-specific and varies as a function of the physiological state and social experience of the individual. However, clues to the neurobiology of social behavior have come from the fact that social bonding is sometimes associated with reproduction. For example, the birth process is stressful in most mammals, and females may form new social bonds with infants present immediately following birth. (Under natural conditions, the infant present in the immediate postpartum period would be the female's own offspring.)

The same hormones that are released around the time of birth are also present at other times and may be capable of influencing the formation of social bonds between adults. Sexual behavior can facilitate social bonding, although mating is not essential for pair bonding. Nonsexual cohabitation or simply living with another individual is also associated with a preference for the familiar partner. However, the tendency to select a familiar partner may be dramatically facilitated by the presence of certain hormones, including hormones that are released during sexual behavior and interactions between adults and infants (Williams et al., 1994; as cited in Carter & Keverne, 2002). Studies conducted primarily over the past decade have implicated small peptide hormones, synthesized in the hypothalamus (i.e., neuropeptides), in social bonding.

A recurrent relationship also exists between stressful events and the formation of social bonds, possibly because under adverse conditions, social relationships may be critical to survival. For example, experiments in male prairie voles have shown that a brief stressor (such as a 3-minute swim) or treatment with stress hormones facilitates the tendency of males to form pair bonds with females (DeVries, DeVries, Taymans, & Carter, 1996; DeVries, Guptaa, Cardillo, Cho, & Carter, 2002). In females, similar stress can actually inhibit the formation of a social bond with a male (DeVries, DeVries, Taymans, & Carter, 1995). However, female prairie voles that have been exposed to a stressful experience are not incapable of forming new social bonds. Following exposure to a stressor, females do develop a preference for other females. This sex difference in the preferred social partner (opposite- vs. same-sex) following a stressful experience illustrates the importance of context in understanding the factors that may regulate social bonding. These studies also highlight an important difference in the way that male and females manage psychological and physical challenges (Carter et al., 1995; Carter & Keverne, 2002).

NEUROENDOCRINOLOGY AND SOCIAL BEHAVIOR

Both selective and nonselective social behaviors are based on physiological processes that are regulated and experienced by the nervous system (Carter & Keverne, 2002). Many of the chemicals that are associated with social behavior are synthesized in the brain and act on the nervous system. As described previously, hormonal processes associated with birth, lactation, sexual behavior, and stress have all been implicated in pair bond formation. In addition, neurotransmitter systems, including dopamine and endogenous opioids, both of which are implicated in "reward," may also play a role in social bonding.

Among the other hormones that have been implicated in social bonding (and pair bonding in particular) are oxytocin, vasopressin, corticotropin-releasing factor (CRF), and adrenal hormones, including corticosterone (Carter & Keverne, 2002). Gonadal steroids, including estrogen and testosterone, also can play a role in social behavior, although it is possible that many of the effects of steroids are mediated indirectly through actions on other systems, including peptide hormones.

The endocrine and social histories of an individual can alter the capacity to form pair bonds. The same hormones that have been implicated in the expression of social behaviors are also capable of playing a role in the development of the nervous system, producing an adaptive "programming" of the nervous system (Carter, 2003; Seckl, 2004; Weaver et al., 2004). Powerful ontogenetic factors, including exposure to hormones from both endogenous and exogenous sources, can contribute to the later expression of species, gender, and individual differences in social behaviors. Some specific examples of the capacity of early or especially powerful experiences to produce long-lasting changes in behavior or physiology are described next.

OXYTOCIN

One mammalian neuropeptide, oxytocin, has a central role in reproduction, including sexual behavior, birth, and lactation, and also modulates the hypothalamic–pituitary–adrenal (HPA) axis. These properties make oxytocin an excellent candidate for the integration of emotional states and feelings with the physiological processes through which social support bestows its benefits (Carter, 1998).

Oxytocin is made primarily in the brain in two hypothalamic nuclei: the supraoptic (SON) and paraventricular (PVN) nuclei. As measured by gene expression, oxytocin is the most abundant peptide in the hypothalamus (Gautvik et al., 1996). Oxytocin is released by social stimuli, especially touch (Uvnas-Moberg, 1998), and during positive social interactions may permit the expression of vulnerable behaviors. Treatment with exogenous oxytocin facilitates positive social behaviors, including social engagement, social recognition, and selective partner preferences and parental behavior (Pedersen & Bocca, 2002; Carter, 1998; Carter & Keverne, 2002; Winslow & Insel, 2004). Important to understanding the benefits of social support is the fact that oxytocin is capable of buffering reactivity to stressful experiences. For example, oxytocin has anxiolytic and analgesic properties (Uvnas-Moberg, 1998). Oxytocin also reduces the release of stress hormones and the reactivity of the autonomic nervous system, including reductions in heart rate and blood pressure (Porges, 2003a, 2003b; Neumann, 2001).

Oxytocin acts on receptors throughout the body, including those found in abundance in the hypothalamus and areas of the nervous system that influence social behaviors and emotion. The integrative effects of oxytocin may be based in part on the fact that this hormone has only one known type of receptor (Gimpl & Fahrenholz, 2001). (Other neurochemicals, such as the related neuropeptide vasopressin, typically have several receptor subtypes, allowing a single molecule to have diverse and varied functions.) Oxytocin receptor binding also is correlated with positive social behaviors throughout life (Parker, Kinney, Phillips, & Lee, 2001;

Francis, Young, Meaneny, & Insel, 2002). The specific neural properties of oxytocin, including its capacity to buffer stress, may help to explain the role of social support as a positive factor in mental and physical health.

VASOPRESSIN

Vasopressin is structurally related to oxytocin, differing by two of nine amino acids. Vasopressin is made in the same hypothalamic nuclei (SON and PVN) but usually not by the same cells that synthesize oxytocin. Small amounts of vasopressin also are synthesized in the amygdala, the bed nucleus of the stria terminalis, and the lateral septum, especially in the presence of androgen (De Vries & Villalba, 1997). Vasopressin has functions throughout the body, acting on three subtypes of receptors, including V1a and V1b, that are found in the nervous system.

SIMILARITIES AND DIFFERENCES
BETWEEN OXYTOCIN AND VASOPRESSIN

Oxytocin and vasopressin have several functions in common, possibly because they have the capacity to influence each other's receptors. Vasopressin has been implicated in social bonding (Winslow, Hastings, Carter, Harbaugh, & Insel, 1993; Cho, DeVries, Williams, & Carter, 1999; Lim, Hammock, & Young, 2004), as well as parental behavior (Marler, Bester-Meredith, & Brainor, 2003; Bales, Kim, et al., 2004). When given exogenously, both peptides may influence social bonds and parental behavior in both sexes (Cho et al., 1999; Bales, Plotsky, et al., 2004). However, males with more endogenous central vasopressin may be more reliant than females on vasopressin (De Vries & Simerly, 2002). In particular, vasopressin seems to play a role in vigilance and mate guarding; these behaviors are seen in both sexes but are most typically associated with male behavior.

Of particular importance to understanding the role of the physiological and emotional consequences of oxytocin and vasopressin may be the differential actions of these peptides on arousal and reactivity to stressors (Engelmann, Wotjak, Neumann, Ludwig, & Landgraf, 1996; Carter, 1998). Vasopressin is sometimes considered a "stress" hormone and a component of the HPA axis and is associated with and released during periods of self-defense and stress. For example, vasopressin may increase the physiological responses of the HPA axis to stress in rats. With regard to the HPA axis, the effects of oxytocin and vasopressin tend to be in opposite directions. The actions of vasopressin (such as increased heart rate and blood pressure) may permit mobilization and self-protection (Porges, 2003a, 2003b).

Oxytocin and vasopressin, of course, do not work alone. Many hormones and neural systems are involved in social behavior and in what we humans call "social support." As one example, there is recent evidence implicating dopamine–oxytocin interactions and dopamine–vasopressin interactions in social bond formation (Aragona et al., 2006). Dopamine may be essential in the development of selective social relationships. Many other hormones, neurotransmitters and neural systems are involved in social behavior and social support, and many of these factors are probably beyond the scope of our current knowledge.

"STRESS" AND HOMEOSTASIS

Traditional stress research has been dominated by studies of the HPA (McEwen, 2003). Such studies have centered on understanding the detrimental effects of high levels of or chronic exposure to glucocorticoids. More recently, stress research has focused on the central nervous system (CNS) and specific central neuroendocrine components of the HPA axis, such as corticotropin-releasing factor (CRF), which plays a major role in the regulation of reactivity to threatening or stressful stimuli. CRF, acting on the CNS, has also been associated with defensive behaviors, anxiety, and negative emotions (Bakshi & Kalin, 2000; Charney & Bremner, 2004). CRF also has been shown to play a role in pair-bond formation (DeVries et al., 2002), further implicating stressful experiences in the regulation of social bonds.

Studies of the biology of stress tend to focus on the sympathetic nervous system and defensive processes. This research often fails to address the contributions of less well identified neural systems that actively promote health, growth, and restoration (Singer & Ryff, 2001). Among these are the parasympathetic components of the autonomic nervous system (ANS) and their representations within the CNS (Porges, 2003a, 2003b). Integral to many functions of the ANS and CNS are neuropeptides (such as oxytocin) that are capable of modulating (and, in some cases, down-regulating) the HPA response (Carter, 1998; Uvnas-Moberg, 1998; Neumann, 2001). These neural systems work in unison with the HPA axis to allow the body to adapt to various challenges.

DEVELOPMENTAL INFLUENCES ON SOCIALITY

Remarkably, during early development the same peptides that are implicated in adult social behaviors appear to be capable of programming tendencies toward different patterns of sociality (Carter, 2003). The capacity to form social bonds depends on genetic differences, including those that are responsible for species-typical and gender-specific patterns of social behavior. However, genetic differences (at least those known at present) are not sufficient to explain individual variations in social behaviors. There is increasing evidence that social experiences, especially in early life, may contribute to enduring changes in patterns of behavioral responses. Among the behaviors and neural systems that are changed by early experience are those necessary for pair-bond formation (Bales & Carter, 2003a, 2003b; Bales, Lewis-Reese, & Carter, 2003; Bales, Kim, Lewis-Reese, & Carter, 2004) and other forms of social behavior (Levine, 2001; Weaver et al., 2004). For example, when prairie voles are deliberately undisturbed during the preweaning period, subsequent tendencies to be either social or exploratory are reduced (Bales et al., 2003). In contrast, animals that receive early handling—possibly mediated by enhanced maternal stimulation—may, later in life, show increases in sociality.

In prairie voles, exposure to exogenous oxytocin during neonatal life has the capacity to facilitate a later tendency to form male–female pair bonds or to be generally social (Bales & Carter, 2003b). Early exposure to oxytocin also may reduce behavioral and neuroendocrine reactivity to a novel environment and may enhance subsequent hypothalamic synthesis of oxytocin (Yamamoto et al., 2004). In contrast, even brief neonatal exposure to an oxytocin receptor antagonist (OTA) may disrupt subsequent social behaviors, including the tendency to form social bonds, to exhibit parental behaviors, and to manage anxiety or stress. Many of the consequences of early peptide manipulations are sexually dimorphic. Ongoing research has revealed that a single exposure to an OTA on the first day of life produced a long-lasting reduction in vasopressin (V1a) receptor binding in the extended amygdala (Bales, Plotsky, et al., 2004) and reductions in vasopressin synthesis in the PVN (Yamamoto et al., 2004) in males. These effects of OTA were not seen in the females. Perhaps even more interesting was our recent finding that a single exposure to oxytocin in early life in male voles produced a long-lasting increase in V1a binding in the ventral pallidum (Bales, Plotsky, et al., 2004), a brain region that also contains receptors for dopamine. A coexistence of vasopressin and dopamine receptors may enhance the rewarding properties of social interactions. This neuroendocrine change (found only in males) is consistent with our earlier finding that neonatally oxytocin-treated males are more likely to form pair bonds (Bales & Carter, 2003b).

WHAT MECHANISMS PERMIT SPECIES, SEX, AND INDIVIDUAL DIFFERENCES IN THE CAPACITY TO FORM PAIR BONDS?

The complete answer to this question, of course, remains to be discovered. Differential availability of peptides or their receptors, including oxytocin and vasopressin, suggest clues to some of these differences. If a hormone does not have an appropriate target (receptor located in a particular brain area), then the effects of these chemicals may "fall on deaf ears." For example, sex differences in the capacity to form pair bonds may be due in part to the developmental programming of the presence or absence of receptors for oxytocin or vasopressin. Hypothalamic vasopressin is androgen dependent and may be particularly important in regulating certain masculine behavioral traits. In our studies in prairie voles, the sexually dimorphic capacity of an OTA to down-regulate both vasopressin receptors and the vasopressin peptide may help to explain the fact that OTA exposure was especially disruptive to male behavior. In contrast, in females (but not males) a single treatment with exogenous oxytocin produced reductions in V1a receptor binding in the lateral septum, medial preoptic area, and ventral pallidum. As mentioned earlier, in males, early oxytocin exposure up-regulated V1a receptors in the ventral pallidum. The colocalization of high levels of vasopressin receptors with dopamine receptors in the ventral pallidum may help to explain the capacity of some species (such as prairie voles) to form social bonds, whereas other species without this colocalization of vasopressin and dopamine do not form such bonds (Young & Wang, 2004; Lim, Hammock, & Young, 2004). Related processes might begin to explain gender and individual differences in behaviors that rely on vasopressin or oxytocin.

DOES VASOPRESSIN ALSO PROGRAM
THE DEVELOPING NERVOUS SYSTEM?

At present we know much less about the developmental effects on social behavior of vasopressin. Preliminary experiments in voles suggested that postnatal exposure to either vasopressin or a vasopressin antagonist did not disrupt the capacity of prairie voles to pair bond. However, animals exposed to neonatal vasopressin, especially males, tended to become more aggressive, whereas aggression was very low in animals exposed prenatally to either control treatments or a vasopressin antagonist (Stribley & Carter, 1999). Thus it is likely that changes in vasopressin also have enduring behavioral effects that are related but not identical to those seen when oxytocin is manipulated.

IMPLICATIONS FOR HUMAN DEVELOPMENT

There is growing evidence that early experiences, including physiological and behavioral changes associated with pregnancy, birth, lactation, and the management of infants during the postpartum period, have the capacity to produce long-lasting changes in human behavior (Teicher et al., 2003). For ethical and practical reasons, most of the research dealing with mechanisms for early experience comes from animal models. However, examples of potential interest also may be drawn from human development. As one example, it is known that human breast milk contains oxytocin and related hormones; these hormones may not be present in infant formulas. Thus the decision to breast-feed could represent an endocrine manipulation with long-lasting consequences for the newborn. Routine endocrine treatments, including the use of exogenous oxytocin (pitocin) during labor and, more recently, the use of oxytocin antagonists (such as a commercial OTA called Atosiban), also hold the potential to influence the parent and offspring in ways that have not been investigated in humans. Based primarily on research in animals, we can hypothesize that touch or other forms of social stimulation, via long-lasting physiological processes, can retune or "program" the nervous system for life (Levine, 2001; Weaver et al., 2004).

Remarkably little is known regarding the role of hormones such as oxytocin in human behavior. Some information may come from the study of lactating women. Compared with bottle-feeding mothers, breast-feeding women are buffered from physiological and psychological stress (see Carter, Altemus, & Chrousos, 2001). For example, we have observed that the amount of cortisol and other stress hormones released following intense exercise is about twice as high in bottle-feeding versus breast-feeding mothers (matched for other variables; Altemus, Deuster, Gallivan, Carter, & Gold, 1995). More recently, Heinrichs, Baumgartner, Kirschbaum, and Ehlert (2003) have shown that both social support and intranasal oxytocin are capable of reducing reactivity in men (measured by salivary cortisol) in a psychosocial stress paradigm.

Of special relevance to human health is the capacity of a perceived sense of social support or the presence of social bonds to reduce fear and overreactivity in the face of stress. Reductions in social behavior and stress management are features of many forms of mental illness, including autism, depression, and schizophrenia (Kirkpatrick, 1997; Insel, O'Brien, & Leekman, 1999). Episodes of certain mental illness, such as anxiety disorders, depression, and even schizophrenia, may be induced or at least exacerbated by social stressors, especially in the absence of social bonds. Furthermore, chronic elevations in sympathoadrenal activity may be detrimental to physical and emotional health, and there is increasing evidence that hormones of the HPA axis have a role in mental illness (Charney & Bremner, 2004). Thus behavioral–physiological processes that buffer the developing nervous system may be of particular importance to good mental health.

SUMMARY

The human nervous system is a product of evolution and shares many features with other mammalian species. It is increasingly clear that social behavior and social experiences have powerful roles in neural development, especially under conditions of challenge or stress. Hormones, including oxytocin, vasopressin, CRF, and corticosterone, have newly identified central roles in behavior and stress management. Each of these hormones also may have the capacity to regulate both the development of the nervous system and the subsequent expression of behavior, in part through their capacity to program the developing nervous system. For both practical and theoretical reasons, it is important to realize that the mechanisms that underlie traits such as the capacity to form social bonds are dynamic and capable of being influenced by early experience, often through effects on the same systems that regulate sociality in adulthood.

Taken together, these and related findings (see Carter, 1998, 2003; Carter & Keverne, 2002) support the general hypothesis that social bonding is regulated in a species-specific, gender-specific, and probably individual-specific manner by both oxytocin and vasopressin (and almost certainly a host of other neurochemicals). Peptide hormones are of particular interest here because they are exceptionally responsive to social experiences and may provide a mechanism through which behavioral experiences, mediated by changes in these hormones or their receptors, could be transmitted across generations. Evidence supporting intergenerational transmission of social experiences via changes in peptides also comes from recent research on maternal behavior in rats (see Pedersen & Boccia, 2002).

Adaptive changes in these neural systems, especially at the level of various peptides and relevant receptors, could begin to explain individual differences in behavior. The capacity of these neuroendocrine systems to undergo long-lasting functional modifications also may help to explain the origins of what has been called "gender," "personality," or "temperament." Furthermore, understanding these systems offers potential insights into the development of pathological or maladaptive behaviors.

ACKNOWLEDGMENTS

Recent studies on voles from my laboratory were sponsored by the National Institutes of Health (especially Grant No. PO1 HD 38490), the Institute for Research on Unlimited Love, and the National Alliance for Autism Research. The contribution of many colleagues whose work is cited below is gratefully acknowledged.

REFERENCES

Altemus, M., Deuster, P. A., Gallivan, E., Carter, C. S., & Gold, P. W. (1995). Suppression of hypothalamic–pituitary–adrenal responses to exercise stress in lactating women. *Journal of Clinical Endocrinology and Metabolism, 80,* 2954–2959.

Aragona, B. J., Liu, Y., Yu, Y. J., Curtis, J. T., Detwiler, J. M., Insel, T. R., et al.

(2006). Nucleus accumbens dopamine differentially mediates the formation and maintenance of monogamus pair bonds, *Nature Neuroscience, 9,* 133–139.

Bakshi, V. P., & Kalin, N. H. (2000). Corticotropin-releasing hormone and animal models of anxiety: Gene–environment interaction. *Biological Psychiatry, 48,* 1175–1198.

Bales, K. L., & Carter, C. S. (2003a). Sex differences and developmental effects of oxytocin on aggression and social behavior in prairie voles (*Microtus ochrogaster*). *Hormones and Behavior, 44,* 178–184.

Bales, K. L., & Carter, C. S. (2003b). Developmental exposure to oxytocin facilitates partner preferences in male prairie voles (*Microtus ochrogaster*). *Behavioral Neuroscience, 117,* 854–859.

Bales, K. L., Kim, A. J., Lewis-Reese, A.D., & Carter, C. S. (2004). Both oxytocin and vasopressin may influence alloparental care in male prairie voles. *Hormones and Behavior, 45,* 354–361.

Bales, K. L., Lewis-Reese, A., & Carter, C. S. (2003) Neonatal handling affects male monogamous behaviors in prairie voles (*Microtus ochrogaster*). *Developmental Psychobiology, 43,* 246.

Bales, K. L., Plotsky, P. M., Young, L. J., Lim, M. M., Grotte, N., & Carter, C. S. (2004). Neonatal manipulations of oxytocin have sexually dimorphic effects on vasopressin receptor binding in monogamous prairie voles. *Society for Neuroscience Abstracts, 758,* 13.

Carter, C. S. (1998). Neuroendocrine perspectives on social attachment and love. *Psychoneuroendocrinology, 23,* 779–818.

Carter, C. S. (2003). Developmental consequences of oxytocin. *Physiology and Behavior, 79,* 383–397.

Carter, C. S., Altemus, M., & Chrousos, G. P. (2001). Neuroendocrine and emotional changes in the postpartum period. *Progress in Brain Research, 133,* 241–249.

Carter, C. S., DeVries, A. C., & Getz, L. L. (1995). Physiological substrates of mammalian monogamy: The prairie vole model. *Neuroscience and Biobehavioral Reviews, 19,* 303–14.

Carter, C. S., and Keverne, E. B. (2002). The neurobiology of social affiliation and pair bonding. In D. Pfaff (Ed.), *Hormones, brain, and behavior* (Vol. 1, pp. 299–335). San Diego, CA: Academic Press.

Charney, D. S., & Bremner, J. D. (2004). The neurobiology of anxiety disorders. In D. S. Charney, & E. J. Nestler (Eds.), *The neurobiology of mental illness* (pp. 605–627). New York: Oxford University Press.

Cho, M. M., DeVries, A. C., Williams, J. R., & Carter, C. S. (1999). The effects of oxytocin and vasopressin on partner preferences in male and female prairie voles (*Microtus ochrogaster*). *Behavioral Neuroscience, 113,* 1071–1080.

DeVries, A. C., DeVries, M. B., Taymans, S. E., & Carter, C. S. (1995). The modulation of pair bonding by corticosterone in female prairie voles. *Proceedings of the National Academy of Sciences of the USA, 92,* 7744–7748.

DeVries, A. C., DeVries, M. B., Taymans, S. E., & Carter, C. S. (1996). Stress has sexually dimorphic effects on pair bonding in prairie voles. *Proceedings of the National Academy of Sciences of the USA, 93,* 11980–11984.

DeVries A. C., Guptaa, T., Cardillo, S., Cho, M., & Carter, C. S. (2002). Corticotropin-releasing factor induces social preferences in male prairie voles. *Psychoneuroendocrinology, 27,* 705–714.

De Vries, G. J., & Simerly, R. B. (2002). Anatomy, development, and function of sexually dimorphic neural circuits in the mammalian brain. In D. Pfaff (Ed.), *Hormones, brain, and behavior* (Vol. 4, pp. 137–192). San Diego: Academic Press.

De Vries, G. J., & Villalba, C. (1997). Brain sexual dimorphism and sex differences in parental and other social behaviors. *Annals of the New York Academy of Sciences, 807,* 273–286.

Engelmann, M., Wotjak, C. T., Neumann, I., Ludwig, M., & Landgraf, R. (1996). Behavioral consequences of intracerebral vasopressin and oxytocin: Focus on learning and memory. *Neuroscience and Biobehavioral Reviews, 20,* 341–358.

Francis, D., Young, L. J., Meaneny, M. J., & Insel, T. R. (2002). Naturally occurring differences in maternal care are associated with the expression of OT and AVP (V1a) receptors: Gender differences. *Journal of Neuroendocrinology, 14,* 349–353.

Gautvik, K. M., de Lecea, L., Gautvik, V. T., Danielson, P. E., Tranque, P., Dopazo, A., et al. (1996). Overview of the most prevalent hypothalamus-specific mRNAs, as identified by directional tag PCR subtractions. *Proceedings of the National Academy of Sciences of the USA, 93,* 8733–8738.

Gimpl, G., & Fahrenholz, F. (2001). The oxytocin receptor system: Structure, function and regulation. *Physiological Review, 81,* 629–683.

Heinrichs, M., Baumgartner, T., Kirschbaum, C., & Ehlert, U. (2003). Social support and oxytocin interact to suppress cortisol and subjective responses to psychosocial stress. *Biological Psychiatry, 54,* 1389–1398.

Hrdy, S. B. (1999). *Mother nature: Maternal instincts and how they shape the human species.* New York: Ballantine Press.

Insel, T. R., O'Brien, D. J., & Leckman, J. F. (1999). Oxytocin, vasopressin, and autism: Is there a connection? *Biological Psychiatry, 45,* 145–157.

Kiecolt-Glaser, J. K., Preacher, K. J., MacCallum, R. C., Malarkey, W. B., & Glaser, R. (2003). Chronic stress and age-related increases in the proinflammatory cytokine interleukin-6. *Proceedings of the National Academy of Sciences of the USA, 100,* 9090–9095.

Knox, S. S., & Uvnas-Moberg, K. (1998). Social isolation and cardiovascular disease: An atherosclerotic pathway? *Psychoneuroendocrinology, 23,* 877–890.

Levine, S. (2001). Primary social relationships influence the development of the hypothalamic–pituitary–adrenal axis in the rat. *Physiology and Behavior, 73,* 255–260.

Lim, M. M., Hammock, E. A. D., & Young, L. J. (2004). The role of vasopressin in the genetic and neural basis of monogamy. *Journal of Neuroendocrinology, 16,* 325–332.

Lim, M. M., Wang, Z. X., Olazabal, D. E., Ren, X. H., Terwilliger, E. F., & Young, L. J. (2004). Enhanced partner preference in a promiscuous species by manipulating the expression of a single gene. *Nature, 429,* 754–757.

Marler, C. A., Bester-Meredith, J. K., & Brainor, B. C. (2003). Paternal behavior and aggression: Endocrine mechanisms and nongenomic transmission of behavior. *Advances in the Study of Behavior, 32,* 263–323.

McEwen, B. S. (2003). Interacting mediators of allostasis and allostatic load: Towards an understanding of resilience in aging. *Metabolism, 52,* 10–16.

Neumann, I. D. (2001). Alterations in behavioral and neuroendocrine stress coping strategies in pregnant, parturient and lactating rats. *Progress in Brain Research, 133* 143–152.

Panksepp, J., Nelson, E., & Bekkedal, M. (1997). Brain systems for the mediation of social separation-distress and social reward. *Annals of the New York Academy of Sciences, 807,* 78–100.

Parker, K. J., Kinney, L. F., Phillips, K. M., & Lee, T. M. (2001). Paternal behavior is associated with central neurohormone receptor binding patterns in meadow voles (*Microtus pennsylvanicus*). *Behavioral Neuroscience, 5,* 1349–1356.

Pedersen, C. A., & Boccia, M. L. (2002). Oxytocin links mothering received, mothering bestowed and adult stress responses. *Stress, 5,* 259–267.

Porges, S. (2003a). The polyvagal theory: Phylogenetic contributions to social behavior. *Physiology and Behavior, 79,* 503–513.

Porges, S. (2003b). Social engagement and attachment: A phylogenetic perspective. *Annals of the New York Academy of Sciences, 1008,* 31–47.

Seckl, J. R. (2004). Prenatal glucocorticoids and long-term programming. *European Journal of Endocrinology, Nov, 151,* (Suppl. 3), U49–U62.

Singer, B. H., & Ryff, C. D. (Eds.). (2001). New horizons in health: An integrative approach. Washington, DC: National Academy Press.

Stribley, J. M., & Carter, C. S. (1999). Developmental exposure to vasopressin increases aggression in adult prairie voles. *Proceedings of the National Academy of Sciences of the USA, 96,* 12601–12604.

Teicher, M. H., Andersen, S. L., Polcari, A., Anderson, C. M., Navlta, C. P., & Kim, D. M. (2003). The neurobiological consequences of early stress and childhood maltreatment. *Neuroscience and Biobehavioral Reviews, 27,* 33–44.

Uchino, B. N., Cacioppo, J. T., & Kiecolt-Glaser, J. K. (1996). The relationship between social support and physiological processes: A review with emphasis on underlying mechanisms and implications for health. *Psychological Bulletin, 119,* 488–531.

Uvnas-Moberg, K. (1998). Oxytocin may mediate the benefits of positive social interaction and emotions. *Psychoneuroendocrinology, 23,* 819–835.

Weaver, I. C., Cervoni, N., Champagne, F. A., D'Alessio, A. C., Sharma, S., Seckl, J. R., et al. (2004). Epigenetic programming by maternal behavior. *Nature Neuroscience, 7,* 847–854.

Winslow, J. T., & Insel, T. R. (2004). Neuroendocrine basis of social recognition. *Current Opinion in Neurobiology, 14,* 248–253.

Winslow, J. T., Hastings, N., Carter, C. S., Harbaugh, C. R., & Insel, T. R. (1993). A role for vasopressin pair bonding in monogamous prairie voles. *Nature, 365,* 545–548.

Yamamoto, Y., Cushing, B. S., Kramer, K. M., Epperson, P. D., Hoffman, G. E., & Carter, C. S. (2004). Neonatal manipulations of oxytocin alter oxytocin and vasopressin in the paraventricular nucleus of the hypothalamus in a gender-specific manner. *Neuroscience, 125,* 947–955.

20

The Quiet Revolution of Existential Neuroscience

Marco Iacoboni

CLARIFYING THE ASSUMPTIONS

In the past two decades, we have witnessed the merging of scientific disciplines into novel, interdisciplinary enterprises. Cognitive science and neuroscience have produced the new and quite successful field of cognitive neuroscience. Social psychology and neuroscience have produced in parallel the new exciting field of social neuroscience. Moreover, in the past decade, social psychologists and cognitive neuroscientists have effectively joined forces to create the fascinating field of social cognitive neuroscience. In this latter field, the scientific approach that dominates is the one that uses functional imaging techniques to study brain–behavior relationships. Other approaches—for instance, lesion studies in neurological patients—are also used to study the neural basis of social cognition but less frequently than the functional imaging approach. In this chapter, I discuss some of the work that has been performed in my lab on mirror neurons, imitation, and social cognition. This work has been carried out mostly using imaging techniques. Before discussing this work, however, I would like to make explicit some tacitly held assumptions in the functional imaging and the social-cognitive neuroscience fields.

The dominant underlying broadly shared assumptions of all the scientific fields mentioned, and particularly of functional neuroimaging—those unsaid but implicitly held concepts that constitute a general framework for data interpretation and, more generally, for what makes sense in the practice of science—are mostly derived from assumptions dominant in classical cognitive science and in what John Haugeland termed "good old-fashioned artificial intelligence" (GOFAI; Haugeland, 1985). The three main assumptions I discuss here are (1) the subject–world and inner–outer dichotomy, (2) the strictly linked assumption of the role of representations in the mind of the cognitive subject contemplating the world, and (3) the assumption, in turn linked to the second one, of the atomism of the input that the cognitive agent should receive from the world. The first two assumptions can be formulated as such: the cognitive agent or subject understands the objects of the world by using internal mental states that represent those objects of the world and, by so doing, produces knowledge. These internal mental states represent the outer objects of the world in an inner mental world; thus these representations do not really depend on the objects they represent. These assumptions naturally fit the experimental setup of brain-imaging studies, in which an individual is isolated in a scanner and presented with various stimuli that he or she must "process," yielding some brain activity that reflects the brains "representations" of the stimuli. Moreover, different kinds of elements (motion, color, or even "social" vs. "nonsocial") of what is presented to the participants are assumed to be processed largely independently of each other (the assumption of the atomism of the input), thus yielding different types of brain activity related to different elements of the input. And this picture seems quite accurate, in that we can reliably induce activations in specific brain areas for specific kinds of stimuli. For instance, area V4 is activated by color, area MT/V5 is activated by motion, the so-called face fusiform area (FFA) is activated by watching a face. Even the empirical work and theoretical approach that challenges the notion that certain kinds of stimuli are processed by localized and specialized neural systems (Haxby et al., 2001) takes the assumption of the atomism of the input for granted.

What I suggest is that one can look at things with different eyes. In fact, some empirical work in the neuroscience of sociality seems to suggest—quietly but resolutely—that the assumptions of the subject–world, inner–outer dichotomy, of representations independent of the things they represent, and of the atomism of the input may not be easily applied in some cases. Thus, rather than the picture of a meaning-giving brain that looks at the outside world and makes sense of it with a reflective and analytical approach, what emerges from some work in social cognitive neuroscience is the view of a human brain that needs a body to exist in a world of shared social norms in which meaning originates from being-in-the-world. This view is reminiscent of motives recurring in at least one flavor of what is called existential phenomenology (Heidegger, 1927). For this reason, I call this view "existential neuroscience."

THE SUBJECT–WORLD, INNER–OUTER DICHOTOMY

One of the most powerful aspects of human behavior is the tendency to imitate others. We do this very early in life (Meltzoff & Moore, 1977), but we also tend to do it throughout adulthood (Chartrand & Bargh, 1999). There is a developmental trajectory according to which a prepotent form of imitation earlier in life (Wapner & Cirillo, 1968) is what one could call "specular" imitation. That is, when the imitator and the model are face-to-face, the imitator tends to imitate the model as if in front of a mirror. Thus, if the model raises the left hand, the imitator raises the right hand. In our imaging work, we had identified a frontoparietal system relevant to imitation (Iacoboni et al., 1999; Koski et al., 2002) that is likely the human homologue of frontoparietal areas in the macaque brain that contain mirror neurons, that is, neurons that fire both when the monkey performs an action and when it sees somebody else performing the same action (Rizzolatti & Craighero, 2004). Within the human frontoparietal mirror system that is activated during imitation (see Figure 20.1), the activity in the frontal area (pars opercularis of the inferior frontal gyrus) seems particularly relevant to aspects of imitation associated with the goal of an action. For instance, a functional magnetic resonance imaging (fMRI) study from our group shows that, when actions with visible goals are imitated, the activity in pars opercularis of the inferior frontal gyrus is higher than when the same movement is imitated in absence of a visible goal (Koski et al., 2002). In a subsequent study, we used frameless stereotaxy to guide repetitive transcranial magnetic stimulation (rTMS) over pars opercularis of the inferior frontal gyrus. The rTMS approach allows experimenters to impair transiently the functions of the cortical areas directly stimulated. While

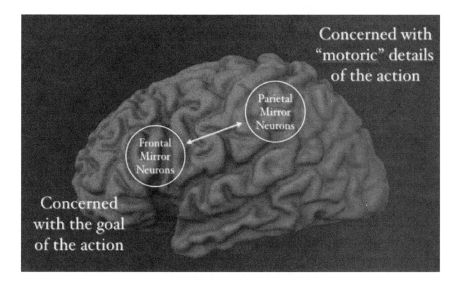

FIGURE 20.1. Three-dimensional view of the lateral wall of the human brain. The two human areas with mirror neuron properties are located in the *pars opercularis* of the inferior frontal gyrus and in the rostral part of the inferior parietal lobule.

being stimulated over pars opercularis of the inferior frontal gyrus, participants had a selective impairment in imitation but not in a visuomotor task in which the motor output was identical to the imitation task (Heiser, Iacoboni, Maeda, Marcus, & Mazziotta, 2003). Importantly, the deficit in imitation was selective for the goal of the action but not for specific aspects of the movement, such as movement time and trajectory. Thus both fMRI and rTMS provide complementary evidence that supports the relevance of pars opercularis of the inferior frontal gyrus with regard to the goal of imitative actions. It turns out that this same cortical region shows higher activity during specular imitation (right-hand imitation of a left-hand action) compared with anatomical imitation (right-hand imitation of a right-hand action; Koski, Iacoboni, Dubeau, Woods, & Mazziotta, 2003). If one considers the relevance of goals for this cortical region, the dominance of specular imitation early in development, and the fact that specular imitation substantially means that both the imitator and the model share the same sector of space during imitative behavior, one is led to hypothesize that a general goal of imitating others seems to be "directed toward" them, a process according to which a certain intimacy between model and imitator is achieved through space and action sharing. What is this intimacy if not the interdependence of both parties, model and imitator, rather than the expression of a separation between the perceiver (the imitator) and the perceived (the model)?

Another example of how the relation between neural activity and space seems to map better on to a concept of *being-amid* rather than on to the concept of a subject–world dichotomy comes from the neurophysiological work in primates of Graziano and collaborators (Graziano, Taylor, Moore, & Cooke, 2002). The classical and intuitive concept of space is that space is a unitary medium through which we move and operate and interact with others (here, a socially relevant practice that seems strongly culture-dependent is the practice of standing the appropriate distance from people; Dreyfus, 1991). This classical and intuitive concept of a unitary space, however, has been challenged in the past two decades by converging observations in clinical neurology and primate neurophysiology. Patients with hemi-inattention tend to neglect things located in the hemispace contralateral to the cerebral lesion. Typically, the lesions associated with hemineglect are located in the right hemisphere, the hemi-inattention occurring for the left hemispace. Some of these patients, however, show a double dissociation, such that some patients show hemineglect only for near space and that some other patients show hemineglect only for far space (Bisiach, Perani, Vallar, & Berti, 1986; Halligan & Marshall, 1991). Near space is practically definable by what is reachable with the hand. The boundaries between near and far space, however, are flexible. In fact, when a patient with near-space neglect is given a long stick to bisect a line in far space, the patient shows the classical rightward bias typical of unilateral neglect also in far space. In contrast, if the patient bisects the line in far space with a light pen, no rightward bias is observed (Berti & Frassinetti,

2000). These data suggest that the use of the stick altered the near-space map, stretching it to a much larger distance from the body of the patient. Neurophysiological data from Iriki and collaborators provide the single-cell mechanism for this phenomenon (Iriki, Tanaka, & Iwamura, 1996). Iriki and colleagues trained monkeys to use a rake to get food. Monkeys were initially clumsy with the rake but eventually learned how to use it proficiently. Single-cell recordings in parietal bimodal neurons with a tactile receptive field at the hand and a visual receptive field around the hand and anchored to this body part demonstrated that, after the monkey had learned how to master the tool, the visual receptive field of the parietal neuron had extended to incorporate the entire length of the rake. These data suggest that the kind of spatial maps provided by the primate brain are pragmatic maps, determined by the kinds of actions that can be performed in that space sector. In fact, the frontoparietal networks associated with near and far space (see Figure 20.2) have physiological properties in line with this concept. The frontoparietal cortical areas relevant to far space are the frontal and parietal eye fields, with neurons having properties associated with ocular movements and with sensory responses to nongraspable stimuli such as light flashes. The frontoparietal cortical areas associated with near space have neurons that are active during reaching and grasping movements, and with sensory responses to three-dimensional, graspable objects (Rizzolatti, Fogassi, & Gallese, 1997; Rizzolatti, Riggio, & Sheliga, 1994).

The work of Graziano and colleagues has initially defined the polysensory properties of premotor and posterior parietal neurons that seem relevant to creating a peripersonal space map (Graziano & Gross, 1998; Graziano, Hu, & Gross, 1997; Graziano, Reiss, & Gross, 1999; Graziano, Yap, & Gross, 1994). Neurons in two polysensory areas in the frontal and parietal lobes that are also well connected anatomically, the ventral intraparietal area (VIP) and the polysensory zone (PZ) in the precentral gyrus, have tactile receptive fields mostly with respect to the arm and the

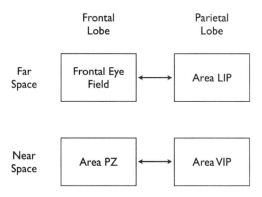

FIGURE 20.2. Schematic diagram of frontoparietal circuits for far and near space.

head. These neurons also respond to visual and auditory stimuli located close to their tactile receptive fields. These properties seem to suggest that these neurons provide a map of the space around us. This space map might well be the map representing a space completely separated from us, albeit close. However, electrical stimulation of these two areas produces complex, coordinated movements that are identical to defensive movements that occur in natural conditions (Cooke & Graziano, 2003, 2004; Cooke, Taylor, Moore, & Graziano, 2003). For instance, a set of polysensory neurons with tactile receptive fields on the face of the monkey and visual receptive fields around the tactile receptive field, when stimulated, produce a defensive posture that includes "a facial grimace, a squinting of the eye, a turning of the head away from the side of the sensory receptive fields, a hunching of the shoulders, a fast thrusting of the hand into the space beside the head, and a turning of the hand such that the palm faced outward, away from the head" (Graziano et al., 2002). The sensorimotor integration properties of these frontal and parietal areas suggest that, rather than implementing an abstract representation of an "outer" near space, these neural ensembles are relevant to a direct sense of *being-amid*, of being-in-the-world. One could argue, however, that, after all, these frontoparietal cortical areas seem relevant to very basic aspects of sensorimotor behavior, but not very relevant to more complex behaviors that may play a more central role in human sociality. The following sections discuss increasingly more complex and more "social" aspects of human behavior to test whether or not we should abandon the mentalistic dominant assumptions I discussed earlier in favor of a more "existential" (remember the dictum "existence precedes essence") approach.

THE ASSUMPTION OF DISEMBODIED INTERNAL REPRESENTATIONS

A corollary of the inner–outer dichotomy is that the outer world must be represented internally, using amodal and abstract symbols that bear arbitrary relations to the perceptual and motor states that produce them (Fodor, 1983). Recent data from different disciplines—from social psychology (Niedenthal, Barsalou, Winkielman, Kauth-Gruber, & Ric, 2005) to neuroscience—suggest that this idea may not be entirely correct. Using TMS, Fadiga and colleagues (Fadiga, Fogassi, Pavesi, & Rizzolatti, 1995) reported for the first time that action observation facilitates corticospinal excitability. They stimulated the primary motor cortex of normal volunteers while recording motor-evoked potentials (MEPs) over muscles of the hand contralateral to the stimulated motor cortex. Fadiga and colleagues recorded greater MEPs while participants observed actions, compared with control experimental conditions. These findings have been replicated in other labs, including ours (Aziz-Zadeh, Iacoboni, Zaidel, Wilson, & Mazziotta, 2004; Aziz-Zadeh, Maeda, Zaidel, Mazziotta, & Iacoboni,

2002; Gangitano, Mottagny, & Pascual-Leone, 2001; Strafella & Paus, 2000). The most commonly accepted explanation for this effect is the following: Watching an action activates inferior frontal mirror neurons in ventral premotor cortex. These neurons have a direct input onto primary motor cortex. Thus the activation in inferior frontal mirror neurons modulates the subthreshold membrane potential of primary motor neurons, such that these neurons are more readily excitable by the transcranial magnetic pulse.

One of the most important aspects of this motor facilitation is that it is muscle-specific. That is, facilitation can be observed only in muscles involved in the observed action, not in other muscles. This is true even for muscles of the same body part. That is, if participants observe the extension of fingers, only muscles involved in finger extension, not muscles involved in finger flexion, will show the facilitation. The muscle specificity of the effect suggests that this motor resonance behavior is a dynamic, embodied, relational process of some form of imitation rather than representing an entity with informational content about the actions of others that is completely independent of those actions. Given that it would be highly inefficient to parrot others continuously, it is likely that there exist neural control mechanisms that suppress such embodied, imitation-like forms of action recognition. In fact, there is evidence that patients with large prefrontal lesions may show uncontrolled imitative behavior (De Renzi, Cavalleri, & Facchini, 1996; Lhermitte, Pillon, & Serdaru, 1986), likely due to the dysfunction of such control mechanisms.

Similar phenomena have been observed even in the domain of language. Listening to speech sounds activates primary motor areas necessary to produce speech sounds, as reported in a recent fMRI study performed in our lab (Wilson, Saygin, Sereno, & Iacoboni, 2004). Moreover, while listening to speech sounds, tongue muscles show facilitation when stimulated with TMS. Once again, this facilitation is specific to the muscles necessary to emit the sounds listened to (Fadiga, Craighero, Buccino, & Rizzolatti, 2002). This evidence suggests that our perception of things involves various forms of mimicry.

This seems to be true even in the domain of emotions and empathy. It is well known that humans have the automatic tendency to imitate each other while interacting socially, the so-called "chameleon effect" (Hatfield, Cacioppo, & Rapson, 1994). It has been shown that the tendency to imitate others in social situations correlates with the tendency to be empathic (Chartrand & Bargh, 1999). At the level of neural systems, it is well known that the limbic system is very important for emotional behavior. In our work on imitation, we had identified a neural architecture for imitation comprising three major cortical systems: the superior temporal cortex, the rostral part of the posterior parietal cortex, and the inferior frontal cortex. Within this architecture, the superior temporal cortex would provide a higher-order visual description of the action, the posterior parietal cortex would provide somatosensory information, and the inferior frontal cortex would code the goal of the action (Iacoboni, 2003, 2005; Iacoboni, Kaplan, & Wilson, in press). Thus we have here two well-identified large-scale neural systems for emotion and imitation; but a strong functional link between the two, as suggested by the behavioral data on mimicry and empathy (Chartrand & Bargh, 1999; Hatfield et al., 1994), suggests that these two systems must interact in an even larger-scale network. Anatomical data on the insula suggest that the dysgranular sector of the insula connects the limbic system to the three major systems that make up the neural architecture for imitation, namely, superior temporal cortex, posterior parietal cortex, and inferior frontal cortex. To test whether these anatomical connections would result in a functionally significant large-scale network, we used fMRI while participants were observing and imitating facial emotional expressions. What we observed (Carr, Iacoboni, Dubeau, Mazziotta, & Lenzi, 2003) was a substantially similar pattern of activated areas during observation and imitation—with greater activity during imitation than during observation—in all the critical areas outlined here, thus suggesting two main concepts: first, that the perception of emotional states in others involves the activation of the same brain areas we use to express those emotions; second, that this activation includes a large-scale neural network comprising cortical areas relevant to imitation, the anterior insula and the limbic system. By the same token, lesion data show impairment in perception of facial emotional expressions when the lesions encompass the insula (Adolphs, Damasio, Tranel, Cooper, & Damasio, 2000; Calder, Keane, Manes, Antoun, & Young, 2000).

THE ASSUMPTION OF THE ATOMISM OF THE INPUT

Another critical assumption that permeates cognitive neuroscience in general and social cognitive neuroscience in particular is what could be called the assumption of the atomism of the input. This basically means that one assumes that the mind can process elements of the world independent of each other and of the context they are in. Thus a given situation can be processed by using some combinatorial strategy over categories of fixed, self-standing, and context-free elements. This assumption has been challenged on logical grounds (Andler, 2000; Taylor, 2000). Here I provide some experimental neuroscience evidence that challenges the assumption of the atomism of the input as well.

In area F5 of the macaque brain there are premotor neurons that fire during object-directed actions such as grasping, manipulating, holding, and tearing (Rizzolatti et al., 1988). Some of these neurons also have sensory properties in that the neurons fire while the monkey is not making any movement but is simply observing certain kinds of stimuli. There are at least two major classes of visuomotor neurons in F5, the so-called *mirror* neurons discussed earlier and *canonical* neurons. Canonical neurons have motor properties identical to mirror neurons, that is, both types of neurons fire during the execution of object-directed actions. Mirror and canonical neurons are distinguished by their sensory properties. As mentioned earlier, mirror neurons fire at the sight of object-directed actions performed by others but not at the sight of pantomimed actions in the absence of the object. Canonical neurons fire at the sight of graspable three-dimensional objects (Gallese, Fadiga, Fogassi, & Rizzolatti, 1996). The commonly accepted interpretation of these sensory properties is that mirror neurons provide some form of action recognition, whereas canonical neurons provide some form of analysis of the affordance of the object, how-to-grab-that-thing. This interpretation is quite reasonable and, at first sight, it does not seem to go against the assumption of the atomism of the input. In fact, it looks as though different kinds of things (actions and objects) are processed by different kinds of neurons. However, there is indeed a problem. Canonical neurons do not fire at the sight of an object-directed action, even though the object is visible. This neural property of canonical neurons—which is not well known—is really problematic for the assumption of the atomism of the input, because there is no apparent reason why canonical neurons should not fire at the sight of a cup that somebody else is going to grasp. After all, these neurons do fire at the sight of the cup when nobody is going to grasp it. Thus the neural activity in F5 while watching somebody grasping a cup—rather than being a combinatorial activity of neurons that respond separately to elements of the scene, that is, of mirror neurons responding to the sight of the action and of canonical neurons responding to the sight of the visible object—mysteriously sums up to firing in mirror neurons and absence of firing in canonical neurons. This firing pattern is not readily explained by an account of processing of self-standing, context-free elements. It is much more readily explained by a holistic stance, which assumes that the nature of any given element is determined only by the "whole" and that this "whole" is never simply determined by the sum of its elements. Thus, when the cup is going to be grasped by somebody, it is no longer simply a cup; it belongs to the grasping action. This concept is reminiscent of the intentional arc of Merleau-Ponty: "From the outset the grasping movement is magically at its completion" (Merleau-Ponty, 1945, p. 119).

A different kind of empirical evidence also seems to support a holistic stance much more than the atomism of the input. In a recent imaging study, we investigated the role of mirror neurons in understanding the intentions of others (Iacoboni et al., 2005). It has been proposed that mirror neurons may provide a neural mechanism for understanding the intentions of other people (Gallese & Goldman, 1998). Most of the evidence on mirror neurons, however, could be interpreted more parsimoniously as suggesting that mirror neurons provide a relatively simple action-recognition mechanism. Such a mechanism is reminiscent of some features of categorical perception (Diehl, Lotto, & Holt, 2004; Liberman, Harris, Hoffman, & Griffith,

1957). In fact, some mirror neurons do not discriminate between stimuli of the same category (i.e., the sight of different kinds of grasping actions can activate the same neuron), but they do discriminate well between actions belonging to different categories, even when the observed actions share several visual features. These properties seem more likely to support an action-recognition mechanism ("that's a grasp") than an intention-coding mechanism. The reason is that the same action can be associated with different intentions. We can grasp a cup in order to drink or in order to clean up the table. Given that there is not a one-to-one mapping between actions and intentions, one might conclude that mirror neurons are exclusively involved in action recognition, or at least in some aspects of it.

Typically, however, the context in which the actions occur is an important clue for clarifying the intentions of others (the "why" of an action). The same action done in two different contexts acquires different meanings and may reflect two different intentions. Thus we investigated whether observing the same grasping action—either embedded in contexts that cued the intention associated with the action or in the absence of a context to cue the observer—elicited the same or differential activity in mirror areas for grasping in the human brain. If mirror neurons for grasping simply code the type of observed action, then the activity in mirror areas should not be influenced by the presence or the absence of context. If, in contrast, mirror neurons code the intention associated with the observed action, then the presence of a context that cues the observer should modulate activity in mirror areas. To test these competing hypotheses, we studied 23 normal volunteers with fMRI while they watched three kinds of stimuli: grasping hand actions without a context, context only (a scene containing objects), and grasping hand actions embedded in contexts. The context cued the intention associated with the grasping action (either drinking or cleaning up) in the condition displaying both action and context. We found that observing grasping actions embedded in contexts yielded greater activity in inferior frontal cortex mirror areas than observing grasping actions in the absence of contexts and in observing contexts only (Iacoboni et al., 2005). This suggests that mirror neurons do not simply provide an action-recognition mechanism but rather represent a neural system for coding the intentions of other people. Again, rather than the combinatorial processing of elements, this neural pattern seems to reflect more a holistic stance toward contexts, actions, and intentions.

A DEFAULT HUMAN STATE: BEING SOCIAL

We are skilled at existing. And skill at existing certainly means having the ability to negotiate a complex network of social interactions into which we are thrown. In spite of this complexity, it seems we are able to understand the social relations between people automatically and effortlessly, even though we briefly glance at interacting people with our peripheral vision while we are engaged in our everyday activities, such as driving, going to the mall, or buying fresh produce at the farmer's market. How do we do this? In a recent study, we asked participants to watch 20-second video clips depicting realistic everyday interactions. The clips were organized such that during the first 12 seconds only one person was shown (the single-person segment), whereas the last 8 seconds showed an interaction between the first person and a second person (the relational segment). When compared with a resting baseline, both the single person and the relational segments yielded activation in areas known to be relevant to socially important stimuli, such as the face fusiform area, inferior frontal mirror areas, and superior temporal areas responding to actions and biological motion. Moreover, two medial cortical areas, the dorsomedial prefrontal cortex and the medial parietal cortex, revealed signal increases compared with the resting baseline. The relational segment of the clip also yielded signal increases in all these areas compared with the single-person segment of the clip (Iacoboni et al., 2004). What is notable here is that the dorsomedial prefrontal and medial parietal cortices belong to a set of areas that are known collectively as the default state areas of the human brain. The reason is that these areas tend to show task-independent deactivation in a wide variety of experimental conditions. This puzzling feature led researchers to assign functions to these regions on the basis of the experimental conditions that deactivated these areas less (Mitchell, Heatherton, & Macrae, 2002). However, this interpretational approach is quite unusual. Typically, functions are assigned to brain systems on the basis of the experimental conditions that increase activity in the neural systems under investigation. What we proposed on the basis of our findings is that one of the default states of humans is to "think socially," explicitly or implicitly, and that the cortical areas mostly engaged with this continuous social thinking are the ones that are deactivated when artificial laboratory tasks with very little ecological validity are used. Other reports have recently supported our suggestion (Greene, Sommerville, Nystrom, Darley, & Cohen, 2001; Mitchell, Macrae, & Banajia, 2004; Rilling, Sanfrey, Aronson, Nystrom, & Cohen, 2004).

Interestingly, these medial prefrontal and medial parietal areas show signal increase in politically sophisticated individuals while these participants respond to political questions. In contrast, political novices (that is, people who know and care little about politics) show decreased activity in these medial areas while responding to political questions (Schreiber & Iacoboni, unpublished observations). These political novices behave like typical participants in a typical cognitive experiment. Taken together, these findings suggest that the activity of these areas truly reflect an existential form of skill. Politically sophisticated people think about politics almost continuously. Politics is certainly one of the fabrics of their lives. We are all skilled at understanding social relationships; we do it all the time. The activity in these medial cortical areas seems to correlate with this existential form of skill. If this is correct, we can predict that people with social problems, such as individuals with autism, should show reduced activity in medial prefrontal and medial parietal cortex while watching social interactions, compared with control participants, as they show reduced activity in mirror neuron areas when observing and imitating facial emotional expressions (Dapretto et al., 2006).

CONCLUSION

In this chapter, I invited the reader to look at things with different eyes. We are so entrenched in our way of doing science that we take for granted assumptions that may need to be rediscussed. Some of these assumptions are so basic that they often mold our own language, making it very difficult to see things differently. I hope I provided some evidence from the neuroscience of social behavior that will invite people to adopt, at least temporarily, a different interpretational perspective. This approach may disclose a whole new world.

ACKNOWLEDGMENTS

This work was supported by the Brain Mapping Medical Research Organization, the Brain Mapping Support Foundation, the Pierson–Lovelace Foundation, the Ahmanson Foundation, Tamkin Foundation, the Jennifer Jones Simon Foundation, the Capital Group Companies Charitable Foundation, the Robson family, the William M. and Linda R. Dietel Philanthropic Fund at the Northern Piedmont Community Foundation, the Northstar Fund, and grants from the National Center for Research Resources (Nos. RR12169, RR13642 and RR08655), the National Science Foundation (No. REC-0107077), and the National Institute of Mental Health (No. MH63680).

REFERENCES

Adolphs, R., Damasio, H., Tranel, D., Cooper, G., & Damasio, A. R. (2000). A role for somatosensory cortices in the visual recognition of emotion as revealed by three-dimensional lesion mapping. *Journal of Neuroscience, 20,* 2683–2690.

Andler, D. (2000). Context and background: Dreyfus and cognitive science. In M. Wrathall & J. Malpas (Eds.), *Heidegger, coping, and cognitive science* (pp. 137–159). Cambridge, MA: MIT Press.

Aziz-Zadeh, L., Iacoboni, M., Zaidel, E., Wilson, S., & Mazziotta, J. (2004). Left hemisphere motor facilitation in response to manual action sounds. *European Journal of Neuroscience, 19*(9), 2609–2612.

Aziz-Zadeh, L., Maeda, F., Zaidel, E., Mazziotta, J., & Iacoboni, M. (2002).

Lateralization in motor facilitation during action observation: A TMS study. *Experimental Brain Research, 144*(1), 127–131.

Berti, A., & Frassinetti, F. (2000). When far becomes near: Remapping of space by tool use. *Journal of Cognitive Neuroscience, 12*(3), 415–420.

Bisiach, E., Perani, D., Vallar, G., & Berti, A. (1986). Unilateral neglect: Personal and extrapersonal. *Neuropsychologia, 24*, 759–767.

Calder, A. J., Keane, J., Manes, F., Antoun, N., & Young, A. W. (2000). Impaired recognition and experience of disgust following brain injury. *Nature Neuroscience, 3*(11), 1077–1078.

Carr, L., Iacoboni, M., Dubeau, M. C., Mazziotta, J. C., & Lenzi, G. L. (2003). Neural mechanisms of empathy in humans: A relay from neural systems for imitation to limbic areas. *Proceedings of the National Academy of Sciences of the USA, 100*(9), 5497–5502.

Chartrand, T. L., & Bargh, J. A. (1999). The chameleon effect: The perception-behavior link and social interaction. *Journal of Personality and Social Psychology, 76*(6), 893–910.

Cooke, D. F., & Graziano, M. S. (2003). Defensive movements evoked by air puff in monkeys. *Journal of Neurophysiology, 90*(5), 3317–3329.

Cooke, D. F., & Graziano, M. S. (2004). Sensorimotor integration in the precentral gyrus: Polysensory neurons and defensive movements. *Journal of Neurophysiology, 91*(4), 1648–1660.

Cooke, D. F., Taylor, C. S., Moore, T., & Graziano, M. S. (2003). Complex movements evoked by microstimulation of the ventral intraparietal area. *Proceedings of the National Academy of Sciences of the USA, 100*(10), 6163–6168.

Dapretto, M., Davies, M. S., Pfeifer, J. H., Scott, A. A., Sigman, M., Bookheimer, S. Y., et al. (2006). Understanding emotions in others: Mirror neuron dysfunction in children with autism spectrum disorders. *Nature Neuroscience, 9*(1), 28–30.

De Renzi, E., Cavalleri, F., & Facchini, S. (1996). Imitation and utilisation behaviour. *Journal of Neurology, Neurosurgery, and Psychiatry, 61*(4), 396–400.

Diehl, R. L., Lotto, A. J., & Holt, L. L. (2004). Speech perception. *Annual Review of Psychology, 55*, 149–179.

Dreyfus, H. L. (1991). *Being-in-the-world: A commentary on Heidegger's* Being and Time, *Division I*. Cambridge, MA: MIT Press.

Fadiga, L., Craighero, L., Buccino, G., & Rizzolatti, G. (2002). Speech listening specifically modulates the excitability of tongue muscles: A TMS study. *European Journal of Neuroscience, 15*, 399–402.

Fadiga, L., Fogassi, L., Pavesi, G., & Rizzolatti, G. (1995). Motor facilitation during action observation: A magnetic stimulation study. *Journal of Neurophysiology, 73*, 2608–2611.

Fodor, J. A. (1983). *The modularity of mind*. Cambridge, MA: MIT Press.

Gallese, V., Fadiga, L., Fogassi, L., & Rizzolatti, G. (1996). Action recognition in the premotor cortex. *Brain, 119*, 593–609.

Gallese, V., & Goldman, A. (1998). Mirror neurons and the simulation theory of mind-reading. *Trends in Cognitive Sciences, 2*, 493–501.

Gangitano, M., Mottaghy, F. M., & Pascual-Leone, A. (2001). Phase-specific modulation of cortical motor output during movement observation. *Neuroreport, 12*(7), 1489–1492.

Graziano, M. S., & Gross, C. G. (1998). Spatial maps for the control of movement. *Current Opinion in Neurobiology, 8*(2), 195–201.

Graziano, M. S., Hu, X. T., & Gross, C. G. (1997). Coding the locations of objects in the dark. *Science, 277*, 239–241.

Graziano, M. S., Reiss, L. A., & Gross, C. G. (1999). A neuronal representation of the location of nearby sounds. *Nature, 397*(6718), 428–430.

Graziano, M. S., Taylor, C. S., Moore, T., & Cooke, D. F. (2002). The cortical control of movement revisited. *Neuron, 36*(3), 349–362.

Graziano, M. S., Yap, G. S., & Gross, C. G. (1994). Coding of visual space by premotor neurons. *Science, 266*, 1054–1057.

Greene, J. D., Sommerville, R. B., Nystrom, L. E., Darley, J. M., & Cohen, J. D. (2001). An fMRI investigation of emotional engagement in moral judgment. *Science, 293*(5537), 2105–2108.

Halligan, P. W., & Marshall, J. C. (1991). Left neglect for near but not for far space in man. *Nature, 350*, 498–500.

Hatfield, E., Cacioppo, J. T., & Rapson, R. L. (1994). *Emotional contagion.* Paris: Cambridge University Press.

Haugeland, J. (1985). *Artificial intelligence: The very idea.* Cambridge, MA: MIT Press.

Haxby, J. V., Gobbini, M. I., Furey, M. L., Ishai, A., Schouten, J. L., & Pietrini, P. (2001). Distributed and overlapping representations of faces and objects in ventral temporal cortex. *Science, 293*(5539), 2425–2430.

Heidegger, M. (1927). *Being and time.* New York: Harper & Row.

Heiser, M., Iacoboni, M., Maeda, F., Marcus, J., & Mazziotta, J. C. (2003). The essential role of Broca's area in imitation. *European Journal of Neuroscience, 17*(5), 1123–1128.

Iacoboni, M. (2003). Understanding intentions through imitation. In S. H. Johnson (Ed.), *Taking action: Cognitive neuroscience perspective on intentional acts* (pp. 107–138). Cambridge, MA: MIT Press.

Iacoboni, M. (2005). Understanding others: Imitation, language, empathy. In S. Hurley & N. Chater (Eds.), *Perspectives on imitation: From mirror neurons to memes* (pp. 77–99). Cambridge, MA: MIT Press.

Iacoboni, M., Kaplan, J., & Wilson, S. (in press). A neural architecture for imitation and intentional relations. In C. Nehaniv & K. Dautenhahn (Eds.), *Imitation and social learning in robots, humans and animals: Behavioural, social and communicative dimensions.* Cambridge, UK: Cambridge University Press.

Iacoboni, M., Lieberman, M. D., Knowlton, B. J., Molnar-Szakacs, I., Moritz, M., Throop, C. J., et al. (2004). Watching social interactions produces dorso-medial prefrontal and medial parietal bold fMRI signal increases compared to a resting baseline. *NeuroImage, 21*(3), 1167–1173.

Iacoboni, M., Molnar-Szakacs, I., Gallese, V., Buccino, G., Mazziotta, J., & Rizzolatti, G. (2005). Grasping the intentions of others with one's own mirror neuron system. *PLoS Biology, 3*(3), e79.

Iacoboni, M., Woods, R. P., Brass, M., Bekkering, H., Mazziotta, J. C., & Rizzolatti, G. (1999). Cortical mechanisms of human imitation. *Science, 286*(5449), 2526–2528.

Iriki, A., Tanaka, M., & Iwamura, Y. (1996). Coding of modified body schema during tool use by macaque postcentral neurones. *Neuroreport, 7*, 2325–2330.

Koski, L., Iacoboni, M., Dubeau, M. C., Woods, R. P., & Mazziotta, J. C. (2003). Modulation of cortical activity during different imitative behaviors. *Journal of Neurophysiology, 89*(1), 460–471.

Koski, L., Wohlschlager, A., Bekkering, H., Woods, R. P., Dubeau, M. C., Mazziotta, J. C., et al. (2002). Modulation of motor and premotor activity during imitation of target-directed actions. *Cerebral Cortex, 12*(8), 847–855.

Lhermitte, F., Pillon, B., & Serdaru, M. D. (1986). Human autonomy and the frontal lobes: Part 1. Imitation and utilization behavior: A neuropsychological study of 75 patients. *Annals of Neurology, 19*, 326–334.

Liberman, A. M., Harris, K. S., Hoffman, H. S., & Griffith, B. C. (1957). The discrimination of speech sounds within and across phoneme boundaries. *Journal of Experimental Psychology, 54*, 358–368.

Meltzoff, A. N., & Moore, M. K. (1977). Imitation of facial and manual gestures by human neonates. *Science, 198*, 74–78.

Merleau-Ponty, M. (1945). *Phenomenology of perception.* London: Routledge.

Mitchell, J. P., Heatherton, T. F., & Macrae, C. N. (2002). Distinct neural systems subserve person and object knowledge. *Proceedings of the National Academy of Sciences of the USA, 99*(23), 15238–15243.

Mitchell, J. P., Macrae, C. N., & Banaji, M. R. (2004). Encoding-specific effects of social cognition on the neural correlates of subsequent memory. *Journal of Neuroscience, 24*(21), 4912–4917.

Niedenthal, P. M., Barsalou, L. W., Winkielman, P., Krauth-Gruber, S., & Ric, F. (2005). Embodiment in attitudes, social perception, and emotion. *Personality and Social Psychology Review, 9*(3), 184–211.

Rilling, J. K., Sanfey, A. G., Aronson, J. A., Nystrom, L. E., & Cohen, J. D. (2004). The neural correlates of theory of mind within interpersonal interactions. *NeuroImage, 22*(4), 1694–1703.

Rizzolatti, G., Camarda, R., Fogassi, M., Gentilucci, M., Luppino, G., & Matelli, M. (1988). Functional organization of inferior area 6 in the macaque monkey: II. Area f5 and the control of distal movements. *Experimental Brain Research, 71*, 491–507.

Rizzolatti, G., & Craighero, L. (2004). The mirror-neuron system. *Annu Rev Neurosci, 27*, 169–192.

Rizzolatti, G., Fogassi, L., & Gallese, V. (1997). Parietal cortex: From sight to action. *Current Opinion in Neurobiology, 7*, 562–567.

Rizzolatti, G., Riggio, L., & Sheliga, B. M. (1994). Space and selective attention. In C. Umiltà & M. Moscovitch (Eds.), *Attention and performance: Vol. 15. Conscious and nonconscious information processing* (pp. 231–265). Cambridge, MA: MIT Press.

Strafella, A. P., & Paus, T. (2000). Modulation of cortical excitability during action observation: A transcranial magnetic stimulation study. *Neuroreport, 11*, 2289–2292.

Taylor, C. (2000). What's wrong with foundationalism? Knowledge, agency, and world. In M. Wrathall & J. Malpas (Eds.), *Heidegger, coping, and cognitive science* (pp. 115–134). Cambridge, MA: MIT Press.

Wapner, S., & Cirillo, L. (1968). Imitation of a model's hand movement: Age changes in transposition of left–right relations. *Child Development, 39*, 887–894.

Wilson, S. M., Saygin, A. P., Sereno, M. I., & Iacoboni, M. (2004). Listening to speech activates motor areas involved in speech production. *Nature Neuroscience, 7*(7), 701–702.

21

Affiliative Responses to Stress
A SOCIAL NEUROSCIENCE MODEL

Shelley E. Taylor and Gian C. Gonzaga

When scientists choose a metaphor to characterize stress, they usually pick "fight or flight." This characterization of stress response seems incomplete when one realizes that humans have few of the physical resources necessary to fight or flee. Humans do not have sharp teeth, claws, or thick skin. We are slow of foot and unable to fly or hide under water. One advantage humans do have is the impulse to affiliate with others, and we propose that this is a core aspect of human responses to stress. Human survival has depended on group living, and manifold evidence shows that under conditions of threat, human beings come together to protect one another (Caporeal, 1997). On the one hand, this observation is so obvious that it scarcely needs documentation. Despite this fact, until recently little attention has been devoted to understanding why humans affiliate under stress and the biological underpinnings of that affiliation.

We begin this chapter by characterizing existing models of stress responses, focusing on the fight-or-flight response. We then describe a biobehavioral model of affiliative responses to stress that our laboratory has been developing over the past few years. From animal studies and our own data, we infer that there is an affiliative system that signals the need for affiliation, especially in response to stress, in some animal species and in humans. We suggest that elevations in the neuropeptide oxytocin (OT) may act as a biological marker, indicating that social affiliations have fallen below an adequate level to meet current challenges. This might occur, for example, if there were chronic gaps in one's social network, such as separation or a loss of companionship, or it might occur in response to externally imposed demands from the environment, such as those resulting from stress or threats. Once signaled, the need for social contacts is met through purposeful social behavior, such as affiliation. Supportive affiliative contacts reduce biological and psychological stress responses, but contact with hostile or nonsupportive others in times of stress can augment these stress responses. The vital importance of quality of social ties in stressful circumstances points to a need to understand the mechanisms that prompt affiliation under stress.

We hypothesize that OT may act, roughly, as a social thermostat that is responsive to adequacy of social resources, which prompts affiliative behavior when social resources fall below an adequate level and which reduces biological and psychological stress responses once positive social contacts are (re)established. Although some of the links in the model are currently speculative, the bones of a model that may characterize affiliative processes, especially in response to stress, appear to be in place.

RESPONSES TO STRESS: FIGHT OR FLIGHT

The dominant conception of human and animal biobehavioral responses to stress has been the fight-or-flight response (Cannon, 1932). Fight or flight has two aspects—a behavioral component and a biological component. The behavioral component of fight or flight is obvious: In response to a threat, one can become aggressive and mount an antagonistic response to the threatening circumstances or one can flee, either literally or metaphorically. Among the responses that contemporary stress researchers interpret as flight behavior are coping strategies such as social withdrawal and patterns of substance use, especially drug and alcohol abuse.

The biological component of fight or flight depends on two interacting stress systems, the sympathetic nervous system and the hypothalamic–pituitary–adrenocortical (HPA) axis. The actions of the sympathetic-adrenomedullary (SAM) system are mediated primarily by the catecholamines norepinephrine and epinephrine, which exert effects on adrenergic receptors in target tissues to produce, among other changes, increases in heart rate and blood pressure, dilation of the airways, and enhanced availability of glucose and fatty acids for energy. These coordinated responses facilitate short-term mobilization of an organism's resources for rapid, intense physical activity. Threatening stressors also engage the HPA axis. Corticotropin-releasing hormone (CRH), produced in the paraventricular nuclei (PVN) of the hypothalamus, stimulates the secretion of adrenocorticotropic hormone (ACTH) by the anterior pituitary, resulting in the release of glucocorticoids, such as cortisol. Glucocorticoids serve an important function at low basal levels by permitting or restoring processes that prime homeostatic defense mechanisms. This integrated pattern of HPA-axis activation modulates a wide range of functions, including energy release and immune activity.

These two systems are important because they account for both the protective effects of stress responses and their long-term costs. Together these systems shunt reserves of energy for fight or flight, and the subjective experience is arousal and often fear or anxiety. As such, these responses have short-term benefits under stressful circumstances because they mobilize the body to meet the demands of pressing situations and then prime homeostatic mechanisms that restore the body to its previous functioning. With repeated or recurrent stress, however, biological stress responses can have long-term costs that have implications for health (McEwen, 1998). For example, excessive or repeated discharge of epinephrine or norepinephrine can lead to the suppression of cellular immune function, produce hemodynamic changes such as chronic increases in blood pressure, and provoke abnormal heart rhythms. Glucocorticoids have immunosuppressive effects, and stress-related increases in cortisol have been tied to an increased susceptibility to infectious disorders (Cohen et al., 2002). More long-lasting elevations in glucocorticoids, such as occur in chronically or recurrently stressful environments, are prognostic for the development of hypertension, cardiovascular disease, and insulin resistance, enhancing risk for diabetes, among other disorders (McEwen & Lasley, 2002).

Research on human responses to stress has focused on fight or flight, both because it was one of the earliest responses to stress identified by research and because the scientific study of stress is based heavily on animal studies, which provide ample evidence for fight or flight. When stress researchers began to study stress in human beings, they borrowed from the animal paradigm in ways conducive to identifying fight-or-flight responses in humans as well (see Taylor et al., 2000, for a review). Although fighting and fleeing are unquestionably in the repertoire of human responses to threats and stress, there are at least two reasons to suspect that they are unlikely to be the only responses, and perhaps not even the dominant responses. First, fighting could leave vulnerable offspring at risk for predation. Fleeing, likewise, may have been impractical because abandoning a young infant would almost always be fatal to the offspring, and fleeing with an infant or young toddler might slow the caregiver down enough to be at enhanced risk for attack. Human beings would not have survived as a species had they not developed stress responses that protected their offspring in times of danger.

Moreover, fighting or fleeing may not be humans' best defense against predators. Humans evolved in small hunter–gatherer groups. Coming together as a group, instead of fleeing or fighting on one's own, would provide more hands for defense and perhaps confuse or intimidate a predator. These groups would have provided advantages in the face of other stressors as well, such as information about resource location. In short, there are good reasons to think humans have evolved to use social relationships as a primary resource to deal with stressful circumstances.

TEND AND BEFRIEND

To address social responses to stress, our laboratory has been working with the metaphor "tend and befriend" (Taylor, 2002; Taylor et al., 2000). Our position is that under conditions of stress, tending to offspring and affiliating with others (what we call befriending) are at least as common responses to stress in humans as fight or flight.

From animal studies and our own data, we infer that there is an affiliative neurocircuitry that prompts affiliation, especially in response to stress, in many animal species, and especially in humans. We suggest that this system regulates social-approach behavior and does so in much the same way as occurs for other appetitive needs. That is, just as people have basic needs, such as hunger, thirst, sexual drives, and other appetites, they also need to maintain an adequate level of protective and rewarding social relationships.

Just as occurs for these other appetites, we suggest that there is a biological signaling system that comes into play if one's affiliations fall below an adequate level. Once signaled, the appetitive need is met through purposeful social behavior, such as affiliation. If social contacts are hostile or unsupportive, then psychological and biological stress responses are heightened. If social contacts are supportive and comforting, stress responses decline. Positive contacts then lead to a decline in need and, in the context of stress, a decline in stress responses. The fact that affiliation may look very much like other appetitive needs is not coincidental. Because biological neurocircuitries tend to be efficient, the dopamine and opioid systems that are recruited for other reward-based systems are likely to be recruited for the satisfaction of affiliative needs, as well (see Depue & Morrone-Strupinksy, 2005).

In building our model, we have focused heavily on OT and the opioid system (see Figure 21.1). We maintain that OT and opioids are released in response to (at least some) stressors, especially those that may trigger affiliative needs; OT prompts affiliative behavior in response to stress, in conjunction with dopaminergic and opioid systems; and OT, in conjunction with positive social contacts, attenuates biological stress responses (SNS, HPA axis) that can arise in response to social threats. This OT–opioid–dopaminergic system is an appetitive system that regulates social approach behavior and recruits the neurocircuitry for reward in its enactment. Finally, we suggest that some of the health benefits associated with social support and social integration may be mediated by this appetitive social-approach system via attenuation of threat responses. We address each of these links.

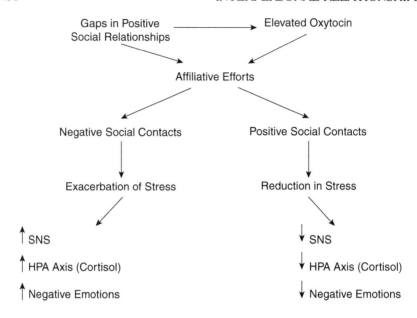

FIGURE 21.1. A model of affiliative responses to stress.

SEPARATION DISTRESS AND OPIOID FUNCTIONING

Affiliation is vital to the survival of human beings. Accordingly, there are likely to be biobehavioral mechanisms that are sensitive to social threats or loss of social contact, resulting in social distress and consequent efforts to remedy the situation. A paradigm for such a system is separation distress, which has been studied primarily in young animals and human infants. When the young are separated from the mother, separation distress in offspring can result, especially during particular developmental periods. The experience of separation leads to distress vocalizations (e.g., crying in human infants or active searching for the caregiver in toddlers) that may prompt the return of the caregiver.

This system appears to depend, in part, on brain opioids. Evidence consistent with this pathway includes the fact that brain opioids reduce separation distress and that drugs such as morphine reduce distress vocalizations in animals (Panksepp, 1998). In experimental animal studies, opioid consumption can be increased by depriving animals of companionship (Alexander, Coambs, & Hadaway, 1978). Mice that lack the μ-opioid receptor gene emit fewer distress vocalizations when separated from their mothers, further suggesting that endogenous opioid binding is a significant basis of infant attachment behavior (Moles, Kieffer, & D'Amato, 2004). From data such as these, researchers have inferred that the neurocircuitry for social pain draws on the neurocircuitry for physical pain, a hypothesis that has recently been lent additional credibility by neuroimaging studies in humans (Eisenberger, Lieberman, & Williams, 2003). Opioids also appear to be involved in the experience of positive social interaction (Panksepp, 1998). OT may underlie some of these processes as well, as we next suggest.

OXYTOCIN AND SOCIAL DISTRESS

OT is a hypothalamic neuropeptide that is implicated in human and animal stress responses (Miaskowski, Ong, Lukic, & Haldar, 1988). Although its exact role in stress processes has not been fully identified, its potential role in modulating psychological and biological stress responses has garnered particular scientific interest (Taylor et al., 2000).

Researchers have theorized that OT is implicated in infant bonding and in processes involving separation and reunification (Panksepp, 1998). For example, Nelson and Panksepp (1996) separated rat pups from their mothers for several hours and then reunited them for half an hour. Before each reunion, the mothers' ventral surface was sprayed with a distinctive odor; control animals were reunited with a cotton pad permeated with the same order. Following 3 days of this testing, the pups were tested for attraction to the conditioned odor. Only pups that had been reunited with the mothers showed selective approach and attraction to the odor. The attraction was blocked in animals that had received an OT antagonist, suggesting that OT is implicated in this pattern. Thus there appears to be a role for OT in the neurocircuitry that underlies separation and reunification.

Our research has focused on the role of OT in social distress in adults. Adults, as well as infants and young children, experience gaps in their social relationships and may experience an analog of separation distress, which may implicate the same biological systems as in the young. OT is known to be released in response to some stressors (Sapolsky, 1992), but, in humans, the kinds of stress that may be associated with OT have, until recently, been largely unknown. Drawing on the literature relating OT to separation distress, we hypothesized that elevated OT may be a marker of the need for positive social contact (Taylor et al., 2006).

To examine these processes, we assessed the stress responses of older women who either were or were not on hormone therapy (Taylor et al., 2006). Levels of OT are strongly augmented by estrogen, and so animal studies that have examined the effects of OT often use estrogen-treated females (McCarthy, 1995). Postmenopausal women are a human analog for this paradigm, because postmenopausal women produce little or no estrogen, whereas women who are on hormone therapy receive a dose of estrogen every day. Accordingly, a sample that has substantial variability in estrogen levels is likely to also produce substantial variability in OT, as was true in our work. As such, one may see what OT's role may be with respect to stress (Taylor et al., 2006).

To test our hypothesis that OT is a marker for social distress, we gave women measures of psychological and social functioning and related their responses to levels of OT. The questionnaires included assessments of gaps in relationships (that is, whether the women had experienced any decline in their contacts with significant others) and assessments of how positive and how negative their relationships with significant others were. For comparative purposes, the women filled out a detailed assessment of psychological distress, the Symptom Checklist–90 (SCL-90; Derogatis & Spencer, 1982), as well as a self-esteem scale (Rosenberg, 1965).

Women who were experiencing gaps in their social relationships had elevated levels of OT, as we had predicted. In particular, women with higher levels of OT were more likely to report reduced contact with their mothers, with their best friends, with a pet, and with the social groups of which they were a part. OT levels were sensitive to the absence of positive relations with the partner, as well. Women who reported that their husbands were not supportive were more likely to have high levels of OT. Specifically, women with high levels of OT reported that their husbands were less likely to understand the way they felt about things and less likely to care for them and that they could not open up to their husbands if they needed to share their concerns. Poor quality of the marital relationship and infrequent display of affection by one's partner were also associated with higher levels of OT. These findings suggest that OT may be sensitive to the absence of positive aspects of significant social relationships.

Similar results were found by Turner and her colleagues (Turner, Altemus, Enos, Cooper, & McGuinness, 1999), who looked at the relation of OT to social relationships in a sample of young women. They found that elevated OT was associated with anxiety over relationships, with perceived coldness or intrusiveness of relationships, and with not being in a primary romantic relationship. Taken together, these two studies (Taylor et al., 2005; Turner et al., 1999) are consistent with the inference that OT may signal gaps or problems in social support.

However, to make this case requires several additional steps. First, one would have to rule out the possibility that OT is simply related to any kind of distress. We found that OT was not related to self-esteem or to general psychological distress, only to gaps in or problems with positive relationships. This evidence for discriminant validity suggests that the distress that OT signals may be distinctively social in nature. A second step for establishing discriminant validity would be to show that OT is related to social distress and that other stress hormones are not. As a comparison, we examined the relation of cortisol to the social indicators that were associated with OT. None of the correlations was significant.

Because we did not manipulate levels of OT, there is a possibility that causality goes in the other direction. Although the alternative direction of causality cannot be entirely ruled out, some data are inconsistent with it. The women with high levels of OT were more likely to have recently lost their mothers or their pets to death, or in the case of their mothers, to mental and physical deterioration. It is unlikely that women high in OT would be more likely than other women to experience the deaths or deterioration of their mothers or their pets. Consequently, it is more likely that elevated OT is a marker of gaps in positive relationships.

Our portrayal of OT as a stress hormone that is naturally elevated in response to social distress conflicts sharply with the characterization of OT that has appeared in some of the scientific literature and much of the popular literature. A substantial amount of research has documented the anxiolytic effects of OT (McCarthy, 1995), tying OT to a relaxed, calm psychological state. This view of the "emotional" underpinnings of OT has also found its way into the popular literature, in which OT has, for example, been characterized as a "feel-good" or "cuddling" hormone (e.g., CBS Evening News, May 19, 2000), among similar characterizations.

There are at least two possible reconciliations of these seemingly opposing views. One possibility is that basal OT reflects social distress but that OT pulsatility is associated with calm and companionable feelings (Turner et al., 1999). OT pulsatility, as induced exogenously and in conjunction with affiliation, may produce the anxiolytic effects of OT that have been so widely documented in the experimental animal literature (McCarthy, 1995). A second possibility stems from the fact that past research has not consistently disentangled the effects of OT from the effects of affiliative contact. The pleasurable feelings credited to OT may be due instead to its positive affiliative consequences and/or to OT's impact on other aspects of the affiliative neurocircuitry, for example, modulation of pathways that implicate reward, such as the mesolimbic dopamine and opioid systems (Depue & Morrone-Strupinsky, 2005; Young, Lim, Gingrich, & Insel, 2001). That is, returning to our model (Figure 21.1), it may be the case that OT initially signals distress and subsequently induces affiliative efforts, which result in affiliative contact. If those contacts are supportive, then affiliation should produce accompanying positive feelings, perhaps underpinned by dopamine and opioid involvement.

RELATION OF OT AND OPIOIDS TO AFFILIATION

If OT is related to social distress, as we suggest, then as an affiliative hormone, OT may provide an impetus for social contact to ameliorate stress. Taylor et al. (2000) raised this possibility in their tend-and-befriend account of female responses to stress. Specifically, we hypothesized that the seeking of social support in response to stress may be mediated, in part, by the release of OT in response to stress.

Manifold evidence, most of which has come from animal studies, relates OT to affiliation. In a typical study, a rat, monkey, or sheep is injected with OT, and the impact on behavior is observed. Exogenous administration of OT has been found to increase maternal behavior in several species (see Carter, Lederhendler, & Kirkpatrick, 1999; Fahrbach, Morrell, & Pfaff, 1985; Kendrick, Keverne, & Baldwin, 1987). Opioid mechanisms are also implicated in these processes. Administration of opioid antagonists, for example, such as naloxone or naltrexone, results in less caregiving and protective behavior toward infants in rhesus monkeys (Martel, Nevison, Rayment, Simpson, & Keverne, 1993), inhibits maternal behavior in sheep (Kendrick & Keverne, 1989), and diminishes the attractive qualities of conditioned maternal cues in rats (Panksepp, Nelson, & Bekkedal, 1999). The facts that OT is elevated in response to at least some stressors and that it provides an impetus for maternal behavior represent important links for the "tending" aspect of the tend-and-befriend model (Taylor, 2002; Taylor et al., 2000). Specifically, it suggests that OT may function both as a stress indicator and as an impetus for protection of offspring.

Animals demonstrate a preference for other animals in whose presence they have previously experienced high brain OT and opioid activity, suggesting that companionship has some of the same biological underpinnings as maternal–infant bonding (Panksepp, 1998). Social contact is enhanced and aggression is diminished following OT treatment in estrogen-treated female prairie voles (Witt, Carter, & Walton, 1990), and the exogenous administration of OT in rats causes an increase in social contact and in grooming (Carter, De Vries, & Getz, 1995; Drago, Pederson, Caldwell, and Prange, 1986; Witt, Winslow, & Insel, 1992).

With reference to humans, Carter (1998) suggested that OT may be at the core of many affiliative contacts, including mother–infant attachments, adult pair bonds, and friendships. However, in humans, the relation of OT to affiliative behavior is somewhat more conjectural, in part because it is hard to get at OT's central nervous system activity in humans. As a result, researchers have related OT to behaviors observed in people with naturally high levels of OT, especially nursing mothers (e.g., Light et al., 2000), or have administered OT exogenously. Despite the complexities of tests in humans, OT is thought to underlie social bonding, including initial formation of adult pair bonds (Panksepp, 1998).

Opioid involvement is implicated in affiliative activity as well. Jalowiec, Calcagnetti, and Fanselow (1989), for example, found that administration of an opioid antagonist suppressed juvenile social behavior. Opioid-blocking agents also lead to reduced social activity and grooming in animals. For example, Martel et al. (1993) administered naltrexone to female rhesus monkeys and observed a decline in social grooming. Opioid mechanisms appear to be implicated in human affiliative responses as well. Jamner, Alberts, Leigh, and Klein (1998) administered naltrexone to college students and found that, in women only, it increased the amount of time that women spent alone, reduced the amount of time they spent with friends, reduced the likelihood that they would contact their friends, and reduced the pleasantness of their interactions with friends. It thus appears that a fairly broad array of affiliative behaviors may be subserved by OT and opioid mechanisms.

OT and opioids, then, are implicated in affiliative behaviors, a fact that takes on particular significance in the context of stress. McCarthy (1995) has suggested that, for animals to exhibit social responses to stress, arousal must be sufficiently controlled to avoid the aggression or flight behavior that might otherwise ensue. Similarly, Taylor (Taylor, 2002; Taylor et al., 2000) has suggested that at least partial inhibition of the fight-or-flight response may be required for tending-and-befriending activities to be initiated. Thus one would expect to see evidence that, over time, OT in conjunction with opioids leads to affiliative contact, which, when positive, leads to reduced stress responses.

RELATION OF OT AND OPIOID FUNCTIONING TO STRESS RESPONSES

OT has been related to reduced autonomic activity and HPA-axis responses to stress. In species as varied as rats, sheep, and prairie voles, exogenous administration of OT or stimulation of OT secretion via stroking has been found to decrease sympathetic reactivity (Uvnäs-Moberg, Ahlenius, Hillegaart, & Alster, 1994), blood pressure (Petersson, Alster, Lundeberg, & Uvnäs-Moberg, 1996), pain sensitivity, and corticosterone levels, among other findings suggestive of a reduced stress response (Carter, 1998; Insel, 1997; Uvnäs-Moberg, 1997; Uvnäs-Moberg et al., 1994).

As noted earlier, a substantial amount of research has also documented the anxiolytic effects of OT (McCarthy, 1995). For example, experimental evidence from animal studies suggests that exogenous administration of OT enhances sedation and relaxation (Uvnäs-Moberg, et al., 1994). OT has also been tied to behavioral signs of reduced fearfulness (such as less freezing and more exploration) among female rodents in open field tests (Mantella, Vollmer, Li, & Amico, 2003; McCarthy, 1995).

Although the stress-reducing properties of OT are less well documented in humans, the existing research is consistent with the evidence from animal studies. High levels of OT or exogenous administration of OT in humans produces decreases in sympathetic activity (e.g. Light et al., 2000; Uvnäs-Moberg, 1997) and inhibits the secretion of adrenocorticotropic hormone (ACTH) and cortisol (Altemus, Deuster, Gallivan, Carter, & Gold, 1995; Chiodera & Legros, 1981). For example, Heinrichs, Baumgartner, Kirschbaum, and Ehlert (2003) administered or did not administer OT to 37 men via nasal spray and found reduced anxiety and lower cortisol levels during the course of a laboratory stress challenge (the Trier Social Stress Task; TSST) among those who had received OT; the reduced cortisol response was especially pronounced in those men who also experienced social support from a friend. Studies comparing breast-feeding mothers (in whom OT levels are high) with bottle-feeding mothers have found lower anxiety among the breast-feeding mothers (Virden, 1988) and lower anxiety, depression, stress, and guilt following breast feeding (which prompts OT release) as compared with bottle feeding (Modahl & Newton, 1979).

The inhibitory action of OT on cortisol secretion may be due to hypophysial inhibition of ACTH release, as well as to effects at the adrenal gland level (Legros, Chiodera, & Geenen, 1988). OT also increases the sensitivity of brain opioid systems. If OT injection is accompanied by naloxone, cortisol levels do not change, but OT administration alone leads to significant reduction in cortisol secretion (Coiro et al., 1985). These findings suggest that some of the antistress properties of OT may be mediated by an opioid pathway.

Thus the evidence that OT attenuates stress responses is strong in animal studies and highly suggestive in human studies. However, as noted earlier, many of the studies that document the stress-reducing qualities of OT have not disentangled the effects of OT from affiliation. We hypothesize that the stress-reducing qualities of OT may depend on rewarding social contact, but that hostile or unsupportive social contacts during stressful times will exacerbate psychological and biological stress responses.

We examined this issue in our recent research (Taylor et al., 2005). We recruited postmenopausal women who were or were not on hormone therapy who completed a laboratory challenge task, specifically the TSST. The TSST involves the preparation and delivery of a speech to an unresponsive audience and performing difficult mental arithmetic under harassing conditions. It reliably increases heart rate, blood pressure, and cortisol responses to challenge (Kirschbaum, Pirke, & Hellhammer, 1995). Blood draws were taken from an indwelling intravenous catheter at three time points to assess oxytocin levels at baseline, postchallenge, and recovery. Eight saliva samples were taken across the stress challenge to assess cortisol, and blood pressure was also taken at these times.

We found that women low in oxytocin showed the expected increase in cortisol in response to stress tasks, followed by a decrease in cortisol during recovery. By contrast, women with high OT levels had significantly higher cortisol levels initially, which decreased early on in the laboratory procedures but which became elevated again following the stress tasks (see Figure 21.2). Cortisol levels then decreased during recovery. Although not definitive, this pattern suggests that elevated OT, in conjunction with relationship distress, is associated with greater, not less, HPA activity. The next section integrates these observations into an overall perspective on affiliation under stress.

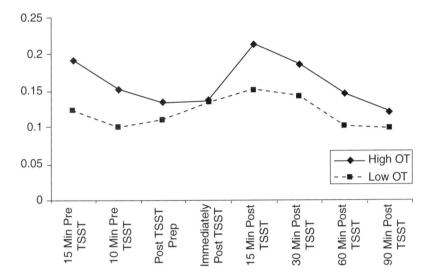

FIGURE 21.2. Cortisol levels across stress task for women with high and low levels of oxytocin.

A MODEL OF AFFILIATION UNDER STRESS

Humans and animals need positive social relationships. Relationships are essential to survival, because others provide the protection needed to maintain both one's own safety and that of offspring. We suggest that humans have evolved a warning system that alerts them to gaps in their relationships that may signal a threat to safety. OT, as well as opioids, is implicated in this process. In our research, OT is distinctively associated with gaps in positive relationships and with an absence of rewarding emotional contact with a partner.

Additional evidence that affiliation engages a biobehavioral social-approach regulatory system that draws on OT, opioids, and the dopamine neurocircuitry is provided in a recent review by Depue and Morrone-Strupinsky (2004). Although their goal was to characterize the trait of affiliation, they suggested, as we have, that affiliation is a reward-based system that has appetitive and consummatory phases, as other reward-based systems have. They suggest that the appetitive phase of affiliation especially implicates dopamine and that opioids are implicated in the consummatory phase of affiliation. Our analysis, although at a different level than that of Depue and Morrone-Strupinsky's (2005), is largely consistent with their model. However, our model departs from theirs in a few respects. First, we believe that the research evidence implicates opioids at both the appetitive and consummatory phases of affiliation. The fact that opioids are involved in separation distress and in seeking affiliative contacts supports this conclusion. Second, we suggest that the physical quiescence often associated with affiliative contact not only is due to opioid involvement at the consummatory phase of affiliation, as Depue and Morrone-Strupinsky (2005) maintain, but also results from attenuation of HPA-axis and sympathetic activity via oxytocinergic and opioid pathways, at least under stressful circumstances and in conjunction with positive social contacts.

Third, we suggest that OT and, as discussed shortly, vasopressin (AVP) have a greater role in affiliation than the relatively modest role accorded them in the Depue and Morrone-Strupinksy (2005) model. Depue and Morrone-Strupinsky suggest that OT and AVP may be implicated primarily in the perception and recognition of and memory for affiliative partners. They point out that affiliation relies on the underlying capacity to experience the rewards elicited by affiliative stimuli and that much social affiliation depends on the establishment of conditioned preferences for specific individuals, which is dependent on their reward capacity. As noted, our model suggests a more central role of OT and, to be discussed shortly, AVP, extending beyond memory for affiliative stimuli and the ability to recognize familiar conspecifics to include the signaling of affiliative needs, the initiation of affiliative activity, and concomitant impact on psychological and biological stress responses. Although one would hardly disagree with the conclusion that some individuals are more rewarding than others, we suggest that the affiliative neurocircuitry is only somewhat dependent on the establishment of conditioned preferences for specific individuals. Indeed, what is notable about human affiliative behavior, especially under stress, is that it occurs not only with familiar others but often with complete strangers. Despite these differences, the model of Depue and Morrone-Strupinsky (2005) and our own model have substantial points of commonality, especially in their overall characterization of affiliative processes as an appetitive system.

BENEFITS OF AFFILIATION UNDER STRESS

What would be the benefits of a biobehavioral system that is sensitive to relationship quality, that prompts affiliation, and that modulates stress responses? Looking at the affiliative system from the standpoint of evolutionary theory suggests clear survival benefits of a biobehavioral mechanism that signals gaps in social support and prompts affiliation for communal responses to stress. Individual safety, as well as the safety of offspring, would be ensured by such a system. What is intriguing, though, is that such a system continues to have such powerful effects on health and survival into the present day. Few of us encounter predators on a daily basis that provide threats to our own safety or to our children. Yet this biobehavioral system, nonetheless, has a major effect on health through social support and social integration.

Research consistently shows that social support reduces psychological distress, such as depression or anxiety (e.g. Fleming, Baum, Gisriel, & Gatchel, 1982; Lin, Ye, & Ensel, 1999), and promotes psychological adjustment to a broad array of stressful conditions (see Taylor, 2007, for a review). Because anxiety and depression are significant predictors of the progression of several chronic diseases, the amelioration of distress via affiliation may represent one pathway by which OT and opioid mechanisms exert effects on health.

In both animal and human studies, social isolation is tied to a significantly enhanced risk of mortality (House, Landis & Umberson, 1988) and a heightened risk of both chronic and acute health disorders (Taylor, 2007). Although not all the mechanisms that explain these strong relationships are known, one key pathway is via stress responses (Cacioppo & Hawkley, 2003). When humans are socially isolated, their sympathetic nervous system and HPA-axis responses to stress may continue unabated, leading to a state of immunological vulnerability. People without social support systems, for example, are more vulnerable to infectious disorders (Cohen, Doyle, Skoner, Rabin, & Gwaltney, 1997). Correspondingly, the positive impact of social ties on health outcomes is as powerful as or more powerful than established (negative) risk factors for diseases, including lipid levels and smoking.

Whether the attenuation of stress responses by OT and opioids is sufficient to produce these clinical effects of social support is, at present, unclear. However, recent animal research on wound healing has suggested that this is a promising avenue for research (Detillion, Craft, Glasper, Prendergast, & DeVries, 2004). Specifically, in this study, Siberian hamsters received cutaneous wounds and were then exposed to immobilization stress. The stressor increased cortisol concentrations and impaired wound healing, but only in socially isolated, not in socially housed, animals. Thus social housing acted as a stress buffer. Removing cortisol via adrenalectomy eliminated the impact of the stressor on wound healing, thereby implicating the HPA axis in the wound-healing process. Of particular relevance to the current arguments, treating the isolated hamsters with OT eliminated the stress-induced increases in cortisol and facilitated wound healing; treating socially housed hamsters with an OT antagonist delayed wound healing. These data strongly imply that social contacts protect against the adverse effects of stress through a mechanism that implicates OT-induced suppression of the HPA axis. Thus there appear to be discernible clinical consequences (wound healing) of OT suppression of the HPA axis.

But social contacts during stressful times are not always positive. Indeed, social stress is one of the most taxing threats that humans experience, significantly engaging the HPA axis (Dickerson & Kemeny, 2004). During stressful times, potentially supportive companions may also be under stress, compromising their ability to be sources of comfort or help.

When this occurs, stress responses may not only not be attenuated by OT, but also may actually be exacerbated. Thus quality of social contacts would appear to be an important factor influencing the relation of OT to stress responses.

POTENTIAL SEX DIFFERENCES IN AFFILIATION UNDER STRESS

Does the model described in this chapter primarily characterize female responses to stress (Taylor et al., 2000), or might it characterize males' responses as well? The fact that OT's effects are strongly influenced by estrogen makes this an important question. Much of the animal evidence on the stress-reducing effects of OT has been conducted with females, especially estrogen-treated females, and much of the data from humans comes from women, as well.

As noted, Heinrichs et al. (2003) administered oxytocin via nasal spray to men and then put them through a laboratory stress challenge (i.e., TSST). They found the same antianxiety effects and reduction in HPA-axis activity in his men as has been found in animal studies. Clearly OT can have stress-reducing effects in men (see also Chiodera & Legros, 1981). However, because Heinrichs et al.'s paradigm used exogenous administration of OT, it showed that OT *can* have these effects in men but not that it necessarily *does*. Because OT secretion is strongly enhanced by estrogen (McCarthy, 1995) and antagonized by androgen in at least some species (Jezova, Jurankova, Mosnarova, Kiriska, & Skultetyova, 1996), OT levels may not typically be high enough in men for their stress-reducing effects to be significant (see Taylor et al., 2000, for a discussion).

Women's consistently stronger affiliative responses to stress, compared with those of men (Tamres, Janicki, & Helgeson, 2002; Taylor, 2002), is also potentially consistent with a greater role for OT in women's than men's stress responses in that OT is consistently tied to affiliative activity. Although the sex difference in affiliation under stress is moderate, it is extremely robust. In addition, the stress literature indicates that men's and women's responses to stress may assume somewhat different forms, with women disproportionately involved in reducing the stress of offspring. At the time when human stress responses evolved, work was largely segregated by sex, with men responsible for hunting and women responsible for food gathering and for child care. This segregation suggests that the selection pressures on females for stress responses that benefit both themselves and their offspring may have been greater than was true for males (Taylor, 2002).

Taking these points together, the biological underpinnings of men's social behavior under stress will likely be somewhat different than those of women. The hormone vasopressin (AVP) has a molecular structure that is very similar to that of OT. Unlike OT, AVP's effects appear to be enhanced in the presence of androgens, and so it has been thought to play a more important role in men's behavior than in women's (Panksepp, 1998). AVP is important to stress responses because it is involved in the maintenance of plasma volume and blood pressure during shock, among other functions. AVP may also be implicated in the modulation of neuroendocrine responses to stress. Exogenous administration of AVP appears to enhance HPA-axis responsivity to stress. In a review of 30 studies, Fehm-Woldsdorf and Born (1991) found that exogenous administration of AVP increased central nervous system arousal and increased anxiety, as well. AVP has also been tied to prosocial responses to stress in male prairie voles—for example, guarding and patrolling of territory, defense of mate, and defense of offspring against intruders (see Carter, 1998; Carter, et al., 1995, for a review). The AVP receptor gene is associated with pair bonding and monogamous behavior in voles (Lim et al., 2004). It is unknown whether AVP underlies men's affiliative responses to stress, and virtually nothing is known about the behavioral implications of vasopressin in humans. Thus a biobehavioral model of men's affiliative behavior under stress remains a work in progress, but a possible role for AVP in these processes would be a logical place to begin.

CONCLUSIONS

The affiliative neurocircuitry is increasingly understood, at least at the molecular level. Social neuroscientists are now beginning to integrate that neurocircuitry with its psychological and behavioral components. The evidence to date suggests that this will be a worthwhile endeavor. A picture of the emerging regulatory role of affiliation in response to stress and its biological underpinnings is coming into view.

OT and opioids appear to be biomarkers of social distress that accompany gaps in or problems with social relationships and that may provide an impetus for affiliation. OT and opioids are implicated in the seeking of affiliative contact, especially in animal studies. This reasoning is consistent with previous arguments that the human tendency to seek social support in response to stress may be mediated, in part, by OT and opioids, as well (Taylor, 2002; Taylor et al., 2000). Linking the signaling function of OT directly to affiliative behavior in humans is an important next step. OT, in conjunction with opioids, also modulates stress responses. In conjunction with positive affiliative contacts, OT attenuates psychological and biological stress responses, but in conjunction with hostile and unsupportive contacts, OT appears to exacerbate psychological and biological stress responses.

Finally, our research underscores the enduring importance of investigating the interplay of social and biological responses to stress. Recently,

great strides have been made in mapping the neurobiological underpinnings
of affiliative behavior (Carter et al., 1999; Depue & Morrone-Strupinsky,
2005; Panksepp, 1998). With each effort, the affiliative neurocircuitry and
its engagement in response to stress come closer to being understood.

ACKNOWLEDGMENT

Preparation of this chapter was supported by National Science Foundation Grant
No. SBR 9905157 to Shelley E. Taylor. Gian C. Gonzaga was supported by
National Institute of Mental Health Training Grant No. MH15750.

REFERENCES

Alexander, B., Coambs, R., & Hadaway, P. (1978). The effect of housing and gender on morphine self-administration in rats. *Psychopharmacology, 58,* 175–
179.
Altemus, M., Deuster, P., Gallivan, E., Carter, C., & Gold, P. (1995). Suppression
of hypothalamic–pituitary–adrenal responses to exercise stress in lactating
women. *Journal of Clinical Endocrinology and Metabolism, 80,* 2954–2959.
Cacioppo, J. T., & Hawkley, L. C. (2003). Social isolation and health, with an
emphasis on underlying mechanism. *Perspectives in Biology and Medicine, 46,*
S39–S52.
Cannon, W. B. (1932). *The wisdom of the body.* New York: Norton.
Caporeal, L. R. (1997). The evolution of truly social cognition: The core configura-
tion model. *Personality and Social Psychology Review, 1,* 276–298.
Carter, C. S. (1998). Neuroendocrine perspectives on social attachment and love.
Psychoneuroendocrinology, 23, 779–818.
Carter, C. S., DeVries, C., & Getz, L. L. (1995). Physiological substrates of mam-
malian monogamy: The prairie vole model. *Neuroscience and Biobehavioral
Reviews, 19,* 303–314.
Carter, C. S., Lederhendler, I. I., & Kirkpatrick, B. (1999). *The integrative neurobi-
ology of affiliation.* Cambridge, MA: MIT Press.
Chiodera, P., & Legros, J. J. (1981). Intravenous injection of synthetic oxytocin
induces a decrease of cortisol plasma level in normal man. *Comptes rendus des
seances de la Societe de biologie et de ses filiales, 175,* 546–549.
Cohen, S., Doyle, W. J., Skoner, D. P., Rabin, B. S., & Gwaltney, J. M., Jr. (1997).
Social ties and susceptibility to the common cold. *Journal of the American
Medical Association, 277,* 1940–1944.
Cohen, S., Hamrick, N., Rodriguez, M. S., Feldman, P. J., Rabin, B. S., & Manuck,
S. R. (2002). Reactivity and vulnerability to stress-associated risk for upper
respiratory illness. *Psychosomatic Medicine, 64,* 302–310.
Coiro, V., Chiodera, P., Rossi, G., Volpi, R., Salvi, M., Camellini, L., et al. (1985).
Effect of naloxone on oxytocin-induced cortisol decrease in normal men. *Acta
Endocrinologica, 108,* 261–265.
Depue, R. A., & Morrone-Strupinsky, J. V. (2005). A neurobiobehavioral model of
affiliative bonding: Implications for conceptualizing a human trait of affilia-
tion. *Behavioral and Brain Sciences, 28,* 313–395.

Derogatis, L. R., & Spencer, P. M. (1982). *The Brief Symptom Inventory (BSI): Administration and Procedures Manual–I.* Baltimore: Clinical Psychometric Research.

Detillion, C. E., Craft, T. K., Glasper, E. R., Prendergast, B. J., & DeVries, C. (2004). Social facilitation of wound healing. *Psychoneuroendocrinology, 29,* 1004–1011.

Dickerson, S. S., & Kemeny, M. E. (2004). Acute stressors and cortisol responses: A theoretical integration and synthesis of laboratory research. *Psychological Bulletin, 130,* 355–391.

Drago, F., Pederson, C. A., Caldwell, J. D., & Prange, A. J., Jr. (1986). Oxytocin potently enhances novelty-induced grooming behavior in the rat. *Brain Research, 368,* 287–295.

Eisenberger, N. I., Lieberman, M. D., & Williams, K. D. (2003). Does rejection hurt? An fMRI study of social exclusion. *Science, 302,* 290–292.

Fahrbach, S. E., Morrell, J. I., & Pfaff, D. W. (1985). Possible role for endogenous oxytocin in estrogen-facilitated maternal behavior in rats. *Neuroendocrinology, 40,* 526–532.

Fehm-Wolfsdorf, G., & Born, J. (1991). Behavioral effects of neurohypophyseal in healthy volunteers: 10 years of research. *Peptides, 12*(6), 1399–1406.

Fleming, R., Baum, A., Gisriel, M. M., & Gatchel, R. J. (1982, September). Mediating influences of social support on stress at Three Mile Island. *Journal of Human Stress,* 14–23.

Heinrichs, M., Baumgartner, T., Kirshbaum, C., & Ehlert, U. (2003). Social support and oxytocin interact to suppress cortisol and subjective responses to psychological stress. *Biological Psychiatry, 54,* 1389–1398.

House, J. S., Landis, K. R., & Umberson, D. (1988). Social relationships and health. *Science, 241,* 540–545.

Insel, T. R. (1997). A neurobiological basis of social attachment. *American Journal of Psychiatry, 154,* 726–735.

Jalowiec, J. E., Calcagnetti, D. J., & Fanselow, M. S. (1989). Suppression of juvenile social behavior requires antagonism of central opioid systems. *Pharmacology, Biochemistry, and Behavior, 33,* 697–700.

Jamner, L. D., Alberts, J., Leigh, H., & Klein, L. C. (1998, March). *Affiliative need and endogenous opioids.* Paper presented at the annual meeting of the Society of Behavioral Medicine, New Orleans, LA.

Jezova, D., Jurankova, E., Mosnarova, A., Kiriska, M., & Skultetyova, I. (1996). Neuroendocrine response during stress with relation to gender differences. *Acta Neurobiologae Experimentalis, 56,* 779–785.

Kendrick, K. M., & Keverne, E. B. (1989). Effects of intracerebroventricular infusions of naltrexone and phentolamine on central and peripheral oxytocin release and on maternal behaviour induced by vaginocervical stimulation in the ewe. *Brain Research, 505,* 329–332.

Kendrick, K. M., Keverne, E. B., & Baldwin, B. A. (1987). Intracerebroventricular oxytocin stimulates maternal behaviour in the sheep. *Neuroendocrinology, 46,* 56–61.

Kirschbaum, C., Pirke K. M., & Hellhammer D. H. (1995). Preliminary evidence for reduced cortisol responsivity to psychological stress in women using oral contraceptive medication. *Psychoneuroendocrinology, 20,* 509–514.

Legros, J. J., Chiodera, P., & Geenen, V. (1988). Inhibitory action of exogenous oxytocin on plasma cortisol in normal human subjects: Evidence of action at the adrenal level. *Neuroendocrinology, 48,* 204–206.

Light, K. C., Smith, T. E., Johns, J. M., Brownley, K. A., Hofheimer, J. A., & Amico, J. A. (2000). Oxytocin responsivity in mothers of infants: A preliminary study of relationships with blood pressure during laboratory stress and normal ambulatory activity. *Health Psychology, 19,* 560–567.

Lim, M. M., Wang, Z., Olazabal, D. E., Ren, X., Terwilliger, E. F., & Young, L. J. (2004). Enahanced partner preference in a promiscuous species by manipulating the expression of a single gene. *Nature, 429,* 754–757.

Lin, N., Ye, X., & Ensel, W. (1999). Social support and depressed mood: A structural analysis. *Journal of Health and Social Behavior, 40,* 344–359.

Mantella, R. C., Vollmer, R. R., Li, X., & Amico, J. A. (2003). Female oxytocin-deficient mice display enhanced anxiety-related behavior. *Endocrinology, 144,* 2291–2296.

Martel, F. L., Nevison, C. M., Rayment, F. D., Simpson, M. J. A., & Keverne, E. B. (1993). Opioid receptor blockade reduces maternal affect and social grooming in rhesus monkeys. *Psychoneuroimmunology, 18,* 307–321.

McCarthy, M. M. (1995). Estrogen modulation of oxytocin and its relation to behavior. In R. Ivell & J. A. Russell (Eds.), *Oxytocin: Cellular and molecular approaches in medicine and research* (pp. 235–245). New York: Plenum Press.

McEwen, B. S. (1998). Protective and damaging effects of stress mediators. *New England Journal of Medicine, 338,* 171–179.

McEwen, B. S., & Lasley, E. N. (2002). *The end of stress as we know it.* Washington, DC: National Academies Press.

Miaskowski, C., Ong, G. L., Lukic, D., & Haldar, J. (1988). Immobilization stress affects oxytocin and vasopressin levels in hypothalamic and extrahypothalamic sites. *Brain Research, 458,* 137–141.

Modahl, C., & Newton, N. (1979). Mood state differences between breast and bottle-feeding mothers. *Proceedings of the Serono Symposia: Vol. 20B, Emotion and reproduction,* (pp. 819–822).

Moles, A., Kieffer, B. L., & D'Amato, F. R. (2004). Deficit in attachment behavior in mice lacking the μ-opioid receptor gene. *Science, 304,* 1983–1985.

Nelson, E. E., & Panksepp, J. (1996). Brain substrates of infant–mother attachment: Contributions of opioids, oxytocin, and norepinephrine. *Neuroscience and Biobehavioral Reviews, 22,* 437–452.

Panksepp, J. (1998). *Affective neuroscience.* London: Oxford University Press.

Panksepp, J., Nelson, E., & Bekkedal, M. (1999). Brain systems for the mediation of social separation distress and social reward. In C. S. Carter, I. I. Lederhendler, & B. Kirkpatrick (Eds.), *The integrative neurobiology of affiliation* (pp. 221–244). Cambridge, MA: MIT Press.

Petersson, M., Alster, P., Lundeberg, T., & Uvnäs-Moberg, K. (1996). Oxytocin causes a long-term decrease of blood pressure in female and male rats. *Physiology and Behavior, 60,* 1311–1315.

Rosenberg, M. (1965). *Society and the adolescent self-image.* Princeton, NJ: Princeton University Press.

Sapolsky, R. M. (1992). *Stress, the aging brain, and the mechanisms of neuron death.* Cambridge, MA: MIT Press.

Tamres, L., Janicki, D., & Helgeson, V. S. (2002). Sex differences in coping behavior: A meta-analytic review. *Personality and Social Psychology Review, 6,* 2–30.

Taylor, S. E. (2002). *The tending instinct: How nurturing is essential to who we are and how we live.* New York: Holt.

Taylor, S. E. (2007). Social support. In H. S. Friedman & R. C. Silver (Eds.), *Foundations of health psychology* (pp. 145–171). New York: Oxford University Press.

Taylor, S. E., Gonzaga, G., Klein, L. C., Hu, P., Greendale, G. A., & Seeman, S. E. (2006). Relation of oxytocin to psychological and biological stress responses in older women. *Psychosomatic Medicine, 68,* 238–245.

Taylor, S. E., Klein, L. C., Lewis, B. P., Gruenewald, T. L., Gurung, R. A. R., & Updegraff, J. A. (2000). Biobehavioral responses to stress in females: Tend-and-befriend, not fight-or-flight. *Psychological Review, 107,* 411–429.

Turner, R. A., Altemus, M., Enos, T., Cooper, B., & McGuinness, T. (1999). Preliminary research on plasma oxytocin in normal cycling women: Investigating emotion and interpersonal distress. *Psychiatry, 62,* 97–113.

Uvnäs-Moberg, K. (1997). Oxytocin-linked antistress effects: The relaxation and growth response. *Acta Physiologica Scandinavica, 640,* 38–42.

Uvnäs-Moberg, K., Ahlenius, S., Hillegaart, V., & Alster, P. (1994). High doses of oxytocin cause sedation and low doses cause an anxiolytic-like effect in male rats. *Pharmacology, Biochemistry, and Behavior, 49,* 101–106.

Virden, S. F. (1988). The relationship between infant feeding method and maternal role adjustment. *Journal of Nurse-Midwifery, 33,* 31–35.

Witt, D. M., Carter, C. S., & Walton, D. M. (1990). Central and peripheral effects of oxytocin administration in prairie voles (*Microtus ochrogaster*). *Pharmacology, Biochemistry, and Behavior, 37,* 63–69.

Witt, D. M., Winslow, J. T., & Insel, T. R. (1992). Enhanced social interactions in rats following chronic, centrally infused oxytocin. *Pharmacology, Biochemistry, and Behavior, 43,* 855–861.

Young, L. J., Lim, M. M., Gingrich, B., & Insel, T. R. (2001). Cellular mechanisms of social attachment. *Hormones and Behavior, 40,* 133–138.

22

The Social Neuroscience of Relationships
AN EXAMINATION OF HEALTH-RELEVANT PATHWAYS

Bert N. Uchino, Julianne Holt-Lunstad, Darcy Uno,
Rebecca Campo, and Maija Reblin

> The recent realization that the leading causes of disability and death in
> Western civilizations have substantial social and behavioral components,
> and the emergence of interest and research on the social and behavioral
> factors related to public health are therefore significant. These
> developments have stimulated interest among social psychologists not
> only in physiological concepts and techniques, but also in questions
> regarding which, when, and how physiological mechanisms moderate the
> effects of social stimuli on individual action, experience, and health.
> —CACIOPPO, PETTY, AND TASSINARY (1989, p. 83)

Social processes are among the more powerful psychological predictors of
physical health outcomes (Berkman, 1995; Cohen, 1988; House, Landis, &
Umberson, 1988; Kiecolt-Glaser & Glaser, 1995; Uchino, 2004). As predictors or mechanisms, social events appear to play important roles in both
the development and exacerbation of physical health conditions (Berkman,
Glass, Brissette, & Seeman, 2000; Kiecolt-Glaser, McGuire, Robles, &
Glaser, 2002). For instance, social support, besides being a consistent epidemiological predictor of mortality in itself (Uchino, 2004), is purported to
be an important pathway in other risk factors, such as socioeconomic status and personality processes (Adler et al., 1994; Smith, 1992). Researchers

interested in social processes and physical health are thus in a unique position to inform the surge of research linking psychological and behavioral factors to health outcomes.

It is important to note that the examination of social processes and health inherently involves differing levels of analysis. This multilevel perspective that "bridges" social and biological perspectives is the hallmark of social neuroscience (Berntson & Cacioppo, 2000; Cacioppo & Berntson, 1992). Social neuroscience is characterized by an examination of the reciprocal influences between social processes and neuroscientific principles and events. The term was put forth in 1992 by Cacioppo and Berntson to characterize the emerging neuroscience literature that included advances in the brain sciences, animal models of psychological processes (e.g., motivation, learning and memory), and neuroendocrine–immune interactions (e.g., stress and relationship processes) that had relevance to social phenomena. Our program of research has been guided by this perspective and acknowledges the importance of physiological principles to inform theory and generate research on health-relevant social-psychological phenomena.

Our laboratory has been interested in the links between social relationships and physical health—the social neuroscience of relationships. It is our view that a social neuroscience perspective is critical to understanding the links between social ties and health outcomes. In fact, physiological measures have served multiple conceptual purposes in our research. First, biological measures have been used as indices of some psychological processes (e.g., stress buffering) to differentiate conceptual predictions. Second, physiological assessments have been important "intermediate endpoints" of health outcomes. In such cases, biological measures become an important part of the theoretical modeling of the phenomenon that can inform us about the type or stage of disease influenced by social processes. For instance, cardiovascular disease has a long-term etiology, and social processes may play a role in the development or exacerbation of diagnosed cardiovascular conditions. Most of our work has focused on the cardiovascular system, so we first provide an overview of such assessments. We next discuss how we have practically applied a social neuroscience perspective to our program of research, followed by an illustrative review of our studies.

OVERVIEW OF CARDIOVASCULAR MEASURES

Cardiovascular disorders (CD) are presently the leading cause of death in the United States for both men and women (American Heart Association, 2003). In fact, they account for about as many deaths as the next seven leading causes of death combined. The most prevalent CD are hypertension (resting blood pressure $\geq$ 140/90 mmHg) and coronary heart disease (e.g., myocardial infarction). Resting blood pressure is an important cardiovascular risk factor, and recent guidelines label systolic blood pressure (SBP) between 120 and 139 mmHg and/or diastolic blood pressure (DBP) between 80 and 89 mmHg as prehypertension. The assessment of ambulatory blood pressure during daily life is also important because it predicts cardiovascular risk above and beyond that of resting assessments (Perloff, Sokolow, & Cowan, 1983; Verdecchia et al., 1994).

Blood pressure and heart rate are among the more common measures used in social neuroscientific studies (see Stern, Ray, & Quigley, 2001). Of course, such general indices are multiply determined, and we routinely examine their underlying determinants because of (1) their potential links to more specific psychological and biological processes (Blascovich & Tomaka, 1996) and (2) their implications for disease processes in their own right (Cacioppo, 1994; Julius, 1993; Binkley, Nunziata, Haas, Nelson, & Cody, 1991).

Blood pressure can be assessed noninvasively via the ausculatory (cuff with a microphone) or oscillometric (cuff with pressure transducer) methods (see Shapiro et al., 1996). Although blood pressure is an important endpoint in itself, measures are also available to model its underlying determinants (Sherwood et al., 1990). Blood pressure is a function of flow (i.e., cardiac output) and resistance (i.e., total peripheral resistance; TPR). Cardiac output can be estimated noninvasively via impedance cardiography. Impedance cardiography is based on Ohm's law: Voltage (V) = Current (I) × Resistance (R). In a system in which I is constant, changes in R (or impedance) varies directly with changes in V. More specifically, blood is a conductor, so an increase in thoracic blood volume following a heartbeat produces an interpretable change in thoracic impedance that can be recorded as a voltage signal. Stroke volume can then be estimated using the Kubicek equation (see Sherwood et al., 1990) and the subsequent cardiac output measured in liters per minute (heart rate × (stroke volume/1000)). Once estimates of cardiac output are obtained, TPR can be calculated (i.e., TPR = [mean arterial pressure/cardiac output] × 80) in resistance units (dynes-second • cm^{-5}).

Heart rate is another common measure in social neuroscience. It is expressed as the number of beats per minute and can be recorded at the surface of the skin via electrocardiography (ECG; see Jennings et al., 1981). It is driven by both the sympathetic nervous system (SNS) and parasympathetic nervous system (PNS). These neural inputs can vary in a reciprocal, coactive, or independent fashion (Berntson, Cacioppo, & Quigley, 1993a). Validated noninvasive measures of both SNS and PNS influences on the heart are available and include pre-ejection period (PEP) and respiratory sinus arrhythmia (RSA), respectively (Cacioppo et al., 1994). PEP is a measure of contractility and is commonly assessed via impedance cardiography. It is operationalized as the time interval in milliseconds of the Q-point of the ECG (onset of ventricular depolarization) to the B-point (onset of blood ejection from the ventricles) of the dZ/dt signal. Thus, PEP is the time interval required from depolarization to generate the necessary force to eject blood from the ventricles. This process is thought to provide a good measure of SNS influences on the heart because the myocardium is primarily innervated by the SNS. Pharmacological blockade studies provide evidence for the validity of this measure, although variations in other confounding factors need to be considered depending on the protocol (e.g., preload and afterload effects; Sherwood et al., 1990).

RSA is the rhythmical fluctuation in heart periods occurring at the respiration band (i.e., 0.12–0.40 Hz) that is associated with a shortening and lengthening of heart periods during inspiration and expiration, respectively (Berntson, Cacioppo, & Quigley, 1993b). Hz is a unit of frequency that corresponds to one cycle per second. Therefore, the 0.12 to 0.40 Hz frequency band of RSA corresponds to heart period fluctuations between 7.2 to 24 cycles (breaths) per minute. RSA reflects the activity of vagal motor neurons as gated through a central respiratory generator. It is evident on the high-frequency component of heart periods (> 0.12 Hz) due to the dynamic characteristics and low-pass filtering properties of parasympathetic effector synapses (Berntson et al., 1993b). Pharmacological blockade studies also provide evidence for the validity of this measure, although variations in confounding factors also need consideration depending on the protocol and method of assessing RSA (e.g., respiratory rate; Grossman, van Beek, & Wientjes, 1990).

Based on these integrated cardiovascular assessments, we have modeled the effects of relationship processes on stress-induced cardiovascular reactivity. Although there is still debate about the health significance of cardiovascular reactivity (Treiber et al., 2003), preliminary evidence exists that stress-induced changes in cardiovascular function may be independent predictors of the development and exacerbation of cardiovascular disease (Kamarck et al., 1997; Krantz et al., 1991; Light, Dolan, Davis, & Sherwood, 1992; Matthews, Woodall, & Allen, 1993; Sheps et al., 2002). Thus relationships may influence cardiovascular disease by reducing (e.g., stress-buffering) or exacerbating (e.g., social stress) cardiovascular reactivity (Uchino, Cacioppo, & Kiecolt-Glaser, 1996).

However, several important issues need to be considered in stress-reactivity paradigms. First, changes in cardiovascular reactivity may reflect several component processes. There are at least two explanations for changes in reactivity during such laboratory protocols: distress and effort. Stress can clearly increase reactivity and is usually the main interest in reactivity-disease protocols. However, differences in task effort or engagement may also influence cardiovascular responding (Wright & Kirby, 2001). If the primary interest is in stress-related processes, researchers will need to pilot tasks, design relevant controls, and/or include ancillary measures of task effort and engagement and stress (also see Blascovich & Tomaka, 1996).

Second, performance differences can complicate the ability to make generalizations of reactivity effects. In many cases, investigators are interested in inferring how physiologically reactive individuals are to stressors in general, rather than just to the exact tasks that are used. For instance, older adults may be more reactive to video-game stressors simply due to a lack of experience with such stimuli, but not to other stressors (e.g., speech task). The use of aggregation across multiple tasks appears helpful in increasing the generalizability and reliability of reactivity protocols (Kamarck et al., 1992). Yet the type of stressor needs to be carefully chosen, and demonstrating that such reactivity differences are not driven by task-specific factors will be necessary if the goal is to draw inferences more generally.

Finally, the work on cardiovascular reactivity suggests that stress may influence either the development and/or the exacerbation of cardiovascular disease. Such differences in disease processes highlight the conceptual role played by physiological measures in the social neuroscience of relationships. Biological measures are an integral part of the theoretical phenomenon that informs the type and stage of disease that may be influenced by relationships. Such information has important implications for the appropriate design of health-relevant interventions that seek to apply social neuroscientific research. Measures of particular physiological processes thus need to be chosen carefully, with a full conceptual consideration of the disease state of interest.

THE APPLICATION
OF A SOCIAL NEUROSCIENCE PERSPECTIVE

One of the authors of this chapter (BU) routinely teaches a graduate social psychology research methods course in which social neuroscientific principles and events are covered. A response from many students is "OK, this seems very important for social psychology, but how do we begin to apply this perspective to our own research?" In order to address this question, students perform the following exercise on their program of research (see Cacioppo & Berntson, 1992). First, identify the phenomenon of interest. That is, what are you trying to explain? Second, list the different levels of analysis that might have an impact on the phenomenon. Attempt to specify the sociocultural, personological, psychological–affective, behavioral, and physiological influences. How specific one gets will be in part determined by the status of the literature (e.g., existing conceptual models) and the ability of the level to shed insight on the phenomenon. Third, at each level of analysis, formulate specific hypotheses linking that level to the phenomenon. Fourth, start at the level that is likely to be more informative and use methods of strong inference (Cacioppo & Tassinary, 1990; Platt, 1964). For instance, within a level, are there competing hypotheses that can be contrasted within the same study? Finally, proceed incrementally across levels, linking or contrasting hypotheses from different levels, thereby fostering more general and integrative theories of the phenomenon.

A brief example of the following exercise from our program of research may be useful. In our laboratory, the phenomenon of interest is the epidemiological links between social relationships and lower mortality rates (House, Landis, & Umberson, 1988). There are multiple factors at different levels of analyses that might influence this phenomenon (Berkman et al., 2000; Cohen, 1988). For instance, at the psychological level, lower perceptions of stress may be one mechanism responsible for the health effects of relationships. In one of our studies we used these levels of analyses to test the pathways responsible for social support and health effects (Uchino, Holt-Lunstad, Uno, & Betancourt, 1999). Consistent with our prior work, we found that low social support was associated with higher resting blood pressure in older adults. Using measures of personality (e.g., hostility), psychological (e.g., perceived stress), and behavioral (e.g., health behaviors) processes, we examined various mediational pathways. Although little evidence was found for a singular pathway, this work aided us in the formation of more focused conceptual and methodological perspectives linking social support to physical health outcomes (see Uchino, 2004).

There are several advantages to this type of multilevel analysis. First, it is integrative. Explicitly modeling the phenomenon at different levels of analyses fosters an examination of the linkages within and between different theories or models that tend to be constrained to one or a few levels of analysis. Thus one begins to form more comprehensive theoretical models of the phenomenon that have the potential for both generality and specificity. A second advantage is that such an approach is generative. It highlights the levels of analysis that need greater attention. With complex social phenomena, it helps researchers to prioritize which levels and links are the most pressing to address. Finally, a multilevel perspective can aid in the process of strong inference. In specifying hypotheses within and across levels of analysis, it makes salient competing hypotheses that can serve as the basis for crucial tests.

One important issue to consider in a social-neuroscientific approach is that few researchers have the training to pursue with equal rigor all levels of analysis (see Taylor, 2004). Collaborative interdisciplinary research is important in this regard, as different areas of expertise can be more efficiently combined. Even then, some researchers may try to learn as much as they can about different physiological systems in their collaboration, whereas others feel quite comfortable leaving that to the biomedical experts on the team. If one chooses collaborators carefully, both approaches can be successful. Our personal preference has been to be as informed as possible on the critical physiological mechanisms. This has helped us (1) identify in a preliminary fashion what questions are feasible, (2) formulate more complex hypotheses within and across levels of analysis, and (3) understand with greater appreciation the complexity of biomedical perspectives on health and disease. This approach is reflected in our program of research, reviewed next.

THE SOCIAL NEUROSCIENCE OF RELATIONSHIPS

The study of relationships and biological function is not new. One of the first psychophysiological inquiries into relationships may have occurred in the 3rd century B.C. (Mesulam & Perry, 1972). In this intriguing case study, a young man had the misfortune of falling in love with his father's new bride. Determined not to show his love, he became sick and was determined to die. Attempts to heal him, of course, came to no avail. However, one particularly astute physician carefully observed the young man when different people visited and noticed that his pulse rate became irregular and that he started to sweat whenever his father's bride came into the room. After several "replications," the diagnosis of lovesickness was made; the father then separated from his bride, and the son returned to health.

In the preceding example, physiological measures were used as indices of a process that was difficult to access via self-report. In fact, many early and contemporary social-neuroscientific studies on relationships have been aimed at tapping into processes that individuals are either unwilling or unable to report (see Berntson & Cacioppo, 2000). In a seminal chapter by Shapiro and Crider (1969), the authors reviewed research that applied this approach to a number of intriguing social paradigms. These paradigms included attempts to examine (1) physiological responses during the psychotherapeutic process, (2) the links between empathy and physiological changes, and (3) social status effects during social interactions (also see Kaplan & Bloom, 1960). Shapiro and Crider (1969) suggested that "By examining information from several levels of response, with the view to determining their mutual lawfulness, the very distinctions between behavioral and physiological, overt and covert, voluntary and involuntary, are likely to give way to more fruitful dimensions of analysis" (p. 4).

Our program of research is based on this perspective and focuses on the large body of epidemiological studies suggesting that both the quantity and quality of one's relationships predicts lower all-cause mortality (see reviews by Berkman et al., 2000; House et al., 1988; Uchino, 2004). The links between social relationships and health are most evident for cardiovascular mortality (Berkman, Leo-Summers, & Horwitz, 1992; Brummett et al., 2001; Orth-Gomér, Rosengren, & Wilhelmsen, 1993), with some studies showing links with lower cancer (Ell, Nishimoto, Medianski, Mantell, & Hamovitch, 1992; Welin, Larsson, Svärdsudd, Tibblin, & Tibblin, 1992) and HIV (Lee & Rotheram-Borus, 2001) mortality. In this chapter we focus on the links between social ties and cardiovascular endpoints. Later in the chapter we return to the implications of our research for other disease processes.

Our modeling of this phenomenon began with a focus on social support. Many studies conceptualize support as the functions that are provided by social relationships. These functions are usually organized along two dimensions: perceived availability of and received support (Dunkel-Schetter & Bennett, 1990). This is an important distinction, as such measures are not highly correlated and are often associated with different effects (Barrera, 2000; Uchino, 2004). Using a laboratory reactivity paradigm, we sought to test the utility of separating the perceived availability and receipt of social support (Uchino & Garvey, 1997). We randomly assigned participants to conditions of no support or perceived-available support from an experimenter while they performed a stressful speech task. Participants in the perceived-available-support condition were instructed that the experimenter would be available to provide support if needed. This manipulation provided a relatively pure manipulation of available support, as participants typically did not seek out support from the experimenter. Results were consistent with our expectations, as individuals for whom support was simply made available showed significantly lower SBP and DBP reactivity during stress (see reviews by Lepore, 1998; Uchino et al., 1996).

The support-availability findings reported here are interesting because elevated cardiovascular reactivity during stress may be linked to gradual increases in blood pressure over time that confer increased vulnerability to cardiovascular disease. We have provided preliminary evidence for this developmental model involving social support, aging, and blood pressure. In one study, resting blood pressure was assessed in men and women between the ages of 20 and 70 (Uchino et al., 1999). As shown in Figure 22.1, we found that age significantly predicted increased resting SBP for individuals low in perceived support; however, individuals high in perceived support had relatively low SBP that did not increase as a function of age. Similarly significant findings were also obtained for resting DBP. These findings replicated and extended our prior research on social support and the biological aging process (e.g., Uchino, Cacioppo, Malarkey, Glaser, & Kiecolt-Glaser, 1995).

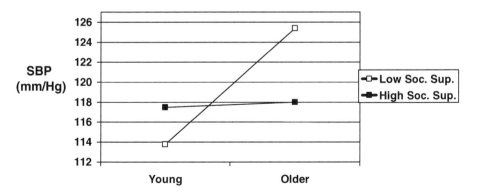

FIGURE 22.1. Predicted SBP as a function of social support and chronological age (plotted 1 *SD* above and below the mean).

The cross-sectional design, however, is a significant limitation and ongoing research is now evaluating the proposed longitudinal associations.

Although social support is clearly an important predictor of health outcomes, we have become interested in a more comprehensive conceptualization of relationships and health given our phenomenon of interest. This interest is fueled by research that shows that positive and negative aspects of relationships tend to be separable dimensions and that both predict important health outcomes (Finch et al., 1989; Friedman et al., 1995; Kiecolt-Glaser & Newton, 2001; Newsom, Nishkishiba, & Morgan, 2002; Rook & Pietromonaco, 1987). In fact, we have argued that the separability of positive and negative aspects of social relationships may have significant conceptual implications for their joint study. The framework depicted in Figure 22.2 suggests that any given social network member may differ in his or her underlying positive and negative basis (Cacioppo & Berntson, 1994; see Uchino, Holt-Lundstad, Uno, & Flinders, 2001). A unique aspect of this conceptualization for the social relationships and health literature is represented in the high-positivity/high-negativity corner. We label such a network member as "ambivalent network tie" (e.g., overbearing parent, volatile romance). The implications of such ambivalent relationships have not been adequately considered, as most prior research on social support has ignored the negative aspects that may cooccur with the positive aspects of relationships (Coyne & DeLongis, 1986; Uchino et al., 2001). This practice needs closer consideration because ambivalent relationships are a common feature of social networks and tend to predict increased psychological distress (Uchino, Holt-Lundstad, Smith, & Bloor, 2004). We have argued that failure of researchers to separate such ambivalent ties from other network types (e.g., purely supportive ties) may obscure reliable associations

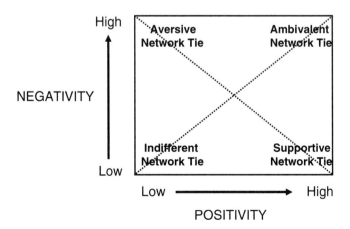

FIGURE 22.2. General conceptual framework incorporating the positive and negative effects of social relationships on health.

between relationships and health outcomes (Holt-Lunstad, Uchino, Smith, Cerny, & Nealey-Moore, 2003; Uchino et al., 2001).

In one study using this general framework, we examined the prediction of age differences in cardiovascular reactivity via these different categories of relationships (Uchino et al., 2001). Of particular interest was the association between ambivalent ties and age differences in cardiovascular function. On the one hand, social networks that contain many such ambivalent ties may be associated with negative outcomes because such ties are a significant source of interpersonal stress (e.g., Sandler & Barrera, 1984). On the other hand, it is possible that networks that contain many ambivalent ties may be associated with relatively beneficial effects on health-related outcomes because individuals might still benefit from positive aspects of these relationships (e.g., Abbey, Abramis, & Caplan, 1985).

In order to test these competing perspectives, men and women between the ages of 30 and 70 performed an acute-stress protocol (Uchino et al., 2001). To assess the different categories depicted in Figure 22.2 we utilized the social relationships index (SRI; see Uchino et al., 2001; Uchino et al., 2004, for scale validation information). The SRI can be used to calculate the total number of individuals in one's network who are in the supportive, ambivalent, aversive, and indifferent categories (see Figure 22.2).

Besides finding cardiovascular evidence for the benefits of having socially supportive ties, significant interactions between age and ambivalent ties were found. Individuals with a relatively high number of ambivalent network ties showed greater heart rate reactivity and a greater shortening of PEP reactivity (indicating greater sympathetic activation of the heart) as a function of age. In comparison, age did not predict heart rate or PEP reactivity for individuals characterized by a relatively low number of ambivalent network members. These results were independent of various demographic variables, task-specific performance or affect, health behaviors, and other categories of relationships (e.g., number of supportive ties). It provided support for the utility of the general model depicted in Figure 22.2, as well as a developmental process involving social ties, aging, and disease. Of course, longitudinal evidence will be needed to provide stronger evidence for such a model.

We also sought to investigate whether these differences occurred in the real world by using ambulatory recording methods (Holt-Lunstad et al., 2003). In this study, healthy men and women underwent a 3-day ambulatory blood pressure (ABP) assessment in which a reading was taken approximately 5 minutes into each social interaction. This event-sampling paradigm was adapted from prior work by Reis and Wheeler (1991). After each interaction, participants completed a standard diary that also included ratings of the quality of the relationship in terms of how positive and negative they normally felt toward the interaction partner.

Analyses were conducted using random regression models that statistically controlled for various extraneous factors (e.g., body mass, posture).

Consistent with our framework, the highest ABP was found when participants were interacting with a person with whom they felt relatively high levels of both positivity and negativity (see Figure 22.3). This significant effect was independent of structural aspects of a relationship, as we also found that simply interacting with family members and romantic partners was associated with lower ABP. The findings again suggest that interactions with ambivalent ties may be stressful. However, it was surprising that interactions with supportive ties were associated with ABP that was comparable to interactions with aversive and indifferent ties. Although more detailed measures of the types of interactions were not available, we speculate that our college-age participants might be engaging in more active interactions with supportive ties (e.g., speaking about positive events vs. more trivial events) that would result in short-term elevations in ABP. Of course, the overall support and familiarity of these relationships should be associated with generally beneficial influences on ABP (see Steptoe, Lundwall, & Cropley, 2000).

As in our prior social-support studies, we have also utilized controlled laboratory manipulations in order to elucidate the more precise mechanisms by which ambivalent ties may be related to health. In one study, women were randomly assigned to bring in a close nonromantic male or female friend whom they had known for at least 6 months (Uno, Uchino, & Smith, 2002). The quality of the friendship was assessed via the SRI and was used to categorize the relationship as purely positive or ambivalent. During the study, participants performed a series of stressful speech tasks while these friends wrote standardized supportive or no-support (neutral) statements. These notes were given to participants between speeches while measures of cardiovascular reactivity were assessed.

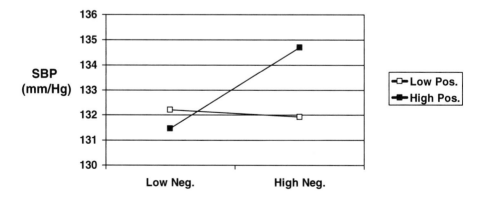

FIGURE 22.3. Predicted SBP levels during social interactions as a function of normally perceived relationship positivity and negativity (plotted 1 *SD* above and below the mean).

Preliminary analyses verified that the notes were perceived as supportive depending on the assigned condition. Importantly, women interacting with ambivalent friends had significantly greater increases in TPR than women interacting with supportive friends. Consistent with this vascular effect, women interacting with ambivalent friends also had marginally higher DBP reactivity compared with those interacting with supportive friends. These effects were moderated by the gender of the support provider, as women interacting with ambivalent female friends were most likely to show greater reactivity and to perceive that friend as more dominant in our support paradigm. These findings are consistent with research suggesting that women may be more sensitive to support processes from other women (e.g., Barbee, Gulley, & Cunningham, 1990).

There are at least two explanations for the links found between ambivalent ties and physiological processes (see Uchino et al., 2001). According to the stress-enhancing hypothesis, interactions with ambivalent friends may entail significant interpersonal stress. An ambivalent network member may be less predictable and thus may be associated with heightened interpersonal stress. On the other hand, the support-interference hypothesis suggests that ambivalent ties may be detrimental to health by interfering with social support in times of need. Despite the positivity that exists in ambivalent relationships, individuals may not be able to benefit from support from such ties because the coexisting negativity may lead them to question the accuracy or sincerity of the support.

We recently tested these competing hypotheses in a preliminary fashion by having men and women discuss positive, negative, and neutral life events with an ambivalent or a supportive friend (Holt-Lunstad, Uchino, Smith, & Hicks, 2006). If ambivalent relationships are general sources of stress, we would expect increased reactivity when individuals are discussing both positive and negative events with an ambivalent friend. However, if individuals do not benefit from support during times of stress then we should see increased reactivity primarily when participants are disclosing negative events to an ambivalent friend.

In this study, individuals completed the SRI in a pretesting session and were randomly assigned to bring in a supportive or an ambivalent friend. The social interaction was structured so that participants spoke in 1-minute periods regarding their personal feelings about the event. The friend also responded for 1-minute periods and was instructed to say what would come naturally to him or her. Preliminary analyses showed that ambivalent friends were again viewed as significantly more dominant than supportive friends. In addition, state anxiety during the study was elevated throughout for individuals who were with an ambivalent friend. No relationship-based differences in reactivity were found when participants discussed a neutral topic with their friends. However, a significant interaction occurred between relationship quality and the event topic on SBP reactivity. As predicted by the support-interference hypothesis, participants exhibited the greatest levels of SBP reactivity when disclosing a negative event to an ambivalent friend.

Although our results appear more consistent with the support-interference hypothesis, it is possible that seeking support from an ambivalent friend during negative life events is in itself stress enhancing and can contribute to support interference. In addition, other results suggested more subtle ways in which ambivalent friends may enhance stress. Analyses of baseline levels of cardiovascular activity showed that participants expecting to interact with ambivalent friends had significantly higher heart rates, an effect driven by lower parasympathetic control of the heart (as indexed by RSA). These data may indicate a reduced ability to regulate aspects of the cardiovascular system in the presence of such ambivalent ties. We are now examining more specific processes responsible for these and related findings at the social (e.g., relationship exchanges, history), psychological (e.g., appraisals), and behavioral (e.g., health behaviors) levels of analysis.

EMERGING ISSUES IN THE SOCIAL NEUROSCIENCE OF RELATIONSHIPS

Our program of research has been aimed at examining the cardiovascular consequences of relationships, with implications for understanding cardiovascular disease. Several emerging themes from the broader literature (some of which we are pursuing) rely on measures from multiple physiological systems, including endocrine and immune processes. Such studies are important, as they highlight how diverse systems are coordinated during social processes and provide a more comprehensive approach to the social neuroscience of relationships and health.

Recent research is turning to oxytocin as a particularly relevant endocrine hormone (Uvnäs-Moberg, 1998; Taylor et al., 2000). Oxytocin is a hypothalamic hormone that is best known for its role in milk ejection during breast feeding and uterine contractions accompanying labor. However, oxytocin also appears to vary according to various social stimuli (e.g., touch, massage) and has antistress effects in both the brain and more peripheral physiological systems (Taylor et al., 2000). For instance, oxytocin release is associated with decreases in cortisol levels, blood pressure, and sympathetic activity and with increases in parasympathetic activity (Uvnäs-Moberg, 1998). It also appears that the antistress effects of oxytocin stimulation become more pronounced over time; thus individuals in stable, fulfilling relationships or social groups should experience the greatest benefits.

Emerging data on immune-related inflammatory processes also provides a promising avenue for greater integration among these diverse physiological systems and disease states. Most research linking social support to immune processes has emphasized its potential role in cancer, HIV, and infectious diseases more generally (Uchino et al., 1996). There is now increased emphasis on how inflammatory immune processes may influence the atherosclerotic processes (Ross, 1999). For instance, immune cells (e.g., macrophages) can accumulate at the site of cholesterol deposits and release hormones that contribute to the formation, development, and subsequent rupturing of plaques in the arterial walls (Libby, Ridker, & Maseri, 2002). IL-6 and C-reactive proteins have received the greatest attention as markers of inflammatory processes and predict a range of health problems, including cardiovascular disease, diabetes, and frailty more generally (Papanicolaou, Wilder, Manolagas, & Chrousos, 1998; Rattazzi et al., 2003). The mechanisms underlying regulation of inflammatory markers such as IL-6 suggest links to the hypothalamic–pituitary–adrenal axis and SNS activation (Papanicolaou et al., 1998). Such findings (including those reviewed here for oxytocin) provide an exciting opportunity for researchers attempting to model how social processes may influence disease outcomes using a conceptually driven biological approach.

CONCLUSIONS

In this chapter we have argued for the importance of a social neuroscientific approach to understanding the health effects of relationships. We have actively used this approach to guide our program of research. This social neuroscience of relationships highlights the different levels of analysis that are relevant for an integrative understanding of social ties and health. It can provide the basis for a sustained, generative program of research with potential integration across disciplinary boundaries. Such interdisciplinary research is now an emerging standard in many areas of inquiry (Anderson, 1998; Taylor, 2004). Indeed, social psychologists are in a unique position to contribute to such interdisciplinary efforts given our conceptual and methodological training at the social, psychological, and behavioral levels of analysis. It provides an opportunity to more fully embrace and integrate diverse perspectives on complex, multiply determined social-psychological phenomena.

ACKNOWLEDGMENTS

This research was generously supported by Grant Nos. R55 AG13968 (James A. Shannon Director's Award) and RO1 AG018903 from the National Institute on Aging, as well as grant number R01 MH58690 from the National Institute of Mental Health and Grant No. R01 HL68862 from the National Heart, Lung, and Blood Institute. We would like to thank David Lozano, Daniel Litvack, John T. Cacioppo, Robert Kelsey, and William Guethlein for their expert technical assistance and for providing us with copies of their data acquisition and reduction software (i.e., ANS suite, Mindware, and ENSCOREL). Many thanks to Fredrick Rhodewalt and John T. Cacioppo for their valuable comments on a draft of this chapter.

REFERENCES

Abbey, A., Abramis, D. J., & Caplan, R. D. (1985). Effects of differential sources of social support and social conflict on emotional well-being. *Basic and Applied Social Psychology, 6,* 111–129.

Adler, N. E., Boyce, T., Chesney, M. A., Cohen, S., Folkman, S., Kahn, R. L., et al. (1994). Socioeconomic status and health: The challenge of the gradient. *American Psychologist, 49,* 15–24.

American Heart Association. (2003). *Heart disease and stroke statistics: 2004 update.* Dallas, TX: American Heart Association.

Anderson, N. B. (1998). Levels of analysis in health science: A framework for integrating sociobehavioral and biomedical research. *Annals of the New York Academy of Sciences, 840,* 563–576.

Barbee, A. P., Gulley, M. R., & Cunningham, M. R. (1990). Support seeking in personal relationships. *Journal of Social and Personal Relationships, 7,* 531–540.

Barrera, M., Jr. (2000). Social support research in community psychology. In J. Rappaport & E. Seidman (Eds.), *Handbook of community psychology* (pp. 215–245). New York: Kluwer Academic/Plenum.

Berkman, L. F. (1995). The role of social relations in health promotion. *Psychosomatic Medicine, 57,* 245–254.

Berkman, L. F., Glass, T., Brissette, I., & Seeman, T. E. (2000). From social integration to health: Durkheim in the new millennium. *Social Science and Medicine, 51,* 843–857.

Berkman, L. F., Leo-Summers, L., & Horwitz, R. I. (1992). Emotional support and survival after myorcardial infaction: A prospective, population-based study of the elderly. *Annals of Internal Medicine, 117,* 1003–1009.

Berntson, G. G., & Cacioppo, J. T. (2000). Psychobiology and social psychology: Past, present, and future. *Personality and Social Psychology Review, 4,* 3–15.

Berntson, G. G., Cacioppo, J. T., & Quigley, K. S. (1993a). Cardiac psychophysiology and autonomic space in humans: Empirical perspectives and conceptual implications. *Psychological Bulletin, 114,* 296–322.

Berntson, G. G., Cacioppo, J. T., & Quigley, K. S. (1993b). Respiratory sinus arrhythmia: Autonomic origins, physiological mechanisms, and psychophysiological implications. *Psychophysiology, 30,* 183–196.

Binkley, P. F., Nunziata, E., Haas, G. J., Nelson, S. D., & Cody, R. J. (1991). Parasympathetic withdrawal is an integral component of autonomic imbalance in congestive heart failure: Demonstration in human subjects and verification in a paced canine model of ventricular failure. *Journal of the American College of Cardiology, 18,* 464–472.

Blascovich, J., & Tomaka, J. (1996). The biopsychosocial model of arousal regulation. In M. P. Zanna (Ed.), *Advances in experimental social psychology* (Vol. 29, 1–51). New York: Academic Press.

Brummett, B. H., Barefoot, J. C., Siegler, I. C., Clapp-Channing, N. E., Lytle, B. L., Bosworth, H. B., et al. (2001). Characteristics of socially isolated patients with coronary artery disease who are at elevated risk for mortality. *Psychosomatic Medicine, 63,* 267–272.

Cacioppo, J. T. (1994). Social neuroscience: Autonomic, neuroendocrine, and immune responses to stress. *Psychophysiology, 31,* 113–128.

Cacioppo, J. T., & Berntson, G. G. (1992). Social psychological contributions to the decade of the brain: Doctrine of multilevel analysis. *American Psychologist, 47,* 1019–1028.

Cacioppo, J. T., & Berntson, G. G. (1994). Relationship between attitudes and evaluative space: A critical review, with emphasis on the separability of positive and negative substrates. *Psychological Bulletin, 115,* 401–423.

Cacioppo, J. T., Berntson, G. G., Binkley, P. F., Quigley, K. S., Uchino, B. N., & Fieldstone, A. (1994). Autonomic cardiac control: II. Basal response, noninvasive indices, and autonomic space as revealed by autonomic blockade. *Psychophysiology, 31,* 586–598.

Cacioppo, J. T., Petty, R. E., & Tassinary, L. G. (1989). Social psychophysiology: A new look. *Advances in Experimental Social Psychology* (Vol. 22, pp. 39–91). New York: Academic Press.

Cacioppo, J. T., & Tassinary, L. (1990). Inferring psychological significance from physiological signals. *American Psychologist, 45,* 16–28.

Cohen, S. (1988). Psychosocial models of the role of social support in the etiology of physical disease. *Health Psychology, 7,* 269–297.

Coyne, J. C., & DeLongis, A. (1986). Going beyond social support: The role of social relationships in adaptation. *Journal of Consulting and Clinical Psychology, 54,* 454–460.

Dunkel-Schetter, C., & Bennett, T. L. (1990). Differentiating the cognitive and behavioral aspects of social support. In B. R. Sarason, I. G. Sarason, & G. R. Pierce (Eds.), *Social support: An interactional view* (pp. 267–296). New York: Wiley.

Ell, K., Nishimoto, R., Medianski, L., Mantell, J., & Hamovitch, M. (1992). Social relations, social support and survival among patients with cancer. *Journal of Psychosomatic Research, 36,* 531–541.

Finch, J. F., Okun, M. A., Barrera, M., Zautra, A. J., & Reich, J. W. (1989). Positive and negative social ties among older adults: Measurement models and the prediction of psychological distress and well-being. *American Journal of Community Psychology, 17,* 585–605.

Friedman, H. S., Tucker, J. S., Schwartz, J. E., Tomlinson-Keasey, C., Martin, L. R., Wingard, D. L., et al. (1995). Psychosocial and behavioral predictors of longevity: The aging and death of the "Termites." *American Psychologist, 50,* 69–78.

Grossman, P., van Beek, J., & Wientjes, C. (1990). A comparison of three quantification methods for estimation of respiratory sinus arrythmia. *Psychophysiology, 27,* 702–714.

Holt-Lunstad, J., Uchino, B. N., Smith, T. W., Cerny, C. B., & Nealey-Moore, J. B. (2003). Social relationships and ambulatory blood pressure: Structural and qualitative predictors of cardiovascular function during everyday social interactions. *Health Psychology, 22,* 388–397.

Holt-Lunstad, J., Uchino, B. N., Smith, T. W., & Hicks, A. (2006). *Social relationships and cardiovascular function: The impact of relationship quality when discussing positive and negative life events*. Manuscript submitted for publication.

House, J. S., Landis, K. R., & Umberson, D. (1988). Social relationships and health. *Science, 241*, 540–545.

Jennings, J. R., Berg, W. K., Hutcheson, J. S., Obrist, P., Porges, S., & Turpin, G. (1981). Publication guidelines for heart rate studies in man. *Psychophysiology, 18*, 226–231.

Julius, S. (1993). Sympathetic hyperactivity and coronary risk in hypertension. *Hypertension, 21*, 886–893.

Kamarck, T., Everson, S., Kaplan, G., Manuck, S., Jennings, R., Salonen, R., et al. (1997). Exaggerated blood pressure responses during mental stress are associated with enhanced carotid atherosclerosis in middle-aged Finnish men. *Circulation, 96*, 3842–3848.

Kamarck, T. W., Jennings, J. R., Debski, T. T., Glickman-Weiss, E., Johnson, P. S., Eddy, M. J., et al. (1992). Reliable measures of behaviorally-evoked cardiovascular reactivity from a PC-based test battery: Results from student and community samples. *Psychophysiology, 29*, 17–28.

Kaplan, H. B., & Bloom, S. W. (1960). The use of sociological and social-psychological concepts in physiological research: A review of selected experimental studies. *Journal of Nervous and Mental Disease, 131*, 128–134.

Kiecolt-Glaser, J. K., & Glaser, R. (1995). Psychoneuroimmunology and health consequences: Data and shared mechanisms. *Psychosomatic Medicine, 57*, 269–274.

Kiecolt-Glaser, J. K., & Newton, T. L. (2001). Marriage and health: His and hers. *Psychological Bulletin, 127*, 472–503.

Kiecolt-Glaser, J. K., McGuire, L., Robles, T., & Glaser, R. (2002). Emotions, morbidity, and mortality: New perspectives from psychoneuroimmunology. *Annual Review of Psychology, 53*, 83–107.

Krantz, D. S., Helmers, K. F., Bairey, N., Nebel, L. E., Hedges, S. M., & Rozanski, A. (1991). Cardiovascular reactivity and mental stress-induced myocardial ischemia in patients with coronary artery disease. *Psychosomatic Medicine, 53*, 1–12.

Lee, M., & Rotheram-Borus, M. J. (2001). Challenges associated with increased survival among parents living with HIV. *American Journal of Public Health, 91*, 1303–1309.

Lepore, S. J. (1998). Problems and prospects for the social support–reactivity hypothesis. *Annuals of Behavioral Medicine, 20*, 257–269.

Libby, P., Ridker, P. M., & Maseri, A. (2002). Inflammation and atherosclerosis. *Circulation, 105*, 1135–1143.

Light, K. C., Dolan, C. A., Davis, M. R., & Sherwood, A. (1992). Cardiovascular responses to an active coping challenge as predictors of blood pressure patterns 10 to 15 years later. *Psychosomatic Medicine, 54*, 217–230.

Matthews, K. A., Woodall, K. L., & Allen, M. T. (1993). Cardiovascular reactivity to stress predicts future blood pressure status. *Hypertension, 22*, 479–485.

Mesulam, M., & Perry, J. (1972). The diagnosis of lovesickness: Experimental psychophysiology without the polygraph. *Psychophysiology, 9*, 546–551.

Newsom, J. T., Nishishiba, M., & Morgan, D. L. (2003). The relative importance of three domains of positive and negative social exchanges: A longitudinal model with comparable measures. *Psychology and Aging, 18*, 746–754.

Orth-Gomér, K., Rosengren, A., & Wilhelmsen, L. (1993). Lack of social support and incidence of coronary heart disease in middle-aged Swedish men. *Psychosomatic Medicine, 55,* 37–43.

Papanicolaou, D. A., Wilder, R. L., Manolagas, S. C., & Chrousos, G. P. (1998). The pathophysiologic roles of interleukin-6 in human disease. *Annals of Internal Medicine, 128,* 127–137.

Perloff, D., Sokolow, M., & Cowan, R. (1983). The prognostic value of ambulatory blood pressure. *Journal of the American Medical Association, 249,* 2793–2798.

Platt, J. R. (1964). Strong inference. *Science, 146,* 347–353.

Rattazzi, M., Puato, M., Faggin, E., Bertipaglia, B., Zambon, A., & Pauletto, P. (2003). C-reactive protein and interleukin-6 in vascular disease: Culprits or passive bystanders? *Journal of Hypertension, 21,* 1787–1803.

Reis, H. T., & Wheeler, L. (1991). Studying social interaction with the Rochester interaction record. In L. Berkowitz (Ed.), *Advances in experimental social psychology* (pp. 269–318). New York: Academic Press.

Rook, K. S., & Pietromonaco, P. (1987). Close relationships: Ties that heal or ties that bind. *Advances in Personal Relationships, 1,* 1–35.

Ross, R. (1999). Mechanisms of disease: Atherosclerosis—An inflammatory disease. *New England Journal of Medicine, 340,* 115–126.

Sandler, I. N., & Barrera, M., Jr. (1984). Toward a multimethod approach to assessing the effects of social support. *American Journal of Community Psychology, 12,* 37–52.

Shapiro, D., & Crider, A. (1969). Psychophysiological approaches in social psychology. In G. Lindsey & E. Aronson (Eds.), *The handbook of social psychology,* (2nd ed., pp. 1–49). London: Addison-Wesley.

Shapiro, D., Jamner, L. D., Lane, J. D., Light, K. C., Myrtek, M., Sawada, Y., et al. (1996). Blood pressure publication guidelines. *Psychophysiology, 33,* 1–12.

Sheps, D. S., McMahon, R. P., Becker, L., Carney, R. M., Freedland, K. E., Cohen, J. D. et al. (2002). Mental stress-induced ischemia and all-cause mortality in patients with coronary artery disease. *Circulation, 105,* 1780–1784.

Sherwood, A., Allen, M., Fahrenberg, J., Kelsey, R., Lovallo, W., & Van Doornen, L. (1990). Methodological guidelines for impedance cardiography. *Psychophysiology, 27,* 1–23.

Smith, T. W. (1992). Hostility and health: Current status of a psychosomatic hypothesis. *Health Psychology, 11,* 139–150.

Steptoe, A., Lundwall, K., & Cropley, M. (2000). Gender, family structure, and cardiovascular activity during the working day and evening. *Social Science & Medicine, 50,* 531–539.

Stern, R. M., Ray, W. J., & Quigley, K. S. (Eds.). (2001). *Psychophysiological recording* (2nd ed.). New York: Oxford University Press.

Taylor, S. E. (2004). Preparing for social psychology's future. *Journal of Experimental Social Psychology, 40,* 139–141.

Taylor, S. E., Klein, L. C., Lewis, B. P., Gruenewald, T. L., Gurung, R. A. R., & Updegraff, J. A. (2000). Biobehavioral responses to stress in females: Tend-and-befriend, not fight-or-flight. *Psychological Review, 107,* 411–429.

Treiber, F. A., Kamarck, T., Schneiderman, N., Sheffield, D., Kapuku, G., & Taylor, T. (2003). Cardiovascular reactivity and development of preclinical and clinical disease states. *Psychosomatic Medicine, 65,* 46–62.

Uchino, B. N. (2004). *Social support and physical health: Understanding the health consequences of our relationships.* New Haven, CT: Yale University Press.

Uchino, B. N., Cacioppo, J. T., & Kiecolt-Glaser, J. K. (1996). The relationship between social support and physiological processes: A review with emphasis on underlying mechanisms and implications for health. *Psychological Bulletin, 119,* 488–531.

Uchino, B. N., Cacioppo, J. T., Malarkey, W., Glaser, R., & Kiecolt-Glaser, J. K. (1995). Appraisal support predicts age-related differences in cardiovascular function in women. *Health Psychology, 14,* 556–562.

Uchino, B. N., & Garvey, T. G. (1997). The availability of social support reduces cardiovascular reactivity to acute psychological stress. *Journal of Behavioral Medicine, 20,* 15–27.

Uchino, B. N., Holt-Lunstad, J., Smith, T. W., & Bloor, L. (2004). Heterogeneity in social networks: A comparison of different models linking relationships to psychological outcomes. *Journal of Social and Clinical Psychology, 23,* 123–139.

Uchino, B. N., Holt-Lunstad, J., Uno, D., & Betancourt, R. (1999). Social support and age-related differences in cardiovascular function: An examination of potential mediators. *Annals of Behavioral Medicine, 21,* 135–142.

Uchino, B. N., Holt-Lunstad, J., Uno, D., & Flinders, J. B. (2001). Heterogeneity in the social networks of young and older adults: Prediction of mental health and cardiovascular reactivity during acute stress. *Journal of Behavioral Medicine, 24,* 361–382.

Uno, D., Uchino, B. N., & Smith, T. W. (2002). Relationship quality moderates the effect of social support given by close friends on cardiovascular reactivity in women. *International Journal of Behavioral Medicine, 9,* 243–262.

Uvnäs-Moberg, K. (1998). Oxytocin may mediate the benefits of positive social interaction and emotions. *Psychoneuroendocrinology, 23,* 819–835.

Verdecchia, P., Porcellati, C., Schillaci, C., Borgioni, C., Ciucci, A., Battistelli, M., et al. (1994). Ambulatory blood pressure: An independent predictor of prognosis in essential hypertension. *Hypertension, 24,* 793–801.

Welin, L., Larsson, B., Svärdsudd, K., Tibblin, B., & Tibblin, G. (1992). Social network and activities in relation to mortality from cardiovascular diseases, cancer and other causes: A 12-year follow-up of the study of men born in 1913 and 1923. *Journal of Epidemiology and Community Health, 46,* 127–132.

Wright, R. A., & Kirby, L. D. (2001). Effort determination of cardiovascular response: An integrative analysis with applications in social psychology. In M. Zanna (Ed.), *Advances in experimental social psychology* (Vol. 33, pp. 255–307). San Diego: Academic Press.

Index